Healthy Healing

AN ALTERNATIVE
HEALING REFERENCE

Linda G. Rector-Page, N.D., Ph.D.

The ninth edition is dedicated to the Sierra Foothills research team,
and to the
health-committed nutritional consultants
in natural food stores all over the United States,
who accurately catalogued and shared the case histories and product experiences
that made this edition possible.

This reference is to be used for educational information.
It is not a claim for cure or mitigation of disease, but rather an adjunctive approach,
supplying individual nutritional needs
that otherwise might be lacking
in today's lifestyle.

First Edition, June 1985. Copywrite req. Nov. 1985.
Second Edition, January 1986.
Third Edition, Revised, September 1986.
Fourth Edition, Revised/Updated, May 1987.
Fifth Edition, November 1987.
Sixth Edition, Revised/Updated, June 1988.
Seventh Edition, Revised/Update, Jan. 1989, Sept. 1989, March 1990.
Eighth Edition, Revised/Updated/Expanded, July, 1990.
Ninth Edition, Revised/Updated/Expanded, Sept., 1992.

What people say about "HEALTHY HEALING".......

✳ "I've been telling everybody I know about "HEALTHY HEALING", because it's the best reference I've seen for personal healing." - J.C., Northampton, MA., retail consumer.

✳ "HEALTHY HEALING" is the most important reference book for working with my customers that has ever been printed. It enables detailed assistance for a wide range of health problems." - F.H., Mgr., Real Foods 2, Ca.

✳ "HEALTHY HEALING" is an extremely high quality resource that I use in my practice a lot. I recommend it to my patients that are interested in self care." - Dr. D.K., D.C., Campbell, Ca.

✳ "HEALTHY HEALING" is so useful that I am sending each of my daughters a copy so they may have them on their kitchen table for daily use. You have made a great, tremendous contribution. Many, many thanks!" - E. K., Claremont, CA., retail customer.

✳ We use the "HEALTHY HEALING" book as a reference tool for our staff as well as our customers. The body work section is very informative, and gives the customers other options." - L.L., Dept. Mgr., Mollie Stones, Redwood City, Ca.

✳ "HEALTHY HEALING" is my Bible." - J.R., Mgr. Lassens Health Foods, Thousand Oaks, Ca.

✳ "We use the "HEALTHY HEALING" book daily, and have sold more than 100 books in 6 months. We and our customers have appreciated the helpful choices available. It is very convincing to the choices in print, and protects us from beng accused of prescribing without a medical license." - L. B., owner, Richardson's Health Foods, Fort Worth, TX.

✳ "HEALTHY HEALING" is the best selling reference guide in our store." - C.M., Gen Mgr. Pilgrims, Seattle, Wa.

✳ "HEALTHY HEALING" is an excellent resource for natural healing." - W. C., M.D., Spokane, Wa.

✳ "HEALTHY HEALING" was one of the first places that I found a clue to my arrhythmia. It subsided and then disappeared, and I haven't had a problem since. I am very grateful for the help your book gave me." - E. S. Gresham, OR., retail consumer.

✳ "Thank you for writing such an amazing book. I consult "HEALTHY HEALING" often and have always been successful in the treatments." - K. T., Santa Cruz, Ca., retail customer.

✳ "HEALTHY HEALING" is the book we always refer to when helping customers." - O. A., Asst. Mgr., Wild Oats, Sante Fe, N.M.

✳ "Our store does over 3 million dollars in sales a year, and "HEALTHY HEALING" is one of the best selling tools we've ever had. Not only does it increase primary sales, but secondary sales as well." - L. B., Vice-President, Sunflower Shoppe, Fort Worth, Tx.

✳ "HEALTHY HEALING" greatly helps our sales." - Zippy, Mgr., Whole Foods, Palo Alto, Ca.

✳ "HEALTHY HEALING" is very informative. My customers love the different approaches to each ailment. It's really the complete approach." - M. B., Wild Oats Mkt., Boulder, CO.

✳ "HEALTHY HEALING" has been added to my library for referral, to maintain our family's good health and happiness. This book is so informative, well-written and comprehensive." - J. N., Seattle, WA., retail customer.

✳ "We have sold over 250 "HEALTHY HEALING" books in the last 10 months. It is a quick reference book for determining vitamin, mineral, herb and nutritional needs in an easy, usable form. Linda Rector-Page's credentials of Naturopathic doctor and Ph.D. in nutrition and herbal research help us take the guesswork out of what to do. Our customer response has been very positive in terms of the nutritional healing benefits that they have received." - R. B., owner, Sunflower Shoppe, Fort Worth, TX.

✳ "HEALTHY HEALING" is our store guide and primary source of nutritional information. Very, very excellent guidebook." - C. M., Artesian Health Foods, Stockton, CA.

✳ "Our whole family uses "HEALTHY HEALING". Incredibly effective healing resource." - L. A., St. Helena, Ca., consumer.

THE HIGHEST CALLING OF THE HEALER
IS TO RALLY THE MIND AND BODY AGAINST THE DISEASE.

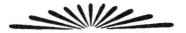

EVEN <u>ONE</u> MIRACLE CURE CAN SHOW THE VALUE OF A THERAPY
WITH THE BODY'S OWN HEALING POWERS. IF THE THERAPY IS NATURAL,
NON-INVASIVE, AND DOES NO HARM, IT CAN BE TRIED WITH
CONFIDENCE AS A VALID CHOICE.

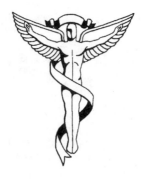

NEITHER DRUGS NOR HERBS NOR VITAMINS ARE A CURE FOR ANYTHING.
THE BODY HEALS ITSELF.
THE HUMAN BODY IS INCREDIBLY INTELLIGENT.
IT USUALLY RESPONDS TO INTELLIGENT THERAPIES.
THE HEALING PROFESSIONAL CAN HELP THIS PROCESS ALONG
BY OFFERING INTELLIGENT CHOICES.

Other Books By
LINDA RECTOR-PAGE, N.D., Ph.D.

"Cooking For Healthy Healing"

"How To Be Your Own Herbal Pharmacist"

&

The Healthy Healing Library Series

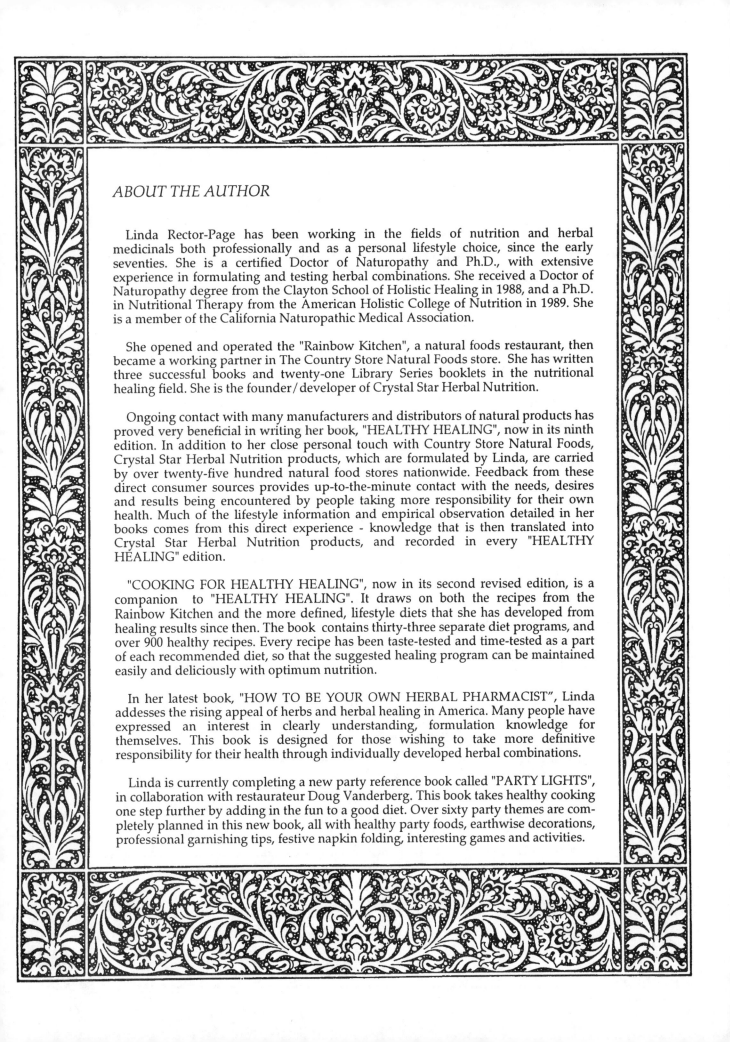

ABOUT THE AUTHOR

Linda Rector-Page has been working in the fields of nutrition and herbal medicinals both professionally and as a personal lifestyle choice, since the early seventies. She is a certified Doctor of Naturopathy and Ph.D., with extensive experience in formulating and testing herbal combinations. She received a Doctor of Naturopathy degree from the Clayton School of Holistic Healing in 1988, and a Ph.D. in Nutritional Therapy from the American Holistic College of Nutrition in 1989. She is a member of the California Naturopathic Medical Association.

She opened and operated the "Rainbow Kitchen", a natural foods restaurant, then became a working partner in The Country Store Natural Foods store. She has written three successful books and twenty-one Library Series booklets in the nutritional healing field. She is the founder/developer of Crystal Star Herbal Nutrition.

Ongoing contact with many manufacturers and distributors of natural products has proved very beneficial in writing her book, "HEALTHY HEALING", now in its ninth edition. In addition to her close personal touch with Country Store Natural Foods, Crystal Star Herbal Nutrition products, which are formulated by Linda, are carried by over twenty-five hundred natural food stores nationwide. Feedback from these direct consumer sources provides up-to-the-minute contact with the needs, desires and results being encountered by people taking more responsibility for their own health. Much of the lifestyle information and empirical observation detailed in her books comes from this direct experience - knowledge that is then translated into Crystal Star Herbal Nutrition products, and recorded in every "HEALTHY HEALING" edition.

"COOKING FOR HEALTHY HEALING", now in its second revised edition, is a companion to "HEALTHY HEALING". It draws on both the recipes from the Rainbow Kitchen and the more defined, lifestyle diets that she has developed from healing results since then. The book contains thirty-three separate diet programs, and over 900 healthy recipes. Every recipe has been taste-tested and time-tested as a part of each recommended diet, so that the suggested healing program can be maintained easily and deliciously with optimum nutrition.

In her latest book, "HOW TO BE YOUR OWN HERBAL PHARMACIST", Linda addesses the rising appeal of herbs and herbal healing in America. Many people have expressed an interest in clearly understanding, formulation knowledge for themselves. This book is designed for those wishing to take more definitive responsibility for their health through individually developed herbal combinations.

Linda is currently completing a new party reference book called "PARTY LIGHTS", in collaboration with restaurateur Doug Vanderberg. This book takes healthy cooking one step further by adding in the fun to a good diet. Over sixty party themes are completely planned in this new book, all with healthy party foods, earthwise decorations, professional garnishing tips, festive napkin folding, interesting games and activities.

TABLE OF CONTENTS

About Alternative Healing & Modern Medicine Today

Much traditional healing knowledge, and personal health empowerment in the general population has dropped away over the years, as medical advances and "letting the doctor do it" have become a way of life in the 20th century. Indeed our society has allowed the entire health care industry to become so powerful and so disproportionately lucrative that it is now in the business of illness rather than health.

In recent years, however, the realization is more prevalent that conventional medical methods can only go so far before major expense outweighs the value of the treatment or the insurance costs, and we see the undeniable fact that the doctor "can't always do it". In addition, respected studies on many wide-ranging aspects of health and healing are now convincing informed people that most illness does not just drop out of the sky and hit them over the head. Health is an ongoing process, and must be approached differently, with different answers.

The 90's are seeing an ever increasing use of alternative therapies, as drug and medical costs, even reasonable medical insurance payments, rapidly go beyond the reach of most families. As orthodox medical treatment becomes more invasive, and less in touch with the person who is ill, people are becoming more willing to take a measure of responsibility for their own health. The best news is that natural remedies work - often far better than current medical prescriptions.

Conventional medicine has always put the emphasis on crisis intervention. This is where it is the most successful of all healing methods. Standard medicine is about doing battle with a disease or an imminent threat to life. It brings up the big guns of surgery and drugs to search out and destroy dangerous organisms. It is the kind of treatment necessary for acute disease, major accidents, emergencies and wartime life-saving (which is indeed where modern medicine developed).

However, it is much less successful in cases of chronic illness - the diseases related to aging and lifestyle - such as arthritis, osteoporosis, lower back pain, high blood pressure, coronary-artery disease, ulcers, hormone imbalances, etc. In these instances the big guns and emergency measures are usually not applicable or tend to overkill, and do not allow the body to heal itself.

Almost all illness is self-limiting. Most recoveries occur naturally. The human body is a healing system beautifully designed to meet most of its problems without outside intervention. And even when outside help is required, our innate resources are of great value in the strategy of treatment. Healing can be enhanced even in serious illness if the patient can be kept free of depression and panic. Panic constricts blood vessels, causing additional burden on the heart. Depression intensifies existing diseases, and opens the door to new ones. There is a direct connection between the mental state of the patient and the ability of the immune system to do its job. Emotional devastation impairs immune function. Freedom from depression and panic increases the body's interleukins, vital immune defense substances.

Medical schools do not teach disease prevention, or proper diet and exercise as a part of health. Doctors receive no reward for health, only for treating illness. The interaction of mind and body are downplayed as of little practical concern, stating that a patient's state of mind does not matter to bacteria or a virus. Objective measures of health are emphasized - the number of white blood cells, blood pressure readings, etc., instead of how the patient *feels*. Doctors are trained to use drugs, surgery, and the latest laboratory technologies. To paraphrase Abraham Maslow, "if all you're trained to use is a hammer, the whole world looks like a nail".

This approach does not sit well with the more health-informed public today, who want more control over their health problems, and intend to be a part of the decision making process about their healing needs.

Modern medicine also teaches that pain means sickness. It does not recognize that pain is also the body's way of informing us that we are *doing* something wrong, not necessarily that something *is* wrong. Pain can tell us that we are smoking too much, eating too much, or eating the wrong things. It can notify us when there is too much emotional congestion in our lives, or too much daily stress. Pain can be a friend with useful information about our health, so that we can successfully address the cause of a problem. But conventional medicine treats it only as a powerful enemy, prescribing a plethora of pills and treatments that often only mask it or drive it underground, usually to resurface later with increased intensity.

In addition, people are constantly pressured by the medical community to have yearly exams with exhaustive tests, to be screened for high cholesterol, high blood pressure, breast lumps, and cancer. If there are acute pains or other symptoms that indicate the need for a doctor, obvious common sense dictates that a doctor should be called, or emergency medical steps taken. However, much of the constant pressure for testing is driven by greed. It has become a well-known fact that many physicians have a financial interest as well as an informational interest in ordering numerous X-rays and blood tests, in performing surgeries and in prescribing certain medications. The fear of malpractice lawsuits also causes doctors to be overly zealous when ordering tests. These practices are forcing many people to realize that regular medical testing can be hazardous to your health - both physically and mentally. Physical hazards include faulty diagnoses, inaccurate tests, botched surgical procedures, dangerous medications and treatments, etc. The more tests a person undergoes, the greater the odds of being told, often incorrectly, that something is wrong. Great mental anxiety is brought on by needless testing, needless medication, needless surgery, and a brusque, uncaring, or rushed doctor. You can literally worry yourself sick when there is nothing particularly wrong.

Not every problem requires costly, major medical attention. There is room and need for alternatives. A sensible lifestyle, with good healthy food, regular moderate exercise and restful sleep is still the best medicine for many problems. We need to be re-educated about our health - to be less intimidated about doctors and disease. Today's health care consumers are not only more aware of alternative healing choices, and more confident in their own healing strength, but also want to do something for themselves to get better. The time has clearly come for a partnership between the health care professional and the patient, so that the healing resources from both sides can be optimally employed.

This book is a reference for the alternative health care choices open to those wishing to take more responsibility for their own well-being. The recommended suggestions are backed up by extensive research into therapies for each specific ailment, and by contributing health care professionals and nutritional consultants from around the country, with many years of eyewitness and hands-on experience in alternative healing results.

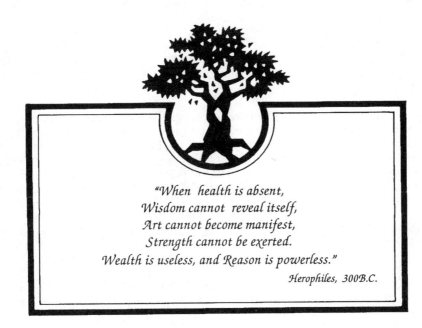

"When health is absent,
Wisdom cannot reveal itself,
Art cannot become manifest,
Strength cannot be exerted.
Wealth is useless, and Reason is powerless."

Herophiles, 300B.C.

How To Use This Book

This is a reference for people at the beginning of a new concept in healing and preventive health care. I call it "Lifestyle Therapy". The natural healing suggestions in this book work <u>with</u> the body functions, not outside them. They don't cause side effects or trauma on the system.
For long-lasting permanent health, the body must do its own work. The natural therapy methods described here will help rebalance specific areas of the body so that it can function normally.

Each person and body is individual, so there are a number of suggestions under each healing category: **FOOD THERAPY, VITAMINS/MINERALS, HERBAL THERAPY, and BODYWORK.** Obviously no one will use everything in any one category, or even use each category - but there is a great deal to choose from, so that each person can put together the best healing program for himself.

The bold print suggestions within each category are those we have found to be the most helpful for the most people. These highlighted recommendations can many times be considered complete programs in themselves, and can be successfully used together.

✦ Where a method has also proven effective for children, a small child's face ☺ appears at the end of the recommendation.
✦ Where a remedy has proven particularly successful for women, a female symbol ♀ appears at the end of the recommendation.
✦ Where a remedy has proven particularly effective for men, a male symbol ♂ appears at the end of the recommendation.

The recommended diets are "real people" diets, used by people with particular health conditions who have related their experiences to us. We have found over the years that diseases change (through mutation, environment, treatment, etc.) and people's immune responses to them change. Therefore, in this and in our other books, the diet programs are continually modified to meet new and changing needs.

The **"foot"** and **"hand"** diagrams on the specific ailment pages graphically show the reflexology pressure points for each body area, so that you can use reflexology when indicated as a viable therapy. In some cases, the points are very tiny, particularly for the glands. They will take practice to pinpoint. The best sign that you have reached the right spot is that it will usually be very tender, denoting crystalline deposits or congestion in the corresponding body part. However, there is often a feeling of immediate relief in the area as the waste deposit breaks up for removal by the body.

All recommendations have been used extensively in our practice and found to be effective. The information comes from real people who have experienced real improvement in their health. The programs are not static, and are constantly being updated with new information in every area. Every edition of "HEALTHY HEALING" offers you the latest knowledge from an ever-widening network of natural healing professionals - nutritional consultants, holistic practitioners, naturopaths, world-widr data bases - and the all-important information from the sufferers themselves, who have taken responsibility for their health with success.

All recommended doses are daily amounts unless otherwise specified.

About Herbal Remedies & How Herbs Work

Plants and people share the most essential element of all: the spark of life. This precious thing can neither be measured nor re-created in a laboratory. Herbs have been used from the time of recorded history for every facet of life - health, healing, energy, creativity, work, love, birth, death, regeneration, meditation, survival, and more. Herbs are all-encompassing and timeless, as nature itself is infinite and eternal. Therapeutic herbs have a unique spirit, with wide-ranging properties, and far-reaching possibilities for medicinal activity. Mankind can look back through thousands of years to herbal medicinals as a safe, readily available, gentle means of healing. Because the history of herbal healing is so rich, it allows us to see that herbs are also perfectly adaptable to today's requirements, with the same focused strength and reliability. We are only beginning to scratch the surface of their forgotten truth.

Herbs are more than a scientific, or even a natural healing system. God seems to show his face through herbs, so that we can see them as an art, tools of metaphysical Nature as well as of Science. Herbs react integrally with each different person. They can help with almost every aspect of human need, and like all great realities of Nature, there is so much more about themthan we shall ever know.
Many informed men and women today realize the value of herbs as alternative therapies that can noticeably improve their lives, and that they themselves can use safely and easily. Herbs are concentrated foods, whole essences, with the ability to address both the symptoms and causes of a problem. As nourishment, herbs can offer the body nutrients it does not always receive, either from poor diet, or environmental deficiencies in the soil and air. As medicine, herbs are essentially body balancers, that work with the body functions, so that it can heal and regulate itself. Hundreds of herbs are regularly available in several usable forms and at all quality levels. Worldwide communications and improved storage allow us to simultaneously obtain and use herbs from different countries and different harvests, an advantage ages past did not enjoy. However, because of the natural variety of soils, seeds, and weather, every crop of botanicals is unique. Every batch of a truly natural herbal formula will, therefore, also be slightly different, and offer its own unique benefits and experience.

Herbs in their whole form are not drugs. Do not expect the activity or response of chemical antibiotics or tranquilizers. These agents only treat the symptoms of a problem. Generally, you have to take more and more of a drug to get the same effect. Herbal medicines work differently. Herbs are nutritional foundation nutrients, working through the glands, nourishing the body's deepest and most basic elements, such as the brain, glands and hormones. Results will seem to take much longer. But this fact only shows how herbs actually work, acting as support to control and reverse the cause of a problem, with more permanent effect. Even so, some improvement from herbal treatment can usually be felt in three to six days. Chronic or longstanding degeneration will, of course take longer. A traditional rule of thumb is one month of healing for every year of the problem. Herbal combinations are not addictive or habit-forming, but are powerful nutritional agents that should be used with care. Balance is the key to using herbal nutrients for healing. It takes a litle more attention and personal responsibility than mindlessly taking prescription drugs, but the extra care is worth far more in the results you can achieve for your body.

As with other natural therapies, there is sometimes a "healing crisis" in an herbal healing program. This is traditionally known as the "Law of Cure", and simply means that sometimes you will seem to get worse before you get better. The body frequently begins to eliminate toxic wastes quite heavily during the first stages of a system cleansing therapy. This is particularly true in the traditional three to four day fast that many people use to begin a serious healing program. Herbal therapy without a fast works more slowly and gently. Still, there is usually some discomfort and weakness as disease poisons are released into the bloodstream to be flushed away. Strength and relief shortly return when this process is over. Watching this phenomenon allows you to observe your own body processes at work toward healing itself - a very interesting experience indeed.

Most herbs, as edible plants, are as safe to take as foods. They have almost no side effects as natural medicines. Occasionally a mild allergy-type reaction may occur as it might occur in response to a food. This could happen because herb quality is poor, because it has been adulterated with chemicals in the growing/storing process, or in rare cases, because incompatible herbs were used together. Or it may be just an individual adverse response to a certain plant. *The key to avoiding an adverse reaction is moderation, both in formulation and in dosagee.* Anything taken to excess can cause negative side effects. Normal common sense, care, and intelligence are needed when using herbs for either food or medicine.

Herbs work better in combination than they do singly. There are several reasons for this.
❶ Each formula compound contains two to five primary agent herbs that are part of the blend for specific purposes. Since all body parts, and most disease symptoms, are interrelated, it is wise to have herbs which can affect each part of the problem. For example, in a prostate healing formula, there would be herbs to dissolve sediment, anti-inflammatory herbs, tissue-toning and strengthening herbs, and herbs with anti-biotic properties.
❷ A combination allows inclusion of herbs that can work at different stages of need. A good example of this is an athlete's formula, where there are herbs for short-term energy, long-range endurance, muscle tone, glycogen and glucose use, and reduction of lactic acid build-up.
❸ A combination of several herbs with similar properties can increase the latitude of effectiveness, not only through a wider range of activity, but also reinforcing herbs that were picked too late or too early, or grew in adverse weather conditions for full potency.
❹ No two people, or their bodies, are alike. Good response is augmented by a combination of herbs.
❺ Finally, some very potent and complex herbs, such as capsicum, lobelia, sassafras, mandrake, tansy, Canada snakeroot, wormwood, woodruff, poke root, and rue are beneficial in small amounts and as catalysts, but should not be used alone.

With these things in mind, we have found that it is best to take herbal capsule combinations in descending strength: 6 the first day, 5 the second day, 4 the third, 3 the fourth, 2 the fifth, and 2 the sixth for the first week. Rest on the 7th day. When a healing base is built in the body, decrease to the daily maintenance dose recommended for each particular formula. Most combinations should be taken no more than 6 days in a row to allow the body to regularly restore its own balance.

Other quick tips on taking herbal mixtures:
❶ A 24 hour juice fast before starting an herbal formula will often produce greater effectiveness.
❷ Take capsules with a warm drink for faster results.
❸ Abstain from alcohol, meat, caffeine and tobacco if possible during use to give the herbs a cleaner environment in which to work.

Therapeutic herbs work best when used on as as-needed basis. Because herbal effects can be quite specific, take the best formula for your particular goal at the right time - *rather than all the time* **- for optimum results. In addition, rotating and alternating herbal combinations according to your changing health needs allows the body to remain most responsive to their effects.**

Herbs also work better when combined with a natural foods diet. Everyone can benefit from an herbal formula, but results increase dramatically when fresh foods and whole grains form the diet basis. Subtle healing activity is more effective when it doesn't have to labor through excess waste material, mucous, or junk food accumulation. (Most of us carry around 10 to 15 pounds of excess density.)
Interestingly enough, herbs themselves can help counter the problems of "civilization foods". They are rich in minerals and trace minerals, the basic elements missing or diminished in today's "quick-grow", oversprayed, over-fertilized farming. Minerals and trace minerals are a basic element in food assimilation. Mineral-rich herbs provide not only the healing essences to support the body in overcoming disease, but also the foundation minerals that allow it to take them in!

Each individual body has its own unique and wonderful mechanism, and each has the ability to bring itself to its own balanced and healthy state. Herbs simply pave the way for the body to do its own work, by breaking up toxins, cleansing, lubricating, toning and nourishing. They work through the glands at the deepest levels of the body processes - at the cause, rather than the effect.

When correctly used, herbs promote the elimination of waste matter and toxins from the system by simple natural means. They support nature in its fight against disease.

Herbal Preparation Methods

**TEAS ❖ CAPSULES ❖ EXTRACTS ❖ BATHS ❖ COMPRESSES
POULTICES ❖ SALVES ❖ OILS ❖ ELECTUARIES**

How To Use Them ✦ Which Form Is Right For You

HERBAL TEAS are the most basic of all natural healing mediums, easily absorbed by the body as hot liquid. While they are the least concentrated of all herbal preparations, many herbs are optimally effective when steeped in boiling water. The brewing water releases herbal energy and volatile oils, and provides flushing action for cleansing toxic wastes that are loosened and dissolved by the herbs. Teas have milder and more subtle effects than capsules or extracts, but they often work synergistically with both of these stronger medicinal forms to boost efficiency and value.

Tips on taking herbal teas:
❶ Use 1 packed small teaball to 3 cups of water for medicinal-strength tea.
❷ Bring water to a boil, remove from heat, add herbs and steep covered, off heat: 10 to 15 minutes for a leaf and flower tea; 15 to 25 minutes for a root and bark tea. Keep teapot lid tightly closed during steeping so the volatile oils will not escape.
❸ Use a teapot of glass, ceramic or earthenware. Do not use aluminum which can negate herbal effectiveness as the metal washes into the hot liquid and gets into the body.
❹ Drink medicinal teas in frequent small sips throughout the day rather than all at once. One half to one cup 3 to 4 times during a sixteen hour period will allow absorption of the liquid without passing before it has a chance to work.
❺ Use distilled water or pure spring water for increased herbal strength and effectiveness.
Note: The cutting of herbs for tea bags creates thousands of facets on the herb structure, causing the loss of essential volatile oils. For best results, gently crumble leaves and flowers, and break roots and barks into pieces before steeping.

   ❧ An infusion is a tea made from leaves, stems and flowers, or powdered herb.
Pour 1 cup of boiling water over 1 tablespoon of fresh herb, 1 teaspoon of dried herb, or 4 opened capsules of powdered herb, ($1/2$ to $3/4$ teaspoon). Cover and let steep 10 to 15 minutes. Never boil. A cold infusion can be made by simply allowing the herbs, especially powders, to stand in cool water for an hour or more.
   ❧ "Sun tea" is a cold infusion where the herbs are placed in a covered jar and allowed to stand in the sun.
   ❧ A decoction is a tea made from roots and bark. Use directions above, or put two tablespoons of cut pieces into one cup of cold water. Bring to a light boil, (over open flame rather than electric heat if possible). Cover, and simmer gently for 20-30 minutes. Strain. For best results, repeat the same process with the same herbs. Strain again and mix both batches.

❧

HERBAL CAPSULES are generally four times stronger than teas, more concentrated in form, and an easy, convenient way to take in the benefits of therapeutic herbs. Capsules can make both oil and water-soluble herbs available to the body through stomach acid and enzyme activity. Capsules are viable carriers of measureable amounts of essential amino acis such as L-Lysine and Tryptophan. Capsules also work well in providing gland and hormone precursor elements, such as phyto-estrogens and progesterones.
We have found that it is best to take herbal capsule combinations in descending strength: six the first day, five the second day, four the third, three the fourth, two the fifth, and two the sixth for the first week. Rest on the 7th day. Most combinations should be taken no more than six days in a row to allow the body to regularly restore its own balance. When a healing base is built in the body, a decrease to the daily maintenance dose is recommended for the particular formula.

❧

HERBAL EXTRACTS are four to eight times stronger than capsules, and are especially effective when taken as drops and held under the tongue, bypassing the digestive system and its acid/alkaline breakdown of substances. Herbs in extract form offer concentrated, easily digestible,

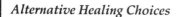

therapeutic foods, which give the body nutritional support it may not receive because of deficient diet, and the increasing environmental pollutants in the water, air and soil.

Their strength and ready availability make extracts efficient emergency measures. Ten to fifteen drops under the tongue, held as long as possible, three to four times daily are effective for the first week of an acute condition. After this first week, the vital force of the body will often have been sufficiently stimulated in its own healing ability, and the dose may be reduced to allow the system to take its own individual route to balance. *As with other forms of herbal mixtures, most extracts should be taken no more than 6 days in a row with a rest on the seventh day, before resuming, to allow the body to do its own work.* As the body increases its ability to right itself, the amount and frequency of the dosage should be decreased, to once a day, then every other day, etc., and lessening from 15 to 5 drops, then to dilutions in water. This is the optimum way in our experience for success with extracts. You may have to adjust time spans and amounts for your own state of health or recurrence of the problem.

Herbs are not addictive or habit-forming even in strong extract form. Very small doses can be used repeatedly over a period of time to help build a healthy base for restoring body balance.

Note about the difference between tinctures and extracts: Tinctures are a diluted way of taking herbs. They usually display a very high alcohol content, and the herb content per fluid ounce is very low. An extract generally displays a low alcohol content, and the herb content per fluid ounce is very high. In value-for-money-terms, an extract is usually the best choice.

Note: Homeopathic formulas in liquid form are not *the same as herbal tinctures or extracts, and their use is different. (See HOMEOPATHIC REMEDIES in this book.)*

HERBAL BATHS are soothing, gentle, alternate ways of absorbing herbal benefits through the skin. In essence, you are soaking in an herbal tea or mineral fluid, and allowing the skin to take in the healing nutrients rather than the mouth and digestive system. Soak for at least 30 to 45 minutes to give the body time to absorb the herbal properties. Use a muslin bath bag, and rub the body with the herbal solids for additional exfoliation and absorbency.

The procedure for taking an effective healing bath is important. There are two good methods to use.
❶ Draw very hot bath water. Put the bath herbs, seaweeds, or mineral crystals into an extra large tea ball or muslin bath bag, (add mineral salts directly to the water). Steep until water cools and is aromatic.
or
❷ Make a strong tea infusion in a large teapot, strain and add to bath water.

HERBAL DOUCHES are an effective method for treating localized vaginal infections. Use one full douche bag for each application. Simply steep the herbs as a strong tea, and pour the strained liquid into the douche bag. Let cool. Sit on the toilet, insert the applicator, and rinse the vagina with the herbal liquid. Most vaginal conditions need douching three times daily for three to seven days. If the problem has not responded in this time, a qualified health professional should be consulted.

HERBAL SALVES AND OINTMENTS are semi-solid preparations that allow absorption of herbal properties through the skin. The skin is, of course, the body's largest organ of ingestion, and topical herbal mediums can be used frequently for allover relief and support. They may easily be made by mixing powdered herbs with cocoa butter or petroleum jelly. Or an herbal tea or oil may be mixed into melted beeswax or lanolin, and then hardened in the refrigerator.

HERBAL COMPRESSES AND FOMENTATIONS also provide a soothing, gentle way to transfer herbal benefits into the body through the skin. Soak clean cotton cloths in a strong tea, and apply them as hot as possible to the affected area. The heat energizes the activity of the herbs, and opens the pores of the skin for fast assimilation. The technique of *alternating hot and cold compresses* is also a successful therapy, stimulating circulation, veins, capillaries and nerve functions. The hot compress should contain the herbs; the cold compress should be plain.

HERBAL POULTICES AND PLASTERS are made from either fresh herbs crushed and blended in the blender with a little olive or wheat germ oil, or dried herbs mixed into a paste with water, cider vinegar or wheat germ oil. Both are spread on a piece of clean cloth or gauze, applied and bound directly on the affected area. The whole thing is then covered with plastic wrap to keep from soiling clothes or sheets, and left on for 24 hours. There is usually some throbbing pain while the poultice is drawing out the infection and neutralizing toxic poisons. This stops when the infection has been drawn out, and signals the time to remove the poultice. A fresh poultice may be applied every 24 hours for several days.

A plaster is made by spreading a thin coat of honey on a clean cloth, and sprinkling it with an herbal mixture such as cayenne, ginger, and prickly ash, hot mustard or horseradish. The cloth is then taped directly over the affected area, usually the chest, to relieve lung and mucous congestion.

HERBAL OILS are used externally for massage, skin treatments, healing ointments, dressings for wounds and burns, and occasionally for enemas and douches.

To make an herbal oil for home use, simply infuse the herb in oil instead of water. Olive, safflower or almond oil are all good bases for an herbal oil.

ELECTUARIES are mediums that mask the bitter taste of an herb, and are usually for children. They are made by grinding or blender blending fresh or dried herbs with a little water into a paste. This paste can be mixed with twice the amount of honey, maple syrup, butter, peanut butter or cream cheese for palatability. You can roll the paste into a ball and stuff it into a piece of bread or a cookie. Or simply open up capsules, or mix a tea or extract drops, into juice, soda, or a sweet dessert if there is taste resistance, or if the child has trouble taking pills.

> ✦ Child dosage is as follows:
> $1/2$ dose for children 10-14 years
> $1/3$ dose for children 6-10 years
> $1/4$ dose for children 2-6 years
> $1/8$ dose for infants and babies

Herbal effectiveness usually goes by body weight. Dose decisions should be based on that premise for adults as well as children. All recommendations in this book are for adults.

☞ Whichever herbal form you choose, it is usually most beneficial to take greater amounts at the beginning of your program, to build a good healing base in the system, and start the body's own vital balancing force more quickly. As the therapeutic agents establish themselves and build in the body, and you begin to notice good response and balance returning, fewer and fewer of the large initial doses should be taken, finally reducing the dosage to longer range maintenance and preventive amounts.

However, and this is very important, we have found over and over again that with **immune deficient, opportunistic, and degenerative diseases,** *it takes a great deal of time to rebuild a healthy system. Even when a good healing program is working, and obvious improvement is being made,* **adding <u>more</u> of the healing agents in an effort to speed benefits can often aggravate symptoms,** *and bring about worse results!*

The immune system is a very fragile entity, and can be overwhelmed instead of stimulated. An afflicting virus can even seem to mutate and be nourished by supplementation, instead of arrested by it. **In this type of case, including Candida Albicans, Multiple Sclerosis, Epstein-Barr Virus, Lupus, and particularly AIDS and ARC, moderate amounts are excellent, mega-doses are not.** *Much better results* can be obtained by giving yourself more time and gentler treatment.

When working with herbs and alternative healing methods, choose the elements that will address your worst problem first. One of the bonuses of a natural healing program is the frequent discovery that other conditions were really complications of the first problem, and often take care of themselves as the body comes into balance.

The body knows how to use herbs. Give them time. They are working.

Vitamins

What They Are ✦ How They Work ✦ Why You Need Them

Vitamins are organic micro-nutrients that act like spark plugs in the body, keeping it "tuned up", and functioning at high performance. *But you cannot live on vitamins. They are not pep pills or substitutes for food. They are not the components of body structure. They stimulate, but do not act as, nutritional fuel.* As catalysts, they work on the cellular level, often as co-enzymes, regulating body metabolic processes through enzyme activity, to convert proteins and carbohydrates to tissue and energy. Notwithstanding their minute size and amount in the body, vitamins are absolutely necessary for growth, vitality, resistance to disease, and healthy aging. Even small deficiencies can endanger the whole body. Unfortunately, it takes weeks or months for signs of some deficiencies to appear as the body uses up its supply, and even then a problem is often hard to pinpoint, because the cells usually continue to function less and less efficiently until they receive proper nourishment or suffer irreversible damage.

Vitamin therapy and supplementation do not produce results overnight. Vitamins fill the nutritional gaps at the deepest levels of the body processes. Regenerative changes in body chemistry usually require as much time to rebuild as they did to decline.

Even though it is impossible to sustain life without them, most vitamins cannot be synthesized by the body, and must be supplied from foods or supplementation. Excess amounts are excreted through the urine, or stored by the body until needed. Consequently, we have found that after a *short period of higher dosage* in which to build a solid foundation, a program of *moderate* amounts over a *longer* period of time brings about better body balance and more permanent results.

A little goes a long way.

Vitamin RDAs were established by the National Academy years ago as a guideline for the amounts of vitamins and minerals needed to prevent the most severe deficiency diseases. Today, because of poor dietary habits, over-processed foods, and agri-business practices, most health professionals recognize that supplemental amounts are often needed to achieve adequate nutrition and health. No dietary survey to date has shown that all recommended RDA nutrient intakes are being consumed through the daily diet. A recent USDA survey of the food intake of 21,500 people over a three day period showed that *not a single person* of those surveyed consumed 100% of the RDA for the nutrients surveyed. Only 3% ate the recommended number of servings from the four food groups. Only 12% ate the RDA for protein, calcium, iron, magnesium, zinc or vitamins A, C, B_6, B_{12}, B_2, and B_1. More importantly, the study noted that focusing solely on efforts to change dietary habits and discounting supplementation as a valuable option, leaves much of the American population at nutritional risk.

Those most affected include:
✦ Women with excessive menstrual bleeding who may need iron supplements.
✦ Pregnant or nursing women who may need extra iron, calcium and folic acid.

✦ The elderly, many of whom do not even eat $2/3$ of the RDA for calcium, iron, vitamin A or C. In addition, the elderly take at least 50% of the total prescribed medications in the U.S. Since 90 out of the 100 most prescribed drugs interfere with normal nutrient metabolism, it is becoming a sad fact that many older people don't absorb much of the nutrition that they do eat.
✦ Others with disorders or diseases, or on medications that interfere with nutrient intake, digestion, metabolism and absorption.
✦ People who are dieting for weight loss with low total calorie intake.
✦ Those at risk for heart and circulatory blockages.
✦ Those who have recently had surgery, or suffer from serious injuries, wounds or burns.
✦ Those with periodontal disease.
✦ Those at risk for osteoporosis.

✦ Some vegetarians, who may not receive enough calcium, iron, zinc or vitamin B_{12}.

✦

As we age, vitamins can be particularly valuable aids to health maintenance of both body and mind. Throughout our lives, vitamins can help us to go beyond average health to optimal health.

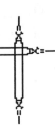

THE MOST ESSENTIAL VITAMINS

❧ **VITAMIN A** - fat soluble, requiring fats and zinc as well as other minerals and enzymes for absorption. Counteracts night blindness, weak eyesight, and strengthens the optical system. Supplementation lowers risk of many types of cancer. Retinoids inhibit malignant transformation, and reverse premalignant changes in tissue. Particularly effective, even in large amounts, against lung cancer. An anti-infective that also builds immune resistance. Helps develop strong bone cells; a major factor in the health of skin, hair, teeth and gums. Deficiency results in eye dryness and the inability to tear, night blindness, rough, itchy skin, poor bone growth, weak tooth enamel, chronic diarrhea, frequent respiratory infection. Long-term use of mineral oil laxatives reduces A absorption.
Effective food sources: vegetables, leafy greens, yams, sweet potatoes, liver, watermelon, fruits, eggs.

❧ **BETA CAROTENE** - a vitamin A precursor, converting to A in the liver as the body needs it. A powerful anti-infective and anti-oxidant for immune health, protection against environmental pollutants, slowing the aging process, and allergy control. Supplementation protects against respiratory diseases and infections. A key in preventing some kinds of cancer, and in developing anti-tumor immunity.
Effective food sources: green leafy vegetables, green pepper, carrots and other range vegetables, sea vegetables.

THE B COMPLEX VITAMINS - the B Complex vitamins are essential to almost every aspect of body function, including metabolism of carbohydrates, fats, amino acids and energy production. B Complex vitamins work together. While they can and do work as partitioned substances for specific problems or deficiencies, they should be taken as a whole for broad-spectrum activity.

❧ **VITAMIN B_1 - Thiamine** - known as the "morale vitamin" because of its beneficial effects on the nervous system and mental attitude. Promotes proper growth in children, aids carbohydrate utilization for energy, and supports the nervous system. Enhances immune response. Helps control motion sickness. Wards off mosquitos and stinging insects. Pregnancy, lactation, diuretics and oral contraceptives require extra thiamine. Smoking, heavy metal pollutants, excess sugar, junk foods, stress and alcohol all deplete thiamine. Deficiency results in insomnia, fatigue, confusion and poor memory, and muscle coordination.
Effective food sources: asparagus, brewer's yeast, brown rice and whole grains, beans, nuts and seeds, wheat germ.

❧ **VITAMIN B_2 - Riboflavin** - commonly deficient in the American diet. Necessary for energy production, and for fat and carbohydrate metabolism. Helps prevent cataracts and corneal ulcers, and benefits vision generally. Promotes healthy skin, especially in cases of psoriasis. Helps protect against drug toxicity and environmental chemicals. Pregnancy and lactation, red meat, excess dairy consumption, prolonged stress, sulfa drugs, diuretics and oral contraceptives require extra riboflavin. Deficiency is associated with alcohol abuse, anemia, hypothyroidism, diabetes, ulcers, cataracts, and congenital heart disease.
Effective food sources: almonds, brewer's yeast, broccoli, green leafy vegetables, eggs, wild rice, mushrooms, yogurt.

❧ **VITAMIN B_3 - Niacin** - broad spectrum of functions, including energy production, cholesterol metabolism, sex hormone synthesis and proper digestion. Promotes healthy skin and nerves. Deficiency results in dermatitis, headaches, gum diseases, sometimes high blood pressure, and negative personality behavior with mental depression. However, because niacin can rapidly open up and stimulate circulation, (a niacin flush is evidence of this), it can act quickly to reverse deficiencies and disorders. Relieves acne, diarrhea and other gastrointestinal disorders, migraine headaches and vertigo attacks. Supplementation is synergistic with chromium, via GTF to improve blood sugar regulation for diabetes and hypoglycemia. Helps reduce serum blood fats, triglycerides and cholesterol, while raising HDLs.
Effective food sources: almonds, avocados, brewer's yeast, fish, organ meats, legumes, bananas, whole grains.

❧ **VITAMIN B_5 - Pantothenic Acid** - an anti-oxidant vital to proper adrenal activity. A precursor to cortisone production and an aid to natural steroid synthesis, therefore important in control and prevention of arthritis and high cholesterol. Fights infection by building antibodies, and defends against stress, fatigue and nerve disorders. A key to overcoming postoperative shock and drug side effects after surgery. Inhibits hair color loss. Deficiency results in anemia, fatigue, muscle cramping and lack of coordination.
Effective food sources: brewer's yeast, brown rice, poultry, yams, whole grains, organ meats, broccoli, legumes.

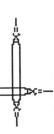

✤ **VITAMIN B6 - Pyridoxine -** a key factor in red blood cell regeneration, amino acid/protein metabolism, and carbohydrate use. A primary immune stimulant, shown in recent studies to have particular effect against liver cancer. Supplementation inhibits histamine release in the treatment of allergies and asthma. Supports all aspects of nerve health including neuropsychiatric disorders, epilepsy and carpal tunnel syndrome. Works as a natural diuretic, especially in premenstrual edema. Controls acne, promotes beautiful skin, alleviates morning sickness, and is a key to anti-aging factors in the body. Protects against environmental pollutants, smoking and stress. Oral contraceptives, thiazide diuretics, penicillin and alcohol deplete B6. Deficiency results in anemia, depression, lethargy, nervousness, water retention, and skin lesions.
Effective food sources: bananas, brewer's yeast, buckwheat, organ meats, fish, avocados, legumes, poultry, nuts.

✤ **VITAMIN B12 - (Cyano) Cobalamin -** an anti-inflammatory and analgesic that works with calcium for absorption. A primary part of DNA synthesis and red blood cell formation. Involved in all immune responses. A specific in blocking sulfite-induced asthma. New research shows success in cancer management, especially in tumor development. Energizes, relieves fatigue, depression, hangover, and poor concentration. Supplied largely animal food sources, B12 is often deficient for vegetarians, and deficiency can take five or more years to appear after body stores have been depleted. Deficiency results in anemia, nervous system degeneration, dizziness, heart palpitations, and unhealthy weight loss. Long term use of cholesterol-lowering drugs, oral contraceptives, anti-inflammatory and anti-convulsant drugs deplete B12.
Effective food sources: cheeses, poultry, sea vegetables, yogurt, eggs, organ meats, brewer's yeast, fish.

✤ **BIOTIN -** a member of the B Complex family, necessary for metabolism of amino acids and essential fatty acids, and in the formation of anti-bodies. Needed for the body to therapeutically use folacin, B12 and pantothenic acid. Oral supplementation has shown good results with in controlling hair loss, dermatitis, eczema, dandruff and seborrheic scalp problems. Improves glucose tolerance in diabetics. New research indicates enhanced immune response in Candida Albicans and CFS. Those taking long term anti-biotics require extra biotin. Deficiencies result in skin disorders and muscle pains.
Effective food sources: poultry, raspberries, grapefruit, tomatoes, tuna, brewer's yeast, salmon, eggs, organ meats.

✤ **CHOLINE -** a lipotropic and B Complex family member. Works with inositol to emulsify fats. A brain nutrient and neurotransmitter that aids memory and learning ability, and is effective against Alzheimers disease and other neurological disorders. Part of a program to overcome alcoholism, liver and kidney disorders. New research indicates success in programs for cancer management. Helps control dizziness, lowers cholesterol, and supports proper liver function.
Effective food sources: organ meats, eggs, fish, unrefined vegetable oils, legumes, soy products.

✤ **FOLIC ACID - Folacin -** an important factor in the synthesis of DNA, enzyme production and blood formation. Essential for division and growth of new cells, it is an excellent supplement during pregnancy (800mcg. daily) to guard against spinal bifida and neural tube defects. Prevents anemia, helps control leukemia and pernicious anemia, and is effective for alcoholism. Effective against some pre-cancerous lesions. Absolutely necessary to counteract the immuno-depression state following chemotherapy with MTX. Deficiency results in malabsorption problems such as Crohn's disease and sprue. Aluminum antacids, oral contraceptives, alcohol, long-term anti-biotics and anti-inflammatory drugs increase the need for folic acid.
Effective food sources: leafy vegetables, liver, peas, brewer's yeast, broccoli, fruits, soy products.

✤ **INOSITOL -** a lipotropic and non-vitamin B Complex family member. Works with biotin and choline to control male pattern baldness, hypertension, and arteriosclerosis. Metabolizes serum blood fats to lower cholesterol and control fatty deposits on the liver. An "inositol cocktail" may be taken as a spring tonic to revive a sluggish system. Helps reduce breast and ovarian cancer risk, and controls estrogen-related premenstrual symptoms. Helps control many of the side-effects occurring with diabetes. Effective for athletes by enhancing oxygen delivery to the tissues.
Effective food sources: almonds, beans, onions, oranges, peanut butter, oats, peas, tomatoes, zucchini.

✤ **PABA - Para-Aminobenzoic Acid -** a B Complex family member and component of folic acid, PABA has sun-screening properties, is effective against sun and other burns, and is used in treating vitiligo, (depigmentation of the skin). Successful with molasses, pantothenic and folic acid in restoring lost hair color. New research shows success against skin cancers caused by UV radiation (lack of ozone-layer protection).
Effective food sources: brewer's yeast, eggs, molasses, wheat germ.

✣ **VITAMIN C - Ascorbic Acid** - a primary factor in immune strength and maintenance. Protects against cancer, viral and bacterial infections, heart disease, arthritis and allergies. A strong antioxidant to prevent free radical damage. New research indicates supplementation helps reduce cancer risk. Safeguards against radiation, heavy metal toxicity, environmental pollutants and early aging. Accelerates healing after surgery, increases infection resistance, and is essential to formation of new collagen tissue. Controls alcohol craving, prevents constipation, and lowers cholesterol. A key factor in treatments for diabetes, high blood pressure, male infertility, and in suppressing the AIDS virus. Supports adrenal and iron insuffiency, especially when the body is under stress. Relieves withdrawal symptoms from addictive drugs, tranquilizers and alcohol. Aspirin, oral contraceptives, smoking and tetracycline inhibit vitamin C absorption and deplete C levels. Supplementation should be considered if these things are part of your lifestyle. Deficiency results in easy bruising and bleeding, receding gums, slow healing, fatigue and rough skin.
Note: The new metabolite form of vitamin C, Ester C™ is biochemically the same as the naturally metabolised C substance in the body. It is both fat and water soluble, and non-acid. Uptake of C is absorbed twice as fast into the bloodstream, and excreted twice as slowly as ordinary vitamin C. This means that vitamin C in the tissues can be up to four times higher than normally possible.
Effective food sources: citrus fruits, green peppers, papaya, tomatoes, kiwi, potatoes, greens, cauliflower, broccoli.

✣ **BIOFLAVONOIDS** - part of the vitamin C complex, and necessary to its proper function. Bioflavs prevent arteries from hardening, enhance blood vessel, capillary and vein strength. They protect connective tissue integrity, control bruising, internal bleeding and mouth herpes. They help lower cholesterol, and stimulate bile production. Bioflavs are anti-microbial against infections. They reduce cataract formation, and guard against diabetic retinopathy. The body does not produce its own bioflavonoidss, which must be obtained regularly from the diet. Strongest supplementary form is quercetin.
Effective food sources: white part beneath the skin of citrus fruits, herbal sources, buckwheat, most vegetables.

✣ **VITAMIN D** - a fat soluble "sunlight vitamin", it works with vitamin A to utilize calcium and phosphorus in building bone structure and healthy teeth. Helps in all eye problems including spots, conjunctivitis and glaucoma. Helps protect against colon cancer. Air pollution, anti-convulsant drugs and lack of sunlight deplete Vitamin D. Deficiency results in nearsightedness, psoriasis, soft teeth, muscle cramps and tics, slow healing, insomnia, nosebleeds, fast heartbeat and arthritic symptoms.
Effective food sources: cod liver oil, herring, halibut, salmon, tuna, eggs, liver.

✣ **VITAMIN E** - an active fat soluble anti-oxidant and important immune stimulant. An effective anticoagulant and vasodilator against blood clots and heart disease. Retards cellular and mental aging, alleviates fatigue and provides tissue oxygen to accelerate healing of wounds and burns. Works with selenium against the effects of aging and cancer by neutralizing free radicals. The most cell protecting form seems to be E succinate (dry E). Improves skin problems and texture. Helps control baldness and dandruff. Deficiency results in muscle and nerve degeneration, anemia, skin pigmentation.
Effective food sources: almonds, leafy vegetables, salmon, soy products, wheat germ/wheat germ oil, organ meats.

✣ **VITAMIN K** - a fat soluble vitamin necessary for blood clotting. Reduces excessive menstruation. Helps heal broken blood vessels in the eye. Aids in arresting bone loss and post-menopausal brittle bones. Helps in cirrhosis and jaundice of the liver. Acts as an anti-parasitic for intestinal worms.
Effective food sources: seafoods, sea vegetables, leafy vegetables, liver, molasses, eggs, oats, crucifers, sprouts.

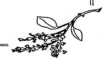

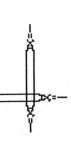

Achieving a healthy life style is not just hard work.
It is also fun.
It feels so worthwhile.
It is one of the most rewarding things you can do.

Minerals & Trace Minerals

What They Are ✦ How They Work ✦ Why You Need Them

Minerals and trace minerals are the building blocks of life. They are the most basic of nutrients, the bonding agents in and between you and food - allowing the body to absorb nutrients. **Minerals** are needed by everyone for good health and an active life. They are especially necessary for athletes and people in active sports, because you must have minerals to run. All the minerals together comprise only about 4% of the body weight, but they are responsible for major areas of human health. **Minerals** keep the body pH balanced - alkaline instead of acid. They are essential to bone formation, and to the digestion of food. They regulate the osmosis of cellular fluids, electrical activity in the nervous system, and most metabolic functions. They transport oxygen through the system, govern heart rhythm, help you sleep, and are principle factors in mental and emotional balance. **Trace minerals** are only .01% of body weight, but deficiencies in even these micro-nutrients can cause severe depression, P.M.S. and other menstrual disorders, hyperactivity in children, sugar imbalances (hypoglycemia and diabetes), nerve and stress conditions, high blood pressure, osteoporosis, premature aging of skin and hair, memory loss and the inability to heal quickly.

Minerals are important. Hardly any of us get enough.

Minerals cannot be synthesized by the body, and must be regularly obtained through our food, drink, or mineral baths. Minerals from plants and herbs are higher quality and more absorbable than from other sources. They work optimally with the body's enzyme production for assimilation. Today's diet of refined foods, red meats, caffeine and fatty foods, inhibits mineral absorption. High stress life styles that rely on tobacco, alcohol, steroids, anti-biotics and other drugs also contribute to mineral depletion. To make matters worse, many minerals and trace minerals are no longer sufficiently present in our fruits and vegetables. They have been leached from the soil by the chemicals and fertilizers used in commercial farming today, and by the sprays and pesticides used on the produce itself. Even foods that still show measureable amounts of mineral composition have lower quality and quantity than we are led to believe, because most testing was done decades ago when sprays and pesticides were not as prolific as they are now.

Organically grown, unsprayed produce is often difficult to obtain on a regular, high quality basis. Because of this, plant minerals from herb sources have become an easy, reliable way to obtain valuable mineral benefits. Herbal minerals are balanced, whole foods that the body easily recognizes and uses. Because of their concentrated nature, herbs can be used as healing agents as well as to maintain nutrient levels in the body. Unlike partitioned or chemically formed supplements, the minerals in herbs are cumulatively active in the body forming a strong, solid base.

Minerals can really give your body a boost. For mineral strength, eat organically grown produce whenever possible, and take a high quality herb or food source mineral supplement.

THE MOST ESSENTIAL MINERALS & TRACE MINERALS

❖ **BORON** - enhances calcium, magnesium, phosphorus and vitamin D use in bone formation and density. Stimulates estrogen production which protects against the onset of osteoporosis. A significant nutritional deterrent to bone loss for athletes.
Effective food sources: most vegetables, fruits, such as apples, pears, grapes and nuts.

❖ **CALCIUM** - most abundant mineral in the body. Needs vitamin D for good absorption. Necessary for synthesis of B12. Works with phosphorus to build sound teeth and bones, with magnesium for cardiovascular health and skeletal strength. Helps blood clotting, lowers blood pressure, prevents muscle cramping, maintains nervous system health, controls anxiety and depression, and insures high quality rest and sleep. Helps prevent colon cancer and osteoporosis. Aluminum-based antacids interfere with calcium absorption. Antibiotics and cortico-steroid drugs increase calcium needs. Calcium citrate has the best record of absorbency.
Effective food sources: green vegetables, milk and dairy products, sea vegetables, tofu, molasses, shellfish.

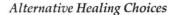

❖ **CHLORINE** - *naturally occurring chlorine* stimulates liver activity, gastric juices, and smooth joint/tendon operation. An electrolyte, it helps maintain body fluid osmotic pressure and acid/alkaline balance. *Effective food sources: seafoods and seaweeds, salt.*

❖ **CHROMIUM** - an essential trace mineral needed for glucose tolerance and sugar regulation. Deficiency means high cholesterol, heart trouble, diabetes or hypoglycemia, poor carbohydrate and fat metabolism, and premature aging. Supplementation can reduce blood cholesterol levels, increase HDL cholesterol levels, and diminish atherosclerosis. Greatest effectiveness as a biologically active form of GTF (chromium, niacin and glutathione) to control diabetes through insulin potentiation. For athletes, chromium supplements are a healthy, safe way to convert body fat to muscle. For dieters, chromium curbs the appetite as it raises body metabolism. 200mcg. to 600mcg. of chromium picolinate appear to be the most biologically active. *Effective food sources: brewer's yeast, clams, honey, whole grains, cheese, liver, corn oil, grapes, raisins.*

❖ **COBALT** - an integral component of vitamin B$_{12}$ synthesis. Aids in hemoglobin formation. *Effective food sources: green leafy vegetables, liver.*

❖ **COPPER** - helps to control inflammatory arthritis/bursitis symptoms. Aids in iron absorption, protein metabolism, bone mineralization, blood clotting and formation. SOD is a copper-containing enzyme that protects against free radical damage. Helps prevent hair from losing its color. Deficiencies result in high cholesterol, anemia, heart arrhythmias and nerves. Excess copper sometimes results in mental depression. *Effective food sources: molasses, raisins, seafoods, high fiber cereals, organ meats, nuts, legumes, eggs.*

❖ **FLUORINE** - as <u>calcium fluoride</u>, (not sodium fluoride as is added to drinking water), increases bone strength, reduces carbohydrate-caused acidity in the mouth, and the incidence of tooth decay. *Effective food sources: widespread in foods and fluoridated drinking water.*

❖ **GERMANIUM** - should be used only as *organic* sesquioxide. Acts as an anti-cancer agent, particularly where there is tumor metastasis, by activating macrophages and increasing production of killer cells. A stimulus to interferon in the body for immune strength. Facilitates oxygen uptake, detoxifies and blocks free radicals. Effective for viral/bacterial and fungal infections, osteoporosis, arthritis, heart, blood pressure and respiratory conditions. Success with leukemia, AIDS, brain, lung, pancreatic/lymphatic cancers. *Effective food sources: Chlorella, garlic, tuna, oysters, green tea, reishi mushroom, aloe vera, ginseng, leafy greens.*

❖ **IODINE** - a major component of good thyroid function and proper metabolism. Deficiency results in goiter, hypothyroidism, cretinism, confused thinking, and menstrual difficulties. Necessary for skin, hair, and nail health, and correct wound healing, iodine also prevents toxicity from radiation. *Effective food sources: seafoods and sea vegetables.*

❖ **IRON** - combines with proteins and copper to produce hemoglobin which carries oxygen throughout the body. Iron deficiency results in fatigue, muscle weakness and anemia. Iron strengthens immunity, and is a key to healing from injury. Important for women using the Pill and during pregnancy. Keeps hair color young, eyes bright, the body strong. However, free un-bound iron is a strong pro-oxidant, and can be toxic at abnormally high levels, resulting in iron overload with harmful free radicals linked to some cancers, heart disease, diabetes, arthritis and endocrine dysfunction. Vitamin E and C with bioflavonoids are used to treat iron overload. Using herbal or food sources as supplements avoids the problem altogether. *Effective food sources: molasses, cherries, prunes, leafy greens, poultry, liver, legumes, peas, eggs, fish, whole grains.*

❖ **LITHIUM** - an earth's crust trace mineral used clinically as lithium arginate. Successful in treating manic-depressive disorders, hyperkinesis in children, epilepsy, alcoholism, drug withdrawal, and migraine headaches. New research is showing therapeutic success with malignant lymphatic growths, arteriosclerosis and chronic hepatitis. Overdoses can cause palpitations and headaches. *Effective food sources: mineral waters, whole grains and seeds.*

❖ **MAGNESIUM** - the critical mineral for osteoporosis and the skeletal system. Necessary for good nerve and muscle function, healthy blood vessels and balanced blood pressure. Athletes need extra magnesium for endurance and exercise capacity. An important part of tooth and bone formation, heart and kidney health, and restful sleep. Counteracts stress, nerves, irregular heartbeat, emotional instability and depression. Calms hyperactive children. Supplemental success with alcoholism, diabetes, and asthma. A co-factor for the absorption and metabolism of carbohydrates, of vitamin C, B complex, and other minerals. Deficien-

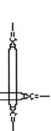

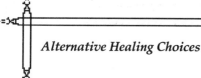

cy results in muscle spasms, cramping and gastro-intestinal disturbances.
Effective food sources: dark green vegetables, seafood, whole grains, dairy foods, nuts, legumes.

✤ **MANGANESE** - nourishes brain, and nerve centers. Aids in sugar and fat metabolism. Necessary for DNA/RNA production. Involved with SOD protection against free radical damage. Enhances immune response. Helps eliminate fatigue, nerve irritability and lower back pain. Reduces seizures in epileptics. Deficiencies result in poor hair and nail growth, loss of hearing, poor muscle/joint coordination. Chemical tranquilizers deplete manganese. The citrate form shows best absorption performance.
Effective foods sources: eggs, green vegetables, legumes, nuts, pineapple, bananas, whole grains and cereals, liver.

✤ **MOLYBDENUM** - a metabolic mineral, necessary in mobilizing enzymes. New research is showing success for esophageal cancers and sulfite-induced cancer.
Effective foods sources: whole grains, brown rice, brewer's yeast, mineral water. Dependent on good soil content.

✤ **PHOSPHORUS** - the second most abundant body mineral. Occurs in ratio balance with calcium. Necessary for skeletal infrastructure, brain oxygenation, and cellreproduction. Maintains acid/alkaline balance. Increases muscle performance while decreasing muscle fatigue. Excessive antacids deplete phosphorus.
Effective food sources: eggs, fish, organ meats, dairy products, legumes., nuts, poultry.

◗ **POTASSIUM** - an electrolyte mineral located in the body fluids. Balances the acid/alkaline system, transmits electrical signals between cells and nerves, and enhances athletic performance. Works with sodium to regulate the body's water balance. Necessary for heart health (hypertension and stroke), normal muscle function, energy storage, nerve stability, enzyme and hormone production. Helps oxygenate the brain for clear thinking and controls allergic reactions. Stress, hypoglycemia, diarrhea and acute mental anxiety all cause potassium deficiency. A potassium broth (page 53) from vegetables is one of the greatest natural healing tools available for cleansing and returned body energy.
Effective food sources: dried fruits, lean poultry and fish, dairy foods, legumes, seeds, vegetables, whole grains.

✤ **SELENIUM** - a component of glutathione, and powerful anti-oxidant. Protects the body from free radical damage and heavy metal toxicity. An anti-cancer and immune stimulant agent. Works with vitamin E to prevent fat and cholesterol accumulation in the bloodstream. Protects against heart weakness and degenerative diseases. Enhances elasticity of skin and body tissue. Deficiency results in aging skin, liver damage, increased oxidation,hypothyroidism, and in severe cases, digestive/eliminative tract cancers. Most effective supplement source is selenomethionine. Should be used only from organic sources.
Effective food sources: brewer's yeast, sesame seeds, garlic, tuna, kelp, wheat germ, oysters, fish, organ meats.

✤ **SILICON** - responsible for connective tissue growth and health. Prevents arteriosclerosis. Necessary for collagen production and synthesis - all healing and rebuilding processes. Can regenerate the body infrastructure, including not only the skeleton, but tendons, ligaments, cartilage, connective tissue, skin , hair and nails. Recent research shows that silicon supplementation can actually bring about bone recalcification.
Beneficial food sources: whole grains, horsetail herb.

✤ **SODIUM** - an electrolyte that helps regulate kidney and body fluid function. Involved with high blood pressure <u>only</u> when calcium and phosphous are deficient in the body.
Beneficial food sources: celery, seafoods, sea vegetables, cheese, dairy products.

✤ **SULPHUR** - the "beauty mineral" for smooth skin, glossy hair, hard nails and collagen synthesis. It is critical to protein absorption, and part of many amino acids.
Effective food sources: eggs, fish, onions, garlic, hot peppers, mustard, horseradish.

✤ **VANADIUM** - a cofactor for several enzymes. Needed for cell metabolism. Deficiency linked to heart disease, poor reproductive ability, and infant mortality.
Effective food sources: whole grains, fish, olives, radishes, vegetables.

✤ **ZINC** - a co-enzyme of SOD that protects against free radicaldamage. Essential to formation of insulin, immune strength, gland, sexual and reproductive health. Critical to immune function. Helps prevent birth defects, enhances sensory perception, accelerates healing. A brain food that helps control mental disorders and promotes mental alertness. Picolinate form is the most absorbable.
Effective food sources: brewer's yeast, eggs, mushrooms, soy foods, wheat germ, sunflower and pumpkin seeds.

ABOUT THE AUTHOR

Linda Rector-Page has been working in the fields of nutrition and herbal medicine both professionally and as a personal lifestyle choice, since the early seventies. She is a certified Doctor of Naturopathy and Ph.D., with extensive experience in formulating and testing herbal combinations. She received a Doctorate of Naturopathy from the Clayton School of Holistic Healing in 1988, and a Ph.D. in Nutritional Therapy from the American Holistic College of Nutrition in 1989. She is a member of both the American and California Naturopathic Medical Associations.

Linda opened and operated the "Rainbow Kitchen," a natural foods restaurant, then became a working partner in The Country Store Natural Foods store. She has written four successful books and a series of special library booklets in the nutritional healing field. She is the founder/developer of Crystal Star Herbal Nutrition.

Broad, continuous research in all aspects of the alternative healing world, from manufacturers, to stores to consumers has been the cornerstone of success for her reference work **"HEALTHY HEALING,"** now in its ninth edition.
Crystal Star Herbal Nutrition products, which are formulated by Linda, are carried by over twenty-five hundred natural food stores nationwide. Feedback from these direct consumer sources provide up-to-the-minute contact with the needs, desires and results being encountered by people taking more responsibility for their own health. Much of the lifestyle information and empirical observation detailed in her books comes from this direct experience - knowledge that is then translated into Crystal Star Herbal Nutrition products, and recorded in every **"HEALTHY HEALING"** edition.

"COOKING FOR HEALTHY HEALING," now in its second revised edition, is a companion to **"HEALTHY HEALING."** It draws on both the recipes from the Rainbow Kitchen and the more defined, lifestyle diets that she has developed from healing results since then. The book contains thirty-three separate diet programs, and over 900 healthy recipes. Every recipe has been taste-tested and time-tested as a part of each recommended diet, so that the suggested healing program can be easily maintained with optimum nutrition.

In **"HOW TO BE YOUR OWN HERBAL PHARMACIST,"** Linda addresses the rising appeal of herbs and herbal healing in America. Many people have expressed an interest in clearly understanding herbal formulation knowledge for personal use. This book is designed for those wishing to take more definitive responsibility for their health through individually developed herbal combinations.

Linda has just completed a new party reference book called **"PARTY LIGHTS"** in collaboration with restaurateur Doug Vanderberg. This book takes healthy cooking one step further by adding in the fun to a good diet. Over sixty party themes are completely planned in this new book, all with healthy party foods, earthwise decorations, professional garnishing tips, festive napkin folding, interesting games and activities.

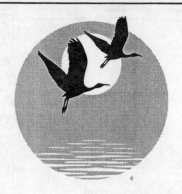

Books by Linda Rector-Page, N.D., Ph.D. available from
Healthy Healing Publications

To order: Call us at
1-(800)-736-6015

or mail this form to:
Healthy Healing Publications
16060 Via Este, Sonora, California, 95370.

BOOKS

☐ **9500.** "HEALTHY HEALING" by Linda Rector-Page, N.D., Ph.D.
An alternative healing reference for both consumer and retailer. SRP - $26.95.

☐ **9600.** "COOKING FOR HEALTHY HEALING" 2nd Edition, by Linda Rector-Page, N.D., Ph.D.
Over 900 recipes and 33 separate diet programs for health and healing. SRP - $27.95.

☐ **9650.** "HOW TO BE YOUR OWN HERBAL PHARMACIST" by Linda Rector-Page, N.D., Ph.D.
An herbal formulating, preparation, and complete reference guide for the consumer. SRP - $15.95.

☐ **9680.** "PARTY LIGHTS" by Linda Rector-Page, N.D., Ph.D. & Doug Vanderberg.
A party reference book & cookbook for healthy party foods and earthwise decorations. SRP - $19.95.

The Library Series Booklets by Dr. Linda Rector-Page, N.D., Ph.D.
A new series of small handbooks on specific health subjects. - Price $2.95 each.

*9301. Menopause & Osteoporosis - Taking Charge of Your Life Change
*9300. Renewing Female Balance
*9311. Cancer - Can Alternative Therapies Help?
*9307. The Energy Crunch & You
*9305. Male Health & Energy
*9306. Body Cleansing, Detoxification & Waste Management
*9308. Stress & Tension Relief & Getting Pain Out of Your Life
*9303. Colds & Flu & You - Building Optimum Immunity
*9304. Fighting Infections with Herbs & About Sexually Transmitted Infections
*9302. Do You Want to Have a Baby? Conception & Natural Prenatal Care

Available in 1995
*9319. Power Plants - Herbal Nutrients That Can Change Your Health
*9315. Do You Have Blood Sugar Blues?
*9312. A Fighting Chance For Weight Loss & Cellulite Control
*9320. Gland & Organ Health; Strengthening Your Body Basics
*9313. Overcoming Arthritis With Natural Therapy
*9314. Candida & Chronic Fatigue Syndrome
*9310. Heart & Circulatory Health; Controlling High Blood Pressure & Cholesterol
*9309. Allergy Control & Management; Overcoming Asthma
*9316. Beautiful Skin, Hair & Nails Naturally
*9317. Don't Let Your Food Go to Waste - Better Digestion & Nutrient Assimilation
*9318. Herbal Therapies For Children

EACH OF DR. PAGE'S BOOKS ARE THOROUGHLY RESEARCHED - THROUGH EMPIRICAL OBSERVATION AS WELL AS FROM INTERNATIONALLY DOCU-MENTED EVIDENCE. STUDIES ARE ONGOING AND UPDATED. FOR MORE INFORMATION ABOUT HER OTHER BOOKS AND PAPERS SEND A SELF-ADDRESSED, STAMPED ENVELOPE WITH YOUR REQUEST TO HEALTHY HEALING PUBLICATIONS, 16060 VIA ESTE, SONORA, CA. 95370.

All books are published by Healthy Healing Publications.

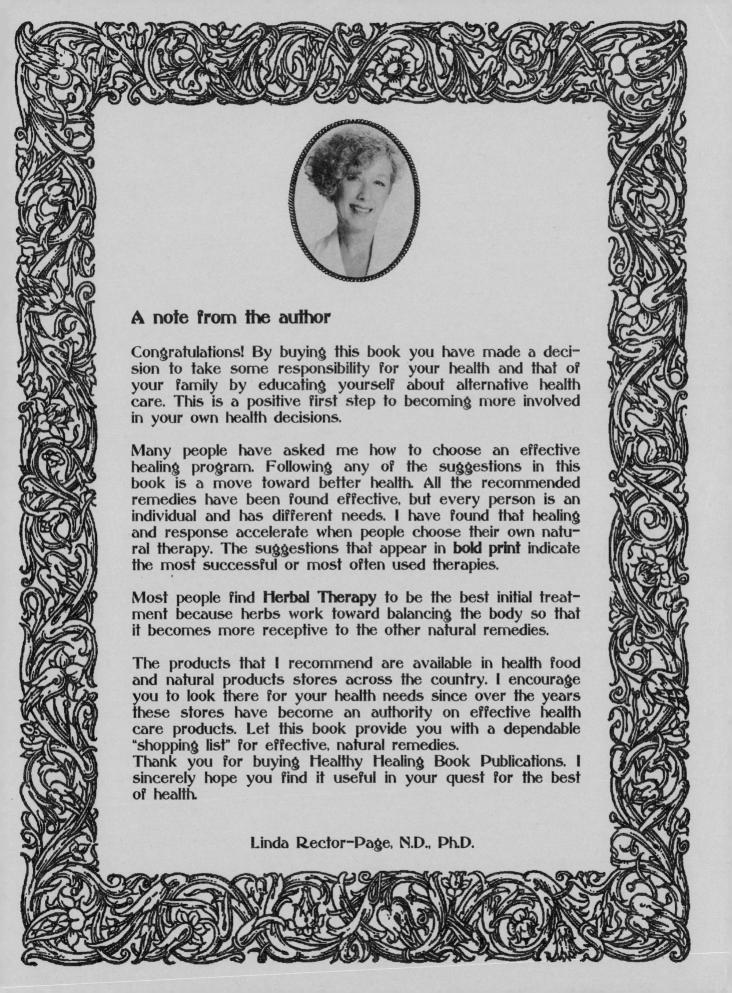

A note from the author

Congratulations! By buying this book you have made a decision to take some responsibility for your health and that of your family by educating yourself about alternative health care. This is a positive first step to becoming more involved in your own health decisions.

Many people have asked me how to choose an effective healing program. Following any of the suggestions in this book is a move toward better health. All the recommended remedies have been found effective, but every person is an individual and has different needs. I have found that healing and response accelerate when people choose their own natural therapy. The suggestions that appear in **bold print** indicate the most successful or most often used therapies.

Most people find **Herbal Therapy** to be the best initial treatment because herbs work toward balancing the body so that it becomes more receptive to the other natural remedies.

The products that I recommend are available in health food and natural products stores across the country. I encourage you to look there for your health needs since over the years these stores have become an authority on effective health care products. Let this book provide you with a dependable "shopping list" for effective, natural remedies.

Thank you for buying Healthy Healing Book Publications. I sincerely hope you find it useful in your quest for the best of health.

Linda Rector-Page, N.D., Ph.D.

TURNING A FIZZLE INTO A SIZZLE

Party Lights:
The Encyclopedia of Home Entertaining

• NIFTY PARTY IDEAS   • 700 DELIGHTFUL RECIPES

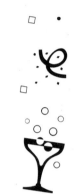

Written by nutrition guru, HEALTH HEALING author and herbal formulator Dr. Linda Rector-Page, and co-authored by party giver for the stars and chef extraordinaire, Doug Vanderberg, this 350-page "Encyclopedia of Home Entertaining" enables the reader to plan and execute the party event of their dreams. From its imaginative suggestions of party themes to its easy-to-follow decorating instructions and over 700 user-friendly recipes, *PARTY LIGHTS* is the definitive guide to affordable, healthy, low-fat, high-fun celebrating.

"We wrote the book with the notion that a little drama should be the keynote of any home event. An evening in your home with friends is more exciting than an empty restaurant or cold theater," Page says.

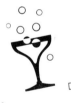

"The difference between a fizzle and a sizzle is the ambience – the attention to detail in your decorations, your food and activities," Vanderberg says. "Bringing it all together is easy with *PARTY LIGHTS*."

Whether you're giving a romantic dinner for two or a costume theme party for 200, *PARTY LIGHTS* provides you with a step-by-step guide to creating the kind of event that will bring praise from your guests and leave you energized rather than exhausted. Sunday brunches, exotic gatherings with an international flair, or just plain down-home country fixings are included with detailed guides to success.

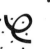

Never again will you scramble for instructions about shopping lists, napkin folding, garnishes, exotic motifs, menu selections, hors d'oeuvres or the right desserts. This book will also help you decide which games are appropriate for adults or children.

PARTY LIGHTS provides complete plans for anniversaries, holiday celebrations, children's parties, weddings, bridal showers, baby showers and fundraisers. Decorations are made from simple things, many of which you probably have around the house, and they're fun and easy to assemble. If you're concerned about health food, watching your budget and wanting to stay conscious of recycling to preserve our precious planet, *PARTY LIGHTS* can guide you with these concerns.

Nothing matters if all the tasks to create your celebration don't enable you to enjoy the event you're giving. So, the bottom-line goal of *PARTY LIGHTS* is to help you have fun as you entertain. Of course, since these ideas and menus have been "party" tested, the authors are certain you, too, will get kudos and applause from your guests when you follow the simple instructions. So, if you have delayed scheduling a family celebration, that special evening with you-know-who, or an all out party-hearty occasion, *PARTY LIGHTS* offers the inspiration to go for it!

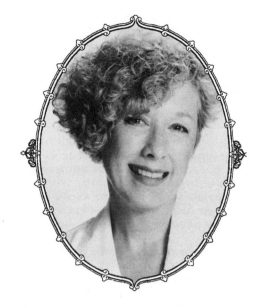

A Guide to the Safe Use of Herbs

by

Dr. Linda Rector-Page, N.D., Ph.D.

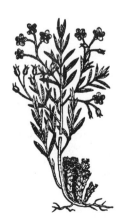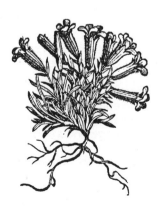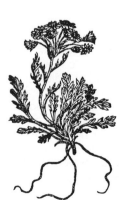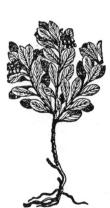

About The Safe Use Of Herbs & How Herbs Work

Herbs are concentrated foods, whole essences, with the ability to address both the symptoms and causes of a problem. As nourishment, herbs can offer the body nutrients it does not always receive, either from poor diet, or environmental deficiencies in the soil and air. As medicine, herbs are essentially body balancers, that work with the body functions, so that it can heal and regulate itself.

Herbal formulas can be broad based for over all strength and nutrient support, or specific to a particular ailment or condition. Herbs work like precision instruments in the body, not like sledge hammers.
❊

Most herbs, as edible plants, are as safe to take as foods. They have almost no side effects as natural medicines. Occasionally a mild allergy-type reaction may occur as it might occur to a food. This could happen because herb quality is poor, because it has been adulterated with chemicals in the growing/ storing process, or in rare cases, because incompatible herbs were used together. Or it may be just an individual adverse response to a certain plant. The key to avoiding an adverse reaction is moderation, both in formulation and in dosage. Anything taken to excess can cause negative side effects. Normal common sense, care, and intelligence are needed when using herbs for either food or medicine.

While many drugs use plant isolates or concentrates, herbs in their whole form are not drugs. Do not expect the activity or response of chemical anti-biotics or tranquilizers. These agents only treat the symptoms of a problem. In general, you have to take more and more of a drug to get the same effect. Herbal medicines work differently. **Herbs are nutritional foundation nutrients**, working through the glands, nourishing the body's deepest, basic elements, such as the brain, glands and hormones. Results will seem to take much longer. But this fact only shows how herbs actually work, acting as support to control and reverse the cause of a problem, with more permanent effect. Even so, some improvement from herbal treatment can usually be felt in three to six days. Chronic or long standing degeneration will, of course take longer. **A traditional rule of thumb is one month of healing for every year of the problem.**
❊

Herbal combinations are not addictive or habit-forming, but are powerful nutritional agents that should be used with care. Balance is the key to using herbal nutrients for healing. Every person is different, with different nutritional needs. It takes a little more attention and personal responsibility than mindlessly taking a prescription drug, but the extra care is worth far more in the results you can achieve for your body.

As with other natural therapies, there is sometimes a "healing crisis" in an herbal healing program. This is traditionally known as the "Law of Cure", and simply means that you may seem to get worse before you get better. The body frequently begins to eliminate toxic wastes quite heavily during the first stages of a cleansing therapy. This is particularly true in the traditional three to four day cleansing fast that many people use to begin a serious healing program. Temporary exacerbation of symptoms can range from mild to fairly severe, but usually precedes good results. Herbal therapy without a fast works more slowly and gently. Still, there is usually some discomfort and weakness as disease poisons are released into the bloodstream to be flushed away. Strength and relief shortly return when this process is over. Watching this phenomenon allows you to observe your body processes at work healing itself...an interesting experience indeed.
❊

✍Herbs work better in combination than they do singly. Like the notes of a symphony, herbs work better in harmony than standing alone.
There are several reasons for this.

❶ Each formula contains two to five primary agent herbs that are part of the blend for specific purposes. Since all body parts, and most disease symptoms, are interrelated, it is wise to have herbs which can affect each part of the problem. For example, in a prostate healing formula, there would be herbs to dissolve sediment, anti-inflammatory herbs, tissue-toning and strengthening herbs, and herbs with anti-biotic properties.
❷ A combination of herbal nutrients encourages body balance rather than a large supply of one or two focused properties. A combination works to gently stimulate the body as a whole entity.
❸ A combination allows inclusion of herbs that can work at different stages of need. A good example of this is an athlete's formula, where there are herbs for short term energy, long range endurance, muscle tone, glycogen and glucose use, and reduction of lactic acid build-up.
❹ A combination of several herbs with similar properties can increase the latitude of effectiveness, not only through a wider range of activity, but also reinforcing herbs that were picked too late or too early, or grew in adverse weather conditions for full potency.
❺ No two people, or their bodies, are alike. Good response is augmented by a combination of herbs.
❻ Finally, some potent and complex herbs, such as capsicum, lobelia, sassafras, mandrake, tansy, canada snake root, wormwood, woodruff, poke root, and rue are beneficial in small amounts and as catalysts, but should not be used alone.

❧Herbs work better when combined with a natural foods diet. Everyone can benefit from an herbal formula, but results increase dramatically when fresh foods and whole grains form the diet basis. Subtle healing activity is more effective when it doesn't have to labor through excess waste material, mucous, or junk food accumulation. (Most of us carry around 10 to 15 pounds of excess density.)

Interestingly enough, herbs themselves can help counter the problems of "civilization foods." They are rich in minerals and trace minerals, the basic elements missing or diminished in today's "quick-grow," over-sprayed, over-fertilized farming. Minerals and trace minerals are a basic element in food assimilation. Mineral-rich herbs provide not only the healing essences to support the body in overcoming disease, but also the foundation minerals that allow it to take them in!

Each individual body has its own unique and wonderful mechanism, and each has the ability to bring itself to its own balanced and healthy state. **Herbs simply pave the way for the body to do its own work,** by breaking up toxins, cleansing, lubricating, toning and nourishing. They work through the glands at the deepest levels of the body processes - at the cause, rather than the effect.

When correctly used, herbs promote the elimination of waste matter and toxins from the system by simple natural means. They support nature in its fight against disease.
❈

Hundreds of herbs are regularly available today at all quality levels. Worldwide communications and improved storage allow us to simultaneously obtain and use herbs from different countries and different harvests, an advantage ages past did not enjoy. However, because of the natural variety of soils, seeds, and weather, every crop of botanicals is unique. Every batch of a truly natural herbal formula will be slightly different, and offer its own unique benefits and experience.

In the herb world, there must be a firm commitment to excellence, because herb quality is never an accident. It is always the result of high intention, sincere effort, intelligent direction, skillful ability, and a willingness to pay for the difference. There is a world of disparity between fairly good herbs and the best. Since herbal combinations are products for problems, superior stock must go into the quality of formula. Herbal product results speak for themselves.

Clearly, American health care consumers are increasing their use of herbs as natural alternatives to drugs and medicines. For therapeutic success herbs must be BIO-ACTIVE and BIO-AVAILABLE. The herbs that I use are the finest quality that I can find because I work with their naturally occurring, biochemical properties. High quality is not only a desired attribute, it is a mandatory element. Superior plants cost far more than standard stock, but sell for proportionally far less - a true value for the alternative health customer.

❧ Here are some of the checkpoints I use to insure top quality and potency:
Most of the herbs I use are organically grown or wildcrafted in the fresh air of the California and Oregon foothills, and on coastal botanical farms. Others come from the Orient, where herb quality is much prized. All combinations are formulated and filled in small batches. Teas are blended on a weekly basis to assure freshness and highest potency.

❶ **Organically grown or wildcrafted herbs are used whenever available.**
❷ Fresh-dried locally grown herbs are bought immediately upon harvest whenever possible, assuring the shortest transportation time and freshest quality.
❸ **Small amounts of herbs are bought more frequently, rather than large amounts that may lose potency before they are used.**
❻ I buy the best. In the medicinal herb world, price is generally a fair measure of quality. Top quality plants can cost far more than standard herb stock or any conventional food supplement. However, even herbs that seem outrageously priced are usually worth it in terms of healing value; and a little goes a long way.
❼ **All herbs are stored in dark-colored, sealed containers, away from light and heat. For the short time the herbs are waiting to be used, they are kept cool and closed.**
❈

❧ How to take herbs correctly for the most benefit:
Herbs are not like vitamins.
People are always asking me to make an herbal multiple, but I believe this would be doing the public an injustice. While herbs are concentrated, they are not partitioned or isolated substances. There value is in their wholeness and complexity, not their concentration.

Herbs should not be taken like vitamins.
Vitamins are usually taken on a daily maintenance basis to shore up nutrient deficiencies. As stated above, except for some food-grown vitamins, vitamins are partitioned substances. They do not combine with the body in the same way as foods or herbs do, and excesses are normally flushed from the system. Herbs combine and work with the body's enzyme activity; they also contain food enzymes, and/or proteolytic enzymes themselves. They accumulate in and combine with

the body. Taking herbs all the time for maintenance and nutrient deficiency replacement would be like eating large quantities of a certain food all the time. The body would tend to have imbalanced nourishment from nutrients that were not in that food. (In my opinion, this is also true of multiple vitamins. They work best when strengthening a deficient or weak system, not as a continuing substitute for a good diet.)

While most vitamins work best when taken with food, it is not necessary to take herbal formulas with food. Unlike vitamins, herbs provide their own digestive enzymes for the body to take them in. In some cases, with herbs for mental acuity, for instance, the herbs are more effective if taken when body pathways are clear, instead of concerned with food digestion.

Most herbal remedies can be taken as needed, then reduced and discontinued as the problem improves.

Therapeutic herbs work best when used as needed. Because herbal effects can be quite specific, take the best formula for your particular goal at the right time - rather than all the time - for optimum results. In addition, rotating and alternating herbal combinations according to your changing health needs allows the body to remain most responsive to their effects. Reduce dosage as the problem improves - always allowing the body to pick up its own work and bring its own vital forces into action.

Best results may be achieved by taking herbal capsule combinations in descending strength: 6 the first day, 5 the second day, 4 the third, 3 the fourth, 2 the fifth, and 2 the sixth for the first week. Rest on the 7th day. When a healing base is built in the body, decrease to the daily maintenance dose recommended for the formula. Most combinations should be taken no more than 6 days in a row to regular restoration of body balance.

✷ Whichever herbal form you choose, it is usually beneficial to take greater amounts at the beginning of your program, in order to build a good healing base in the system, and start the body's vital balancing force more quickly. As the therapeutic agents establish in the body, and you begin to notice good response and balance returning, less and less of the large initial doses should be taken, finally reducing the dosage to longer range maintenance and preventive amounts.

Take only one or two herbal combinations at the same time.

When working with herbs and alternative healing methods, choose the elements that will address your worst problem first. Take the herbal formula for that problem - reducing dosage and alternating on and off weeks as necessary to allow the body to thoroughly use the herbal properties. One of the bonuses of a natural healing program is the frequent discovery that other conditions were really complications of the first problem, and often take care of themselves as the body comes into balance.

Herb effectiveness usually goes by body weight. Base dose decisions on weight for both adults and children.
Child dosage is as follows:

$1/2$ dose for children 10-14 years

$1/3$ dose for children 6-10 years

$1/4$ dose for children 2-6 years

$1/8$ dose for infants and babies

Herbs are effective in building and strengthening the immune system.

However, I have found over and over again that with immune deficient, opportunistic, and degenerative diseases, it takes a great deal of time to rebuild health. Even when a good healing program is working, and obvious improvement is being made, adding <u>more</u> of the medicinal agents in an effort to speed healing can aggravate symptoms and bring about worse results!

The immune system is a very fragile entity, and can be overwhelmed instead of stimulated. A virulent virus can seem to mutate and be nourished by supplementation, instead of arrested by it. Even for serious health conditions, moderate amounts are the way to go, mega-doses are not. Much better results can be obtained by giving yourself more time and gentler treatment.

Healing herbs are a gift to mankind.
Give them time.

The body knows how to use herbs.
They are working.

Amino Acids

What They Are ✦ How They Work ✦ Why You Need Them

Amino acids are the building blocks of protein in the body. Protein is absolutely necessary to life and growth. It in turn, is composed of, and depends upon the correct supply of amino acids. There are 29 of them known, from which over 1600 basic proteins are formed, comprising <u>over 75%</u> of the body's solid weight. The basic proteins are used by the body to manufacture thousands of structural, contractile, and blood protein. Amino acids also constitute an important part of body fluids, anti-bodies to fight infection, and hormone/enzyme systems to regulate growth and digestion. The liver produces about 80% of all needed amino acids; the remaining 20% must be regularly obtained from our foods. But poor diet, unhealthy habits and environmental pollutants mean that the "**essential amino acids**", (those which the body cannot produce on its own) are often not sufficient in the body to produce the "**non-essentials**", (those formed by metabolic activity). This can be corrected by increasing intake of protein foods and supplementation. (For best absorption, use a food-source or pre-digested supplement. These balanced, full spectrum supplements are absorbed more quickly than dietary amino acids from protein.)

Amino acids are responsible for the growth, maintenance and repair of our bodies throughout our lives. They are valuable sources of energy, play a vital role in rapid brain function and mood elevation, are critical to quick healing, and necessary buffering agents for proper acid/alkaline balance. Indeed the central nervous system cannot function without amino acids, which act as neurotransmitters throughout the body.

Individual amino acid therapies are making great impact in alternative medicine as a way of strengthening the body against disease. Research is finding that specific amino acids can produce specific pharmacological effects in the body. By understanding these effects we can use them to "target" particular nutritional healing goals.

THE MAIN AMINO ACIDS

❖ **ALANINE - non-essential -** helps maintain blood glucose levels, particularly as an energy storage source for the liver and muscles.

❖ **ARGININE - semi-essential -** a prime stimulant for growth hormone and immune response in the pituitary and liver. A specific for athletes and body builders, increasing muscle tone while decreasing fat. Promotes healing of wounds, blocks formation of tumors, and increases sperm motility. Helps lower blood serum fats, and detoxifies ammonia. Curbs the appetite, and aids in metabolizing fats for weight loss. Herpes virus, and schizophrenia can be retarded by "starving" them of arginine foods, such as nuts, peanut butter, cheese, etc.
Nutrient co-factors: mang., magnes., vitamin B₆, zinc. Take with cranberry or apple juice for best results.

❖ **ASPARTIC ACID - non-essential -** abundant in sugar cane and beets; used mainly as a sweetener. A precursor of threonine, it is a neuro-transmitter made with ATP that increases the body's resistance to fatigue. Clinically used to counteract depression and in drugs to protect the liver.

❖ **BRANCH CHAIN AMINOS - Leucine, Isoleucine, Valine (BCAAs) - essential -** called the stress amino acids, they must be taken together in balanced proportion. Easily converted into ATP, critical to energy and muscle metabolism. Aid in hemoglobin formation. Help to stabilize blood sugar and lower elevated blood sugar levels. Used to treat severe amino acid deficiencies caused by addictions. Excellent results in tissue repair from athletic stress, rebuilding the body from anorexia deficiencies, and in liver restoration after surgical trauma.

❖ **CARNITINE - non-essential -** helps regulate fat metabolism through enzyme stimulation. Decreases ischemic heart disease by preventing fatty build-up, and providing muscle energy to

the heart. Speeds fat oxidation for weight loss, and increases the use of fat as an energy source. Helps reduce excess triglycerides in the blood, and aids prostaglandin metabolism. Because it decreases ketone levels, it is valuable to diabetics.
Nutrient co-factors: vitamin C, B6, niacin, lysine, methionine.

✤ **CYSTEINE - semi-essential -** works with vitamins C, E and selenium as an anti-oxidant to protect against radiation toxicity, cancer carcinogens, and free radical damage to skin, and arteries. Stimulates white cell activity in the immune system. Plays an active role in healing treatment from burns and surgery. and renders toxic chemicals in the body harmless. Taken with evening primrose oil, cysteine protects brain and body from alcohol and tobacco effects. (Effective in preventing hangover.) Used successfully in cases of hair loss, psoriasis, skin tissue diseases. Relieves bronchial asthma relief through breakdown of mucous plugs. Helps prevent dental plaque formation. Aids in body uptake of iron.
Nutrient co-factors: vitamins B6, C, B12, magnesium, folacin. Note: Take vitamin C in a 3:1 ratio to cysteine for best results.

✤ **CYSTINE - semi-essential -** the oxidized form of cysteine, and like it, promotes white blood cell activity and healing of burns and wounds. The main constituent of hair. Essential to formation of skin. Cumulative in the body, can sometimes be harmful to the kidneys, and should generally not be used clinically.
Nutrient co-factors: vitamins B6, C, B12, magnesium, folacin.

✤ **GABA - Gamma-Aminobutyric Acid - non-essential -** shows excellent results in treating brain and nerve dysfunctions, such as anxiety, depression, extreme nervous tension, high blood pressure, insomnia, schizophrenia, Parkinson's disease, Alzheimer's disease and hyperkinesis in children. Acts as a natural, non-addictive tranquilizer. Improves depressed sex drive. Used with glutamine and tyrosine to overcome alcohol and drug abuse. Used with niacinimide as a relaxant.

✤ **GLUTAMIC ACID - non-essential -** important for nerve health and function, and in metabolizing sugars and fats. Over 50% of the amino acid composition of the brain is represented by glutamic acid and its derivatives. A prime fuel for the brain because of its transportation of potassium across the blood/brain barrier. Detoxifies ammonia by turning into glutamine in the brain. Helps correct mental and nerve disorders, such as epilepsy, muscular dystrophy, mental retardation, and severe insulin reaction.

✤ **GLUTAMINE - non-essential -** converts readily into 6-carbon glucose, and is therefore one of the best nutrients and energy sources for the brain. Supplementation rapidly improves memory retention, recall, sustained concentration, and alertness. Improves mental performance in cases of retardation, senility, epileptic seizure and schizophrenia. Reduces alcohol and sugar cravings, protects against alcohol toxicity, and controls hypoglycemia reactions. Increases libido and helps overcome impotence. Aids in better mineral absorption, and thus protects against peptic ulcers.
Nutrient co-factors: vitamin B6, magnesium, folacin.

✤ **GLUTATHIONE - non-esssential -** works with cysteine and glutamine as a glucose tolerance factor and anti-oxidant to neutralize radiation toxicity and inhibit free radicals. Assists white blood cells in killing bacteria. Helps detoxify from heavy metal pollutants, cigarette smoke, alcohol and drug (especially PCP) overload. Cleans the blood from the effects of chemotherapy, x-rays and liver toxicity. Works with vitamin E to break down fat peroxides and protect against stroke, chronic kidney failure and cataract formation. Stimulates prostaglandin metabolism and balance.

✤ **GLYCINE & DI-METHYL-GLYCINE (B15) - non-essential -** releases growth hormone when taken in large doses. Converts to creatine, which retards nerve and muscle degeneration, and is thus therapeutically effective for myasthenia gravis, gout, and muscular dystrophy. Helps detoxify the liver. A key factor in regulating hypoglycemic sugar drop, especially when taken upon rising. Used as an antacid ingredient for hyperacidity.

DMG - Di-Methyl-Glycine - once commonly known as B15 - a powerful anti-oxidant and energy stimulant. Used successfully to improve Down's Syndrome and mental retardation cases, and to curb craving in alcohol addiction. DMG is a highly reputed energizer and stimulant whose effects can be attributed to its conversion to glycine. Has been successfully used as a control for epileptic seizure and immune stimulation. Notable therapeutic results in treatment of atherosclerosis, rheumatic fever, rheumatism, emphysema

and liver cirrhosis. Sublingual forms are most absorbable.
Nutrient co-factors: zinc, niacin, B6, folacin. For best results, take before sustained exercise. Note: Too much DMG disrupts the metabolic chain and causes fatigue. The proper dose produces energy, overdoses do not.

❖ **HISTIDINE - semi-essential in adults, essential in infants** - because histimine is formed from histidine, this amino acid becomes a precurser to good immune response, to effective defense against colds, respiratory infections, and in countering allergic reactons. Strong vasodilating and hypotensive properties effective for cardio-circulatory diseases, anemia and cataracts. Abundant in hemoglobin and a key in the production of both red and white blood cells. Synthesizes glutamic acid, aids copper transport through the joints, and removes heavy metals from the tissues, making it successful in treating arthritis. Raises libido in both sexes.

❖ **INOSINE - non-essential** - stimulates ATP energy release. Helps provide muscle endurance and strength when the body's own glycogen reserves run out. Take on an empty stomach with an electrolyte drink before exercise for best results.

❖ **LYSINE - essential** - a primary treatment for the herpes virus; can be used topically or internally for relief. (High lysine foods, such as corn, poultry and avocados should be added if there are recurrent herpes breakouts.) Helps rebuild muscle and repair tissue after injury, surgery or illness. Important for calcium uptake for bone growth, and in cases of osteoporosis, and in reducing calcium loss in the urine. Helps the formation of collagen, hormones and enzymes. Supplementation is effective for Parkinson's disease and hypothyroidism.
Nutrient co-factors: vitamin B6, vitamin C, copper, iron.

❖ **METHIONINE - essential** - an anti-oxidant and free radical de-activator. A major source of organic sulphur for healthy liver activity, lymph and immune health. Protective against chemical allergic reactions. An effective "lipotropic" that keeps fats from accumulating in the liver and arteries, thus keeping high blood pressure and serum cholesterol low. Effective against toxemia during pregnancy. An important part of treatment for rheumatic fever. Supports healthy skin and nails; prevents hair loss.
Nutrient co-factors: vitamin B6, vitamin C, B12, folacin. Take with choline for best results.

❖ **ORNITHINE - non-essential** - works with arginine and carnitine to metabolize excess body fat; with the pituitary gland to promote growth hormone, muscle development, tissue repair, and endurance. An excellent aid to fat metabolism through the liver. Builds immune strength, and helps scavenge free radicals. Detoxifies ammonia, and aids healing.
Nutrient co-factors: manganese, magnesium., vitamin B6, zinc. Not indicated for children.

❖ **PHENALALANINE - essential** - a tyrosine precurser that works with B6 as an anti-depressant and mood elevator on the central nervous system. Successful in treating manic, post-amphetamine, and schizophrenic depression. Aids in learning and memeory retention. Relieves menstrual, arthritic and migraine pain. A thyroid stimulant that helps curb the appetite by increasing the body's production of CCK.
Contra-indications: phenylketonurics (elevated natural phenalalanine levels) should avoid aspartame sweeteners. Pregnant women and those with blood pressure imbalance, skin carcinomas, and diabetes should avoid phenalalanine.
Contra-indications: tumors and cancerous melanoma growths have been slowed through dietary reduction of tyrosine and phenalalanine. Avoid if blurred vision occurs when using.

❖ **DL-Phenalalanine - DLPA** - a safe, effective pain reliever and anti-depressant with an endorphin effect for arthritis, lower back and cerebro-spinal pain. Increases mental alertness, and improves the symptoms of Parkinson's disease.
Contra-indications: avoid DLPA if you have high blood pressure, are pregnant, or diabetic.

❖ **TAURINE - non-essential** - a potent anti-seizure nutrient. A neurotransmitter that helps control hyperactivity, nervous system imbalance after drug or alcohol abuse, and epilepsy. Normalizes irregular heartbeat. Helps prevent circulatory and heart disorders, hypoglycemia, hypothyroidism, water retention and hypertension. Aids in lowering cholesterol levels. Found in high concentrations in bile, mother's milk, shark and abalone. Supplementation is necessary for therapy.
Nutrient co-factors: vitamins B6, B12, magnesium, zinc.

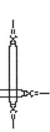

▶ **THREONINE - essential -** works with glycine to aid in overcoming depression, and neurologic dysfunctions such as genetic spastic disorders and M.S. Works with aspartic acid and methionine as a lipotropic to prevent fatty build-up in the liver. Helps to control epileptic seizures. An immune stimulant and thymus enhancer. Important for the formation of collagen, elastin and enamel.

♣ **TRYPTOPHAN - essential -** a precurser of the neurotransmitter serotonin, which is involved in mood and metabolism regulation. A natural, non-addictive tranquilizer for restful sleep. Used successfully, through blood vessel dilation, to decrease hyperkinetic, aggressive behavior, migraine headaches, and schizophrenia. Counteracts compulsive overeating, smoking and alcoholism. An effective anti-depressant, raises abnormally low blood sugar, and reduces seizures in petit mal epilepsy. Produces nicotinic acid (natural niacin) which is being studied to counteract the effects of nicotine from cigarettes.

Nutrient co-factors: vitamin B6, niacin.
Note: At the time of this writing, L-Tryptophane has been recalled by the FDA, and is not available until a safe source is found. It is recommended in this book as an effective sleep aid and relaxant, with every expectation of its safe return to the public.

♣ **TYROSINE - a semi-essential, formed from phenalalnine -** helps to build the body's natural store of adrenalin and thyroid hormones. Is rapidly metabolized as an anti-oxidant throughout the body, and is effective as a source of quick energy, especially for the brain. Converts to the amino acid L-Dopa, which improves brain function, making it a safe therapy for depression, hypertension, parkinson's disease, in controlling drug abuse and aiding drug withdrawal. Increases libido and low sex drive. A growth hormone stimulant. Helps reduce appetite and body fat in a weight loss diet. Part of the production of melanin in the body for skin and hair pigment.

Nutrient co-factors: vitamin C, vitamin B6, magnesium, manganese copper.
Contra-indications: tumors and cancerous melanomas have been slowed through dietary reduction of tyrosine and phenalalanine.

Other indications to consider when using amino acid therapy:

❶ Amino acids work very well with other natural healing agents, such as herbs, minerals and vitamins. We have found that they may be taken together, often with synergistic effect.

❷ Take amino acids with *extra* water or other liquid for optimum absorption by the body.

❸ If using individual free form amino acids, add a full spectrum amino acid compound sometime during the same day for increased results.

❹ Since many free form amino acids compete for uptake by the brain, take free forms separately from each other for maximum results.

❺ Take individual free form amino acids with their nutrient co-factors for best metabolic uptake.

❻ Take free form amino acids, except those for brain stimulation, before meals for best results.

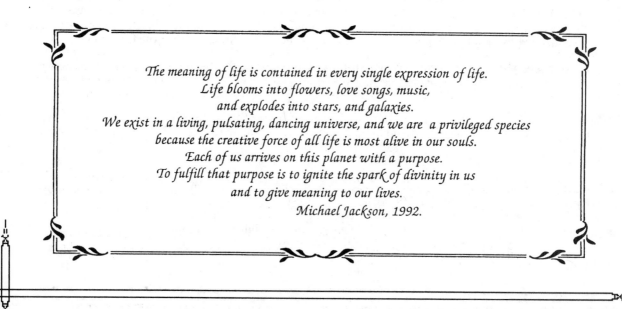

The meaning of life is contained in every single expression of life.
Life blooms into flowers, love songs, music,
and explodes into stars, and galaxies.
We exist in a living, pulsating, dancing universe, and we are a privileged species
because the creative force of all life is most alive in our souls.
Each of us arrives on this planet with a purpose.
To fulfill that purpose is to ignite the spark of divinity in us
and to give meaning to our lives.
Michael Jackson, 1992.

Raw Glandular Extracts

What They Are ✦ How They Work

The organs and glands communicate chemically to the physiological needs of the body with micro-nutrients and polypeptides. Only minute amounts are required to have positive effects. Raw glandular tissues contain intrinsic factors distinct from vitamins, minerals, or enzyme micronutrients. Glandular, or cellular therapy, is based on the premise that glandular substance is biologically active in humans, and that **"like cells help like cells"**. Raw glandulars provide nutrients that aid the reproduction of cells for the particular organ or gland. It is a technique that helps the deepest levels of the body to function as close to normal as possible. For serious diseases, such as cancer, that debilitate the glands and organs, glandular therapy can be very helpful in augmenting the body's own substance so that it can better heal itself.

A very small amount of glandular tissue from an animal gland can be picked up in the bloodstream to support, augment and normalize the corresponding gland or organ in a human being. While glandular therapy is only one part of most holistic treatment, current research is showing that it is valid, effective and safe. Predigested, soluble gland tissue can provide all the benefits of whole fresh glands. Raw liquid glandulars should be taken under the tongue for ready absorption. Freeze-dried, de-fatted, dehydrated concentrates are also available and effective. The highest quality of preservation is obviously essential, since heat processing or salt precipitation render the glands useless.   When one of the glands is not functioning properly, other glands and organs can be affected. Therefore, individual raw glandulars work more effectively when accompanied in the same formula by a small supporting amount of multi-gland compound.

Raw glandulars work particularly well when combined with free form amino acids. Every gland seems to be stimulated by a particular amino acid, which enables it to function more effectively. So a combination of a raw glandular and a harmonizing amino acid provides the human gland with more ability to produce its hormone secretions.

THE MOST ESSENTIAL GLANDULARS

♣ **RAW ADRENAL** - helps stimulate and nourish exhausted adrenals. Aids in adrenal cortex production to reduce inflammation in arthritis and ulcers. Increases body tone and endurance without synthetic steroids. Helps protect against Chronic Fatigue Syndrome and Candida albicans through a normal increase of metabolic rate. Overcomes allergic reactions associated with poor adrenal function. Works with vitamins C and B Complex to control both hypoglycemic and dibetic reactions, and menopause imbalance effects. Increases resistance to infections.

♣ **RAW BRAIN** - improves brain chemistry; testing has shown that the learning process has a biochemical basis. Helps prevent memory loss, chronic mental fatigue, and senility onset. Encourages better nerve stability and restful sleep. Beneficial support during alcoholism recovery.

♣ **RAW FEMALE COMPLEX (usually including raw ovary, pituitary, uterus)** - re-establishes hormonal balance, especially that of estrogen/progesterone. Helps regulate the menstrual cycle, and stimulates delayed or absent menstruation. Normalizes P.M.S. symptoms, and controls cramping. Beneficial for low libido or frigidity. Works with vitamins A and E to increase fertility.

♣ **RAW HEART** - improves heart muscle activity and reduces low density lipoproteins in the blood. Works synergistically with vitamin E, magnesium and zinc.

♣ **RAW KIDNEY** - aids in normalization of kidney/urinary disorders, and improves waste filtering functions. Helps normalize blood pressure. Maintains body fluid and acid/alkaline balance. Works synergistically with vitamin C to maintain mineral balances in the body.

♣ **RAW LIVER** - helps restore the liver from abuse, disease and exhaustion. Improves metabolic activity, and filtering of wastes and toxins like alcohol and chemicals. Aids fat metabolism. In-

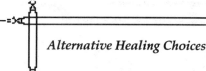

creases healthy bile flow and glucose regulation. Works synergistically with vitamin C and B Complex to purify the blood and restore acid/alkaline balance. Supplementation is effective for jaundice, hepatitis, toxemia and alcoholism.

✤ **RAW LUNG** - supports the lungs against respiratory dysfunctions such as asthma, emphysema, congestion, bronchitis and pneumonia.

✤ **RAW MALE COMPLEX (usually including raw orchic, pituitary, and prostate)** - re-establishes hormonal balance, especially that of testosterone/progesterone/estrogen. Helps normalize the functions of diseased or damaged male organs. Works with zinc and vitamin E to support male body growth, fat distribution and psychic development. Improves sperm count, virility, and chances of fertilization.

✤ **RAW MAMMARY** - helps in healing mastitis and nipple inflammation. Helps control profuse menstruation, period pain, and normalizes too-frequent cycles, especially at the onset of menopause. Excellent support of insufficient milk during lactation.

✤ **RAW ORCHIC**- helps increase male sexual strength and potency by stimulating testosterone production and building sperm count. Also beneficial against male depression and low blood sugar. Supplementation can bring noticeable improvement in athletic performance.

✤ **RAW OVARY** - normalizes estrogen/progesterone balance. Helps correct endometrial misplacement and overgrowth, P.M.S. symptoms and menstrual cramping. Supports hormone production slow down during menopause against hot flashes and mood swings.

✤ **RAW PANCREAS** - the pancreas is a triple function gland producing pancreatin for digestion, and insulin and glucagon for glucose metabolism and balanced blood glucose levels. Pancreas glandular supports enzyme secretions for fat metabolism, hormone balance and food assimilation. Works with B Complex and chromium to secrete hormones that keep intestinal immune response strong against harmful bacteria.

✤ **RAW PITUITARY** - the "master gland", operates in a feedback communications system with the other glands. Made up of three lobes that store and control amazingly myriad and diverse hormones. Works with the hypothalamus in releasing hormone secretions into the body. Stimulates overall body growth through electrolyte metabolism in the ovaries, testes, adrenals and skin. Plays a major role in reproduction, estrogen secretion, blood sugar metabolism, kidney function, skin pigmentation, water retention, and bowel movements. Supplementation can help in cases of hypoglycemia, stress, and infertility. Especially effective for athletes and body builders in controlling excess body stress, sugar balance and fatigue. Works synergistically with vitamin B Complex and beta-carotene.

✤ **RAW SPLEEN** - aids in the building and storage of red blood cells to promote strength and good tissue oxygenation. As a lymphoid organ, filters injurious substances from the bloodstream.Increases absorption of calcium and iron. Protects against immune and arterial deficiency. Supplementation enhances immune function by increasing white blood cell activity.

✤ **RAW THYMUS** - a key factor to growth and disease susceptibility, the thymus stimulates and strengthens the immune system against foreign organisms and toxins. Supplementation helps activate T-cells in the spleen, lymph nodes and bone marrow. Also minimizes problems that occur from aging, since the thymus gland normally shrinks with age. (Zinc supplementation can help regenerate thymic tissue.)

✤ **RAW THYROID** - the thyroid is the main energy-producing and metabolic-regulating gland. Raw thyroid supports these functions, increasing circulation, and controlling obesity and sluggishness caused by thyroid deficiency. Supplementation helps mental alertness, hair, skin and reproductive/sexual problems. Works synergistically with tyrosine and natural iodine. (Be sure to use a compound that is thyroxin-free.)

✤ **RAW UTERUS** - helps support against menses dysfunctions such as amenorrhea, habitual abortion, infertility and irregular periods. Acts as a preventive measure against sub-acute inflammation and infection of the cervical canal and vagina. Aids in calcium use for improved bone cell and muscle functions. Improves tissue growth and repair. Supplementation can help overcome birth control side effects. Works synergistically with raw ovary for best balance, particularly when organs are displaced or prolapsed.

Enzymes & Enzyme Therapy

What They Are ✦ How They Work ✦ Why You Need Them

Enzymes are highly specialized protein molecules which act as catalysts, enhancing the rate of specific chemical reactions in the body. Enzyme activity is truly holistic; most enzymes act together as co-enzymes, or as co-factors with vitamins, minerals and trace minerals for optimum body efficiency. Enzymes exist in all living things. They possess biological as well as chemical properties, and are involved with every single function of the body. Without them we could not breathe, digest food, or even move a muscle. There is even an enzyme, cathepsin, which is stored in our systems for our death, to break down cells and tissue for the body's return to the earth's organic matrix.

There are three categories of enzymes: metabolic enzymes, which run the body processes, repair damage and decay, and heal disease; our own digestive enzymes, which assimilate carbohydrates, proteins and fats into the body, and enzymes in raw foods, which start food digestion, and aid the body's digestive enzymes so they don't have to carry the whole load. Within these categories, there are over 1,000 different kinds of acid, alkaline or neutral enzymes that are quite specific in their functions, acting only on a specific substance, or a group of chemically related substances. Yet enzyme activity and integration is so marvelously efficient that it works in milliseconds, with one hundred percent productivity. In fact, digestive enzymes in human beings are stronger than any of the body's other enzymes, and more concentrated than any other enzyme combination found in nature. A very good thing, since our processed, overcooked, nutrient-poor diets demand a great deal of enzymatic work!

There are three interesting facts about food enzymes:
   ❶ All food, whether plant or animal, has its own enzymes that served it in life. When eaten, these become the property of the eater, are now *its* food enzymes, and begin immediately to work for the eater's digestive benefit.
   ❷ All animal organisms have the proteolytic enzyme cathepsin, which comes into play after death, and becomes the prime factor for autolysis. In other words, the food helps in *its own breakdown* for the good of the eater.
   ❸ Only enzymes found in whole, unprocessed foods give the body the vital force it needs to work properly, to replace cells, and to rebuild in healing. Humans cannot independently assimilate food; our bodies must also have the help of the food itself.

Enzyme therapy has recently evolved from the ability of science to isolate metabolic enzymes. Many naturopaths and chiropractors now use enzyme-containing medicines to clean wounds, dissolve blood clots, and control allergic reactions. Certain diseases, such as cancer, leukemia, anemia, and heart disease can even be diagnosed by measuring the amount of various enzymes in the blood and body fluids. Proteolytic enzymes are being used successfully as anti-inflammatory agents for sports injuries, respiratory problems, degenerative diseases, and healing from surgery. Anti-oxidant co-enzymes, such as glutathione peroxidase, and superoxide dismutase, (SOD), an anti-oxidant enzyme that works with catalase, scavenge and neutralize cell-damaging free radicals by turning them into stable oxygen and H_2O_2, and then into oxygen and water.

The most significant function of enzymes for most of us is the food assimilation process. Digestion is the enzymatic process of mechanically breaking down food, and then chemically converting it for absorption by the body. Digestive enzymes are found mainly in pancreatic juices, the saliva and the small intestine.
Digestive action begins in the mouth when the saliva enzymes ptyalin and maltase act on starch and maltose conversion. In the stomach, gastric juices secrete the enzymes pepsin, lipase and rennin to start the breakdown of proteins, fats (including cholesterol), and milk products. In the small intestine, pancreatic juices secrete the enzymes trypsin, steapsin, and amylopsin to further the digestion of fats, proteins and starches. Several other small intestine enzymes complete the final process. The remaining five percent of the original meal then proceeds to the colon where water and electrolyte salts are extracted, and enzymes stimulate colonies of bacteria to feed on the

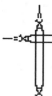
waste. This final stage is where many nutritional deficiencies are manifested in colon and bowel problems. If these bacteria are not called into play, unabsorbed food waste will not be decayed for elimination, and auto-intoxication results.

Note: Besides enzymes, hydrochloric acid and bile activity are essential parts of good digestion. HCl sterilizes and acidifies foods in the stomach, working with pepsin and water to make chyme. The chyme is then neutralized by highly alkaline juices from the pancreas and the intestine, and by bile from the liver and gall bladder. Bile also works with lipase to emulsify fats and convert them to beneficial fatty acids.

THE MOST IMPORTANT ENZYMES FOR DIGESTION

Digestive enzymes are categorized by the function they perform, plus the ending "ase"; e.g. lactase breaks down milk sugar into glucose and galactose.

- **Amylase** - digests starches.
- **Bromelain** - a proteolytic, anti-inflammatory food enzyme from pineapple. Aids digestion of fats.
- **Catalase** - works with SOD to reduce free radical production.
- **Cellulase** - digests cellulose, the fibrous component of most vegetable matter.
- **Chymotrypsin** - helps convert chyme. (see above).
- **Diastase** - a potent vegetable starch digestant.
- **Lactase** - digests lactose, or milk sugar, (almost 65% of humans are deficient).
- **Lipase** - digests fats.
- **Mycozyme** - a single-celled plant enzyme for digestion of starches.
- **Pancreatin** - a broad spectrum, proteolytic digestive aid, derived from secretions of animal pancreas; important in degenerative disease research.
- **Papain and chymopapain** - proteolytic food enzymes from unripe papaya; a vegetable pepsin for digestion of proteins. (Biotec BIOGESTIN is an excellent source of these enzymes, helping to loosen necrotic and encrusted waste material from the intestinal walls.)
- **Pepsin** - a proteolytic enzyme that breaks down proteins into peptides. Can digest 3500 times its weight in proteins.
- **Protease** - digests proteins.
- **Rennin** - helps digest cow's milk products.
- **Trypsin** - a proteolytic enzyme.
  The best natural sources of enzymes are bananas, mangos, sprouts, unripe papayas, avocados and pineapples.

Two final words about maximizing your own enzyme production.

➥ Enzymes are extremely sensitive to heat. Even low degrees of heat can destroy food enzymes and greatly reduce digestive ability. Fresh, raw foods not only require much less digestive work from the body, they can provide many more of their own enzymes to work with yours. Have at least one fresh salad every day.

➥ Many nutrient deficiencies result from the body's inability to absorb them, not from the lack of the nutrients themselves. While science has not been able to manufacture enzymes synthetically, many have been isolated in pure crystalline form and can be used by man to support enzyme deficiencies. Supplemental digestive enzymes and acids such as HCl and bile, help insure assimilation, and maximize utilization of core nutrients for health and healing. If you can't make them, take them.

About Co-enzyme Q10:

CoQ10 is a vital enzyme catalyst in the creation of cellular energy. Found in rice bran, wheat germ, beans, nuts, fish and eggs, it is synthesized in the liver. The body's ability to assimilate food source CoQ10 declines with age. Supplementation has a long history of effectiveness in boosting immunity, increasing cardiac strength, reversing high blood pressure, promoting natural weight loss, inhibiting aging and overcoming periodontal disease.

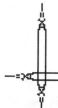

Homeopathic Medicines

What They Are ✦ How To Use Them

Homeopathy is a medical philosophy that recognizes disease as an energy imbalance, a disturbance of the body's "vital force" expressed by disease symptoms. It bases its healing techniques on the fact that the body is a *self healing entity*, and that symptoms are the expression of the body attempting to restore its own balance. **Homeopathic remedies** are based on the principle of stimulating and increasing this inherent curative ability. Each remedy has a number of symptoms that make it unique, just as each person has traits that make him or her unique. Homeopathic physicians are trained to match the patient's symptoms with the precise remedy, which are mild and non-toxic. Even the highest potencies do not create the side effects of allopathic drugs. The remedies themselves neither cover up nor destroy disease, but stimulate the body's own action to rid itself of the problem.

Homeopathic medicine is based on three prescription principles:
   1) The Law Of Similars: "like curing like". From the tiny amount of the active principle in the remedy, the body learns to recognize the hostile microbe and its "modus operandi", a process similar to DNA recognition. This "law" is the reason that a little is better than a lot, and why such great precision is needed.

   2) The Minimum Dose Principle: the dilution of the "like" substance to a correct strength for the individual; strong enough to stimulate the "vital force" without overpowering it. Dilutions, usually in alcohol, are shaken or succussed, a certain number of times (3, 6, or 12 times in commercial use) to increase therapeutic power through the vibratory effect. Each successive dilution *decreases* the actual amount of the substance in the remedy. In the strongest dilutions, there is virtually none of the substance remaining, yet potentiation is the highest for healing effect.

   3) The Single Remedy Principle: where only one remedy is administered at a time.

Although homeopathic treatments are specific to the individual in private practice, we have found two things to be true about the remedies found in most stores today:

➡ They work on the **"antidote"** principle. So more is *not better* in this case. Small amounts over a period of time are far more effective. Frequency of dosage is determined by individual reaction time, increasing as the first improvements are noted. When substantial improvement is evident, indicating that the body's healing force is stimulated, the remedy should be discontinued.
➡ They work on the **"trigger"** principle. A good way to start a healing program is with a homeopathic medicine. The body's electrical activity, stimulated by the remedy, can mean much more rapid response to other, succeeding therapies.

Homeopathy differs from traditional allopathy in two significant ways:
   ❶ Allopathic medicines influence the body to simply mask or reduce the symptoms of a disease without addressing the underlying problem. Homeopathic remedies act as catalysts to the body's immune system to wipe out the root cause.
   ❷ Although both medicinal systems use weak doses of a disease-causing agent to stimulate the body's immune defense against that illness, homeopathy uses plants, herbs and earth minerals for this stimulation, and allopathy uses viruses or chemicals.

The recent worldwide rise in popularity for homeopathy is due to its effectiveness in treating epidemic diseases, such as AIDS, HIV-positive and other life-threatening viral conditions. Many tests are showing that homeopathy not only treats the acute infective stages, but also helps reduces the intake of antibiotics and other drugs that cause side effects, and further weaken an already deficient immune system. In significant 1991 tests, Internal Medicine World Magazine reports six HIV-infected patients who became HIV-negative after homeopathic treatment. Since this and other reports, success with AIDS is being widely experienced by homeopaths as follows:
   ✦ *Prevention* - generating resistance to the virus and subsequent infection;
   ✦ *Treatment during acute illnesses* - reducing their length and severity.
   ✦ *Restoration of health* - revitalizing so that overall health does not deteriorate.

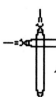

THE MOST POPULAR HOMEOPATHIC REMEDIES

✦ **APIS** - macerated bee tincture. Relieves stinging after bee sting or insect bite

✦ **ARNICA** - excellent for pain relief and speeding healing, particular from sports injuries,such as sprains, strains, stiffness or bruises. May be applied topically or used internally.

✦ **ACONITE** - for children's earaches. Helps the body deal with the trauma of sudden fright or shock.

✦ **ARSENICUM ALBUM** - for food poisoning accompanied by diarrhea; for allergic symptoms such as a runny nose; for asthma and colds.

✦ **BELLADONNA** - Excellent for sudden fever or sunstroke.

✦ **BRYONIA** - for the swelling, inflammation and redness of arthritis when the symptoms are worse with movement and better with cold applications, effective for headache, flu and respiratory infection.

✦ **CANTHARIS** - for treating bladder infections and problems of the uro-genital tract, especially where is burning and urgency to urinate. Also good for burns.

✦ **CHAMOMILLA** - for calming irritable, fussy children, when they are crying because of pain. Particularly effective for teething pain.

✦ **GELSEMIUM** - for energizing people with chronic lethargy; for overcoming dizziness.

✦ **IGNATIA** - a female remedy to relax emotional hypertension; especially during times of great grief or loss.

✦ **LACHESIS** - for premenstrual symptoms that improve once menstrual flow begins. For menopausal hot flashes.

✦ **LEDUM** - for bruises. May be used folowing arnica treatment to fade the bruise after it becomes black and blue.

✦ **LYCOPODIUM** - increases personal confidence. Also favored by estheticians to soothe irritated complexions and as an antiseptic.

✦ **MAGNESIUM PHOS** - for abdominal cramping or spasmodic back pain; particularly for menstrual cramps.

✦ **NUX VOMICA** - for gastrointestinal tract problems, such as upset stomach, abdominal bloating, peptic ulcer and heartburn. A prime remedy for hangover, recovering alcoholics and drug addiction.

✦ **OSCILLOCOCCINUM** - a premiere remedy for flu.

✦ **PODOPHYLLUM** - helps diarrhea.

✦ **PULSITILLA** - for childhood asthma, allergies and ear infections, when the child is tearful and passive.

✦ **RHUS TOX** - a poison ivy derivative; for pain and stiffness in the joints and ligaments when the pain is worse with cold, damp weather.

✦ **SEPIA** - effective in treating herpes, eczema, hair loss and PMS.

How to Take Homeopathic Remedies

For maximum effectiveness, take $1/2$ dropperful under the tongue at a time, and hold for 30 seconds before swallowing; or dissolve the tiny homeopathic lactose tablets under the tongue. These remedies are designed to enter the bloodstream directly through the mouth's mucous membranes. For best absorption, do not eat, drink or smoke for 10 minutes before or after taking. Do not use with chemical medicines, caffeine or alcohol. These things will overpower homeopathy's subtle stimulus.

The basic rule for dosage is to repeat the medicines as needed.

Occasionally, aggravation of symptoms may be noted at first as the body restructures and begins to rebuild its defenses, much the same as healing crises occur with other natural cleansing therapies. This effect usually passes in a short period of time.

The negative side effects and hazards of habituation from drugs are causing many people to turn to the risk-free therapy of homeopathy. Healing can be quite long lasting. The right homeopathic remedy can restore health on all levels.

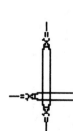

Homeopathic Cell Salts

What They Are ✦ How To Use Them

Mineral, or tissue salts in the body can be used as healing agents for particular health problems. Homeopathic doctor, William Schuessler, discoverer of the **twelve cell salts**, and the Biochemic System of Medicine, felt that every form of illness was associated with imbalances of one or more of the indispensable mineral salts. In addition, his research indicates that homeopathically prepared minerals help to maintain mineral balance in the body, and are used by the body as core, building nutrients at the cellular level. As with other homeopathic remedies, mineral salts are used to stimulate corresponding body cell salts toward normal metabolic activity and health restoration. They "re-tune" the body to return it to a healthy balance.

Cell salts are based on homeopathic remedies and may be used in healing programs with other homeopathic treatment. Only very small amounts are needed to properly nourish the cells.

THE TWELVE CELL SALTS

Many of today's cell salts are now extracted from organic plant sources. These medicines are available in tinctures and as tiny lactose-based tablets that are easily dissolved under the tongue.

✤ **CALCAREA FLUOR - calcium fluoride -** contained in the elastic fibers of the skin, blood vessels, connective tissue, bones and teeth. Used in the treatment of dilated or weakened blood vessels, such as those found in hemorrhoids, varicose veins, hardened arteries and glands.

✤ **CALCAREA PHOS - calcium phosphate -** abundant in all tissues. Strengthens bones, and helps build new blood cells. Deficiency results in anemia, emaciation, slow growth, poor digestion and general weakness.

✤ **CALCAREA SULPH - calcium sulphate -** found in bile; promotes continual blood cleansing. When deficient, toxic build-up occurs in the form of skin disorders, respiratory clog, boils and ulcerations, and slow healing.

✤ **FERRUM PHOS - iron phosphate -** helps form red blood corpuscles to oxygenate the bloodstream. Treats congestive colds and flu and skin inflammation. The biochemic remedy for the first stages of all inflammations, and infective wounds.

✤ **KALI MUR - potassium chloride -** found throughout the body. Deficiency results in coating of the tongue, glandular swelling, scaling of the skin, and excess mucous discharge. Used after Ferrum Phos for inflammatory arthritic and rheumatic conditions.

✤ **KALI PHOS - potassium phosphate -** found in all fluids and tissues. Deficiency is characterized by intense odor from the body. Used to treat mental problems such as depression, irritability, neuralgia, dizziness, headaches, and nervous stomach.

✤ **KALI SULPH - potassium sulphate -** a particular oxygen-carrier for the skin. Deficiency causes a deposit on the tongue, and slimy nasal, eye, ear and mouth secretions.

✤ **MAGNESIA PHOS - magnesium phosphate -** a constituent of the infrastructure of the body. Deficiency impairs muscle and nerve fibers, causing cramps, spasms and neuralgia pain, usually accompanied by prostration and profuse sweat.

✤ **NATRUM MUR - sodium chloride -** found throughout the body; regulates the moisture within the cells. Deficiency causes fatigue, chills, craving for salt, bloating, profuse, secretions from the skin, eyes and mucous membranes, excessive salivation, and watery stools.

✤ **NATRUM PHOS - sodium phosphate -** regulates the acid/alkaline balance. Catalyses lactic acid and fat emulsion. Imbalance is indicated by a coated tongue, itchy skin, sour stomach, loss of appetite, diarrhea and flatulence.

✤ **NATRUM SULPH - sodium sulphate -** an imbalance produces edema in the tissues, dry skin with watery eruptions, poor bile and pancreas activity, headaches, and gouty symptoms.

✤ **SILICEA - silica -** essential to the health of bones, joints, skin, and glands. Deficiency produces catarrh in the respiratory system, pus discharges from the skin, slow wound healing, and offensive body odor. Very successful in the treatment of boils, pimples and abscesses, for hair and nail health, blood cleansing, and rebuilding the body after illness or injury.

About Ayurvedic Medicine, Hypnotherapy, Guided Imagery & Biofeedback

Ayurveda, considered the most ancient existing medical system, is a 4,000 year-old Indian method of healing that includes diet, natural therapies and herbs dependent on body type. In Sanskrit, Ayurveda means "the science of lifespan". Its chief aim is longevity and improved quality of life. It attempts to maximize homeostasis, energy balance and the body's own self-repair mechanisms. Still widely practiced in India, Ayurveda is now enjoying a strong revival in the West. An ayurvedic treatment usually includes music, herbs, massage, steams, facials and aromatherapy. Its key elements include the following:

➡ Body Typing - the basic component in both treatment and diagnosis is biologic individuality. Ayurvedic physicians first determine the patient's psycho-physiological body type.

➡ Herbal Therapy - Ayurveda has a vast, documented legacy for thousands of herbal preparations that are now being scientifically validated. Reserpine for hypertension, digitalis for heart stimulation, and aloe vera all stem from Ayurvedic treatments. New research is being conducted on herbal formulas for tumor reduction in cancer, and on anti-inflammatory compounds such as Boswellia with anti-arthritic properties. Gum Guggul extract is becoming widely recognized in helping to normalize body weight, and cholesterol levels.

➡ Diet - foods are classified according to their effects on the specific body types, and diets are tailored to the patient's body types and individual imbalances.

➡ Behavior and Lifestyle - patients are asked to follow daily and seasonal routines that will help them better integrate with the biological rhythms of nature.

Hypnotherapy is finally being realized for the valuable healing tool it is. In clinical practice, hypnosis stimulates the limbic system - the region of the brain linked to emotion and involuntary responses like adrenal spurts and blood pressure. Habitual patterns of thought and reaction are temporarily suspended during a hypnotic trance, rendering the brain capable of responding to healthy suggestions. Hypnosis does not claim to cure physical ills, but studies indicate that it can help people heal faster, give up smoking, feel less pain and lose weight through suggestion; even long after the hypnotic session ends. One study has shown that burn victims heal considerably faster with less pain and fewer complications if they are hypnotized shortly after they are injured. Hypnotherapy works best as a partnership between doctor and patient in achieving a trance. Resistance to hypnosis accounts for the fact that one in ten people are not hypnotic suggestible.

Guided Imagery therapists use a near-trance condition, induced through spoken suggestion. Patients are asked to visualize their immune systems as an energy force battling their disease. Their immune responses to the particular ailment are studied in great detail. They are then asked to join forces with the immune system, by mentally envisioning the illness and imagining the antibodies and white cells overcoming the foe. Imagery has its roots in the ancient Greek understanding of the mind influencing the subconscious body. The technique, under many different names, has been used throughout the history of medicine, to reduce stress by quieting the mind and therefore speeding healing. It has been employed in modern times to encourage athletes, musicians and other performers to better performance. In healing, it has been successful in overcoming chronic pain or persistent infections, and in shrinking tumor growths. It is also used before minor surgery to help patients recover faster with less pain. Even serious, degenerative illness such as cancer has responded to guided imagery, with patients showing heightened immune activity.

Biofeedback uses an electronic machine to measure skin temperature, or electrodermal response. The patient is wired with sensors and learns to control what are usually involuntary responses, such as circulation to the extremeties, tension in the jaw, heartbeat rates, etc. Biofeedback is now used by medical professionals as a useful tool for controlling several health problems, including asthma, chronic fatigue, epilepsy, drug addiction and chronic pain. It is a successful specific in the treatment of migraines, cold extremities, and psoriasis. Biofeedback is used in relaxation therapy to help overcome insomnia and anxiety. Patients are taught to recognize tension in the forehead through audible/ visual feedback from an EMG (electromyograph). When they can control the forehead muscles, they learn a similar process to produce alpha brain waves that precede sleep.

Aromatherapy

What It Is ✦ How To Use It

Aromatherapy is an ancient science; a part of herbal medicine that uses essential plant oils to produce strong physical and emotional effects in the body. The oils act on different levels. They have a healing action on the physical plane. They restore energy balance. They have deep subconscious effects on emotions. They are elevating and soothing on the spiritual plane.

The oils are distilled from different parts of herbs and flowers by rushing steam through the plant material. The resulting condensed fluids are not really oils, but volatile, non-oily essences that have molecules so small they can penetrate the skin's tissue. As part of a healing treatment, aromatherapy oils are usually combined with massage, a bath or steam to promote cell regeneration, rid the body of toxins and relieve tension. Aromatherapy techniques are now reaching both the home and workplace with air diffusers and inhalers to relieve mental and physical stress.

WAYS TO USE AROMATHERAPY IN HEALING

Remember that essential oils are very concentrated, and should only be used in 1 to 5 drop doses.

Skin Care - *floral waters are the easiest way to use essential oils on the skin. They are mild, well-suited for sensitive and inflamed skin, they may be used effectively by all skin types, and have the same healing properties as the essential oil itself. Make floral waters in a spray bottle if possible, for best application and convenience. To make a therapeutic floral water, simply blend 5 to 10 drops of the essential oil into 4 oz. distilled water. Put in a spray bottle and use as needed.*

- Oils for general skin care - camomile, geranium, lavender, lemon, ylang ylang.
- Oils for dry, or aging skin - rose, carrot seed, rosemary, jasmine, red sage, sandlewood.
- Oils for oily skin - lavender, eucalyptus, geranium,ylang ylang, basil, camphor, lemon.
- Oils for sensitive skin - chamomile, neroli, rose.
- Oils for wrinkled skin - lemon,fennel, palmarosa, carrot seed, myrrh.
- Oils for inflamed skin - chamomile, lavender, neroli, rosewood, geranium, cedarwood.

Note: A drop of any of these may be put on a cotton swab and applied directly to the affected area. Particularly effective for treating a blemish that is just erupting.

- Oils for acne - eucalyptus, juniper, lavender, cajeput, palmarosa, tea tree.
- Oils for eczema or psoriasis - cedarwood, patchouly, lavender, chamomile.

Note: The above oils may also be added to your regular lotions and moisturizers for therapeutic skin benefits. However because the oils are volatile, you cannot make the up the preparation in advance. Pour some lotion into your hand; add 3 drops of oil and apply.

- Lemongrass steam - relaxes face muscles, balances overactive oil glands, oxygenates the blood through the respiratory system. *Simply add a few drops of lemongrass oil to a bowl of steaming water. Put your face 6 to 10 inches above the water, and tent a towel over your head.*
- Oils for skin washes - peppermint, antiseptic (5 drops); eucalyptus, bacteriacidal (5 drops); chamomile, soothing/healing (1 drop); sage, antiseptic tonic (2 drops). *Note: Simply add the recommended number of drops <u>each</u> to 4 ounces of liquid soap and use normally.*

Hair Care

- Brushing oil - to balance, heal, shine, and scent hair and scalp. Blend equal amounts of rosemary and lavender in a container. Place 2 drops on a brush and run several times through hair.
- Oils for dry hair - cedarwood, lavender
- Oils for oily hair - lemongrass, rosemary
- Oils for dandruff - rosemary, cedarwood
- Oils to reduce hair loss - cedarwood, lavender, rosemary, sage, juniper.

Note: The easiest way to use the above oils therapeutically is simply to mix 1/8 oz. of oils into an 8 oz. bottle of your favorite shampoo or conditioner. For scalp diseases, make a scalp rub with 1/8 oz. rosemary, sage or cedarwood oil in 2 oz. grain alcohol or sweet almond oil.

Oral Hygiene

- For fresh breath and better digestion - apply 1 drop peppermint oil on the tongue; or blend 5 drops oil with 1 oz. of cider vinegar and 3 oz. water, and use as a regular mouthwash.

- For a toothache - blend 20 drops clove oil with 1 oz. brandy and apply with a cotton swab.
- For gum problems - Put a few drops of sage or tea tree oil on a cotton swab and apply to gums.

Mental, Emotional and Spiritual Applications - *for best results, apply through massage oil, use a diffuser, take an aromatic bath, or inhale the aromas straight from the bottle.*
- Oils fo refreshment and invigoration - sage, lemon, lime, pine, eucalyptus, vervain.
- Oils to calm nervous tension and emotional stress - sage, pine, geranium, rosemary, pennyroyal.
- Oils for pleasant dreams and insomnia - anise, chamomile, ylang ylang.
- Oils for libido - ylang ylang, patchouly, sandalwood, cinnamon.
- Oils for stimulating intellect and memory - rosemary, petitgrain.
- Oils for serenity and calmness - lavender, pine, camomile, orange.
- Oils for positive motivation - peppermint, lemon, eucalyptus.
- Oils for anxiety and depression - sandalwood, petitgrain, bergamot, geranium, camomile, patchouly.
- Oils for energy and uplifting the spirits - sage, ylang ylang, geranium, palmarosa, rosewood .

Healing Applications - *generally, essential oils will only be a part of the complete treatment.*
Body cleansing and rejuvenation - massage the skin with an oil blend of 15 drops geranium, 35 drops neroli and 1 ounce vegetable oil. Promotes cell regeneration, helps rid the body of toxins and relieves tension. *Note: Blend just before using for most effectiveness.*
Antiseptic oils - lemon, clove, eucalyptus, pine, cinnamon, rosemary, thyme, tea tree.
Note: These are excellent in a diffuser to keep harmful bacteria count down. Effective for upper respiratory infections, colds and flu. Use approx. 30 to 50 drops oils, and let diffuser run for 30 minutes twice a day.
Skin abrasions - Apply one drop of sage or lavender oil to speed healing. *If used for first aid to cuts or bruises, put a few drops on a cotton swab and apply to area.*
Sore throat and cough - Oils such as eucalyptus and tea tree may be applied topically to the throat. Cypress may be taken as a "tea", at a dose of 1 drop to a cup of hot water every hour.
Chest congestion - Make a vapor rub, using 50 drops eucalyptus, 15 drops peppermint, and 10 drops wintergreen to 1 oz. vegetable oil. Rub into chest for relief.
Allergy and asthma relief - Add a few drops of eucalyptus, lavender, sage, peppermint or wintergreen oil to a pot of boiling water or a vaporizer.
Bladder problems - Make a bladder "tea", using 2 drops of lavender, juniper, tea tree, or thyme oil in a cup of hot water. Drink 8 glasses of water a day.
Indigestion - Take 1 to 2 drops with meals of either rosemary, peppermint or lemon oil.
Intestinal or bowel irritation - Use a "tea" with 1 drop geranium oil to a cup of hot water.
Sunburn - use 1 part tea tree oil to 1 part aloe vera gel and apply.
Headache - Apply 1 drop of lavender, peppermint or rosemary oil to back of the neck and temples.
Analgesic rub for sore joints and muscles - Use 20 drops <u>each</u> of clove, eucalyptus, tea tree, and wintergreen oils in 1 oz. vegetable oil. Rub into affected area, or add 1/4 oz. to a bath.

➡ Essential oils are herbs in their most concentrated form. As with other herb forms, blends are often more efficacious than single oils. Never apply straight essential oils, or more than five drops of purchased undiluted oils to the skin. Oils should always be diluted when applied near the eyes, nose mouth or genitals. Use patch testing if there is hypersensitivity to an oil. If any irritation results, discontinue use of that oil. Keep oils out of the reach of children.

➡ Since essential oils are usually quite expensive, many that are sold in stores are adjusted after manufacture, to maintain a certain quality standard at a lower cost. Smaller, reputable companies generally use quality components of natural origin to adjust the strength of their oils with little loss of potency. Oils that have been extended with fatty oils, ketones, terpenes or alcohol will have altered aroma and effects. Synthetic oils, made in a laboratory, may smell similar to essentials, but have no therapeutic impact and should not be used to treat health or beauty problems.

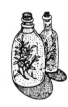

Alternative Healing Bodywork Techniques

REFLEXOLOGY ❖ ACUPUNCTURE ❖ ACUPRESSURE
CHIROPRACTIC ❖ MASSAGE THERAPY ❖ OVERHEATING THERAPY

What They Are ✦ Why You Should Consider Them

Reflexology, today an important part of massage therapy treatment, is a natural science dealing with the reflex points in the hands and feet that correspond to every organ and part of the body. Its goal is to clear the pathways of energy flow throughout the body, and thus return energy and increase immune defenses. The nerves are very like an electrical system, and contact can be made through the feet and hands with each of the ten electro-mechanical zones in the body, allowing location of the reflex points. Proper stimulation of these points through pressure and/or stroking can relieve circulatory and congestive problems at the body's deepest levels. Reflex pressure to a particular meridian point has a definite effect in bringing about better function in all parts of that zone, no matter how remote the point is from the body part in need of healing. The ten reflexology zone meridians connect all the organs and glands in the body, culminating in the hands and feet (see illustration).

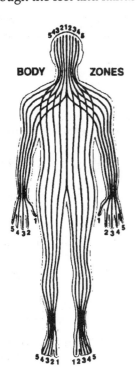

BODY ZONES

Fifteen pounds of applied force can send a surge of energy to the corresponding body area, to remove obstructive crystals, restore normal circulation, and clear congestion. The nerve reflex point on the foot for the afflicted area will be tender or sore indicating crystalline deposits brought about by poor capillary circulation of fluids. Pressure on the known corresponding foot or hand zone can be used for accurate self-diagnosis and treatment. The amount of soreness on the foot point can also indicate the size of the crystalline deposit, and the amount of time it has been accumulating. Pressure point therapy is effective in removing this obstructive congestion, and in relaxing nerve constriction. We have found that pressing on the sore point three times for 10 seconds each time is effective. The treatment may be applied for twenty to thirty minute sessions at a time, about twice a week. Sessions more often than this will not give Nature the chance to use the stimulation or do its necessary repair work. Most people notice frequent and easy bowel movement in the first twenty-four hours after zone therapy as the body throws off released wastes.

For individual use in this book, it is helpful to understand the hand and feet as the body's control panels. The "**foot**" and "**hand**" diagrams on the specific ailment pages will graphically show the pressure points for each area, so that you can use reflexology when indicated. In some cases, the points are very tiny, particularly for the glands. They will take practice to pinpoint. The best rule for knowing when you have reached the right spot is that it will usually be very tender, denoting crystalline deposits or congestion in the corresponding organ. However, there is often a feeling of immediate relief in the area as waste deposits break up for removal by the body.

❋

Acupuncture and acupressure are ancient systems of natural healing from the Orient, that are now reaching their due attention and respect in the western world. As we have noted, the human body is made up of a complex of meridians or "energy pathways". As in reflexology, the meridian points are connected to specific organs and body functions. The pathways regulate and coordinate the body's well-being by distributing "Chi" energy throughout it. When the balance and flow of this energy is upset or obstructed, illness often follows. Acupuncture and acupressure are a painless, non-toxic therapy for redirecting and restoring Chi energy.

Acupuncture uses hair thin needles and/or electrodes to direct and rechannel the energy. Western research has shown that the needles stimulate nerve cells to release endorphins, the body's inherent pain-relieving substances.

❀

Acupressure uses finger pressure on these meridians or massage and stroking to restore the energy.
Both methods are safe and effective for relief of many health problems, including arthritis, chronic pain, carpal tunnel syndrome, and the pain of withdrawal from smoking, alcoholism, and other addictions. Since both methods are free of toxic or additive side effects, they have become an alternative to people who used to live on Motrin, Advil and other pain pills that harmed the liver. We are also realizing their value as part of disease prevention care in the way that they are used in the Orient. Both methods are also effective for animals, and are often recommended for hip dysplasia and arthritis. As with other natural therapies, the aim is to regulate, balance and normalize so the body can function normally. Surgery and drugs can often be avoided, and there are sometimes immediate spectacular results. Traditional western doctors are even finding that these therapies work well *with* conventional medicine. In any case, acupuncture and acupressure can certainly influence the therapeutic course of even serious problems, and should be considered as a means of mobilizing a person's own healing energy and balance.

❀

Chiropractic and massage therapy are body manipulative techniques that relieve pain and returns energy by adjusting the spinal vertebrae, and re-aligning the spine. Most chiropractic work involves spinal subluxations, which occur when one of the vertebrae becomes locked in a fixed position, and is unable to move as it should. Serious fixations cause a host of other problems such as inflamed nerves, tight muscles and spasmodic pain. A chiropractor locates the fixated area of the spine, makes a spinal adjustment, and corrects the subluxation. Other problems aggravated by the fixation usually begin to heal immediately. (Most chiropractors today are no longer "back crackers", but instead use a hand-held "activator" that delivers a controlled, light, fast thrust to the problem area. The thrust is so quick that it accelerates ahead of the body's tightening up and resistance to the adjustment. The gentleness of this method makes adjustments far safer and more comfortable for the patient.) Almost every nerve in the body runs through the spine, and stress-caused constriction tends to accumulate in the lower back, neck and shoulders. Chiropractic adjustments therefore, can address many seemingly unrelated dysfunctions, both physical and subconscious.
Massage therapy is a more over all treatment that also includes reflexology techniques which address whole body harmony. Both massage therapists and some chiropractors regularly treat chronic headaches, PMS, chronic fatigue syndrome, candida albicans, gastro-intestinal conditions, epilespy, psoriasis and skin problems in addition to traditional spinal/nerve problems. Many use a holistic approach with diet correction, nutritional supplements, and enzyme therapy in a personally developed program for their patients.

❀

Overheating Therapy (Hyperthermia) is one of the most powerful natural healing methods available for treating serious disease. It has been used at least since the time of the ancient Greek physicians, and is based on the natural immune defense mechanism of raising body temperature to kill infective organisms, and retard their multiplication. Even slight temperature increases lead to considerable reduction in virus replication in the body. The high body temperature speeds up metabolism, inhibits the growth of the infective organism, and literally burns the "enemy" with heat. Overheating therapy has been used successfully against acute infectious diseases such as flus and cancer, arthritis and other rheumatic conditions, and most recently, against AIDS.
CNN recently showed on camera a blood-overheating procedure for an AIDS patient in the treatment of sarcoma, (the cancer common to AIDS patients that produces the severe skin lesions). The sores vanished in about four months, along with other symptoms. Since then, other AIDS sufferers with sarcoma lesions have undergone hyperthermia, have experienced the same success, and in some cases the blood has even tested negative for the AIDS virus. Since only blood hyperthermia has been tried for AIDS and cancer, the virus may still be in the bone or marrow and may resurface, but there is obvious reduction of symptoms. Despite the great skepticism on the part of the medical community for overheating therapy, it is now faced with the drastic disease of AIDS, for which a drug related cure has not been found. Hyperthermia may once again become known for the valuable healing tool that it is.
Note: Simple overheating therapy imay be used in the home. See page 50 for method and technique.

❀

Optimal Healing After Surgery

**Strengthening Your Body For Surgery ✦ Accelerating Healing
Cleaning Out Drug Residues ✦ Getting Over The Side Effects**

Traditional medicine and its technology can do things that should be appreciated and never forgotten. It can stabilize a life-threatening condition, and arrest life-threatening disease long enough to give the body an opportunity to fight, and a chance to heal itself. But surgery and major medical treatment are always traumatic on the body. You can do much to strengthen your system, alleviate body stress, and increase your chances of rapid recovery and healing.

Before you go to the hospital:

Strengthen the immune system. Include daily:
- ✓ Beta-carotene 25,000IU, and vitamin E 200IU w/ selenium 100mcg. as antioxidants.
- ✓ Vitamin C 1000mg. with bioflavonoids and rutin for tissue integrity.
- ✓ B Complex 100mg. with pantothenic acid 500mg. for adrenal strength.

Eat a high vegetable protein diet. You must have protein to heal.
- ✓ Take a full spectrum, pre-digested amino acid compound, capsules or drink, 1000mg. daily.
- ✓ Eat plenty of brown rice for B vitamins and other whole grains for complex carbohydrates.
- ✓ Take a potassium juice (page 53), potassium supplement liquid, and/or a protein drink every day.

Strengthen body defense measures. Include daily:
- ✓ Bromelain 750mg. (with Quercetin 250mg. if there is inflammation)
- ✓ Germanium 30mg. capsules, (or dissolve 1 gm. Nutricology germanium powder in 1 qt. water, and take 2 to 3 TBS. daily).
- ✓ Sun CHLORELLA 20 tablets, 1 packet of powder, or Crystal Star ENERGY GREEN™.
- ✓ Gotu kola capsules 2 caps 2x daily for one month.
- ✓ Crystal Star GINSENG 6 DEFENSE RESTORATIVE™ TEA, 2x daily.

Note: because the medical community generally uses information and testing results on synthetic, rather than naturally occurring vitamin E sources (such as wheat germ and soy), many doctors insist that no vitamin E be taken four weeks prior to surgery in an effort to curb prolonged post-operative bleeding. We have not found this to be the case with natural vitamin E, but we suggest that you consult your physician if you are in doubt.

✦

When you return home:

Eat a very nutritious diet. Include frequently:
- ✓ Organ meats and/or sea vegetables for absorbable vitamin B_{12}.
- ✓ Seafoods and baked or broiled fish.
- ✓ Brown rice and other whole grains with tofu.
- ✓ Fresh fruits and vegetables.
- ✓ Yogurt and other cultured foods for friendly intestinal flora
- ✓ A potassium broth or juice, (pg. 53), green drink or hot energy tonic.
- ✓ A high protein drink such as Nature's Plus SPIRUTEIN or NutriTech ALL 1.

Clean the body and vital organs, to counteract infection. Include daily for one month:
- ✓ High potency multi-culture compound such as DOCTOR DOPHILUS, or Natren LIFE START 2, 1 teasp. in juice or water with each meal.
- ✓ Crystal Star LIV-ALIVE™ capsules, tea or extract.
- ✓ George's ALOE VERA JUICE with herbs - 1 glass daily in the morning
- ✓ Astragalus capsules or extract with Siberian Ginseng and Reishi mushroom to overcome toxicity, and provide deep body tone.
- ✓ Shark Liver oil or shark cartilage capsules for leukocyte formation to fight infection.
- ✓ Enzyme therapy such as Rainbow Light DETOX-ZYME.
- ✓ Fresh carrot juice or Beta Carotene 50 -100,000IU as anti-infectives.

Build the body and tissues up. Include daily for one month:
- ✓ Futurebiotics VITAL K or other food source absorbable potassium liquid.
- ✓ Crystal Star SYSTEM STRENGTH™ drink, and/or BODY REBUILDER™ with ADR-ACTIVE™ capsules.

✓ Vitamin C with bioflavonoids and rutin 500mg. *only,* <u>with</u> pantothenic acid 500-1000mg.
✓ Vitamin E 400IU w/ Selenium, or carnitine 250mg. <u>with</u> CoQ 10mg. as anti-oxidants.
✓ Zinc 30-50mg. **or** Alta Health SIL-X CAPSULES to help rebuild tissue.
✓ Vitamin B_{12} sublingually, or Ener-B VIT. B_{12} INTERNASAL GEL.
✓ Enzymatic Therapy LIQUID LIVER with GINSENG capsules, **or** Country Life ENERGIX vials.
✓ Aloe vera or calendula gel to heal scars and lesions, or puncture a vitamin A & D oil capsule.

Other recuperation information:
❖ If you are taking antibiotics, take them <u>with</u> Bromelain for better effectiveness, and supplement with B Complex, Vitamin C, Vitamin K and calcium.
❖ If you are taking diuretics, add Vitamin C, potassium and B complex.
❖ If you are taking aspirin, take with vitamin C for best results.
❖ If you are taking antacids, supplement with Vitamin B_1 and/or calcium.
❖ If you smoke, add Vitamin C 500mg., E 400IU, Beta-Carotene 50,000IU, and niacin to an optimal diet.
❖ If you are considering chelation therapy, remember that it goes through the body like a magnet collecting heavy metals and triglycerides. It is not recommended if you have weak kidneys, because too many toxins are dumped into the elimination system too fast, putting unneeded stress on the healing body.

❖

Normalizing The Body After Chemotherapy & Radiation

Chemotherapy and radiation treatments are widely used by the medical community for several types, stages and degrees of cancerous or malignant cell growth. While some partial successes have been proven, the aftereffects are often worse than the disease in terms of healthy cell damage, body imbalance, and lowered immunity. Many doctors and therapists recognize these drawbacks to chemotherapy, but under current government and insurance restrictions, neither they nor their patients have alternatives.

No other treatments except surgery, radiation and chemotherapy have been officially approved by the FDA in the United States for malignant disease. The costs for these treatments are beyond the financial range of most people, who, along with physicians and hospitals must rely on their health insurance to pay these expenses. Medical insurance will not reimburses doctors or hospitals if they use other healing methods. Thus, exorbitant major medical costs and special interest regulation have bound medical professionals, hospitals, and insurance companies in a vicious circle where literally no alternative measure may be used for controlling cancerous growth. Everyone, including the patient, is caught in a political and bureaucratic web, where it all comes down to money instead of health.

New testing and research is also abnormally expensive, and lags for lack of funding. Moreover, when a valid treatment is substantiated, there is not even the reasonable investment certainty that government (and therefore health insurance) approval can be achieved through the maze of red tape and political lobbies. This is doubly unfortunate, since there is much research, and many alternative therapies, being used successfully in Europe and other countries to which Americans are denied access.

Nutritional counselors, holistic practitioners, therapists and others involved in natural healing have done a great deal of testing and work toward minimizing the damage, and rebuilding the body after chemotherapy and radiation. These efforts have had notable success, and may be used with confidence by those recovering both from cancer and its current medical treatment.

For three months after chemotherapy or radiation, take the following daily:
✓ One packet Barley Green granules, or Crystal Star SYTEM STRENGTH™ drink - 1 TB. in hot water.
✓ Mega CoQ 10 capsule - 30mg.
✓ Germanium 30mg. (or dissolve 1 gm. Germanium powder in 1 qt. water and take 3 TBS. daily)
✓ Ener -B vitamin B_{12} INTERNASAL GEL - 1 dose every other day.

✓ Hawthorne extract - $1/2$ dropperful under the tongue 2 x daily as a circulatory tonic.
✓ Crystal Star LIV-ALIVE™ casules and tea, or other good herbal liver cleanser.
✓ Astragalus capsules or extract - 2x daily; and/or Crystal Star GINSENG 6 DEFENSE RESTORATIVE™ TEA, 2x daily.

✓ Ascorbate Vitamin C crystals w/ bioflavonoids, $1/4$ teasp. in liquid every hour = 5-10,000mg, daily.
✓ Floradix HERBAL IRON 1 teasp. 3 x daily, or Crystal Star ENERGY GREEN™ drink.
✓ 800mcg. folic acid daily if MTX (methotrexate) has been used in your treatment. Ask your doctor.
✓ Crystal Star ANTI-FLAM™ caps, or Strength Systems FIRST AID if there is swelling/inflammation.

The Basics Of Beginning A Healing Program

DETOXIFICATION ❖ FASTING ❖ BLOOD CLEANSING

Environmental toxins, secondary smoke inhalation, alcohol, prescription and pleasure drug abuse, "hidden" chemicals and pollutants in our food that cause allergies and addictions, caffeine overload, poor diet, junk foods, and daily acid-causing stress, are all becoming more and more a part of our lives. All of these things result in great strain and depletion to the immune system which eventually results in debilitation and serious disease. Lowered immunity has become a prime factor in today's "civilization and opportunistic" diseases, such as Candida albicans, Chronic Fatigue Syndrome (EBV), Cancer, Lupus, AIDS & ARC.

In the past, detoxification was used either clinically for recovering alcoholics/drug addicts, or individually as a once-a-year 'spring cleaning' for general health maintenance. Today, detoxification is becoming more and more necessary not only to health, but for the quality of our lives, surrounded as we are by so much involuntary toxicity. Optimally, one should seriously cleanse and detoxify the body 2-3 times a year, especially in the Spring, Summer and early Fall, when the body can get an extra boost in this effort from sunlight and natural Vitamin D.

A good detoxification program should be in three stages:

♣ CLEANSING ♣ REBUILDING ♣ MAINTAINING

The first step is to cleanse the body of waste deposits, so you won't be running with a dirty engine or driving with the brakes on. All disease, physical and psychological, is created or allowed by the saturation and accumulation of toxic matter in the tissues, throwing defense mechanisms off, and vitality out of balance. Many years of experience with body cleansing have convinced us that a moderate 3 to 7 day juice fast is the best way to release toxins from the system. Shorter fasts can't get to the root of a chronic or major problem. Longer fasts upset body equilibrium more than most people are ready to deal with except in a controlled, clinical situation.

A well-thought-out moderate fast can bring great advantages to the body by: cleansing it of excess mucous, old fecal matter, trapped cellular, and non-food wastes; and by "spring cleaning the pipes" of uncirculated systemic sludge such as inorganic mineral deposits.

A few days without solid food can be a refreshing and enlightening experience about your life style. A short fast increases awareness as well as available energy for elimination. Your body will become easier to "hear". It can tell you what foods and diet are right for your needs, via legitimate cravings such as a desire for protein foods, B vitamins or minerals, for example. Like a "cellular phone call", this is natural biofeedback.

Fasting works by self-digestion. During a cleanse, the body in its infinite wisdom, will decompose and burn only the substances and tissue that are damaged, diseased or unneeded, such as abscesses, tumors, excess fat deposits, and congestive wastes. Even a relatively short fast can accelerate elimination from the liver, kidneys, lungs and skin, often causing dramatic changes as masses of accumulated waste are expelled. Live foods and juices can literally pick up dead matter from the body and carry it away.

You will be very aware of this if you experience the short period of headaches, fatigue, body odor, bad breath, diarrhea or mouth sores that commonly accompany accelerated elimination. However, digestion usually improves right away as do many gland and nerve functions. Cleansing can also help release hormone secretions that stimulate the immune system, and encourage a disease-preventing environment. In a couple of weeks the body will start rebalancing, energy levels will rise physically, psychologically and sexually, and creativity will begin to expand. You will start feeling like a "different person" - and of course you are.

Outlook and attitude have changed, because through cleansing and improved diet, your actual cell make-up has changed.

You really are what you eat.

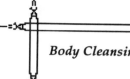

Stage 1: Internally Cleansing The Body

*Three separate **liquid fasting diets** are included in this section to focus on whole-body cleansing: **the first** is specifically aimed at cleansing excess mucous from the lung and respiratory system; **the second** is a colon and bowel cleanse aimed at removing toxins from the elimination system; **the third** is a short 24 hour juice fast for beginning a cleanse when time is a factor. Each diet can help the body release trapped, excess waste matter and alkalize the bloodstream, so that more efficient healing can take place.*

Cleansing diets may be used before and during any therapeutic program, unless the person is weak and pale, with very low energy, or when immediate emergency measures are indicated. Results are usually well worth the effort.

➡ Have a small fresh salad the night before beginning a liquid fast, with plenty of intestinal "sweepers and scourers", such as beets, celery, cabbage, broccoli, parsley, carrots, etc.
Elimination will begin as soon as the first meal is missed. Use organically grown fresh fruits and vegetables for all juices if possible.

➡ End your fasting period gently, with small simple meals. Have toasted wheat germ or muesli, or whole grain granola for your first morning of solid food, with a little yogurt, apple, or pineapple/coconut juice. Take a small fresh salad for lunch with Italian or lemon/oil dressing. Have a fresh fruit smoothie during the day. Fix a baked potato with a little butter and a light soup or salad for dinner. Rebuilding starts right away with the nutrition-rich foods you are taking in.
You are on your way with a fresh, clean system.

Mucous Cleansing: *A 3 to 7 day liquid diet*

On rising: take a glass of *fresh-squeezed* lemon juice and water, (add 1 TB. maple syrup if desired).

Breakfast: take a glass of grapefruit juice if the system is over-acid; or cranberry/apple or pineapple juice.

Mid-morning: have a cup of herb tea, such as fresh comfrey or dandelion leaf, or wild cherry bark; <u>or</u> a tea specifically blended to clear mucous congestion, such as Crystal Star X-PECT-T™, an expectorant to aid mucous release, or RSPR TEA™, an aid in oxygen uptake.

Lunch: take a glass of carrot juice, or a potassium broth or essence (page 53).

Mid-afternoon: have a green drink (page 54), or a packet of Chlorella granules in a glass of water; <u>or</u> a greens and sea vegetable mix, such as Crystal Star ENERGY GREEN DRINK™.

Supper: take a glass of apple juice or papaya/pineapple juice.

❧ **For best results,** break the fast with a small fresh salad on the last night of the cleanse.

Before retiring: take a hot broth with 1 teasp. VEGEX extract for relaxation and strength the next day.
❧ Drink 8 glasses of water daily **in addition** to juices, to thin mucous secretions and aid elimination.

Supplements and Herbal Aids for the Mucous Cleansing Diet:

✜ Take 10,000mg. of ascorbate vitamin C crystals with bioflavonoids daily for the first three days; just dissolve 1/4 - 1/2 teasp. in water or juice throughout the day, until bowel tolerance is reached, and tissues are flushed. Take 5,000mg. daily for the next four days.
✜ Take 1 teasp. 3x daily of garlic/onion syrup. Mash several garlic cloves and a large slice of onion in a bowl, and stir with 3 TBS. of honey. Cover, and let macerate for 24 hours, then remove garlic and onion and take only the honey/syrup infusion.

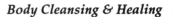

Bodywork Suggestions for the Mucous Cleansing Diet:
❖ Take a brisk 1 hour walk each day of the cleanse; breathe deeply to help lungs eliminate mucous.
❖ Take an enema the first and last day of your fasting diet to thoroughly clean out excess mucous.
❖ Apply wet ginger/cayenne compresses to the chest to increase circulation and loosen mucous.
❖ Take a hot sauna, or long warm baths followed by a brisk rubdown, to stimulate circulation.

Colon and Bowel Elimination Cleanse: *A 3 to 10 day liquid diet*
Bowel elimination problems are often chronic, and may require several rounds of cleansing. This fast may be done all at once or in two periods of five days each.

➡ The night before you begin, take a gentle herbal laxative, either in tea or tablet form, such as HER-BALTONE, Wisdom of the Ancients YERBA MATÉ tea, Crystal Star LAXA-TEA™ or FIBER & HERBS COLON CLEANSE™ capsules.
➡ Soak some dried figs, prunes and raisins in water to cover, add 1 TB. unsulphured molasses, and let soak overnight in a covered bowl.
➡ Six to 8 glasses of pure water daily are necessary for the success of this cleanse.

On rising: take 1 teasp. Sonné LIQUID BENTONITE, **or** 2 teasp. psyllium husks in juice or water; **or** 1 heaping teasp. Crystal Star CHO-LO FIBER TONE™ DRINK MIX (either flavor) in water.

Breakfast: discard fruits from their soaking water and take a small glass of the liquid.

Mid-morning: take a glass of George's ALOE VERA JUICE with herbs.

Lunch: take a small glass of potassium broth or essence (page 53); **or** a glass of fresh carrot juice.

Mid-afternoon: take a large glass of fresh apple juice;
or an herb tea such as alfalfa, fennel, or red clover;
or Crystal Star CLEANSING & PURIFYING™ tea to enhance elimination and provide energy support.

About 5 o' clock: take another small glass of potassium broth or essence; **or** another fresh carrot juice; **or** a green drink (page 54), **or** Green Foods BARLEY GREEN MAGMA granules, or Crystal Star ENERGY GREEN™ drink in water;

Supper: take a large glass of apple juice or papaya juice.
❧ **Break the fast** with a small raw foods meal on the last night of the cleanse.

Before Bed: repeat the body cleansing liquids that you took on rising, **and** take a cup of peppermint or spearmint tea.

Supplements and Herbal Aids for the Bowel Elimination Cleanse:

❖ Take 4-6 Crystal Star FIBER & HERBS COLON CLEANSE™ caps, to help increase systol/diastol activity of the colon, and tone bowel tissue during heavy elimination.
❖ Take a catnip or diluted liquid chlorophyll enema every other night during the cleanse.

Bodywork Suggestions for the Bowel Elimination Cleanse:

❖ Take a brisk daily walk for an hour every day during the fast.
❖ Take several long warm baths during the fast to speed cleansing. A lower back and pelvis massage and dry skin brushing will help release toxins coming out through the skin.

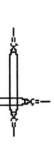

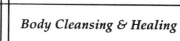
24 Hour Juice Cleanse:

A short 24 hour liquid cleanse is often enough to start a good healing program.
"Beginning" s usually the hardest part of a fast. You have to set aside a block of time, gather all the ingredients for your diet, alter eating times and patterns; in essence change your life style and that of those you live with for a while. This is very difficult to do for many people, and can delay a needed program. The following 24 hour juice and herb tea fast makes things a lot easier. It is a quick cleanse; not with the depth of vegetable juices, or satisfactory for major or chronic problems. But it is often enough, and definitely better than no fast at all.
It will make a difference in the speed of healing.

The night before your fast: have a small fresh green salad with lemon/oil dressing.

On rising: take a glass of 2 fresh squeezed lemons, 1TB. maple syrup and 8 oz. water..

Midmorning: take a glass of cranberry juice from concentrate.

Lunch: take a glass of fresh apple juice, **or** apple/alfalfa sprout juice with 1 packet of chlorella or BARLEY GREEN MAGMA granules dissolved in it.

Midafternoon: take a cup of Crystal Star CLEANSING & PURIFYING™ TEA or MEDITATION™ TEA.

Dinner: take a glass of papaya/pineapple juice to enhance enzyme production, or another glass of apple juice with 1 packet Sun CHLORELLA or Green Foods GREEN MAGMA granules.

Before bed: have a cup of mint tea, **or** 1 teasp. Vegex yeast paste extract in a cup of hot water for relaxation and strength the next day.

✒Break your fast the next morning with fresh fruits and yogurt. Eat light, raw foods during the day, and have a simply prepared, low fat dinner.
✒Drink plenty of pure water throughout the day to flush the system.

Bodywork Suggestions:

✤ Take a long walk during the day.
✤ Use a dry skin brush to help release toxins coming out through the skin, and take a long, warm relaxing bath before retiring.

One Week Brown Rice Cleanse:

Macrobiotic principles may be used for this six day brown rice cleanse. This diet is very successful for dropping a few quick pounds, and balancing the body when it's just feeling low energy or out-of-sorts.

The diet is very simple, easy to take, and easy to fit in with your life style.

➡ Simply drink mixed vegetable juice throughout the day whenever you like. Use the "Personal Best V-8 Juice" recipe on page 55, or Knudsen's VERY VEGGIE JUICE, or regular V-8.
➡ Have steamed brown rice and mixed vegetables for dinner. Any blend of your favorite vegetables if fine. Have at least a cup of rice and several cups of vegetables if you like.
➡ Add any non-fat seasonings to your own taste, (no butter or oil drsssings).
That's all there is to it. Follow this regimen for 6 days. Results in weight, body definition and body chemistry change are noticeable almost immediately. You need the six days to set up an ongoing balance.

Stage Two: Rebuilding & Restoring the Body: *A 2 to 6 week program*

The second part of a good cleansing and detoxification program is to rebuild healthy tissue and restore body energy. It is usually begun after 3 to 10 days of waste and toxin elimination from the blood, lungs and bowels. This phase allows the body's regulating powers to become active with obstacles removed, so it can rebuild at optimum levels.

The rebuilding diet emphasizes raw, fresh, and simply prepared foods. It should be very low in fat, with little dairy, and no fried foods. Avoid alcohol, caffeine, tobacco, and sugars; avoid meats except fish and sea foods.

On rising: take a vitamin/mineral/protein drink, such as Nutri-Tech ALL 1, Nature's Plus SPIRU-TEIN, or Crystal Star SYSTEM STRENGTH™ DRINK with apple or other fruit juice;
or 2 lemons squeezed in water with honey; **or** 2 TBS. apple cider vinegar in water with a little honey.

Breakfast: have some fresh citrus fruit, especially grapefruit or oranges;
or soy milk or low fat yogurt with fresh fruit; **or** a fresh fruit smoothie with a banana;
or whole grain cereal with a little apple juice.

Mid-morning: take a glass of fresh carrot juice, or potassium broth (pg. 53);
or a cup of Siberian Ginseng tea, or Crystal Star FEEL GREAT™ TEA, or chamomile tea;
or a small bottle of mineral water with a packet of CHLORELLA or GREEN MAGMA granules;
or Crystal Star ENERGY GREEN DRINK™ mix in water to deodorize and freshen the GI tract.

Lunch: have a fresh green salad with lemon/oil dressing;
or steamed tofu with fresh greens and dressing;
or steamed vegies such as broccoli, carrots, onions or zucchini with Bragg's LIQUID AMINOS,
or miso, or other Oriental clear soup with Ramen noodles;
and/or a light vegetarian sandwich on whole grain bread.

Mid-afternoon: have a green drink; **or** Crystal Star BIOFLAV., FIBER & C SUPPORT™ drink;
or some raw vegie snacks with kefir cheese or soy cheese and a small bottle of mineral water;
or a cup of herb tea, such as peppermint or red clover, **or** Crystal Star HIGH ENERGY™ TEA.

Dinner: have a baked potato with Bragg's LIQUID AMINOS or soy sauce;
or steamed vegies with brown rice and tofu;
or baked or broiled white fish with a lemon/oil sauce;
or a whole grain vegetarian casserole; **or** a whole grain or vegetable pasta salad, hot or cold.

Before bed: a relaxing cup of herb tea, such as chamomile, or Crystal Star GOOD NIGHT™ TEA.

🍃 Continue with plenty of pure water and other fluids to maximize system activity.

Supplements and Herbal Aids for the Rebuilding Diet:
❖ Take a potassium broth at least once a week, or Crystal Star SYSTEM STRENGTH™ drink.
❖ Take acidophilus liquid or capsules with meals to encourage friendly bacteria in the GI tract.
❖ Take vitamin B$_{12}$, either sublingually or internasally, for healthy cell development.
❖ Take ascorbate or Ester vit. C 3-5000mg. with bioflavonoids for interstitial tissue/collagen growth.
❖ Take Crystal Star ADR-ACTIVE™ **with** BODY REBUILDER™ capsules, 2 **each daily**, to encourage healthy gland activity and strength. Take HEARTSEASE/ANEMI-GIZE™ capsules to help build hemoglobin and increase liver, spleen and lymph function. Take FEEL GREAT™ capsules or tea for stamina and endurance. Use HAWTHORNE extract, 1 dropperful two times daily as a body tonic.

Bodywork Suggestions for the Rebuilding Diet:
❖ Take some mild exercise every day.
❖ Get some sunlight on the body every day possible. Light builds strength along with food. Eating out of doors is especially beneficial. Consider a short camping trip.

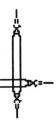

Stage 3: Maintaining A Healthy Immune System:

*The final part of a good cleansing program is keeping your body clean and toxin-free - **very important** after all the hard work of detoxification. Modifying lifestyle habits to include high quality nutrition from both food and supplement sources is the key to a strong resistant body.*
The foods for this maintenance diet should rely heavily on fresh fruits and vegetables for cleansing and soluble fiber; cooked vegetables, grains and seeds for strength, endurance and alkalinity; sea foods, eggs, and low fat cheeses as alternate sources of protein; and lightly cooked sea foods and vege-tables with a little dinner wine for circulatory health.

The following *"GOOD PROTECTION TEST"* can help you monitor your support-system health on a regular basis. Essentially it is a fiber check; enough soluble fiber in the diet to make the stool float, is the protective level against such problems as colitis, constipation, hemorrhoids, diverticulitis, vari-cose veins, and bowel cancer.

➡ **The bowel movement should be regular and effortless.**
➡ **The stool should be almost odorless.**
➡ **There should be very little flatulence.**
➡ **The stool should float rather than sink.**

Supplement & Herbal Suggestions For Maintenance & Disease Prevention:

❖ Keep tissue oxygen levels high with 1-3000mg. vitamin C with bioflavonoids, vitamin B_{12}, interna-sally or sublingually, and vitamin E 4-800IU with selenium daily.
❖ Keep a good level of potassium in the body with high potassium foods, such as broccoli, leafy greens, bananas, and sea vegetables, or a weekly potassium broth or juice; or a potassium supplement such as Twin Lab LIQUID K PLUS, Crystal Star ENERGY GREEN™ drink.
❖ Take unsprayed bee pollen granules, 2 teasp. daily for essential amino acids; and/or high potency royal jelly, 2 teasp. daily for natural pantothenic acid.
❖ Immune enhancing supplements can include bee propolis liquid extract, beta carotene 25,000IU, CoQ10 10mg., zinc 30-50mg., raw thymus extract (during high risk seasons), and Crystal Star HERBAL DEFENSE TEAM™ extract, tea or capsules.
❖ High chlorophyll food supplements fortify immunity, enhance healthy cell development and body balance, and insure alkalinity; chlorella, Green Foods GREEN MAGMA, spirulina, Nature's Plus SPI-RUTEIN, or Crystal Star ENERGY GREEN™ drink.
❖ Foundation multiple vitamins and minerals should be from food or herbal sources for best absor-bency. Some of the best are from Living Source, Mezotrace, New Chapter, and Floradix. Crystal Star makes several combinations high in concentrated herbal minerals; IRON SOURCE, CALCIUM SOURCE™ and MINERAL SOURCE COMPLEX extracts and capsules.
❖ Enzymes and lactobacillus acidophilus are important for good assimilation and adequate intestinal flora. The most effective supplements have multiple complex living organisms that can easily unite with the body. Good maintenance products include DR. DOPHILUS or D.D.S. ACIDOPHILUS; for children, Nature's Plus JR. DOPHILUS chewable wafers or DOCTOR DOPHILUS powder. Crystal Star SYSTEM STRENGTH™ instant drink is full of naturally occuring minerals, enzymes, and amino acids.
❖ High soluble fiber supplementation can insure a fully active elimination system, digestive regula-tion, and cholesterol/blood sugar balance. Some of the most effective and convenient include guar gum capsules before meals, psyllium husks, 2 teasp. in water in the morning and evening, or a high fi-ber drink such as Yerba Prima COLON CARE, or Crystal Star CHO-LO FIBER TONE™ drink or cap-sules.

Bodywork Suggestions For Disease Prevention:

❖ Daily exercise is one of the most important things to do for your life. It increases oxygen uptake in the body to improve metabolism, circulation, and respiratory activity. Every walk you take, every se-ries of stretches you do, strengthens and lengthens your life and health.
❖ Get early morning sunlight on the body every day possible for regular vitamin D.

Blood Cleansing and Purifying Diet for Serious Immune Deficient Diseases:

There is usually a great deal of blood toxicity, fatigue and lack of nutrient assimilation in serious degenerative conditions. A liquid fast is therefore *not recommended*, since iit is often too harsh for an already weakened system. The initial diet should, however, be as pure as possible, in order to be as cleansing as possible - totally vegetarian - free of all meats, dairy foods, fried, preserved and refined foods, and above all, saturated fats. This diet may be followed for 1 to 2 months, or longer if the body is still actively cleansing, or needs further alkalizing. The diet may also be returned to when needed, to purify against relapse or additional symptoms.

On rising: take 2-3 TBS. cranberry concentrate in 8 oz. water with $1/2$ teasp. ascorbate vitamin C crystals, or use a green tea blood cleansing formula, such as Crystal Star GREEN TEA CLEANSER™;
or cut up $1/2$ lemon (with skin) and blend in the blender w. 1 teasp. honey, and 1 cup distilled water;
and $1/2$ teasp. Natren LIFE START 2 lactobacillus complex or Alta Health CANGEST in 8 oz. aloe vera juice.

Take a brisk exercise walk, and get some early morning sunlight every day.

Breakfast: have a glass of fresh carrot juice, with 1 TB. Bragg's LIQUID AMINOS added;
and whole grain muffins or rice cakes with kefir cheese;
or whole grain cereal or pancakes with yogurt and fresh fruit;
or a cup of soy milk or plain yogurt mixed in the blender with a cup of fresh fruit, some walnuts and $1/2$ teasp. Natren LIFE START 2 lactobacillus complex.

Mid-morning: take a weekly colonic irrigation. On non-colonic days, take a potassium broth or essence (pg. 53) with 1 TB. Bragg's LIQUID AMINOS, and $1/2$ teasp. ascorbate vitamin C crystals;
and another fresh carrot juice, or pau de arco tea with $1/2$ teasp. Natren LIFE START 2 added.

Lunch: have a green leafy salad with lemon/flax oil dressing; add sprouts, tofu, avocado, nuts and seeds;
or have an open-face sandwich on rice cakes or a chapati, with soy or yogurt cheese and fresh vegies;
or have a cup of miso soup with rice noodles or brown rice;
or have some steamed vegetables with millet or brown rice and tofu;
and a cup of pau de arco tea or aloe vera juice with $1/2$ teasp. ascorbate vitamin C and $1/2$ teasp. Natren LIFE START 2 lactobacillus complex.

Mid-afternoon: have another carrot juice with 1 TB. Bragg's LIQUID AMINOS;
and a green drink, such as Sun CHLORELLA, GREEN MAGMA or Crystal Star ENERGY GREEN™.

Dinner: have a baked potato with Bragg's LIQUID AMINOS or lemon/oil dressing and a fresh salad;
and another potassium broth, or black bean or lentil soup;
or fresh spinach or artichoke pasta with steamed vegetables and a lemon/flax oil dressing;
or a Chinese steam/stir fry with shiitake mushrooms, vegetables and brown rice;
or a tofu and vegie casserole with yogurt or soy cheese.
☙ Sprinkle $1/2$ teasp. Natren LIFE START 2, or Alta Health CANGEST powder over any cooked food at this meal.

Before Bed: take another 8 oz. glass of aloe vera juice with $1/2$ teasp. ascorbate vitamin C with bioflavs;
and another carrot juice, or papaya juice with $1/2$ teasp. Natren LIFE START 2 lactobacillus powder.

Watchwords for Blood Cleansing and Diet Purification:
✓ All produce should be fresh and organically grown when possible.
✓ A good juicer is really necessary. The investment is well worth it.
✓ Avoid canned, frozen prepackaged foods, and refined foods with colors, preservatives and flavor enhancers. Avoid sodas and artificial drinks.
✓ Avoid concentrated sugars, and sweeteners. Keep table salt use to a minimum.

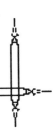

✓ No fried foods of any kind.

✓ Unsweetened mild herb teas and bottled mineral water (6 to 8 glasses) are recommended throughout each day, to hydrate, alkalize, and keep the body flushed of toxic wastes.

✓ $1/2$ teasp. ascorbate vitamin C crystals with bioflavonoids may be added to any drink throughout the day to bowel tolerance for optimum results.

Supplements for the Blood Purifying Diet:
Because such vigorous treatment is necessary, supplementation is desirable at all stages of healing.

❖ Anti-oxidants, such as germanium 100-150mg. with astragalus, Vitamin E 1000IU with selenium 200mcg., CoQ 10 30mg. and octacosonal 1000mg. daily can strengthen white blood cell and T-cell activity, and help overcome side effects and nerve damage from many of the drugs prescribed for these conditions.
◆ Take the above **with** Quercetin Plus and Bromelain 500mg. 3x daily, to prevent auto-immune reactions, **and** high potency digestive enzymes, such as Rainbow Light DETOX-ZYME capsules.

❖ Egg yolk lecithin, highest potency, for active lipids that make the cell walls resistant to attack.

❖ Acidophilus culture complex with bifidus - refrigerated, highest potency, 3 teasp. daily, with biotin 1000mcg., and/or $1/2$ teasp. Lexon B BLEND powder.

❖ Aged aloe vera juice, 2 to 3 glasses daily, to block virus spreading from cell to cell.

❖ Shark liver oil or cartilage, echinacea or pau de arco extract, $1/2$ dropperful 3x daily, to stimulate production of interferon, interleukin and lymphocytes.

❖ Marine-carotene 100,000IU daily as an anti-infective, with Vitamin E 800IU to fight cell damage.

❖ Carnitine 500mg. daily for 3 days. Rest for 7 days, then take 1000mg. for 3 days. Rest for 7 days. Take with high Omega 3 fish or flax oils, 3-6 daily, and evening primrose oil 1000mg. 3x daily.

❖ H_2O_2 - food grade Care Plus OXYGEL, rubbed on the feet morning and evening, or 3% solution taken orally, 1 TB. in 8 oz. water 3 x daily. *Alternate use for best results; one week on and one week off. Note: You can take a simple blood-color test to monitor your own blood cleansing improvement. Make a small, quick, sterilized razor cut on your finger, or prick it with a needle. If the blood is a dark, bluish-purplish color it is not healthy. A bright red color indicates healthy blood. H_2O_2 treatment has been successful in this test by oxygenating the blood.*

❖ Crystal Star LIV-ALIVE™ capsules and LIV-ALIVE™ tea to detoxify the liver.

❖ St. John's Wort extract or Crystal Star ANTI-VI™ extract for antiviral activity.

Bodywork for the Blood Purifying Diet:

❖ Take a colonic irrigation or a Sonné Bentonite clay cleanse once a week to remove lymph congestion infected feces from the intestinal tract.

❖ Overheating therapy has been successful against many of these diseases, by speeding up metabolism, and inhibiting replication of the invading virus. (See page 38.)

❖ Get some morning sunlight on the body every day possible.

❖ Exercise daily. The aerobic oxygen intake alone can be a very important nutrient.

Bodywork Techniques For Successful Cleansing

BATHS ❖ WRAPS ❖ HYDROTHERAPY ❖ ENEMAS ❖ COMPRESSES ❖ OVERHEATING THERAPY

THERAPEUTIC BATHS: Clinics and spas are famous all over the world for their mineral, seaweed and enzyme baths. The skin is the body's largest organ of ingestion, and can assimilate the valuable nutrients from a therapeutic bath in a pleasant, stress-free way. Bathe at least twice daily during a cleanse to remove toxins coming out through the skin. The procedure for taking an effective healing bath is important. In essence, you are soaking in an herbal tea or mineral fluid, and allowing the skin to take in the healing nutrients instead of the mouth and digestive system.

There are two good ways to take a therapeutic bath:
❶ Draw very hot bath water. Put the herbs, seaweeds, or mineral crystals into a large tea ball or muslin bath bag. Add mineral salts directly to the water. Steep until water cools and is aromatic.
❷ Make a strong tea infusion in a large teapot, strain and add to bath water.

➡ Soak as long as possible to give the body time to absorb the healing properties. Rub the body with the solids in the muslin bag during the bath for best results.
➡ All over dry skin brushing before the bath for 5 minutes with a natural bristle brush will help remove toxins from the skin and open pores for better assimilation of nutrients.
➡ After the bath, use a mineral salt rub, such as Crystal Star LEMON BODY GLOW™, a traditional spa "finishing" technique to make your skin feel healthy for hours.

Note: Food grade 35% H_2O_2 may be used as a detoxifying rejuvenation bath to increase tissue oxygen via the skin. Use $1^1/_2$ cups to a full tub of water, and soak for 30 minutes. Or, add $1/_2$ cup H_2O_2, $1/_2$ cup sea salt, and $1/_2$ cup baking soda to bath, and soak $1/_2$ hour.

HERBAL WRAPS: The best European and American spas use herbal wraps as restorative body-conditioning techniques. Wraps are also body cleansing techniques that can be used to elasticize, tone, alkalize and release body wastes quickly. They should be used in conjunction with a short cleansing program, and 6-8 glasses of water a day to flush out loosened fats and toxins. Crystal Star makes two wraps for home use: TIGHTENING & TONING™ to improve muscle, vein and skin tone, and ALKALIZING ENZYME™ to replace and balance important minerals, enhance metabolism and alkalize the system.

HOT AND COLD HYDROTHERAPY: This technique helps open and stimulate the body's vital healing energies. Alternating hot and cold showers, are very effective in many cases for getting the body started on a positive track toward healing. Spasmodic pain and cramping, circulation, muscle tone, bowel and bladder problems, system balance, relaxation, and energy all show improvement with hydrotherapy. The form of hydrotherapy included here is easy and convenient for home use.
  Instructions: Begin with a comfortably hot shower for three minutes. Follow with a sudden change to cold water for 2 minutes. Repeat this cycle three times, ending with cold. Follow with a full or partial massage, or a brisk towel rub and mild stretching exercises for best results.

COMPRESSES: These are used to draw out waste and waste residue, such as cysts or abscesses through the skin, or to release them into the body's elimination channels. Use alternating hot and cold compresses for best results. Apply the herbs to the hot compress, and leave the ice or cold compress plain. We regularly use cayenne, ginger and lobelia effectively for the hot compresses.
  Instructions: Add 1 teasp. powdered herbs to a bowl of very hot water. Soak a washcloth and apply until the cloth cools. Then apply a cloth dipped in ice water until it reaches body temperature. Repeat several times daily. Green clay compresses, effective for growths, may be applied to gauze, placed on the area, and left for all day. Simply change as you would any dressing when you bathe.

ENEMAS: Enemas are a very important therapeutic aid to a congestion cleansing regimen. They increase the release of old, encrusted colon waste, encourage discharge of parasites, freshen the G.I. tract, and make the whole cleansing process easier and more thorough. Enemas should be used during both mucous and colon cleansing diets for optimum results. They are particularly helpful during a healing crisis, or after a serious illness or drug-treated hospital stay to speed healing. Even some headaches and inflammatory skin conditions can be relieved with enemas.

➡ **Herbal Enemas** can immediately alkalize the bowel area, help control irritation and inflammation, and provide local healing action for ulcerated tissue. There are several herbs particularly helpful for enemas. Use 2 cups of very strong brewed tea or solution to 1 qt. of water per enema.

✦ *Garlic,* to help kill parasites and cleanse harmful bacteria, viruses and mucous. (Blend six garlic cloves in two cups cold water and strain. For small children, use 1 clove garlic to 1 pint water.)
✦ *Catnip,* for stomach, digestive problems, cramping, and for childhood disease.
✦ *Pau de Arco,* when tsystem chemistry is imbalanced, as in chronic yeast and fungal infections.
✦ *Spirulina,* when both blood and bowel are toxic.
✦ *Lobelia,* in cases of food poisoning, especially when vomiting prevents antidotal herbs being taken by mouth.
✦ *Aloe Vera,* to heal tissues in cases of hemorrhoids, irritable bowel and diverticulitis.
✦ *Lemon Juice internal wash,* to rapidly neutralize an acid system, cleanse the colon and bowel.
✦ *Acidophilus powder,* mix 4 oz. powder in 1 qt. water - for relief from gas, yeast infections, and candidiasis.

➡ **Coffee Enemas** have become a standard in natural healing for liver and blood related cancers. Caffeine used in this way stimulates the liver and gallbladder to remove toxins, open bile ducts, encourage increased peristaltic action, and produce necessary enzyme activity for healthy red blood cell formation and oxygen uptake. Use 1 cup of **regular** strong brewed coffee to 1 qt. water.

How to take a detoxifying, colonic enema:
Place the enema solution in a water bag, and hang or hold about 18 inches higher than the body. Attach colon tube, and lubricate with vaseline or vitamin E oil. Expel a little water from the tube to let out air bubbles. Lying on the left side, slowly insert the tube about 18 inches into the colon. *Never use force.* Rotate tube gently for ease of insertion, removing kinks, so liquid will flow freely. Massage the abdomen, or flex and contract stomach muscles to relieve any cramping. When all solution has entered the colon, slowly remove the tube and remain on the left side for 5 minutes. Then move to a knee-chest position with the weight of the body on the knees and one hand. Use the other hand to massage the lower left side of the abdomen for several minutes. Massage releases encrusted fecal matter. Roll onto the back for another 5 minutes, massaging up the descending colon, over the transverse colon to the right side, and down the ascending colon. Then move onto the right side for 5 minutes, so that each portion of the colon is reached. Get up and quickly expel fluid into the toilet. Sticky grey or brown mucous, small dark incrusted chunks, or long, tough ribbon-like pieces are frequently loosened and expelled during an enema. These poisonous looking things are usually the obstacles and toxins interfering with normal body functions. The good news is that they are no longer in **you**. You may have to take several enemas before there is no more evidence of these substances.

HERBAL IMPLANTS: Implants are more concentrated solutions for more serious health problems, such as colitis, arthritis or prostate inflammation. Prepare for the implant by taking a small enema with warm water to clear out the lower bowel, which allows you to hold the implant longer. Mix 2 TBS. of your chosen powder, such as spirulina, or wheat grass in $1/2$ cup water. Lubricate the tip of a syringe with vaseline or vitamin E oil, get down on your hands and knees and insert the nozzle into the rectum. Squeeze the bulb to insert the mixture, *but do not release pressure on the bulb before it is withdrawn,* so the mixture will stay in the lower bowel. Hold as long as you can before expelling.

OVERHEATING THERAPY: Overheating, or stimulating a slight fever in the body, is a powerful natural healing tool against serious disease. Fever is a natural defense and healing force of the immune system, created and sustained by the body to rid itself of harmful pathogens and to restore health. The high body temperature speeds up metabolism, inhibits the growth of the harmful virus or bacteria, and literally burns the invading organism with heat. Fever has long been known to be an effective, protective healing measure against colds and simple infections, and also against serious diseases such as cancer and leukemia. Today, artificially induced fevers are used in many biological, holistic clinics for treating acute infectious diseases, arthritic conditions, skin disorders and much more. The newest research indicates that AIDS and related syndromes are also responding to blood heating. (See page 38 for more about clinical hyperthermia.)

A moderate, natural version may be effectively used in the home. It has the beneficial effect of stimulating the body's immunological mechanism, without the stress of fever-inducing drugs.

How to take an overheating bath:

❶ Do not eat for two hours before treatment. Empty bladder and colon if possible.

❷ Obtain a good thermometer so that water temperature may be correctly measured. The bath temperature must be monitored at all times.

❸ Use as large a tub as possible. Plug the emergency outlet to raise the water to the top of the tub. The patient must be *totally covered with water* for therapeutic results - with only nose, eyes and mouth left uncovered. Start slowly running water at skin temperature. After 15 minutes raise temperature to 100 degrees, then in 15 minutes to 103 degrees. Although the water temperature is not high, when the patient is totally covered, no heat escapes from the body and its temperature will rise to match that of the water, creating a slight healing fever.

❹ The length of the treatment should be about 1 hour. If the patient is ill, constant supervision is necessary. The patient's pulse should not go over 130 or 140. Watch the patient's reaction closely. If he/she experiences discomfort, raise to a sitting position for 5 minutes.

❺ Gentle massage with a skin brush during the bath is helpful in stimulating circulation. It helps bring the blood to the surface of the skin, and relieves the heart from undue pressure.

SAUNA HEAT THERAPY

A sauna is another way to use the overheating therapy principles. A long sauna not only induces a healing, cleansing fever, but also causes profuse therapeutic sweating. The skin, in overheating therapy, acts as a "third kidney" to eliminate body wastes through perspiration.

➡ As with the overheating therapy bath, a sauna speeds up metabolism, and inhibits the replication of pathogenic organisms.

➡ All vital organs and glands are stimulated to increased activity.

➡ The body's immune system is supported and its healing functions accelerated.

➡ The detoxifying and cleansing capacity of the skin is dramatically increased by profuse sweating.

Although it is possible to make a do-it-yourself sauna, the procedure is cumbersome. Professional saunas are available in every health club and gym as part of the membership, and the new home-installed models are not only adequate but reasonable in price. For optimum skin cleansing and restoration, take a sauna once or twice a week. Finish each sauna with a cool shower and a brisk rubdown to remove toxins that have been eliminated through the skin.

Note: Although induced fever is a natural, constructive means of biological healing, supervision and advice from an expert practitioner are recommended. A heart and general vitality check is advisable. Also some people who are seriously ill lose the ability to perspire, and this should be known before using overheating therapy.

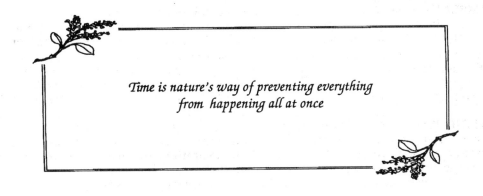

Time is nature's way of preventing everything from happening all at once

Light Macrobiotic & 'New Age' Eating

Macro (long) - biotic (life) stems from the Eastern philosophy of life, and considers the seasons, climate, farming methods, traditional customs, and a person's health condition and activity level in determining the way to eat. Other aspects of the macrobiotic way of life include daily exercise, avoiding synthetic clothing, aluminum, teflon cookware and microwave ovens, expressing gratitude, living positively, and an "early to bed and early to rise" habit. Proper orientation to these considerations, according to this philosophy, leads to happiness, health, freedom and appreciation for the bounties and boundaries of life.

The macrobiotic diet is designed in the Orient to prevent illness and degenerative disease. **In America, macrobiotics has rightly become popular as a therapeutic diet**, encouraging harmony and balance in the body. Thousands of people suffering from cancer, heart disease, diabetes, arthritis and other illnesses are using the macrobiotic system as part of their approach to healing. It is non-mucous forming, low in fat, high in vegetable proteins and fiber, and very alkalizing. Refined foods and those with flavor or coloring additives are avoided. Brown rice, other whole grains, and fresh in-season foods are the mainstays.

A macrobiotic diet is not a set pattern, but very flexible for a person's individual needs. In general this way of eating consists of about 45 to 55% whole grains and beans for good complex carbohydrates and plant protein, 25 to 30% vegetables, 10% soy foods such as tofu, tempeh, tamari and miso, 5% sea vegetables, nuts and seeds, 5% fruit, and 5% cultured foods, such as kefir, kefir cheese and yogurt, with occasional fish and eggs. Condiments and seasonings are an important part of macrobiotic cooking, not only to enhance flavor, but to promote good enzyme and digestive avtivity.

Favorite macrobiotic seasonings include gomashio (sesame salt), kuzu starch, sea salt, daikon radish, ginger pickles, umeboshi plums, tamari soy sauce, tekka, brown rice vinegar, toasted sesame and corn oils, wasabi horseradish, and occasional maple syrup, rice syrup or barley malt for sweetening.

A macrobiotic diet is stimulating to the heart and circulatory systems by keeping the body alkaline and high in natural iodine and potassium. Its emphasis on foods such as miso, bancha tree tea, kukicha twig tea, shiitake and reishi mushrooms, sea vegetables, tofu, other soy foods, and umeboshi plums, make it a diet resistant to disease. In strict form; macrobiotics is a way of eating that is cleansing and balancing at the same time. In a modified, lighter form, it is a way of eating you can live with in health on a lifetime basis.

❂

However, as we learn more about "New Age" ways of eating; macrobiotics, fruit cleansing diets, juice fasting, mono diets, etc., we find that caution must be used if you are not in a controlled clinical environment. **In their <u>strict cleansing/healing form</u>, these diets should be used only as short term programs.**

There must be balance to your diet. It is largely "civilization" foods and a lack of balance that get us into trouble, that lower immunity and resistance to disease. Vitamin B_{12} from animal or dairy products is necessary for cell growth, immunity and energy. Protein is neeeded for healing and strength. Complex carbohydrates are essential for endurance and stamina. Minerals are necessary for assimilation and building blocks, and soluble food fiber is integral to effective body cleansing, and weight maintenance. For the best route to long term health, find out what foods have the elements you need in their natural state, and include them in your diet, raw or simply cooked, on a regular basis.

For more on this optimum way of eating, see **"COOKING FOR HEALTHY HEALING"**, by **Linda Rector-Page.**

Therapeutic Drinks, Juices, Tonics & Broths

Fasting and cleansing foods should be fresh, organically grown, and eaten raw for best results. Raw foods retain the full complement of food nutrients, and help to stabilize and maintain the acid/alkaline balance of the body. Liquids have long been considered an easy way to take absorbable, usable nutrients into the body.

Drinks are the least concentrated form of nutrition, but have the great advantage of rapid assimilation. They can break down and flush out toxins quickly, and provide lubrication to the system. The tissues can be flooded with therapeutic, values in a gentle, and often delicious way. In fact, the body often craves what it needs most, and recognizes natural medicinal drinks as rich in qualities it lacks, such as minerals, proteins, and chlorophyll. Therapeutic liquids can sometimes taste better than anything else.

Many are high in vitamin C, B vitamins and minerals to neutralize the effects of pesticides, environmental pollutants and heavy metals, as well as toxins from the overuse of drugs, caffeine and nicotine.

For both fruits and vegetables, a high quality juicer is the best way to get all the nutrients. However, we have used a regular food processor and blender attachments with moderately good results.

Use organically grown produce whenever possible.

Note: Any of the drinks, juices, tonics and broths in this section can be a part of your increased liquid intake during cleansing or illness.

◖ POTASSIUM JUICE

The single most effective juice for cleansing, neutralizing acids, and rebuilding the body. It is a blood and body tonic to provide rapid energy and system balance.
For one 12 oz. glass:

Juice in the juicer
3 CARROTS
1/2 BUNCH SPINACH
opt. 1 to 2 teasp. Bragg's LIQUID AMINOS

1/2 BUNCH PARSLEY
3 STALKS CELERY

Nutritional analysis: per serving; 69 calories; 3gm. protein; 15gm. carbohydrate; 6gm. fiber; trace fats; 0 cholesterol; 100mg. calcium; 2mg. iron; 52mg. magnesium; 788mg. potassium; 144mg. sodium; 1mg. zinc.

◖ POTASSIUM ESSENCE BROTH

If you do not have a juicer, make a potassium broth in a soup pot. While not as concentrated or pure, it is still an excellent source of energy, minerals and electrolytes.
For a 2 day supply:

Cover with water in a soup pot
3 to 4 CARROTS
2 POTATOES, with skins
1 ONION
3 STALKS CELERY

1/2 BUNCH PARSLEY
1/2 HEAD CABBAGE
1/2 BUNCH BROCCOLI

٭Simmer covered 30 minutes. Strain and discard solids.
٭Add 2 teasp. Bragg's LIQUID AMINOS, or 1 teasp. miso. Store in the fridge, covered.

Nutritional analysis: per serving; 100 calories; 6gm. protein; 22gm. carbohydrate; 9gm. fiber; trace fats; 0 cholesterol; 141mg. calcium; 4mg. iron; 60mg. magnesium; 147mg. sodium; 1mg. zinc; 944 mg. potassium.

GREEN DRINKS, VEGETABLE JUICES & BLOOD TONICS

Green drinks are chlorophyll rich. The molecular composition of chlorophyll is so close to that of human hemaglobin that these drinks can act as "mini-transfusions" for the blood, and tonics for the brain and immune system. They are an excellent nutrient sources of vitamins, minerals, proteins and enzymes. They contain large amounts of vitamin C, B1, B2, B3, pantothenic acid, folic acid, carotene and choline. They are high in minerals, particularly potassium, calcium, magnesium, iron, copper, phosphorus and manganese. They are full of enzymes for digestion and assimilation, some containing over 1000 of the known enzymes necessary for human cell response and growth. Green drinks also have anti-infective properties, alkalize the body, and are excellent for mucous cleansing. They can help clear the skin, cleanse the kidneys, and clean and build the blood.

Fresh vegetable juices carry off acid wastes, and neutralize body pH. They are rich in vitamins, minerals, and enzymes that satisfy the body's nutrient needs, yet don't come burdened by the fats that accompany animal products.

Green drinks and vegetable juices are potent fuel in maintaining human energy and good health. Those included here have been used with therapeutic success for many years. You can have confidence in their nutritional healing and regenerative ability.

❧ KIDNEY FLUSH

A purifying kidney cleanser and diuretic drink, with balancing potassium and other minerals.
For four 8 oz. glasses:

4 CARROTS
4 BEETS with tops
4 CELERY STALKS with leaves

1 CUCUMBER with skin
8 to 10 SPINACH LEAVES, washed
opt. 1 teasp. Bragg's LIQUID AMINOS

Nutritional analysis: per serving; 69 calories; 3gm. protein; 15gm. carbohydrates; 5gm. fiber; trace fats; 0 cholesterol; 81mg. calcium; 2mg. iron; 62mg. magnesium; 760mg. potassium; 143mg. sodium; 1mg. zinc.

❧ PERSONAL BEST V-8

A delicious high vitamin/mineral drink for body balance. A good daily blend even when you're not cleansing.
For 6 glasses:

6 to 8 TOMATOES; or 4 CUPS TOMATO JUICE
$1/2$ GREEN PEPPER
2 STALKS CELERY with leaves
$1/2$ BUNCH PARSLEY
3 to 4 GREEN ONIONS with tops
2 CARROTS
$1/2$ SMALL BUNCH SPINACH, washed, or $1/2$ HEAD ROMAINE LETTUCE
2 LEMONS peeled; or 4 TBS. LEMON JUICE
opt. 2 teasp. Bragg's LIQUID AMINOS and $1/2$ teasp. ground celery seed

Nutritional analysis: per serving; 57 calories; 2 gm. protein; 13gm. carbohydrate; 4gm. fiber; trace fats; 0 cholesterol; 43mg. calcium; 36mg. magnesium; 2mg. iron; 606mg. potassium; 63mg. sodium; 1mg. zinc.

❧ STOMACH/DIGESTIVE CLEANSER

For one 8 oz. glass:

Juice $1/2$ CUCUMBER with skin, 2 TBS. APPLE CIDER VINEGAR and a PINCH of GROUND GINGER. Add enough cool water to make 8 oz.

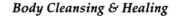

◖ CARROT JUICE PLUS

For 2 large drinks:

4 CARROTS   1/2 CUCUMBER with skin
1 TB. CHOPPED DRY DULSE   2 STALKS CELERY with leaves

Nutritional analysis: per serving; 84 calories; 2gm. protein; 20gm. carbohydrate; 6gm. fiber; trace fats; 0 cholesterol; 88mg. calcium; 1mg. iron; 52mg. magnesium; 706mg. potassium; 119mg. sodium; 1mg. zinc.

◖ SKIN TONIC

Deep greens to nourish, cleanse and tone skin tissue from the inside.
For 1 drink:

1 CUCUMBER with skin   1/2 BUNCH PARSLEY
1 TUB (4 OZ.) ALFALFA SPROUTS   3 to 4 SPRIGS FRESH MINT

◖ EVER GREEN

A personal favorite for taste, mucous release and enzymatic action.

1 APPLE with skin 1 teasp. SPIRULINA or
1 TUB (4 OZ.) ALFALFA SPROUTS   CHLORELLA GRANULES
1/2 FRESH PINEAPPLE skinned/cored 3 to 4 SPRIGS FRESH MINT

◖ HEALTHY MARY COCKTAIL

A virgin mary is really a healthy green drink when you make it fresh..
For 4 drinks:

3 CUPS WATER   1 SLICE GREEN PEPPER
2 TOMATOES   1 STALK CELERY
1 GREEN ONION with tops   12 SPRIGS PARSLEY
1 TB. CHOPPED DRY SEA VEGETABLES, such as WAKAME or DULSE, or 1 teasp. KELP POWDER

◖ SPROUT COCKTAIL

This high protein juice is particularly good for ending a fast.
For 2 drinks:

Juice 3 cored APPLES with skin,
1 TUB (4 oz.) ALFALFA SPROUTS, and 3 to 4 SPRIGS fresh MINT.

Nutritional analysis: per serving; 138 calories; 3gm. protein; 34gm. carbohydrate; 7gm. fiber; 1gm. fats; 0 cholesterol; 37mg. calcium; 1mg. iron; 26mg. magnesium; 303mg. potassium; 6mg. sodium; trace zinc.

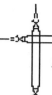

CLEANSING PURIFYING FRUIT DRINKS

*Fruits are wonderful for a quick system wash and cleanse. Their high water and sugar content speeds up metabolism to release wastes quickly and help reduce cravings for sweets. Fresh fruit juices have an alkalizing effect on the body, and are high in vitamins and minerals. However, because of their rapid metabolism, pesticides, sprays and chemicals on fruits can enter the body rapidly. **Eat organically grown fruits whenever possible.** Wash fruit well if commercially grown. **Fruits and fruit juices have their best nutritional effects when taken alone. Eat them before noon for best energy conversion and cleansing benefits** .*

❦ BLOOD BUILDER
A blood purifying drink with iron enrichment.

2 BUNCHES of GRAPES; or 2 CUPS GRAPE JUICE
6 ORANGES, peeled; or 2 CUPS ORANGE JUICE
8 LEMONS peeled; or 1 CUP LEMON JUICE
Stir in: 2 CUPS WATER and 1/4 CUP OF HONEY

❦ STOMACH CLEANSER & BREATH REFRESHER

1 BUNCH of GRAPES; or 1 CUP GRAPE JUICE   1 BASKET STRAWBERRIES
3 APPLES cored; or 1 CUP APPLE JUICE   4 SPRIGS OF FRESH MINT

❦ ENZYME COOLER
An intesinal balancer to help lower cholesterol, cleanse intestinal tract, and allow better assimilation of foods.

1 APPLE, cored and sliced; or 1/2 CUP APPLE JUICE
1 PINEAPPLE, skinned and cored; or 1 1/2 CUPS PINEAPPLE JUICE
2 LEMONS, peeled; or 1/4 CUP LEMON JUICE

❦ DIURETIC MELON MIX
A good morning drink with diuretic properties. Take on an empty stomach - 3 to 5 glasses daily.

For 1 quart: Juice in the blender
3 CUPS WATERMELON JUICE
1/2 CUP PERSIAN MELON JUICE
1/2 CUP HONEYDEW MELON JUICE

❦ GOOD DIGESTION PUNCH
Natural sources of papain and bromelain for enzyme activity, and ginger to break up excess stomach acids.

1 PAPAYA, peeled and seeded; or 1 CUP PAPAYA JUICE
1 PINEAPPLE, skinned and cored; or 1 1/2 CUPS PINEAPPLE JUICE
1 to 2 ORANGES, peeled; or 1/4 - 1/2 CUP ORANGE JUICE
1/4" SLICE FRESH GINGER

❦Other good fasting fruit juices: black cherry juice for gout conditions; cranberry juice for **bladder** and kidney infections; grape and citrus juices for high blood pressure; watermelon juice for **bladder** and kidney malfunction, celery for nerves, and apple juice to overcome fatigue.

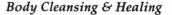

CLEANSING BROTHS & HOT TONICS

Clear broths are a very satisfying form of nutrition during a cleansing fast. They are simple, easy, inexpensive, can be taken hot or cold, and provide a means of "eating" and being with others at mealtime without going off a liquid program. This is more important than it might appear, since solid food, taken after the body has released all its solid waste, but before the cleanse is over, will drastically reduce the diet's success. Broths are also alkalizing, and contribute toward balancing body pH.

Hot tonics are neither broths nor teas, but unique hot combinations of vegetables, fruits and spices with purifying and energizing properties. The ingredients provide noticeable synergistic actiivty when taken together - with more medicinal benefits than the single ingredients alone. Take them morning and evening for best results.

❦ ONION & MISO BROTH

A therapeutic broth with antantibiotic and immune-enhancing properties.
For 6 small bowls of broth:

❧Saute 1 CHOPPED ONION in 1/2 teasp. SESAME OIL for 5 minutes. Add 1 STALK CELERY WITH LEAVES, and saute for 2 minutes. Add 1 QUART WATER or VEGETABLE STOCK. Cover and simmer 10 minutes.
❧Add 3 to 4 TBS. LIGHT MISO. Remove from heat.
❧Add 2 GREEN ONIONS with tops, and whirl in the blender.

Nutritional analysis: per serving; 42 calories; 7gm carbohydrate; 1gm. fat; 2gm. protein; 2mg. iron; 0 cholesterol; 27mg. calcium; trace iron; 12mg. magnesium; 121mg. potassium; 410mg. sodium; trace zinc.

❦ PURIFYING DAIKON & SCALLION BROTH

A clear cleansing drink with bladder flushing activity.
For one bowl.

Heat gently together for 5 minutes
4 CUPS VEGETABLE BROTH
ONE 6" PIECE DAIKON RADISH, peeled and cut into matchstick pieces
2 SCALLIONS, with tops
1 TB. TAMARI, or 1 TB. BRAGG'S LIQUID AMINOS
1 TB. FRESH CHOPPED CILANTRO
PINCH PEPPER

Nutritional analysis: per serving; 25 calories; 1 gm. protein; 2gm. fiber; 0 fat; 1 gm. carbohydrate; 0 cholesterol; 31mg. calcium; trace iron; 15mg. magnesium; 172mg. potassium; 194mg. sodium; trace zinc.

❦ ONION/GARLIC BROTH

A therapeutic broth with anti-biotic properties to reduce and relieve mucous congestion.
For 1 bowl:

❧Sauté 1 ONION and 4 CLOVES GARLIC in 1/2 teasp. SESAME OIL til very soft.
❧Whirl in the blender with a little vegetable broth. Eat in small sips.

Nutritional analysis: per serving; 103 calories; 3gm. protein; 18gm. carbohydrate; 3gm. fiber; 3gm. fats; 0 cholesterol; 56mg. calcium; 1mg. iron; 20mg. magnesium; 315mg. potassium; 7mg. sodium; trace zinc.

COLD DEFENSE CLEANSER

Make this broth the minute you feel a cold coming on.
Heat for 2 drinks:

1 1/2 CUPS WATER
1 teasp. GARLIC POWDER
1 teasp. GROUND GINGER
1 TB. LEMON JUICE

1 TB. HONEY
1/2 teasp. CAYENNE
3 TBS. BRANDY

Simmer gently 5 minutes. Drink in small sips for best results.

Nutritional analysis: per serving; 95 calories; trace protein; 19gm. carbohydrate; trace fiber; trace fats; 10mg. calcium; trace iron; 6mg. magnesium; 53mg. potassium; 7mg. sodium; trace zinc.

COLDS & FLU TONIC

This drink really opens up nasal and sinus passages fast.
For 2 drinks:

Toast in a dry pan til aromatic
4 CLOVES MINCED GARLIC
1/4 teasp. CUMIN POWDER
1/4 teasp. BLACK PEPPER
1/2 teasp. HOT MUSTARD POWDER

Add
1 CUP WATER
1 teasp. TURMERIC
1/2 teasp. SESAME SALT
1 TB. FRESH CILANTRO
1 CUP COOKED SPLIT PEAS
or 1 CUP FRESH FROZEN PEAS

Add 1 TB. OIL and stir in. Toast a little more to blend.
Simmer gently for 5 minutes, and whirl in blender. Very potent.

MUCOUS CLEANSING BROTH

Your Mother was right. Hot chicken broth really does clear out congestion faster.
For 4 bowls:

Use 1 QT. <u>HOMEMADE</u> CHICKEN STOCK (boil down bones, skin and trimmings from 1 fryer in 2 qts. water, and skim off fat).
In a large pot, saute 3 CLOVES MINCED GARLIC, 1 teasp. HORSERADISH, and a PINCH of CAYENNE til aromatic for 5 minutes.
Add chicken stock and simmer for 7-10 minutes. Top with NUTMEG and SNIPPED PARSLEY.

MINERAL RICH ENZYME BROTH

For 6 cups of broth:

Put in a large soup pot
3 SLICED CARROTS
1 CUP CHOPPED FRESH PARSLEY
1 LARGE ONION, chopped

2 POTATOES
2 STALKS CELERY with tops

Add 1 1/2 QTS. WATER, and bring to a boil. Reduce heat and simmer for 30 minutes. Strain and serve with 1 TB. Bragg's LIQUID AMINOS.

❧ ALKALIZING APPLE BROTH

This drink alkalizes, gives a nice spicy energy lift and helps lower serum cholesterol.
For 4 drinks:

❧Saute $1/2$ CHOPPED RED ONION and 2 CLOVES MINCED GARLIC in 1 teasp. OIL til soft.
❧While sautéing, blend in the blender
1 SMALL RED BELL PEPPER
2 TART APPLES cored and quartered
1 LEMON partially peeled, with some peel on
2 TBS. FRESH PARSLEY
2 CUPS KNUDSEN'S VERY VEGGIE-SPICY (or any good spicy tomato juice)
❧Add onion mix to blender and puree. Heat gently and drink hot.

❧ STOMACH & DIGESTIVE CLEANSER

For one 8 oz. glass:

Whirl in the blender
$1/2$ CUCUMBER WITH SKIN   2 PINCHES GROUND GINGER
2 TBS. APPLE CIDER VINEGAR   ENOUGH WATER TO MAKE 8 OZ.

❧ WARMING CIRCULATION TONIC

Immediate body heat against aches, shakes and chills
For 4 drinks:

1 CUP CRANBERRY JUICE   1 CINNAMON STICK
1 CUP ORANGE JUICE   4 TBS. RAISINS
2 TBS. HONEY   4 TBS. ALMONDS chopped
4-6 WHOLE CLOVES   1 teasp. VANILLA
4-6 CARDAMOM PODS

❧Heat all gently for 15 minutes. Remove cloves, cardamom and cinnamon stick. Serve hot.

❧ REVITALIZING TONIC

Very good for a "morning after hangover". Effective hot or cold. Works every time.
Enough for 8 drinks:

Mix in the blender.
ONE 48 OZ. CAN TOMATO JUICE or KNUDSEN'S SPICY VEGIE JUICE
1 CUP MIXED CHOPPED ONIONS
2 STALKS CHOPPED CELERY   2 teasp. HOT PEPPER SAUCE
1 BUNCH OF PARSLEY, chopped   1 teasp. ROSEMARY LEAVES
2 TBS. CHOPPED FRESH BASIL, or 2 teasp. dry $1/2$ teasp. FENNEL SEEDS
$1^1/2$ CUPS WATER   1 teasp. BRAGG'S LIQUID AMINOS
❧Pour into a large pot. Bring to a boil and simmer for 30 minutes.

Representative nutritional analysis for hot tonics: per serving: 42 calories; 2gm. protein; 10gm. carbohydrate; 2gm. fiber; trace fat; 41mg. calcium; 2mg. iron; 26mg. magnesium; 487mg. potassium; 637mg. sodium.

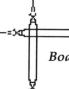

HERB TEAS & HIGH MINERAL DRINKS

Herb teas and high mineral drinks during a liquid fast can provide energy and cleansing without having to take in solid proteins or carbohydrates for fuel.

Herbal teas are the most time-honored of all natural healing mediums. Essentially body balancers, teas have mild cleansing and flushing properties, and are easily absorbed by the system. Herbs and the important volatile oils in them, are released by the hot brewing water, and when taken in small sips throughout the cleansing process, they flood the tissues with concentrated nutritional support to accelerate regeneration, and the release of toxic waste. ❦ See page 13 for the way to take herb teas for therapeutic results. In general, herbs are more effective in combination than when used singly, providing a broader range of activity when taken together in a blend.

❦ Effective Herbs For Blood Cleansing:
Echinacea (Angustifolia and Purpurea), Red Clover, Chaparral, Pau de Arco, Licorice, Burdock, Sarsaparilla, Ginger Rt., Oregon Grape Root, Dandelion, Garlic.
    A sample tea combination for blood cleansing might include: Red Clover, Hawthorne, Pau de Arco, Nettles, Sage, Alfalfa, Milk Thistle Seed, Echinacea, Horsetail, Gotu Kola, and Lemon Grass.

❦ Effective Herbs For Mucous Cleansing:
Garlic, Chlorella, Mullein, Elecampane, Ephedra, Comfrey Root, Pleurisy Root, Fenugreek, Ginger, Cayenne, Hawthorne, Licorice.
    A sample tea combination for mucous cleansing might include: Mullein, Comfrey, Ephedra, Marshmallow, Pleurisy Root, Rosehips, Calendula, Boneset, Ginger, Peppermint, and Fennel Seed.

❦ Effective Herbs For Colon and Bowel Cleansing:
Psyllium Seeds, Flax Seed, Butternut Bark, Cascara Sagrada, Rhubarb, Fennel, Acidophilus, Senna Leaf & Pod, Peppermint.
    A sample tea combination for cleansing the bowel and digestive system might include: Senna Leaf, Papaya Leaf, Fennel Seed, Peppermint, Lemon Balm, Parsley Leaf, Calendula, Hibiscus, and Ginger Root.

❦ Effective Herbs For Bladder Cleansing:
Uva Ursi, Cleavers, Dandelion Leaf, Buchu, Parsley Leaf, Ginger Root, Couchgrass, Juniper Berry, Cornsilk, Gravel Root, Watermelon Seed.
 - **A sample tea combination for gentle bladder and kidney flushing might include:** Uva Ursi, Juniper Berries, Ginger Rt., and Parsley Leaf.

❦ Effective Herbs For Respiratory Cleansing:
Fenugreek Seed, Comfrey, Mullein, Licorice Root, Eucalyptus, Lobelia, Marshmallow Root, Hyssop, Pleurisy Root, Rosehips.
    A sample tea combination for clogged chest and sinuses might include: Marshmallow Root, Rosehips, Mullein Leaf, and Fenugreek Seed.

❦ Effective Herbs For Stomach & Digestive Cleansing:
Dandelion, Hibiscus, Chlorophyll-rich herbs, Catnip, Rosemary, Peppermint, Fennel, Papaya Lf.
    A tea combination for good digestion might include: Peppermint, Hibiscus, Papaya Leaf, Rosemary.

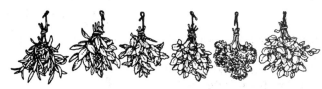

High mineral drinks are food-source mineral supplements, with basic building blocks to balance the acid/alkaline system, regulate body fluid osmosis and electrical activity in the nervous system, and to aid in digestion and regularity. They are vigorous sources of proteins and amino acids with whole cell availability and without animal fats.

❧ MINERAL-RICH AMINOS DRINK
This is an easy, short version of the Crystal Star Herbal Nutrition SYSTEM STRENGTH™ drink. It is a complete, balanced food-source vitamin/mineral supplement that is rich in greens, amino acids and enzyme precursors.

Make up a dry batch in the blender, then mix about 2 TBS. powder into 2 cups of hot water for 1 drink. Let flavors bloom for 5 minutes before drinking. Add 1 teasp. BRAGG'S LIQUID AMINOS to each drink if desired. Sip over a half hour period for best assimilation.
Enough for 8 drinks:

4 to 6 PACKETS MISO CUP SOUP POWDER (Edwards & Son Co. makes a good one)
1 TB. CRUMBLED DRY SEA VEGETABLES (Kombu or Wakame)

¹/₂ CUP SOY PROTEIN POWDER	1 TB. BREWER'S YEAST FLAKES
1 PACKET INSTANT GINSENG TEA GRANULES	2 TBS. BEE POLLEN GRANULES
1 PKT. SPIRULINA or CHLORELLA GRANULES	1 teasp. ACIDOPHILUS POWDER
2 TBS. FRESH PARSLEY LEAF	

❧Add 1 teasp. BRAGG'S LIQUID AMINOS for more flavor.

Nutritional analysis: per serving; 85 calories; 9gm. protein; 10gm. carbohydrate; 2gm. fiber; 2.5gm. fats; 24% calories from fat; 0 cholesterol; 21mg. calcium; 1mg. iron; 8mg. magnesium; 179mg. potassium; 383mg. sodium.

❧ MINERAL-RICH ALKALIZING ENZYME DRINK
This blend is an exceptional source of minerals, trace minerals and enzymes for good assimilation and digestion, and for all cell functions. It helps alkalize body pH for better body balance.

Put the following vegetables in a pot. Add 1¹/₂ quarts of cold water. Simmer for 30 minutes. **Strain,** and take hot or cold. Add 1 teasp. BRAGG'S LIQUID AMINOS to each drink if desired.

2 POTATOES, chunked	1 CUP CARROTS, sliced
1 CUP SLICED CELERY with LEAVES	1 CUP FRESH PARSLEY LEAVES
1 CUP ONION, chunked	

❧Optional additions: 2 TBS. soaked flax seed or oat bran if there is chronic constipation of poor peristalsis.

❧ MINERAL-RICH ENERGY DRINK
This is an easy, simplified version of the Crystal Star Herbal Nutrition ENERGY GREEN™ drink. It is rich in chlorophyllins, with substantial amounts of plant betacarotene, B vitamins, choline, essential fatty acids with GLA, DGLA and linoleic acid, and octacosonal for tissue oxygenation. It contains complex carbohydrates, complete minerals, trace minerals, proteins, and a full-pectrum amino acid complex.

Mix in the blender, then mix about 2 TBS. into 2 cups of hot water for 1 drink. Let flavors bloom for 5 minutes before drinking. Add 1 teasp. BRAGG'S LIQUID AMINOS to each drink if desired.
Enough for 4 drinks:

¹/₂ CUP AMAZAKE RICE DRINK	1 TB. CRUMBLED DULSE
¹/₂ CUP OATS	1 TB. DANDELION LEAF
2 TBS. BEE POLLEN GRANULES	2 TBS. GOTU KOLA HERB
1 PACKET INSTANT GINSENG TEA GRANULES	2 TBS. ALFALFA LEAF
2 PACKETS BARLEY GRASS or CHLORELLA GRANULES	
1 teasp. VITAMIN C CRYSTALS with BIOFLAVONOIDS	

❧Add 1 teasp. LEMON JUICE for flavor if desired.

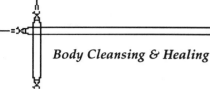
PROTEIN DRINKS & ENERGY TONICS

You must have protein to heal, and the new breed of protein drinks are a wonderful way to get protein without meat or bulk or excess fat. These drinks obtain protein from several sources so that a balance with carbohydrates and minerals is achieved, and a real energy boost felt.

❧ NON-DAIRY MORNING PROTEIN DRINK

For 2 drinks:

1 CUP STRAWBERRIES or KIWI, sliced
1 BANANA, sliced
1 CUP PAPAYA or PINEAPPLE, chunked
8 OZ. SOFT TOFU
or 1 CUP AMAZAKE RICE DRINK

2 TBS. MAPLE SYRUP
1 CUP ORGANIC APPLE JUICE
1 teasp. VANILLA
1 TB. TOASTED WHEAT GERM
1/2 teasp. GINGER POWDER

Nutritional analysis: per serving; 156 calories; 6gm. protein; 28gm. carbohydrate; 3gm. fiber; 3gm. fats 18% calories from fat; 0 cholesterol; 90mg. calcium; 4mg. iron; 85mg. magnesium; 12mg. sodium; 417mg. potassium.

❧ HEAVY DUTY PROTEIN DRINK

Blender blend all. A training drink for optimal athletic performance.
For 2 drinks:

1 CUP WATER
6 TBS. DRY NONFAT MILK
1 BANANA
1 EGG
2 TBS. PEANUT BUTTER
1 TB. CAROB POWDER

1 CUP YOGURT (ANY FLAVOR)
2 TBS. BREWER'S YEAST
1 TB. TOASTED WHEAT GERM
1 teasp. SPIRULINA POWDER
2 teasp. BEE POLLEN GRANULES

Nutritional analysis: per serving; 241 calories; 17gm. protein; 28gm. carbohydrate; 5gm. fiber; 10gm. fats; 283mg. calcium; 2mg. iron; 78mg. magnesium; 774mg. potassium; 156mg. sodium.

❧ DIETER'S MID-DAY MEAL REPLACEMENT PROTEIN DRINK

This drink is good-tasting, filling and satisfying. It is full of foods that help to raise metabolism, cleanse and flush out wastes, balance body pH, and stimulate enzyme production.

Blend a dry batch in the blender. Use 1 TB. powder per glass. Drink slowly.

Makes enough for 12 drinks.:

6 TBS. RICE PROTEIN POWDER
4 TBS. OAT BRAN
2 TBS. FLAX SEED
2 TBS. BEE POLLEN GRANULES
2 teasp. SPIRULINA POWDER

1 teasp. ACIDOPHILUS POWDER
1 teasp. LEMON JUICE POWDER
2 teasp. FRUCTOSE (or to taste)
1/2 teasp. GINGER POWDER

Nutritional analysis: per serving; 45 calories; 4gm. protein; 7gm. carbohydrate; 2gm. fiber; 2gm. fats; 29% calories from fat; 21mg. calcium; 1mg. iron; 17mg. magnesium; 124mg. potassium; 23mg. sodium, trace cholesterol.

About Water

Water is second only to oxygen in importance for health. It makes up 65-75% of the body, and every cell requires water to perform its essential functions. Water maintains system equilibrium, lubricates, flushes wastes and toxins, hydrates the skin, regulates body temperature, acts as a shock absorber for joints, bones and muscles, adds needed minerals, and transports nutrients, minerals, vitamins, proteins and sugars for assimilation. Water cleanses the body inside and out. When the body gets enough water, it works at its peak. Fluid and sodium retention decrease, gland and hormone functions improve, the liver breaks down and releases more fat, and hunger is curtailed. To maintain this wonderful internal environment, you must drink plenty of water every day - at least six to eight glasses to replace lost electrolytes and metabolic waste fluid.

Thirst is not a reliable signal that your body needs water. Thirst is an evolutionary development designed to indicate **severe dehydration.** You can easily lose a quart or more of water during activity before thirst is even recognized. The thirst signal also shuts off before you have had enough for well-being. You have to pay conscious attention to getting enough water every day.

Plain or carbonated cool water is the best way to replace lost body fluid. Second best are unsweetened fruit juices diluted with water or seltzer, and vegetable juices. Alcohol and caffeine-containing drinks are counterproductive in replacing water loss because of their diuretic activity. Drinks loaded with dissolved sugars or milk *increase* water needs instead of satisfying them.

Unfortunately, most of our tap water today is chlorinated, fluoridated, and treated to the point where it can be an irritating, disagreeable fluid instead of a valuable benefit. Regular city tap water may contain as many as 500 different disease-causing bacteria, viruses and parasites. Many toxic chemicals and heavy metals used by industry and agriculture have found their way into ground water, adding more pollutants. Some tap water is now so bad, that without the enormous effort our bodies use to dispose of these chemicals, we would have ingested enough of them to turn us to stone by the time we were thirty! *Fluoridated water increases absorption of aluminum from deodorants, pots and pans, etc. by 600%.* Concern about this lack of purity is leading more and more people to bottled water.

For a healing program, several types of water are worth consideration.

Mineral water usually comes from natural springs with varying mineral content and widely varying taste. The naturally occurring minerals are beneficial to digestion and regularity, and in Europe this form of bottled water has become a fine art. It is not U.S. government regulated for purity except in California and Florida.

Distilled water can be either from a spring or tap source, but is "de-mineralized" so that only oxygen and hydrogen remain. Distilling is accomplished by reverse osmosis, filtering or boiling, then converting to steam and recondensing. It is the purest water available, and ideal for a healing program.

Sparkling water comes from natural carbonation in underground springs. Most are also artificially infused with CO_2 to maintain a standard fizz. This water is an aid to digestion, and is excellent in cooking to tenderize and give lightness to a recipe.

Artesian well water is the Cadillac of natural waters. It always comes from a deep pure source, has a slight fizz from bubbling up under rock pressure, and is tapped by a drilled well. Artesian water never comes in contact with ground contaminants.

❋ **Note:** Beyond buying bottled water, you can also take steps as an individual to conserve water and diminish pollution: ❧ Use biodegradable soaps and detergents. ❧ Don't use water fresheners in your toilets. ❧ Avoid pouring hazardous wastes such as paint, solvents, and petroleum based oils into drains or sewers. ❧ Use natural fertilizers such as manure and compost in your garden. ❧ Avoid using non-biodegradable plastics and polystyrene ❧ Conserve water with conscious attention to what you really need for a shower, bath, laundry or cooking.

About Food Nutrients & Your Health

A Glossary of Healing Foods, Mega-Foods, Nutraceuticals and Pharmafoods

Your diet can be constructed to meet your specific health needs. As we learn more about the health-promoting effects of specific foods and herbs, we are finding that food nutrients are truly "the best medicine". Genetic plant research is showing that unprocessed foods and herbs contain a rich array of important substances produced by the plant's metabolism; and that these substances have a far greater range of health benefits than previously imagined. It is also taking giant strides in producing medicinal foods from natural botanical products, using isolated vitamins, minerals, fatty acids, phospholipids, bioflavonoids and amino acids to make neutraceuticals or pharmafoods for therapeutic use. The foods and nutrients listed in this section are particularly suited to a healing diet.

☛ **ACIDOPHILUS CULTURE COMPLEXES, including lactobacillus, bulgaricus, and bifida bacterium** - beneficial bacteria that synthesize nutrients in the intestinal tract, counteract pathogenic micro-organisms and maintain healthy intestinal environment.

☛ **ALOE VERA,** *Aloe Barbadensis* - long in use for burns and skin care in gel form, aloe juice is now becoming widely known for its digestive and soothing laxative properties.

☛ **AMARANTH** - an ancient Aztec grain-like seed, now being rediscovered in America, amaranth contains very high quality protein, as well as a high concentration of the amino acid lysine. Amaranth has been found compatible with a diet to control Candida albicans yeast overgrowth, and may be used like a grain in grain-free breads and desserts.

☛ **AMAZAKE** - a thick, rich pudding-like mixture made from fermented sweet brown rice. It can be eaten like pudding, used as a base for desserts, or as a high protein, satisfying beverage.

☛ **ARROWROOT** - powdered cassava plant, used as a thickener when a shiny sauce is desired. It may be used as a less processed substitute for cornstarch, without the digestive, elimination and vitamin loss problems cornstarch can cause.

☛ **ASTRAGALUS** - a strong immune enhancer and body tonic. It is a strong antiviral agent, working to produce extra interferon in the body. It is an efficient immune stimulant, and can counteract immune-suppressng effects of cancer drugs and radiation. Vasodilating properties help significantly lower blood pressure, reduce excess fluid retention, and improve circulation. Also used as a kidney-toning diuretic. Chinese research indicates that astragalus is a valuable anticlotting agent in preventing coronary heart disease.

☛ **BARLEY FLOUR**- a low gluten flour with a slightly sweet malty taste. Use it as part of a flour and whole grain mix to lend a nice chewy texture to cookies and muffins.

☛ **BARLEY GRASS -** See *About Green Superfoods*, pg. 87.

☛ **BARLEY MALT SYRUP** - a mild natural sweetener made from barley sprouts and water, and cooked to a syrup. It has a pleasant flavor that is delicious in cookies, muffins and quick breads, and is only 40% as sweet as sugar. (See *About Sweeteners in a Healing Diet*, pg. 77.)

☛ **BASMATI RICE** - a uniquely delicious aromatic whole grain rice, originally from India, but now also being grown as a hybrid in Texas. In our opinion, this is the Cadillac of rice; better for you than white rice, lighter, easier to digest than brown rice.

☛ **BEE POLLEN** - collected by bees from male seed flowers, mixed with secretion from the bee, and formed into granules. Bee pollen is a highly concentrated, perfectly balanced food, notable for possessing all the essential amino acids. It is often used as an antidote during allergy season. 2 teasp. daily is the usual dose. (See *About Bee Pollen, Propolis & Royal Jelly*, pg. 89.)

☙ **BEE PROPOLIS** - a product collected by bees from the resin under the bark of certain trees. It is an antibacterial and antibiotic substance that stimulates the thymus gland and thus boosts immunity, and resistance to infection. (See *About Bee Pollen, Propolis & Royal Jelly*, pg. 89.)

☙ **BENTONITE** - a natural clay substance used for internal cleansing; absorbs toxins and bacteria.

☙ **BLACK BEANS** - Black beans are an excellent source of absorbable protein - particularly good as an alkalizing soup.

☙ **BRAN** - often called miller's bran, the outside shell of the grain, well known these days for its fiber content. Use it as part of a flour mix for texture. One to 2 tablespoons a day with liquid is plenty for regularity and digestion.

☙ **BREWER' S YEAST** - an excellent source of protein, B vitamins, amino acids and minerals. Because it is chromium-rich brewer's yeast can be a key food factor in significantly improving bloood sugar metabolism, and in substantially reducing serum cholesterol and raising HDL's. It helps speed wound healing through an increase in the production of collagen. It has anti-oxidant properties to allow the tissues to take in more oxygen for healing. The B vitamin and mineral content improves both skin texture and blemishes. (May be successfully used in a natural facial mask.) Brewer's yeast is *not* the same as Candida albicans yeast. It is one of the best-immune-enhancing supplements available in food form.

☙ **BUCKWHEAT -** a non-wheat grain. When this grain is roasted, it is known as kasha, a nutty seed popular in casseroles and pilafs. Use the flour as part of a baking mix for milder taste.

☙ **CANOLA OIL** - from the rapeseed plant; high in mono-unsaturated fats, with 10% omega 3 fatty acids, and half the amount of saturated fat found in other vegetable oils. (See *About Fats & Oils*, pg. 80.)

☙ **CAROB POWDER -** a sweet powder with 45% natural sugars, made from the seed pods of a Mediterranean tree. It has a flavor similar to chocolate, but contains less fat and no caffeine. It may be used raw or roasted as a substitute for cocoa in recipes. It does not hinder calcium absorption.

☙ **CHARCOAL, ACTIVATED** - a highly absorbable natural agent that relieves gas and diarrhea. An antidote for almost all poisons.

☙ **CHEESE** - (See *About Milk & Dairy Products During Healing*, pg. 74, for information on low fat, raw, and non-dairy cheeses). Rennet-free cheeses use a bacteria culture, instead of calves' enzymes to separate curds and whey. Goat cheese (chevre) and sheep's milk cheese (feta) are both lower in fat than cow's milk cheeses, and are more easily digestible. Authentic mozzarrella cheese is made from buffalo milk, and is now becoming available on the west coast and in New York - low fat and absolutely delicious! Low sodium cheeses are made in almost every type of cheese, and are a better choice for a healing program.

☙ **CHLORELLA** - a tiny one-celled algae plant, known and grown as a superfood; full of proteins, high chlorophyllins, fiber, beta carotene and many other high quality nutrients. The list of chlorella benefits is long and almost miraculous, from detoxification to energy enhancement, to immune system restoration. (See *About Green Superfoods*, pg. 87.)

☙ **CHROMIUM PICOLINATE** - an exceptionally bio-active source of the mineral chromium. It is a combination of chromium and picolinic acid, a natural substance secreted by the liver and kidneys. Picolinic acid is the body's best mineral transporter. It combines with elements such as iron, zinc and chromium to move them quickly and efficiently into the cells. Chromium plays a vital role in "sensitizing" the body to insulin. Excess body weight in the form of fat tends to impair insulin sensitivity, making it harder to lose weight. This form of chromium also has other benefits. It builds muscles without steroid side effects, promotes healthy body growth in children, speeds wound healing, and decreases proneness of plaque accumulation in the arteries.

☙ **CO-ENZYME Q10** - an essential catalyst nutrient for cellular energy in the body that declines with age. Supplementation provides wide ranging therapeutic benefits. Successful in combatting angina, and degenerative heart function. A vital link in the energy chain, crucial in the prevention and treatment of congestive heart and arterial diseases. Reduces high blood pressure without other medication. Also used in the treatment of inflammatory gum disease. (See *Enzymes & Enzyme Therapy*, pg. 29.)

❧ **CSA, Chondroitin Sulfate A** - an anti-inflammatory agent from bovine cartilage. May be used both topically and internally for a wide range of problems, from anti-aging, anti-stress, and anti-allergen uses to circulatory and orthopedic therapy. Also effective for cardiovascular disease and arthritis.

❧ **CREAM of TARTAR** - tartaric acid, a leavening agent in baking, helps incorporate egg whites. One half teasp. cream of tartar and $1/2$ teasp. baking soda can be substituted for 1 teasp. baking powder.

❧ **DAIKON RADISH** - a mild, almost sweet radish used in macrobiotic and Japanese cooking; it may be eaten shredded fresh or stir fried, and has the therapeutic benefit of gentle diuretic action.

❧ **DASHI** - a healing soup stock and broth used in macrociotic and Japanese cooking. Make it by simmering a 6" peice of kombu sea weed with 2 sliced shiitake mushrooms and 2 teasp. tamari in water.

❧ **DATE SUGAR** - ground up dates. When used in baking, mix with water and then add to recipe to prevent burning. Use as a sweet topping after removing from the oven or stove. (See *About Sweeteners in a Healing Diet*, pg. 77.)

❧ **DULSE** - the most often eaten sea vegetable, with excellent taste and good alkalizing properties. Crumble over vegetables, soups and salads, use in seasonings and savory dishes, or as an effective dieting tea. (See *About Sea Vegetables and Iodine Therapy*, pg. 85.)

❧ **EDTA, (ethylene-diamine-tetra-acetic acid - an amino acid)** - used in chelation therapy to remove toxic and clogging minerals from the circulatory system - particularly those that impair membrane function and contribute to free radical damage. EDTA puts these minerals into solution where they can be excreted by the kidneys.

❧ **EGG REPLACER** - a combination of starches and leavening agents used to replace those qualities of eggs in baking. It is a vegetarian product, cholesterol free.

❧ **ELECTROLYTE DRINKS** - quickly absorbable drinks to replace lost electrolytes and increase energy and endurance. Electrolytes are the soluble minerals in the body fluids and bloodstream. They are easily lost through perspiration and other fluid loss and need constant replacement. They are essential to cell function and maintain the pH balance in the body.The human body runs on electrical energies. Electrolytes transport this energy throughout the body, and allow it to work. When electrolytes are low, we tire easily. When they are adequate we almost instantly experience increased energy. Electrolyte drinks are particularly beneficial for athletes and those doing hard physical work.

❧ **ESSENE BREAD** - a sprouted bread of wheat or rye, with no flour, oil, sweetener, salt or leavening. Perfect for those on a very restricted diet for allergies, food intolerances or candida albicans.

❧ **ESSENTIAL FATTY ACIDS, Linoleic Acid, Alpha Linoleic Acid, Gamma Linoleic Acid, Linolenic Acid, Arachidonic Acid** - major components of all cell membranes; without them, the membranes are unable to function. EFAs are transformed into prostaglandins, hormone-like cell messengers. They are instrumental in energy production, vital to circulation health, and integral to proper metabolism.
  GLA, Gamma Linoleic Acid - obtained from evening primrose oil, black currant, and borage seed oil. A source of energy for the cells, electrical insulation for nerve fibers, a precursor of prostaglandins which regulate hormone and metabolic functions. Therapeutic use is wide ranging from control of PMS and menopause symptoms, to help in nerve transmission for M.S. and muscular dystrophy.

❧ **FLAX SEED OIL** - a high omega 3 oil that has medicinal and cooking uses. An excellent source of unsaturated fatty acids. (See *About Fats & Oils*, page 80.)

❧ **FRUCTOSE** - a highly refined sweetener that is twice as sweet as sugar. It is, however, absorbed more slowly into the bloodstream than sugar and does not require insulin for assimilation. Use *half*

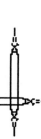

the amount of sugar in cooking. If you are hypoglycemic or diabetic, fructose is still sugar and deserves careful use. (See *About Sweeteners in a Healing Diet*, pg. 77.)

● **GARLIC** - a broad-spectrum therapeutic food with anti-biotic, anti-fungal, anti-parasitic and anti-viral activity. Used extensively for disease prevention; internally against infection of all kinds; externally for eye, ear, nose and throat infections, and because of thiamine content, to prevent mosquito bites. Garlic has a measureable amount of germanium, an antioxidant for endurance and wound healing.

● **GINGER** - a flavorful, aromatic, spicy herb. Both fresh and dried ginger have therapeutic properties for digestive, hypertension, haedaches and other problems. There is an easy way to have fresh ginger on hand without spoilage. Peel fresh roots, chop in the blender, put in a plastic bag, and freeze. Ginger thaws almost immediately. In less than 10 minutes, it's ready for use.

● **GINKGO BILOBA** - the leaf extract of an ancient Chinese tree, used therapeutically to combat the effects of aging. It improves circulation throughout the body, helps send more blood and oxygen to the brain for increased memeory and mental alertness, and protects the brain against mental disorders that can cause senility. Is effective against vertigo, dizziness and ringing in the ears. As an anti-oxidant, it protects the cells against damage from free radicals, and reduces blood cell clumping which can lead to congestive heart disease. Helps return elasticity to cholesterol-hardened blood vessels. Reduces inflammation in the lungs leading to asthmatic attack.

● **GINSENG** - the most effective adaptogen of all tonic herbs. Ginseng has measurable amounts of germanium, provides energy to all body systems, promotes regeneration from stress and fatigue, and rebuilds foundation strength. Particularly nourishing to the male reproductive and circulatory systems. Ginseng is useful for women as a stimulant for brain and memory centers. Ginseng benefits are cumulative in the body. Taking this herb for several months to a year is far more effective than short term doses.

● **GLYCERINE, VEGETABLE** - a naturally-occurring substance found in several sources, often today expressed from coconut. It is metabolized in the body like a carbohydrate, not a fat or oil, and is used regularly in natural cosmetics as a smoothing agent.

● **GOMASHIO** - a mixture of sesame seeds and sea salt. Originally only used in oriental cooking, it is a delicious lower sodium alternative to table salt, and an excellent cooking and baking salt.

● **GREEN MAGMA** - from Green Foods Corp. (See *About Green Superfoods*, pg. 87.)

● **GUAR GUM** - an herbal product that provides soluble digestive fiber and absorbs undesirable intestinal substances. Used therapeutically to lower cholesterol, and flatten the diabetic sugar curve.

● **GUM GUGGUL** - an Indian herb used as a natural alternative to drugs for reducing cholesterol. Gum guggul also decreases platelet stickiness and normalizes blood clotting (and assisting the body in breaking up clots), thus helping to prevent strokes as well as heart attacks.

● **GYMNEMA SYLVESTRE** - an herb that reduces blood sugar levels after sugar consumption. Gymnema has a molecular structure similar to that of sugar that can block absorption of up to 50% of dietary sugar calories. Both sugar and gymnema are digested in the small intestine, but the larger molecule of gymnema cannot be fully absorbed. Taken before sugar, the gymnema molecule blocks the passages through which sugar is normally absorbed, so that fewer sugar calories are assimilated. The remaining sugar is eliminated as waste.
A taste test shows how gymnema works. Taste something sweet, then swish a sip of gymnema sylvestre tea around in your mouth. Now taste something sweet again. You will not be able to taste the sugar, because gymnema has blocked the taste of the sugar in your mouth in the same way it blocks sugar in digestion. Used for hyperinsulinism. Take *with* GTF Chromium to stabilize blood sugar levels.

● **KASHI** - a delicious 7 grain pilaf mix, available puffed for a cold cereal, and cooked as a grain base for almost any rice or pasta type dish. It has a chewy, nutty texture, and a taste unlike any single grain.

Kashi is an excellent source of protein, complex carbohydrates and fiber. Ground into a flour, it is healthy and delicious for all baked goods.

- **KEFIR** - a fermented milk product, it comes plain or fruit-flavored, and may be taken as a liquid or used like yogurt or sour cream. Kefir provides friendly intestinal flora.

- **KUZU** - a powdered thickening root for Japanese dishes and macrobiotic diets. Superior for imparting a shine and sparkle to stir-fried foods and clear sauces. (See *About Dairy Foods on a Healing Diet*, pg. 74.)

- **LECITHIN -** a soy derived granular product, used as a stabilizer and emulsifier to improve smoothnesss. May be substituted for one-third of the oil in recipes for a healing diet. It is also a therapeutic food, for mental and nerve function. Two teasp. daily may be added to almost any food to increase superior phosphatides, choline, inositol, potassium and linoleic acid.

- **MILLET** - a quick-cooking, balanced, gluten-free grain, rich in amino acids, alkalizing to the stomach, and acceptable for those with wheat allergies and Candida albicans yeast.

- **MISO** - is a fermented soybean paste that is a basic medicinal food. It is very alkalizing to the system, lowers cholesterol, represses carcinogens, helps neutralize allergens, pollutants, and the effects of smoking on the body, and provides an immune-enhancing environment. Miso is also a tasty base for soups, sauces, dressings, dips, spreads and cooking stock, and is a healthy substitute for salt or soy sauce. There are many kinds, strengths and flavors of miso, from chickpea (light and mild) to hatcho (dark, and strong). **Natto miso** is the sweetest, a chunky mix of soybeans, barley and barley malt, kombu, ginger and sea salt. Delicious as a relish, sandwich spread, chutney with grains and many other uses. Unpasteurized miso is preferred for a healing diet, since beneficial bacteria and other enzymes, as well as flavor is still intact.
Miso is very concentrated; use no more than $1/2$ to 1 teasp. of dark miso, or 1 to 2 teasp. of light miso per person. Dissolve in a small amount of water to activate the beneficial enzymes before adding to a recipe. Omit salt from the recipe if you are using miso.

- **MOCHI** - is a chewy rice "bread" made from sweet brown rice. It is baked very hot, at 450º and puffs up to a crisp biscuit that can be filled, used as big croutons in soup, or as a delicious casserole topping. It is acceptable for Candida albicans diets.

- **MOLASSES** - blackstrap, unsulphured - although a byproduct of the sugar refining process, molasses has very high mineral content, particularly iron and potassium. It can be taken plain as a supplement for hair regrowth and color, or used in baking and cooking for distinctive flavor.

- **MUSHROOMS -** There are three mushroom species with specific healing properties:
  Shiitake - often called **oyster mushrooms** when fresh, they are usually sold dry. These mushrooms have also been linked to cures for cancers and tumors. They apparently produce a virus which stimulates interferon in the body. Use them frequently - just a few each time. A little goes a long way.
  Reishi - a rare, tree, shiitake-type mushroom from the Orient, now cultivated in America. Reishi, or ganoderma has tonic activity that increases vitality, enhances immunity and prolongs a healthy life. It is an anti-oxidant, used therapeutically for a wide range of serious conditions, including anti-tumor and anti-hepatitis activity. It helps reduce the side effects of chemotherapy for cancer. New research is showing success against chronic fatigue syndrome. Reishi helps regenate the liver, lowers cholesterol and triglycerides, reduces coronary symptoms and high blood pressure, and alleviates allergy symptoms. It calms the nervous system and relieves insomnia.
  Poria Cocos - an American and Chinese mushroom, reduces and regulates excess water retention; purifies body fluids and prevents build-up of toxins.

- **NUTRASWEET** - combines the amino acids phenlalanine and aspartic acid. It is 200 times sweeter than sugar, and has been linked to several problems involving sugar use in the body, such as PKU seizures, high blood pressure, headaches, insomnia and mood swings. Nutrasweet has taken the place of saccharin in pre-prepared foods, and that means we get a lot of it. Be careful of Nutrasweet if you have sugar sensitivities. (See *About Sweeteners in a Healing Diet*, pg. 77.)

👉 **OATS & OAT BRAN** - an excellent fiber grain source, to help lower cholesterol and promote regularity. An excellent addition to any grain or flour mix.

👉 **OCTACOSANOL** - a wheat germ derivative, used therapeutically to counteract fatigue and increase oxygen utilization when exercising. Its anti-oxidant properties are helpful in the treatment of muscular dystrophy and M.S.

👉 **OILS, NATURAL VEGETABLE** - these should be unrefined, either cold or expeller pressed, and stored in the refrigerator after opening. Natural oils provide vitamins A, E, lecithin and essential fatty acids. **Olive Oil** is superior for a healing diet. There are several grades to choose from.
👉*Extra Virgin* - from the first pressing - no additives; highest quality, with the best flavor and aroma.
👉*Fine Virgin* - good flavor, no additives, but with higher acid content.
👉*Plain Virgin* - slightly off flavor and the highest acidity.
👉*Pure* - from the second pressing with additives to mellow bitter taste; includes pulp, pit and skin.

👉 **OMEGA 3 OILS** - Clinical results show a long list of benefits for Omega oils: smoother skin, smoother muscle action, stronger cardiovascular performance, and better functioning of the digestive system. These essential fatty acids not only provide fuel for the heart, but also help prevent blood clotting and high cholesterol and triglyceride levels. In weight loss dieting, these oils eliminate binging and food addiction, help to burn off fats and increase stamina. They help overcome food allergies, promote clearer thinking by lowering blood fats and cholesterol, and improve stamina. *See About Fats & Oils*, pg. 80, for more information on the benefits of these oils. Results are often visible quite rapidly. For cooking purposes, flax oil and olive oil have the best LDL reducing properties.

👉 **PASTA** - versatile, whole grain, vegetable, low fat, low calorie - quick and easy to make, compatible with Oriental, Italian, modified macrobiotic, and very healthy diets. Japanese noodles made from buckwheat (Soba), whole wheat (Udon and Somen), rice (Rice Sticks and Saifun), and combination grain ramens can all be part of a healing diet. High complex carbohydrate Italian pastas include sesame, spinach, artichoke, and soy, in all sorts of shapes and sizes.

👉 **PSYLLIUM HUSKS** - a lubricating, mucilagenous, fiber herb, with drawing, cleansing and laxative properties. Acts as a "colon broom" for chronic constipation; effective for inflammatory diverticulitis; a lubricant for ulcerous intestinal tract tissue.

👉 **PYCNOGENOL** - a concentrated, highly active bioflovonoid extract from pine bark, grapeseed and other fruits. A powerful anti-oxidant, it is 50 times stronger than vitamin E, 20 times stronger than vitamin C. It helps the body resist inflammation, blood vessel and skin damage caused by free radicals. It strengthens the entire arterial system and improves circulation. It reduces capillary fragility, develops skin smoothness and elasticity, and is used in Europe as an "oral cosmetic". It stimulates collagen-rich connective tissue against atherosclerosis and helps joint flexibility in arthritis. It has been used successfully for diabetic retinopathy, varicose veins and hemorrhoids. It is one of the few dietary antioxidants that readily crosses the blood-brain barrier to directly protect brain cells and aid memory.

👉 **QUERCETIN** - a powerful bioflavonoid, and cousin of rutin, quercetin is isolated from blue-green algae. Its primary therapeutic use has been in controlling allergy and asthma reactions, since it suppresses the release and production of the two inflammatory agents that cause asthma and allergy symptoms - histimines and leukotrienes. Always take quercetin with bromelain for best bioavailability and synergistic anti-inflammatory activity.

👉 **QUINOA** - an ancient Inca supergrain, containing complete protein from amino acids, and good complex carbohydrates. It is essentially gluten-free, light and flavorful, and can be used like rice or millet as a diet staple.

👉 **RICE** - There is a taste for everybody in brown rice - all healing, high in B vitamins, and all good. Use a mix of rices for a more complex and individual flavor. Long grain is dry and fluffy; short grain is soft and sticky (good for molds and shaping). Sweet brown can be used for desserts, wehani for its nutty light texture, basmati for aroma, and wild rice for its distinctive chewiness.

● **RICE SYRUP** - a subtle sweetener, both rice syrup and malt syrup come in many different consistencies and flavors, easily digestible, with slow, steady energy-producing complex carbohydrates. (See *About Sweeteners in a Healing Diet*, pg. 77.)

● **ROYAL JELLY** - the milk-like secretion from the head glands of the queen bee's nurse-workers. It is a powerhouse of vitamins, minerals, enzyme precursers and amino acids. It is a natural anti-biotic, a stimulant to the immune system, and has been found effective for many health problems. (See *About Bee Pollen, Propolis & Royal Jelly*, pg. 89 , for more information.)

● **SEA VEGETABLES** - **Arame, Bladderwrack, Dulse, Hijiki, Kelp, Kombu, Nori, Sea Palm, and Wakame** - these foods have superior nutritional content; a rich source of proteins, carbohydrates, minerals and vitamins. They are good alkalizers for the body, and can be used in place of salt or other seasonings. Sea vegetables are the mainstay of iodine therapy. (See *About Sea Vegetables & Iodine Therapy*, pg. 85 for more information on healing properties from food sources.)

● **SOY MILK - SOY CHEESE** - See *About Dairy Free Foods During Healing*, pages 74.

● **SPIRULINA** - another of the high protein algae-source superfoods; spirulina is also rich in B vitamins and beta-carotene. The high chlorophyll content enhances enzyme production and digestion. (See *About Green Superfoods*, pg. 87, for more information.)

● **SPELT & KAMUT** - both high gluten grains - forms of wheat that are richer in amino acids, food enzymes, protein and nutrients than ordinary wheat. Many people with wheat allergies can tolerate these grains.

● **SPROUTS** - **Alfalfa, Red Clover, Mung Bean, Radish, Sunflower** - delicious, highly nutritious, inexpensive food. Sprouts are a wonderful source of protein in the form of amino acids, chlorophyll, enzymes and plant hormones. They are good sources of vitamins A, C, B, and E, with balanced minerals and trace minerals. Sprouts are easy to grow in a sprouting jar or trays at home. Use quality organic seeds for best nutritional results.

● **SUCANAT** - the trade name for a natural sweetener made from dried granulated cane juice. Use 1 to 1 in place of sugar. Nothing is added, only the water removed; all sucanat is from organically grown cane. It is still a concentrated sweetener, however. Use carefully if you have sugar balance problems. (See *About Sweeteners in a Healing Diet*, pg. 77.)

● **TAHINI** - ground sesame butter, that can be used in healthy candies and cookies, and on toast in place of peanut butter, or as a dairy replacement in soups and dressings or sauces without the cholesterol and all the protein.

● **TAMARI** - a wheat free soy sauce, lower in sodium and richer in flavor than soy sauce. Bragg's LIQUID AMINOS, a wonderful energizing protein broth, is also of the tamari family, but unfermented, lower in sodium, and with 8 essential amino acids.

● **TEAS, BLACK & GREEN** - Black teas contain caffeine and tannins, but differ from coffee in the amount and kind of caffeine they have, and in the way they are processed. Black teas, do not raise blood cholesterol levels, or lower vitamin C levels in the body and can be useful in counteracting depression. Cold wet tea bags placed over the eyelids are proven eye brighteners, and help clear red, tired eyes. See *About Black & Green Teas*, pg. 84 , for information relating to a healing diet.

● **TEMPEH** - a meaty Indonesian fermented soy food, containing complete protein and all essential amino acids. It has a robust texture and mushroom-like aroma. Tempeh is also a pre-digested product due to the enzyme action in the culture process, making its nutrients highly absorbable.

● **TOFU** - a delicious soy food, made from soybeans, water, and nigari, a mineral-rich seawater precipitate. Tofu is a convenient, nutritious meat replacement. Combined with whole grains, tofu yields a complete protein that is much less expensive than protein from animal sources. It provides dairy and egg richness without the fat or cholesterol, but with all the calcium and iron. It is cholesterol free.

It is a highly versatile, stress-free, virtually success-guaranteed food. Fresh tofu has a light, delicate character that can take on any flavor perfectly, from savory to sweet. In addition to its culinary talents, tofu is a nutritionally balanced healing food. It is easily substituted for many cholesterol loaded meats and dairy products. It is easy on the digestive system, full of soluble fiber, and a non-mucous-forming way to add richness and creamy texture to recipes.
   ✳ Tofu is low in calories. Eight ounces has only 164 calories.
   ✳ Tofu is rich in organic calcium. Eight ounces supplies the same amount of calcium as eight ounces of milk, but with far more absorbability.
   ✳ Tofu is high in iron. Eight ounces supplies the same amount of iron as 2 oz. of beef liver or 4 eggs.
   ✳ Tofu has high quality protein. Eight ounces supplies the same amount of protein as $3^1/_4$ oz. of beef steak, or $5^1/_2$ oz. of hamburger, or $1^2/_3$ cups of milk, or 2 oz. of regular cheese, or 2 eggs; but it is lower in fat than any of these.
   ✳ Tofu is a nutritionally adequate source of complex carbohydrates, minerals and vitamins.
As tofu's popularity has risen in America, so has the variety of ways you can buy, prepare and eat it. Tofu comes firm-pressed in cubes, in a soft, delicate form, or silken with a custard-like texture. It comes smoked and pre-cooked in seasonings to give it a cheese-like flavor and firmnes, and freeze-dried so that it can be stored at room temperature and reconstituted; (suitable for camping and travel). It comes in deep-fried pouches called age (pronounced "ah-gay") that are hollow inside for filling.
Note: For those with sensitivity to beans and legumes, tofu may be simmered in water-to-cover for 15 minutes before using. This precooks the soybeans so that they won't bother sensitive digestion.

☛ **TORTILLAS** - both whole wheat and corn make good light nutritious pizza crusts, nachos, and wrappers for Mexican-style sandwiches.

☛ **TRITICALE** - a hybrid flour of wheat and rye berries, containing the best properties of both and higher in protein than either.

☛ **TURBINADO SUGAR** - refined sugar without all the molasses removed. (See *About Sweeteners in a Healing Diet*, pg. 77.)

☛ **UMEBOSHI PLUMS** - pickled Japanese apricots with alkalizing, bacteria-killing properties; part of a good macrobiotic diet.

☛ **VINEGARS - Brown Rice, Balsamic, Apple Cider, Herb, Raspberry, Ume Plum** - vinegars have been used for 5000 years as healthful flavor enhancers and food preservers. As part of condiments, relishes or dressings, they help digest heavy foods and high protein meals. The most nutritious vinegars for health are not overly filtered, and still contain the "mother" mixture of beneficial bacteria and enzymes in the bottle. They look slightly cloudy.

☛ **WHEAT GERM & WHEAT GERM OIL** - wheat germ is the embryo of the wheat berry - rich in B vitamins, proteins, vitamin E, and iron. It goes rancid quickly. Buy only in nitrogen-flushed packaging. Wheat germ oil is a good vitamin E source and body oxygenator. One tablespoon provides the antioxidant equivalent of an oxygen tent for 30 minutes.

☛ **WHEAT GRASS** - one of the "chlorophyll superfoods" used for treating cancerous growths and other degenerative diseases. Dr. Ann Wigmore states that 15 pounds of fresh wheatgrass has the nutritional value of 350 pounds of vegetables. We have seen particular success with wheatgrass rectal implants in colon cancer cases.

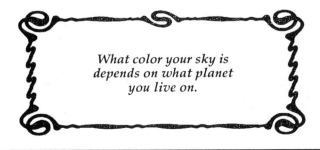

What color your sky is depends on what planet you live on.

About Natural Wines

Naturally fermented wine is more than an alcoholic beverage. It is a complex biological fluid possessing definite physiological values. Wine is still a living food, and can combine with, and aid the body like yogurt or other fermented foods. Many small, family owned wineries make chemical and additive free wines that retain inherent nutrients, imcluding absorbable B vitamins, and minerals and trace minerals such as potassium, magnesium, organic sodium, iron, calcium and phosphorus.

Wine is a highly useful drink for digestion, and in moderation, is a sedative for the heart, arteries and blood pressure. Tests have shown that a glass or two of white wine with dinner can cut heart disease risk by 50%. Because of its high density lipoproteins, wine can free the circulation, relieve pain and reduce acid production in the body. It is superior to tranquilizers or drugs for relief of nervous stress and tension. Its importance should not be overlooked in a weight loss or fitness program, because a glass or two of wine relaxes. When you are relaxed, you tend to eat less.

Recent studies at U.C. Berkeley have shown that red wine is rich in the new class of polyphenols, including the potent anti-carcinogen quercetin, a chemical that can reverse tumor development. Another new study on hepatitis A by the Epidemiology Journal has shown that alcohol can even prevent virus replication.

ALWAYS USE IN MODERATION. *Note: Liquor other than wines is not recommended, even for cooking, when you are involved in a healing program. Although most people can stand a little hard spirits without undue effect, and alcohol burns off in cooking, the concentrated sugar residues won't help a recovering body.*

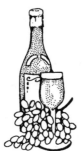

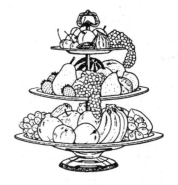

About Fresh Fruits

Fresh fruits are nature's way of smiling.

Fruits are wonderful for a quick system wash and cleanse. Their high natural water and sugar content speeds up metabolism to release wastes rapidly.
Fresh fruit has an alkalizing effect in the body, and is high in vitamins and nutrition. The easily convertible natural sugars transform into quick non-fattening energy that speeds up the calorie burning process.

But these advantages are only true of **fresh** fruits. With fruit, the *way* that you eat it is as important as *what* you eat.
Fruits have their best healing and nutritional effects when eaten alone or with other fruits as a fruit salad, separately from grains and vegetables. With a few exceptions, both fruits and fruit juices should be taken before noon for best energy conversion and cleansing benefits.
Cooking fruits changes their alkalizing properties to acid-forming in the body. This is also true of sulphured, dried fruit, and the combination of fruit with vegetables or grains. Eating fruits in these fashions causes digestion to slow down, and gas, as the high fruit sugars stay too long in the stomach allowing rapid fermentation instead of assimilation.

Eat organically grown fruits whenever possible. The quick metabolism of fruits allows pesticides to enter the body very rapidly.

About A Low Salt Diet

In the past generation, Americans have consumed more NaCl than ever before; too much restaurant food, too many processed and refined foods, too many animal foods. Most people are aware that excessive salt causes heart disease, hypertension, and blood pressure problems. Circulation is constricted, kidneys malfunction, fluid is retained, and migraines occur frequently. Too much salt can produce hyperactivity, aggressive behavior, and poor glandular health.

A salt free diet is obviously desirable for someone who eats too much salt. However, once the body's salinity normalizes, some salt should be brought back into the diet quickly. Adequate salinity is needed for good intestinal tone, strong blood, tissue transportation of nutrients, healthy organs and glands. Too little, or no salt can lead to lack of vitality, stagnated blood and loss of clear thinking.

Regular table salt is almost totally devoid of nutritional value, but there are many other ways to get the good salts that the body needs. Tamari, soy sauce, shoyu, misos, umeboshi plums, sea vegetables, washed, sun-dried sea salt, herb salts and seasonings, sesame salt, and naturally fermented foods such as pickles, relishes and olives all have enzymes and alkalizing properties that make salts usable and absorbable.
LOW SALT, NOT NO SALT, is best for a permanent way of eating.

About Red Meat and a Healing Diet

Eating red meats puts us a step away from environmental harmony. Human digestive systems are not easily carnivorous. The body has to struggle to transmute red meat energy. Eating red meat is a lot like extracting oil out of the ground. It often costs more to get the oil out than it is worth on the market. Thus meat protein, which the body can use, is often cancelled out by the length of digestion time, and the after-dinner lethargy as a disproportionate amount of energy goes to the task of assimilation. Frequent intake of red meat's highly concentrated protein can also create toxicity from unused nitrogens, that are hard for the elimination system to cope with or excrete. A common example of this is the frequent instance of kidney stone formations in heavy red meat eaters.

Animals are also closer to us on the bio-scale of life. They experience fear when killed. They don't want to be eaten. Unlike eating plants, there is no uplifting transmutation of energy. Instead our bodies become denser, with more internal fermentation and body odor. In addition to avoiding red meats for humanitarian reasons, and an awareness of what meats do to the body, the red meats available today are shot through with hormones and slow-release anti-biotics, and preserved with nitrates or nitrites. All these are passed into your body at the dinner table. The stockyard animals we eat now are often sick and overmedicated, and their meat is tainted, chemicalized and adulterated. Red meat is the biggest contributor of excess protein and saturated fat. No one argues that less fat in the diet is healthier, or that saturated fats are the most harmful. Avoidance of red meat considerably reduces dietary saturated fat and concentrated calories. Cooked red meats are acid-forming in the body, and when cooked to well-done can create chemical compounds capable of causing many diseases.

Finally, meat eating promotes more aggressive behavior - a lack of gentleness in personality, and arrogance. From a spiritual point of view, red meat eating encourages ties to the material things in life, expansion of territory, and the self-righteous intolerance that makes adversaries.

People who do not eat red meats have a well documented history of lower risk for heart disease, obesity, diabetes, osteoporosis, and several types of cancer. These people also play an active role in conserving precious water, topsoil, and energy resources that are wasted by an animal-based diet. Avoiding red meats has become one of the most important things you can do for your own health and that of the planet.

About Milk & Dairy Products During Healing

We do not recommend drinking or using cow's milk in cooking when on a healing program, because of its clogging and mucous forming properties. Pasteurized milk is a relatively dead food as far as nutrition is concerned, and even raw milk can be difficult to assimilate for someone with allergies or respiratory problems.

For almost 25% of Americans, dairy intolerance can cause allergic reactions, poor digestion, and abnormal mucous build-up in the body. The human system in general does not easily process cow's milk, cream, ice cream or hard cheese. We tend to throw off excess from these foods, causing continuous, cumulative strain on eliminative organs, and system clogging as the unused matter turns to mucous. Dairy foods can interfere with the cleansing/healing process because of density and high saturated fats. Even people with no noticeable sensitivity to dairy products report a rise in energy when they stop using them as main foods. Because of high dairy fats, reduced intake usually means effective weight loss, and lower blood pressure and cholesterol levels. In addition, women do not handle building foods such as dairy products, as well as men. Their systems back up more easily. Many female problems, such as fibrous growths, bladder, and kidney ailments can be improved by avoiding dairy foods.

Contrary to advertising, dairy products are not even the most desirable source of calcium. Absorbability is poor because of pasteurizing, processing, high fat content, and unbalanced relationship with phosphorus. Hormone residues and additives from current cattle-raising practices, also indicate that calcium and other minerals will be incompletely absorbed. In tests with animals, calves given their own mother's milk that had first been pasteurized, didn't live six weeks.
Many other foods, such as vegetables, nuts, seeds, fish and sea vegetables, contain calcium that is easier for the body to use. Soy cheese, tofu, soy milk, and nut milks may all be used in place of dairy products. Kefir and yogurt, although made from milk, are usually free of the assimilation problems of dairy products. Unless lactose intolerance is very severe, these foods do not cause allergic reactions, and are beneficial to healing because of their friendly bacteria cultures.

Dairy foods should be avoided entirely during a cleansing diet. For building and maintenance diets, consider most dairy products as wonderful for taste, but questionable for premium nutrition. A little is fine - a lot is not. Rich quality can still be achieved without cream, milk, butter, eggs or cheese. Some small changes in cooking habits and point of view are all it takes - mostly a matter of not having these products around the house, and substituting in your favorite recipes with dairy free alternatives. (See next page.) Soon you won't feel deprived at all. Just remember the easy weight you'll lose by not eating saturated dairy fats.

See COOKING FOR HEALTHY HEALING by Linda Rector-Page for delicious, healthy , non-dairy recipes that can be used on almost any healing plan without sacrificing richness or taste.

When dairy foods *are* used, purchase low fat or non-fat products, and goat's milk or raw milk and cheeses, instead of pasteurized. Whole and full fat dairy foods are clearly not good if there is lactose intolerance or if you are on a mucous cleansing diet. Unfortunately for cheese lovers, the saturated fat concentrations in cheese make it particularly hard on the success of a healing diet. These fats are detrimental to both digestion and metabolism. Commercial cheeses, even though often labeled "natural", often contain bleaches, coagulants, emulsifiers, moisture absorbants,mold inhibitors, and rind waxes and dyes that visibly leak into the cheese itself. Many restaurant and pizza cheeses add synthetic flavorings, coloring and preservatives. Processed cheese foods obtain their texture and structure from artificially hydrogenated fats rather than natural fermentation.

Even if you are not on a healing diet, limit cheese consumption to small amounts of low fat and raw cheeses. These cheeses provide usable proteins, with a good calcium/phosphorus/sodium ratio. There is a world of difference in taste. Raw, fresh cream cheese is light years ahead of commercial brands with gums, fillers and thickeners. Raw mozzarrella, farmer cheese, ricotta and cheddar are also superior in taste to pasteurized cheeses and cheese foods, that have higher salts and additives.

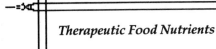

Non-Dairy Options - Alternatives to Milk, Cream, Eggs, and Cheese

➤ **Almond Milk** - a rich non-dairy liquid that can be used as a base for cream soups, sauces, gravies and protein drinks. Use one to one in place of milk in baked recipes, sauces or gravies. For 1 cup almond milk, put 1 CUP ALMONDS in the blender with 2 to 4 CUPS WATER depending on the consistency desired. Add 1 teasp. honey, and whirl until smooth.

➤ **Yogurt** - a good intestinal cleanser that helps balance and replace friendly flora in the G.I. tract. Even though yogurt is dairy in origin, the culturing process makes it a living food, and beneficial for health. Mix equal parts of yogurt with water, chicken or vegetable broth, white wine or sparkling water, and use cup for cup instead of milk in cooking. Make sure you use yogurt with viable cultures.

➤ **Yogurt Cheese** - very easy to make, much lighter in fat and calories than sour cream or cream cheese, but with the same richness and consistency. **Here is how to make it:** Use a piece of cheesecloth or a sieve-like plastic funnel, (available from kitchen catalogs or hardware stores). Simply spoon in as much plain yogurt as you want (usually use about 16 oz.) and hang the cheesecloth over the sink faucet, or put the funnel over a large glass. It takes about 14 -16 hours for the whey to drain out (whey is delicious used as part of the liquid in soups and stews), and voila! you have yogurt cheese. Stored in a covered container in the refrigerator, it will keep for 2 to 3 weeks.

➤ **Kefir** - a cultured food made by adding kefir grains (naturally formed milk proteins) to milk and letting the mix incubate overnight at room temperature to milkshake consistency. Kefir has 350mg. of calcium per cup.
Use the plain flavor cup for cup as a replacement for whole milk, buttermilk or half and half; the fruit flavors may be used in sweet baked dishes.

➤ **Kefir Cheese** - an excellent replacement for sour cream or cream cheese in dips and other recipes, kefir cheese is low in fat and calories, and has a slightly tangy-rich flavor that really enhances snack foods. Use it cup for cup in place of sour cream, cottage cheese, cream cheese or ricotta.

➤ **Soy Milk** - nutritious, versatile, smooth and delicious, soy milk is vegetable-based, lactose/cholesterol free, with unsaturated or polyunsaturated fat. Some studies have shown that using soy milk in the diet can help reduce serum cholesterol. Soy milk contains less calcium and calories than milk, but more protein and iron. It adds a slight rise to baked goods. Use it cup for cup as milk for cooking; plain flavor for savory dishes, vanilla flavor for sweet dishes and on cereal.

➤ **Soy Cheese** - made from soy milk, this cheese is free of lactose and cholesterol. The small amount of calcium caseinate (a milk protein) added allows it to melt. Mozzarrella, cheddar, jack and cream cheese types are widely available. Use it cup for cup in place of any low fat or regular cheese.

➤ **Soy Ice Cream, Frozen Desserts and Soy Yogurt** are now available in a variety of flavors. **Soy Mayonnaise** has also finally been developed with the taste and consistency of dairy mayonnaise.

➤ **Tofu** - a white, digestible curd made from soybeans, tofu is one of the supreme replacements for dairy foods, in texture, taste, and nutritional content. It is high in protein, low in fat and contains no cholesterol. It is available in several varieties, is extremely versatile, and may be used in place of eggs, sour cream, cheese and cottage cheese.

➤ **Miso** - a good dairy substitute in macrobiotic and cleansing/alkalizing diets. Light chickpea miso mixed with vegetable or onion stock is a tasty replacement for milk and seasonings.

➤ **Lecithin** - a high phosphatide soy product, low in fat and cholesterol that can help thicken and emulsify ingredients without using dairy foods. It can make many recipes extra rich and smooth. (See the *Healing Foods Glossary* for information on the therapeutic activity of lecithin.)

➤ **Sesame Tahini** - a rich, smooth, creamy product made from ground sesame seeds. Tahini may be used successfully in place of cream or sour cream in dips, sauces and gravies. Mixed with water to milk consistency, it may be used as a high protein milk substitute in baking. It is an excellent complement to greens and salad ingredients. Mix tahini with oil and other ingredients for salad toppings.

About Low Fat Cottage Cheese - a low fat, cultured dairy product, cottage cheese is beneficial for those with only slight lactose intolerance. It is a good substitute for ricotta, commercial cream cheese, and processed cottage cheese foods that are full of chemicals. Mix with non-fat or low fat plain yogurt to add the richness of cream or sour cream to recipes without the fat.

About Butter - Surprise! Butter is okay in moderation. Although butter is a saturated fat, it is relatively stable and the body can use it in small amounts for energy. Its make-up, like that of raw cream, is a whole and balanced food, used by the body better than its separate components. When butter is needed, use raw, unsalted butter, never margarine, pasteurized butter or shortening. Don't let it get hot enough to sizzle or smoke. If less saturation is desired, use clarified butter. Simply melt the butter. Skim off the top foam. Remove from heat. Let rest a few minutes, and spoon off the clear butter for use. Discard whey solids that settle to the bottom of the pan.

➡ High quality **vegetable oil** may almost always be substituted for butter without loss of taste in a sauté.
➡ **Soy margerine** is an acceptable vegetarian alternative in baking.

About Eggs - More good news! "Experts" are finally realizing what many of us in the whole foods world have long known. Although high in cholesterol, eggs are also high in balancing lecithins and phosphatides, **and do not increase the risk of atherosclerosis.** Nutrition-rich fertile eggs from free-run-and-scratch chickens are a perfect food. The difference in fertile eggs and the products from commercial egg factories is remarkable; the yolk color is brighter, the flavor definitely fresher, and the workability in recipes better. The distinction is particularly noticeable in poached and baked eggs, where the yolks firm up and rise higher. Eggs should be lightly cooked for the best nutrition, preferably poached, soft-boiled, or baked, never fried. As concentrated protein, use them with discretion.

➡ **Egg Replacer** made from potato starch and tapioca flour is a viable egg substitue for baking needs.

➡ **Tofu** may be used in place of eggs in quick breads, cakes, custard-based dishes and quiches.

➡ **Flax Seeds and Water** can replace eggs in quick breads, pancakes and muffins. Use $1/4$ cup flax seeds to $3/4$ cup water. Mix in the blender until <u>thoroughly</u> crushed, and add to batter in place of 3 eggs. Flax seeds are healthful in themselves as a source of soluble and insoluble fiber, and an aid to regularity. They are also rich in lignans. High levels of lignans in the digestive tract have been associated with the reduced risk of colon and breast cancer.

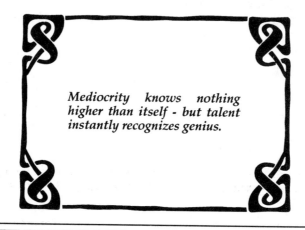

Mediocrity knows nothing higher than itself - but talent instantly recognizes genius.

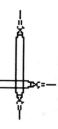

About Sugar & Sweeteners in a Healing Diet

Sugar in America is synonymous with fun, good times and snacking. Our culture instills the powerful urge for sweetness from an early age. But in reality, refined sugar is sucrose, the ultimate naked carbohydrate - stripped of all nutritional benefits. Sugars include raw, brown, natural, yellow D, sucanat, and white sugar. All can be physically addictive, and add nothing but calories to your body. Excessive sugar consumption has many detrimental effects, but the interest in this book is that sugar can be a major interference in a healing program.

Regular sugar intake is known to play a negative part in a host of common diseases: diabetes, hypoglycemia, heart disease, high cholesterol, obesity, nearsightedness, eczema, psoriasis, dermatitis, gout, indigestion, yeast infections, and tooth decay. It provides a breeding ground for staph infection. Sugar is addictive, and like a drug or alcohol it affects the brain first, offering a false energy lift that eventually lets you down lower than when you started.

◆Sugar requires the production of insulin for metabolism - a process that promotes the storage of fat. Metabolized sugar is transformed into fat globules, and distributed over the body where the muscles are not very active, such as on the stomach, hips and chin. Every time you eat sugar, some of those calories become body fat instead of energy.

◆Excess sugar can upset mineral balances in the body. It particularly drains away calcium, overloading the body with the acid-ash residues that are responsible for much of the stiffening of joints and limbs in arthritic conditions. Sugar ties up and dissolves B vitamins in the digestive tract, so that they cannot act. Skin, nerve and digestive problems result.

◆Sugar also plays a part in many negative psychological reactions. It is a food that we eat to "cope" in times of stress and tension. It seems to satisfy a hole in our palates and our psyches. In reality, it produces an over-acid condition in the body, stripping out stabilizing B vitamins. Satisfaction is the very thing you can't get from eating sugar. But as our lives move faster and faster and become more and more stressful, sugar often becomes a bigger and bigger part, pushed on us in many convenience foods. Too much sugar becomes harder and harder to avoid.

◆Finally, excess sugar consumption has been shown to depress the body's immune response and resistance to disease, by inhibiting the release of growth hormone. It also lowers disease control, a proven fact for those with diabetes and hypoglycemia, and now becoming known as well for people with high triglycerides and blood pressure.

The good news is that just because you follow a sugar-free diet doesn't mean you have to give up good taste or the comforts of sweetness. Naturally-occurring whole food sweeteners, such as honey, molasses, maple syrup, fruit juice or barley malt can satisfy the sweet need. They can be handled and metabolized easily by the body in its regular processes.

The following chart can help you convert favorite recipes that use sugar to the correct substitutions for natural sweeteners.

☛☛ If you have serious blood sugar regulation problems, such as diabetes or hypoglycemia, consult the appropriate sections in this book, or your healing professional, about the kind and amount of sweets your body can handle.

☛Amounts are for each cup of sugar.

Sweetener	Amount	Reduce Liquid in the Recipe
*Fructose	1/3 to 2/3 cup	------------
*Maple Syrup	1/3 to 2/3 cup	1/4 cup
*Honey	1/2 cup	1/4 cup
*Molasses	1/2 cup	1/4 cup
*Barley Malt/Rice Syrup	1 to 11/4 cups	1/4 cup
*Date Sugar	1 cup	------------
*Sucanat	1 cup	------------
*Apple or Other Fruit Juice	1 cup	1/4 cup

*Stevia Ribaudiana (Sweet Herb) - 25 times sweeter than sugar. Make a strong liquid infusion. Store tightly covered in the refrigerator. Use sparingly in beverages and recipes.

Products and substances that affect body sugar regulation can have major impact, both good and bad, on a healing program. Therefore, some information about their properties and functions is worthwhile.

The inability to properly process glucose, the number one energy source in the body, affects millions of Americans today. At least twenty million of us suffer from diabetes (high blood sugar) or hypoglycemia (low blood sugar). While seeming to be opposite problems, these two conditions really stem from the same cause - an imbalance between glucose and oxygen in the system which puts the body into a stress state, and leads to gland exhaustion. Poor nutrition is a common cause of both disorders, and both can be improved with a high mineral, high fiber diet, adequate usable protein, small frequent meals, and regular mild exercise.

☛ For people with these sugar imbalances there must be diet and lifestyle change for there to be a real or permanent cure. Alcohol, caffeine, refined sugars and tobacco must be avoided.

☞ **Hypoglycemia** is one of the most widespread disorders in "civilized" nations today. It is a direct effect of excess intake of refined sweets, low fiber foods, and other processed carbohydrates. The pancreas reacts to this overload by producing too much insulin to reduce the blood sugar, and hypoglycemia results.

☞ **Diabetes** is also a disease of "civilization", in which people regularly eat too much sugar, refined carbohydrates and caffeine. These excess carbohydrates are not used correctly, and blood sugar stays too high because too little balancing insulin is produced. The pancreas becomes damaged and exhausted, and glucose cannot enter the cells to provide body energy. Instead it accumulates in the blood, resulting in various symptoms from mental confusion to coma.

Note: Even though poor blood sugar metabolism is the cause of both diabetes and hypoglycemia, the different effects of each problem call for specific modifications. More rapid body response can be attained by approaching low blood sugar and high blood sugar diets separately. See Diabetes and Hypoglycemia pages in this book.

Recent clinical testing with crystalline fructose, and the herbs stevia rebaudiana and gymnema sylvestre have produced some valid good news for sugar reaction disorders. These substances may be seen as blood sugar balance heros, especially in the effort to control sugar intake and sugar cravings, but **they do not eliminate hypoglycemia or diabetes reactions**. Only diet improvement along with regular exercise can make a permanent difference.

➔ **Crystalline Fructose** is a commercially produced sugar with the same molecular structure as that found in fruit. It is low on the glycemic index, meaning that it releases glucose into the bloodstream slowly. It is metabolized by the liver and kidneys in a process that is not regulated by insulin supply; and thus produces liver glycogen rapidly making it a more efficient energy supply than other sweeteners. It is almost twice as sweet as sugar, so less is needed for the same sweetening power, especially in cold foods like desserts.

Fructose can be a sweetener of choice in a weight loss diet. In clinical tests before meals, subjects who drank liquids sweetened with fructose ate 20 to 40% *fewer calories* than normal, more than compensating for the 200 calories in the fructose. Those who drank liquids sweetened with table sugar ate 10 to 15% fewer calories; those who drank liquids sweetened with NutraSweet or aspartame ate the same amount of calories as normal. **Fructose also seems to make eaters pick foods with less fats.**

In dental health studies, less dental plaque was reported with fructose than with sugar. It is reactive to heat, and lower cooking temperatures should be used. If you are hypoglycemic or diabetic, fructose is still sugar and deserves careful use.

➔ **Stevia Rebaudiana**, also known as "sweet herb", is a South American sweetening leaf. It is totally non-caloric, and approximately 25 times sweeter than sugar when made as a concentrated infusion of 1 tsp. leaves to 1 cupful of water. Two drops equal 1 teaspoon of sugar in sweetness. In baking, 1 teaspoon of finely ground stevia powder is equal to 1 cup of sugar. Clinical studies indicate that stevia is safe to use even in cases of severe sugar imbalance.

➔ **Gymnema Sylvestre** is an herb that reduces blood sugar levels after sugar consumption. Gymnema has a molecular structure similar to that of sugar that can block absorption of up to 50% of dietary sugar calories. Both sugar and gymnema are digested in the small intestine, but the larger molecule of gymnema cannot be fully absorbed. Taken before sugar, the gymnema molecule blocks the passages through which

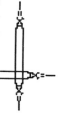

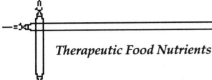

sugar is normally absorbed, so that fewer sugar calories are assimilated. A person who eats a 400 calorie, high sugar dessert will only absorb 200 of the sugar calories. The remaining sugar is eliminated as waste.

A taste test shows how gymnema works. Taste something sweet, then swish a sip of gymnema sylvestre tea around in your mouth. Now taste something sweet again. You will not be able to taste the sugar, because gymnema has blocked the taste of the sugar in your mouth in the same way it blocks sugar in digestion. Used for hyperinsulinism. Take with GTF Chromium to stabilize blood sugar levels.

↞ **About Aspartame** - an artificial sweetener that combines the two amino acids phenylalanine and aspartic acid. Both have neurotransmitter activity. Aspartame is 200 times sweeter than sugar, and has been linked to several problems involving sugar use in the body, such as PKU (phenylketonuria) seizures, high blood pressure, headaches, insomnia and mood swings. Several studies have shown immediate, serious reactions to aspartame, including severe headaches, extreme dizziness, throat swelling and other allergic effects, and retina deterioration. The retina damage is attributed to methyl alcohol, a substance released when aspartame breaks down. Aspartame has also been linked to brain damage in fetuses.
Aspartame has taken the place of saccharin in pre-prepared foods and drinks, and that means we get a lot of it. It's major brand names are NutraSweet and Equal. Be careful of these sweeteners if you have sugar sensitivities. Fortunately, adverse effects are reversible when consumption is stopped. Pregnant and lactating women, very young or allergy-prone children, and those with PKU, (the inability to process phenylalanine) should avoid aspartame products.

↞ **Barley Malt or Rice Syrups** - mild natural sweeteners made from barley sprouts, or rice and water, and cooked to a syrup. They have a pleasant flavor that is delicious in cookies, muffins and quick breads, and is only 40% as sweet as sugar. Their activity is a slow, complex carbohydrate type release in the body that does not bring on high/low insulin levels.

↞ **Blackstrap Molasses** - the leftover sludge after sucrose extract in the sugar making process. Rich in minerals and vitamins. Molasses has more calcium, ounce for ounce than milk, more iron than eggs, and more potassium than and other food. It contains all the B-complex vitamins, and vitamin E. The amounts of pantothenic acid, iron, and inositol make it an excellent treatment for restoring thin and fading hair.

↞ **Sucanat** - the trade name for a natural sweetener made from dried granulated cane juice, and available in health food stores. It has a mild taste, and may be used it 1 to 1 in place of sugar. Nothing is added, only the water is removed. All sucanat is from organically grown cane. It is still a concentrated sweetener, however. Use carefully if you have sugar balance problems.

↞ **A word about honey** - honey is almost twice as sweet as sugar and should be avoided by those with candidiasis and diabetes, and used with great care by those with hypoglycemia. However, it is a raw, natural sweetening substance with proven bioactive antibiotic and antiseptic properties. Along with its sweetening power, honey contains all the vitamins and enzymes necessary for the proper metabolism and digestion of glucose and other inherent sugar molecules.

Recent research is beginning to show that some of the current beliefs about sugar have been overstated. In regard to weight gain, for instance, sugar in candy, cookies and desserts, etc. is far less a fattening culprit than fat. Fat not only contributes more calories, but the calories are metabolized differently in the body, causing much more weight gain than sugar. For more information about sweeteners, check the *Glossary of Healing Foods* on page 64.

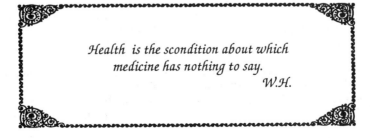

*Health is the scondition about which
medicine has nothing to say.*
W.H.

About Fats & Oils in a Healing Diet

We all know that there is a direct relationship between the quantity of fat we consume and the quality of health we can expect. During this century, Americans have increased their intake of fat calories by over 33%. The link between high salt and fat intake has also become clear. Excess salt inhibits the body's capacity to clear fat from the bloodstream. Warnings and discussions about fat have filled the media in America for a decade. But much of the information is contradictory and inaccurate. This section should simplify the confusion, especially as it relates to choices made for a healing diet.

✤

Saturated & Unsaturated Fats:
All foods contain saturated and unsaturated fats in various proportions, (the difference is in molecular structure) with animal foods higher in saturated fat, and except for palm and coconut oil, vegetable foods higher in unsaturated fat. Saturated fats are solid at room temperature, as in butter or meat fat. They are the culprits that clog the arteries, and lead to heart and degenerative disease. Unsaturated fat, (mono or polyunsaturated) is liquid at room temperature, as in vegetable or nut oils. Although research supports unsaturates as helping to reduce serum cholesterol, just switching to unsaturated fats without increasing dietary fiber will not bring about improvement. In fact, consuming moderate amounts of both kinds of fats, *coupled with a high fiber diet* will benefit most people.

✤

Hydrogenated fats:
Hydrogenation is the process of taking a poly-unsaturated oil and bubbling hydrogen through it to cause reconstruction of the chemical bonds and delay rancidity. It makes unsaturated fats such as corn oil into saturated fats such as margerine. Much testing has shown that these altered fats are comparable to animal fats in terms of saturation and poor utilization by the body. A good alternative to margarine or shortening, much lower in saturated fat, is a combination of equal amounts of warm butter with vegetable oil.

✤

Omega 3 & Omega 6 Fatty Acids:
Omega 3 oils are a family of fatty acids high in EPA (eicosapentaenoic acid), DHA (dihomogam-malinolenic acid), and GLA (gamma linleic acid). They include cold water fish oils, walnut oil, canola oil, wheat germ oil, evening primrose oil and flax oil. Research has indicated that treatments for P.M.S, high blood pressure and rheumatoid arthritis benefit from the use of these fatty acids. Omega 3 oils are also a specific for the 30% of the population trying to keep serum cholesterol levels low.
Omega 6 oils are the group of fatty acids high in linoleic and arachidonic acids, and include sesame, sunflower, safflower and corn oil. Both Omega 3 and Omega 6 fatty acids stimulate the formation of prostaglandins.
Prostaglandins are produced by every cell in the body, and control such things as reproduction and fertility, inflammation, immunity and communication between cells. They also inhibit the over-production of thromboxane, a substance in the body that promotes clotting. Therefore, because blood tends to clot in narrowed arteries, (the major cause of heart attacks) prostaglandins are essential to health.

✤

Lipids: Cholesterol & Triglycerides:
Lipid is an inclusive term for a group of fats and fat-like substances essential to human health. Lipids are found in every cell, and are integral to membrane, blood and tissue structure, hormone/prostaglandin production, and nervous system functions. **Triglycerides** are dietary fats and oils, used as fuel by the body, and as an energy source for metabolism. **Phospholipids** are fats such as lecithin, and cholesterol, vital to cell membranes, nerve fibers and bile salts, and a necessary precursor for sex hormones.

✤

HDLs & LDLs (High and Low Density Lipo-proteins):

Lipoproteins are water-soluble, protein-covered bundles, that transport cholesterol through the bloodstream, and are synthesized in the liver and intestinal tract. "Bad cholesterol", LDLs (low density lipo-proteins) carries cholesterol through the bloodstream for cell-building needs, but leaves behind any excess on artery walls and in tissues. "Good cholesterol", HDLs (high density lipo-proteins) helps prevent narrowing of the artery walls by removing the excess cholesterol and transporting it to the liver for excretion as bile.

♣

Mono & Polyunsaturated fats:

Olive oil is a mono-unsaturated fat that reduces the amount of LDL in the bloodstream. Research shows that it is even more effective in this process than a low fat diet. Another oil high in mono-unsaturated fats is canola or rapeseed oil.

Poly-unsaturated vegetable oils are the chief source for the "essential fatty acids" (linoleic, linolenic and arachidonic) necessary to proper cell membrane function, balanced prostaglandin production and many other metabolic processes. Good poly-unsaturates include sunflower, safflower, sesame oil, and flax oil, one of the best sources of essential fatty acids.

♣

Vegetable oils:

All vegetable oils are free of cholesterol, but some contain synthetic preservatives and are heavily refined, bleached and deoderized with chemical solvents. Others are simply mechanically pressed, filtered and bottled. The highest quality fresh vegetable oils are rich in Omega fatty acids and essential to health in their ability to stimulate prostaglandin levels.

Unrefined oils that are expelled or mechanically pressed go through the least processing and are the most natural. (Cold pressing applies only to olive oil.) They are dark with some sediment, and a taste and odor of the raw material used.

Solvent extracted oil is a second pressing from the first pressing residue. Hexane is generally used to enable the most efficient extraction, and is then burned off at about 300º to evaporate the hexane. Even though small amounts of this petroleum chemical remain, it is still considered an unrefined oil.

Refined oils go through several other processing stages, such as degumming, which keeps the oil from going rancid quickly, but also removes many nutrients, including vitamin E. Refined oils are de-pigmented through charcoal or clay, clarified through deodorizing under high temperatures, and chemically preserved with additives. Refinement means that the oil is clear, odorless, and almost totally devoid of nutrients.

♣

♦Remember that natural, unrefined oils are fragile and become rancid quickly. They should be stored in a dark cupboard or in the refrigerator. Purchase small bottles if you don't use much oil in your cooking.

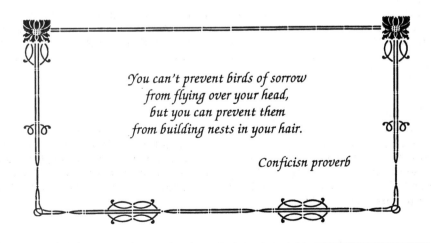

*You can't prevent birds of sorrow
from flying over your head,
but you can prevent them
from building nests in your hair.*

Conficisn proverb

About Caffeine in a Healing Diet

Like most of mankind's other pleasures, there is good news and bad news about caffeine. Moderate use of caffeine has been hailed for centuries for its therapeutic benefits. Every major society uses caffeine in some food form to overcome fatigue, handle pain, open breathing, control weight gain and jump-start circulation. Caffeine is a plant-derived neutraceutical - a part of both foods and medications - coffee, black tea, colas, sodas, chocolate and cocoa, analgesics such as Excedrin, and over-the-counter stimulants such as Vivarin, to name a few.

There is solid evidence for the positive effects of caffeine on mental performance, clearer thinking, and shortened reaction times. Caffeine stimulates serotonin, a brain neurotransmitter produced by tryptophan, that increases the capacity for intellectual tasks, and decreases drowsiness. In modest doses, it improves mood and increases alertness through the release of adrenaline into the bloodstream. It mobilizes fatty acids into the circulatory system, facilitating greater energy production, endurance and work output. It has a direct potentiating effect on muscle contraction for both long and short-term sports and workout activity.

Caffeine also has analgesic properties. Taking aspirin or an herbal pain reliever *with* a caffeine drink will increase the pain relieving effects.

Its benefits for weight loss have long been known since caffeine promotes enhanced metabolism and the conversion of stored body fat to energy. Recent research shows that overweight dieters have subnormal heat production during dieting as the body reacts to lower food intake and metabolic changes. Caffeine causes thermogenesis (calorie burning). In fact, after eating, obese and post-obese people respond to caffeine with *greater thermogenesis* than lean people.

Relatively small, commonly consumed doses of caffeine can significantly influence calorie use by the body. One recent study showed that a single dose of 100mg. of caffeine (the amount in one cup of coffee) increased the metabolic rate almost 4% for two to three hours. When this same amount was consumed at two-hour intervals for 12 hours, the metabolic rate increased 8 to 11%. While these increased metabolic rates seem small, monitoring over several months showed slow, steady, substantial reductions in body weight. This same study also indicated that low doses of caffeine are a successful aid in keeping weight under control after initial weight loss, by keeping metabolism optimally active, and calorie-burning efficient.

Some of the health problems of caffeine are also well known - headaches and migraines, irritability, stomach and digestive problems, anxiety and high blood pressure. As an addictive stimulant, it works as a drug, causing jumpiness and nerves, heart disease, heart palpitations.

Caffeine, **in excessive amounts,** can produce oxalic acid in the system, causing a host of problems waiting to become diseases. It can lodge in the liver, restricting proper function, and constrict arterial blood flow. It leaches out B vitamins from the body, particularly thiamine (for stress control). It depletes some essential minerals, including calcium and potassium. (Moderate amounts do not cause calcium depletion or contribute to bone loss.) Excessive caffeine affects the glands, particularly the adrenals, to exhaustion, causing hormonal imbalances to the point of becoming a major factor in the growth of breast and uterine fibroids in women, and prostate trouble in men. It has been indicated in PMS symptoms, bladder infections, and hypoglycemic/diabetic sugar reactions.

However the carcinogenic effects often blamed on caffeine are now thought to be caused by the roasting process used in making coffee, tea and chocolate. Since decaffeinated coffee has been implicated in some forms of organ cancer, conclusions are being drawn that caffeine is not the culprit - the roasted hydrocarbons are.

✦

Specific areas of health and the effects of caffeine include:

❖ **Caffeine and Pregnancy** - caffeine should be avoided during pregnancy. Like alcohol, it can cross the placenta and affect the fetus' brain, central nervous system and circulation. Recent studies have shown, however that there is *no* relationship between moderate caffeine intake and infertility.

❖ **Caffeine and Breast Disease** - there is official uncertainty about the link between caffeine and breast fibroids, but our own direct experience indicates almost immediate improvement when caffeine intake is decreased or avoided.

❖ **Caffeine and Heart Disease** - heavy coffee drinking (more than 4 cups a day), has been directly implicated in heart disease and high cholesterol. However, many of those early tests were flawed - HDLs (good cholesterol) rose proportionately with LDLs so that risk of heart disease did not increase.

❖ **Caffeine and High Blood Pressure** - excessive caffeine can elevate blood pressure significantly and produce nervous anxiety. This is particularly true when caffeine is combined with phenyl-propanolamine, the appetite suppressant in commercial diet pills.

❖ **Caffeine and Sleep Quality** - caffeine consumed late in the day or at night jeopardizes the quality of sleep by disrupting brain wave patterns. It also means you will take longer to get to sleep.

❖ **Caffeine and Ulcers** - caffeine stimulates gastic secretions, sometimes leading to a nervous stomach or heartburn. However, it is the key "bitter" in the western diet, stimulating bile secretions needed for good digestion. Caffeine *has not* been linked to either gastric or duodenal ulcers.

❖ **Caffeine and Headaches** - caffeine definitely causes headaches in some people - and causes withdrawal headaches when avoided after regular use. As a traditional remedy for temporary relief of migraines, the inherent niacin content of coffee *increases* when the beans are roasted.

❖ **Caffeine and PMS** - caffeine causes congestion through a cellular overproduction of fibrous tissue and cyst fluids. However, low-dose caffeine intake can improve memory and alertness during the menstrual phase. Reducing, rather than avoiding caffeine during menses may offer the best of both worlds.

❖ **Caffeine and Cancer** - recent world-wide studies on breast and bladder cancer have shown no cause relationship between these diseases and caffeine. However, the acidic body state promoted by caffeine is not beneficial to the healing process as the body works to alter its chemistry during healing.

Caffeine is just as difficult as any other addiction to overcome, but if you have any of the above-mentioned health problems, it is worth going through the temporary withdrawal symptoms. Improvement in the problem condition is often noticed right away.

There are good foods to help break the caffeine habit: herb teas, delicious coffee substitutes such as Roma, carob treats instead of chocolate, plain aspirin in place of Excedrin, and energy supportive herbal pick-me-ups with no harmful stimulants of any kind. Use green tea and kola nut as bio-active forms of caffeine for weight loss and mental clarity. Neither has the heated hydrocarbons of coffee that are known to be carcinogenic. (See *About Natural Stimulants & Energizers* in this book.)

✤

The following chart shows amounts of caffeine in common foods so you can make an informed choice.

FOOD	APPROX. AMT. of CAFFEINE
Coffee, one 5 oz. cup	
Decaf	4mg.
Instant	65mg.
Percolated	100mg.
Drip	125mg.
Tea, one 5 oz. cup	
Bag, brewed for 3 minutes	40mg.
Loose, black, brewed for 3 minutes	50mg.
Loose, green, brewed for 3 minutes	45mg.
Iced	30mg.
Cola Drinks, 12 oz. glass	45mg.
Chocolate/Cocoa, 5 oz. cup	5mg.
Milk chocolate, 1 oz.	5mg.
Bittersweet Chocolate, 1 oz.	30mg.

About Green & Black Teas

All black, green and Oolong teas come from *thea sinensis* an evergreen shrub that ranges from the Mediterranean to the tropics, and from sea level to 8000 feet. It can be harvested every 6-14 days depending on the area and climate, and yields tea leaves for 25-50 years. The kind of tea produced is differentiated by the manner in which the leaves are procressed. For green tea, the first tender leaves of spring are picked, then partially dried, rolled, steamed, crushed and dried with hot air. Oolong tea leaves have been allowed to semi-ferment for an hour. Black teas are partially dried, rolled on tile, glass or concrete, and fermented for 3 hours to strengthen aroma and flavor, and reduce bitterness. Black teas are often scented during fermentation with fresh flower blossoms or spices.

Tea nomenclature can be confusing. Names like oolong, black or jasmine tea refer to how the tea was processed. Names such as Assam, Darjeeling or Ceylon, etc., refer to the country or region where the tea was grown. Names such as pekoe, orange pekoe, etc., refer to the leaf size.

- **Bancha Leaf** - the tender spring leaves of the Japanese tea plant, containing unprocessed, bio-active caffeine for mental clarity and weight loss, and theophylline for asthmatic conditions. This is the green tea with the best therapeutic properties.
- **Kukicha Twig** - a smooth, roasted Japanese tea, made from the twigs and stems rather than the leaves of the tea plant. Containing much less caffeine and acidic oils than the leaves, this tea is a favorite in macrobiotic diets for its blood cleansing qualities, high calcium content, and roasted mellow flavor.
- **Darjeeling** - the finest, most delicately flavored of the black Indian teas.
- **Earl Grey** - a popular hearty, aromatic black tea that has been sprayed with bergamot oil.
- **English Breakfast** - a connoisseur's rich, mellow, fragrant black tea with Chinese flavor. It is a combination of Assam flowery orange pekoe and Ceylon broken orange pekoe.
- **Ceylon** - a tea grown in Sri Lanka with a intense, flowery aroma and flavor.
- **Irish Breakfast** - a combination of Assam flowery orange pekoe and Ceylon orange pekoe.
- **Jasmine** - a black tea scented with white jasmine flowers during firing.
- **Lapsang Souchong** - a fine black tea with a strong, smoky flavor.
- **Oolong** - a delicate tea with complex flavo that is semi-fermented and fired in baskets over hot coals.

✦

Green tea has the most dramatic effects in recent laboratory studies, and is preferred for therapeutic use. The leaves are not fermented, but steamed or simply dried after harvest, and therefore fully enzyme-active for asthma or weight loss and cleansing. Green tea is a vasodilator and smooth muscle relaxant in cases of bronchial asthma. It is rich in flavonoids that have anti-oxidant and anti-allergen activity. It has a long history as a beneficial fasting tea, providing energy support and clearer thinking during cleansing.

Recent research in Japan is showing that several cups of green tea on a regular daily basis are effective in reducing lung cancer death rates even in men who smoked two packs of cigarettes a day. Other studies in Tokyo are indicating the same success with stomach and liver cancer rates. Green tea testing shows indications of the ability to reduce serum cholesterol levels. It has also shown definite evidence of tumor and skin cancer prevention in animals, even when exposed to ultraviolet radiation.

Both black and green teas contain enough naturally-occurring fluoride to prevent tooth decay. Both contain polyphenols (not tannins as commonly believed) that act as anti-oxidants, yet do not interfere with iron or protein absorption. As with other anti-oxidants from plants, such as beta carotene and vitamin C, they appear to work at the molecular level, combatting free radical damage to protect against degenerative diseases.

About Sea Vegetables & Iodine Therapy

Sea vegetables have superior nutritional content. They transmit the energies of the sea as a rich source of proteins, complex carbohydrates, minerals and vitamins. Ounce for ounce, along with herbs, they are higher in vitamins and minerals than any other food group. **Sea vegetables** are one of nature's richest sources of vegetable protein, and they provide full-spectrum concentrations of beta carotene, chlorophyll, enzymes and soluble fiber. The distinctive salty taste is not just "salt", but a balanced, chelated combination of sodium, potassium, calcium, magnesium, phosphorus, iron and trace minerals. They convert inorganic ocean minerals into organic mineral salts that combine with amino acids. Our bodies can use this combination as an ideal way to get usable nutrients for structural building blocks. In fact, sea vegetables contain all the necessary trace elements for life, many of which are depleted in the earth's soil.

Sea vegetables are almost the only non-animal source of Vitamin B_{12} necessary for cell growth and nerve function. Their mineral balance is a natural tranquilizer for building sound nerve structure, and proper metabolism.

Sea vegetables alkalize the body, reduce excess stores of fluid and fat, and work to transform toxic metals in the system *(including radiation)*, into harmless salts that the body can eliminate. They purify the blood from acidity effects of the modern diet, allowing for better absorption of nutrients. They strengthen the body against disease.

In this era of processed foods and iodine-poor soils, **sea vegetables and sea foods** stand almost alone as potent sources of natural iodine. Iodine is essential to life, since the thyroid gland cannot regulate metabolism without it. It is an important element of alert, rapid brain activity, and a prime deterrent to arterial plaque. Iodine is also a key factor in the control and prevention of many endocrine deficiency conditions prevalent today, such as breast and uterine fibroids, tumors, prostate inflammation, adrenal exhaustion, and toxic liver and kidney states. Pregnant women who are deficient in iodine are more prone to giving birth to cretin babies, a form of retardation.

Iodine Therapy treatment for these conditions is addressed on the specific pages in this book, but **preventive measures** may be taken against iodine deficiency problems by just adding 2 tablespoons of chopped, dried sea vegetables to the daily diet.

Sea vegetables are delicious, and convenient to buy, store, and use as needed in their sun-dried form. Store them in a moisture proof container and they will keep indefinitely. A wide variety of sea vegetables is available today, both in macrobiotic and regular quality. These include: **Agar Agar, Arame, Bladderwrack, Dulse, Hijiki, Irish Moss, Kelp, Kombu, Nori, Sea Palm, Spirulina, and Wakame.** They may be crushed, chopped or snipped into soups and sauces, crumbled over pizzas, and used as toppings on casseroles and salads. If you add sea vegetables, no other salt is needed, an advantage for a low salt diet.

Here is a delicious salad, soup and topping blend to add sea veggies to your diet. Just *barely whirl in the blender so there are still sizeable chunks.* They will expand in any recipe with liquid, and when heated will return to a beautiful ocean green color.

❧ OCEAN THERAPY SPRINKLE
3/4 CUP CHOPPED DRIED DULSE
1/4 CUP CHOPPED DRIED WAKAME
1/4 CUP DRIED NORI OR SEA PALM
1/4 CUP CHOPPED DRIED KOMBU
1/2 CUP TOASTED SESAME SEEDS

❧

Seaweed baths are Nature's perfect body/psyche balancer. Remember how good you feel after a walk in the ocean? Seaweeds purify ocean pollutants, and they can do the same for your body.

Rejuvenating effects occur when toxins are released from the body. A hot seaweed bath is like a wet-steam sauna, only better, because the kelps and sea greens balance body chemistry instead of dehydrate it. The electrolytic magnetic action of the seaweed releases excess body fluids from congested cells, and dissolves fatty wastes through the skin, replacing them with depleted minerals, particularly potassium and iodine. Iodine boosts thyroid activity, taming the appetite and increasing metabolism so that food fuels are used before they can turn into fatty deposits. Eating sea vegies regularly also has this effect. Vitamin K is another key nutrient in seaweeds. This precursor vitamin helps regulate adrenal function, meaning that a seaweed bath can also help maintain hormone balance for a more youthful body.

How to take a seaweed bath:

If you live near the ocean, gather kelp and seaweeds from the water, (not the shoreline) in clean buckets or trash cans, and carry them home to your tub. If you don't live near the ocean, the dried kelp, sea vegies or whole dulse leaves available in most herb sections of health food stores can be a good alternative. Dried sea greens granules are also available from spa and natural body care firms, such as La Costa and Zia Cosmetics.

Whichever form you choose, run very hot water over the seaweed in a tub, filling it to the point that you will be covered when you recline. The leaves will turn a beautiful bright green if they are fresh. The water will turn a rich brown as the plants release their minerals. Add an herbal bath oil, if desired, to help hold the heat in, and pleasantly scent the water. Let the bath cool enough to get in. As you soak, the smooth gel from the seaweed will transfer onto your skin. This coating will increase perspiration to release toxins from your system, and replace them by osmosis with minerals. Rub the skin with the seaweed leaves during the bath to stimulate circulation, smooth the body, and remove wastes coming out on the skin surface. When the sea greens have done their therapeutic work, the gel coating will dissolve and float off the skin, and the leaves will shrivel - a sign that the bath is over. Each bath varies with the individual, the seaweeds used, and water temperature, but the gel coating release is a natural timekeeper for the bath's benefits. Forty five minutes to an hour is usually long enough to balance the acid/ alkaline system, and encourage liver activity and fat metabolism. Skin tone and color, and circulatory strength are almost immediatly noticeable from the iodine and potassium absorption. After the bath, take a capsule of cayenne and ginger powder to put these minerals quickly through the system.

Note: Overheating and iodine therapy are two of the most effective treatments in natural healing. They are powerful and should be used with care. If you are under medical supervision for heart disease or high blood pressure, check with your physician to determine if a seaweed bath is all right for you.

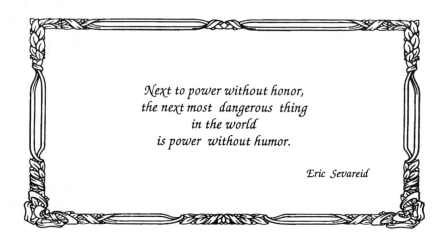

Next to power without honor,
the next most dangerous thing
in the world
is power without humor.

Eric Sevareid

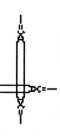

About Green Superfoods

Green foods are rich sources of essential nutrients. We are all adding more salads and green vegetables to our diets. However, because of the great concern for the nutritional quality of produce grown on mineral depleted soils, green superfoods, such as chlorella, spirulina, barley green, wheat grass and alfalfa have become popular. They are nutritionally more potent than regular foods, and are carefully grown and harvested to maximize vitamin, mineral and amino acid concentrations.

Green, and blue-green algae, (phyto-plankton), have been called perfect superfoods, with abundant amounts of high quality, digestible protein, fiber, chlorophyll, vitamins, minerals and enzymes. They are the most potent source of beta carotene available in the world today. They are the richest food source of vitamin B_{12}, higher than liver, chlorella or sea vegetables. Their protein yield is greater than soy beans, corn or beef. They are the only foods sources, other than mother's milk, of GLA, (gamma-linolenic acid). GLA is an essential fatty acid, a precursor to the body's master hormones. Deficiencies in GLA contribute to obesity, heart disease, and PMS. Phyto-plankton are also used therapeutically to stimulate the immune system, improve digestion and assimilation, detoxify the body, enhance growth and tissue repair, accelerate healing, protect against radiation, help prevent degenerative disease and promote longer life.

❧

Chlorella contains a higher concentration of chlorophyll than any other known plant. It is a complete protein food, contains all the B vitamins, vitamin C and E and many minerals actually high enough to be considered supplementary amounts. The cell wall material of chlorella has a particular effect on intestinal and bowel health, detoxifying the colon, stimulating peristaltic activity, and promoting the growth of beneficial bacteria. Chlorella is effective in eliminating heavy metals, such as lead, mercury, copper and cadmium. Antitumor research shows it as an important source of beta carotene in healing. It strengthens the liver, the body's major detoxifying organ, so that it can free the system of infective agents that destroy immune defenses. It reduces arthritis stiffness, lowers blood pressure, relieves gastritis and ulcers. Its rich nutritional content has made it effective in weight loss programs, both for cleansing ability, and in maintaining muscle tone during lower food intake. But its most important benefits seem to come from a combination of molecules that biochemists call the *Controlled Growth Factor*, a unique composition that provides a a noticeable increase in sustained energy and immune health when eaten on a regular basis.

❧

Spirulina is the original green superfood, an easily produced algae with the ability to grow in both ocean and alkaline waters. It is ecologically sound in that it can be cultivated in extreme environments which are useless for conventional agriculture. It can be cultivated on small scale community farms, doubling its bio-mass every two to five days, in such a variety of climates and growing conditions that it could significantly improve the nutrition of local populations currently on the brink of starvation. Research has shown that spirulina alone could double the protein available to humanity on a fraction of the world's land, while helping restore the environmental balance of the planet. Acre for acre, spirulina yields *20 times* more protein than soybeans, *40 times* more protein than corn, and *400 times* more protein than beef. It is a complete protein, providing all 21 amino acids, and the entire B complex of vitamins, including B_{12}. It is rich in beta carotene, minerals, trace minerals, and essential fatty acids. Digestibility is high, stimulating both immediate and long range energy.

❧

Aloe Vera has long been known as an effective skin moisturizer and healer. Its medicinal uses for the skin range from cuts, sunburn, bruises and insect bites, to the healing of ulcerated skin sores, acne, exzema and serious burns. It is a natural antiseptic and astringent for infections both internal and external. It is a natural oxygenator, increasing the body's uptake of oxygen. The juice has become a specific for colon cleansing and colon problems. Recent research is indicating even more wonderful healing results from this superfood - for arthritis, skin cancers, hemorrhoids and varicose veins. Aged aloe vera juice is being widely used in AIDS treatment to block the HIV virus movement from cell to cell.

The green grasses contain all the known mineral and trace mineral elements, a balanced range of vitamins, and hundreds of enzymes for digestion and absorption. The small molecular proteins in these plants can be absorbed directly into the blood for cell metabolism. They are highly therapeutic from the chlorophyll activity absorbed directly through the cell membranes.

Barley Grass contains a broad spectrum of concentrated vitamins, minerals, enzymes, proteins and chlorophyllins. It has eleven times the calcium of cow's milk, five times the iron of spinach, and seven times the amount of vitamin C and bioflavonoids as orange juice. One of its most important contributions is to the vegetarian diet with 80mcg of vitamin B_{12} per hundred grams of powdered juice. Research on barley grass shows encouraging results for DNA damage repair and anti-aging activity. It is an ideal food-source anti-inflammatory agent for healing stomach and duodenal ulcers, hemorrhoids, and for pancreas infections.

Wheat Grass has great curative powers for many degenerative "incurable" diseases when taken as a fresh liquid. Fifteen pounds of fresh wheat grass are equal in nutritional value to 350 pounds of the most choice vegetables. In tablet or powder form it provides highly concentrated food for both people and animals who need more dietary greens and roughage.

Alfalfa is one of the world's richest mineral foods, pulling up earth sources from root depths as great as 130 feet! It is the basis for liquid chlorophyll, with a balance of chemical and mineral constituents almost identical to human hemoglobin. It is used therapeutically for arthritis, a wide range of intestinal and skin disorders, liver problems, breath and body odor, and even cancer.

In essence, eating any of the above green superfoods is like giving yourself a little transfusion to help treat illness, enhance immunity and sustain well-being. They have a synergistic and beneficial effect when added to a normal diet. The green superfoods are valuable in almost all of the healing diets. Over the years we have found the incredible claims about their valuable benefits to have substance and truth.

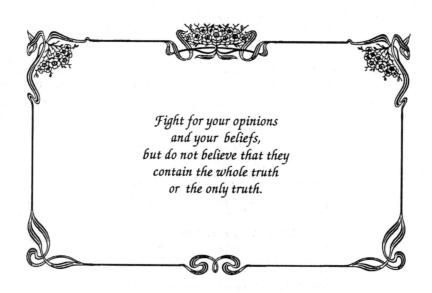

Fight for your opinions
and your beliefs,
but do not believe that they
contain the whole truth
or the only truth.

About Bee Pollen, Royal Jelly & Propolis

❀ **BEE POLLEN** - collected by bees from male seed flowers, mixed with secretion from the bee, and formed into granules. A highly bio-active, tonic nutrient rightly known as a "superfood". Completely balanced for vitamins, minerals, proteins, carbohydrates, fats, enzyme presursors, and all essential amino acids. Bee pollen is a full-spectrum blood building and rejuvenative substance, particularly beneficial for the extra nutritional and energy needs of athletes and those recuperating from illness. It is often used as a tree pollen and spore antidote during allergy season. Bee Pollen also relieves other respiratory problems such as bronchitis, sinusitis and colds. Like royal jelly, pollen helps balance the endocrine system, showing especially beneficial results in menstrual and prostate problems. The enzyme support in bee pollen normalizes chronic colitis and constipation/diarrhea syndromes. Recent research has shown that pollen helps counteract the effects of aging, and increases both mental and physical capability. Two teaspoons daily is the usual dose. Use only unsprayed pollen for therapeutic applications.

❀ **ROYAL JELLY** - the milk-like secretion from the head glands of the queen bee's nurse-workers. It is a powerhouse of B vitamins, the minerals calcium, iron, potassium and silicon, enzyme precursors, a sex hormone and the eight essential amino acids. In fact, it contains every nutrient necessary to support life. It is a natural anti-biotic, stimulates the immune system, deep cellular health and longevity, and has been found effective for a wide range of health benefits.
Royal jelly supplies key nutrients for energy, mental alertness and general well-being. It is one of the world's richest sources of pantothenic acid, known to combat stress, fatigue and insomnia, and is a necessary nutrient for proper digestion and healthy skin and hair. It has been found effective for gland and hormone imbalances that reflect in menstrual and prostate problems.
The highest quality royal jelly products are preserved in their whole, raw, "alive" state, which promotes ready absorption by the body. As little as one drop of pure, extracted fresh royal jelly can deliver an adequate daily supply. If capsules are used, best results are achieved from the freeze dried substance.

❀ **BEE PROPOLIS** - a product collected by bees from the resin under the bark of certain trees. As the first line of defense against beehive micro-organisms, it is a natural antibiotic, antiviral and antifungal substance. In humans it stimulates the thymus gland and thus boosts immunity and resistance to infection. Propolis is rich in bioflavonoids and amino acids and a strong source of trace minerals such as copper, magnesium, silicon, iron, manganese and zinc. It is high in B vitamins, C, E and Beta-carotene. Like all bee products, it has strong antibiotic properties. It is also a powerful anti-viral that is effective against pneumonia and similar viral infections.
Propolis has a wide range of successful therapeutic uses. It is used to treat stomach and other intestinal ulcers. It speeds the healing of broken bones, and accelerates new cell growth. It is part of almost every natural treatment for gum, mouth and throat disorders. Research on propolis and serum blood fats has confirmed its traditional reputation for lowering high blood pressure, reducing arterioscleriosis and lessening the risks of coronary heart disease. New testing is currently being done on propolis and its healing effects on certain skin cancers and melanomas.
Propolis is available in several medicinal forms: a thick, concentrated tincture for applying to warts, herpes lesions or other sores, a lighter, more soluble concentration to mix with liquids and take internally, and in chewable lozenges for mouth, throat and gum healing. The normal dosage is 300mg. daily.

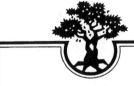

Life gives you surprises,
and
surprises give you life.

About Food Grade Hydrogen Peroxide

Much controversy has surrounded the use of H_2O_2 Food Grade Hydrogen Peroxide for therapeutic anti-infective and anti-fungal applications. Our experience with this source of nascent oxygen has been successful in many areas, **but a great deal of that success is predicated on the way H_2O_2 is used. Directions with this therapeutic product are very specific as to dosage and ailment. Read the bottle label carefully before embarking on a program that includes H_2O_2 to insure success.** Food Grade H_2O_2 is available in two refrigerated forms in health food stores.

✻ **35% FOOD GRADE** - is the strongest available solution and **must be diluted** before external or internal use. **Mix 1 oz. of 35% solution with 11 oz. distilled water for 12 oz. of 3% H_2O_2.**
☞ *Note: At the time of this writing, Vital Health, the main supplier for 35% H_2O_2 has been constrained by the FDA from shipping this form. However, a kit with instructions from Vital Health is available for public use.*
☞ *Note: Do not use H_2O_2 if you have had a heart transplant.*

The **3% dilute solution** may be used internally for serious complaints where higher tissue oxygen is needed to control disease growth. Particular response has been noted for asthma, emphysema, arthritis, Candida albicans, Epstein-Barr virus, certain cancerous growths, and other degenerative conditions such as AIDS and ARC. Other applications for a **3% dilute solution** include athlete's foot, and other fungal conditions; as a douche for vaginal infections; and as an enema or colonic solution during cleansing. It may be used as a mouthwash, skin spray, or on cotton balls to replace the skin's acid mantle that has been removed by soap. Like many antibiotics, H_2O_2 will also kill friendly bacterial culture in the digestive tract. Take an acidophilus supplement or eat some plain yogurt after taking H_2O_2.

✻ **FOOD GRADE GEL** - (Care Products OXY-PLUS GEL), combined with aloe vera juice, vegetable glycerine, and red seaweed extract, is the most popular form for general application, both as an antiseptic and antifungal. It may be applied topically to affected areas on the skin, or massaged into the soles of the feet where the pores are large. It can reach most parts of the body through them. It may also be taken internally for detoxification, using $1/2$ teaspoon of the gel and $1/4$ teasp. powdered ascorbate Vitamin C to an 8 oz. glass of water.
One teaspoon of peroxide gel combination provides 15 drops of 35% H_2O_2.

External and topical uses:
- For athlete's foot, minor cuts, burns and bruises, and insect bites, apply from the bottle.
- For a colon cleansing colonic: use $1/2$ pint of 3% dilute solution to 5 gallons water.
- For a vaginal douche: use 6 TBS. of 3% dilute solution to 1 qt. water.
- For pet health, use 1 oz. 3% H_2O_2 to 1 qt. water; for large animals, use 2 oz. to 1 gallon water.
- For plant health and growth, use 1 oz. 3% solution in 1 qt. water.

Oxygen baths are valuable detoxifying agents, and can noticeably increase body energy and tissue oxygen uptake. Vital Health brand **food grade 35% hydrogen peroxide** is a popular, effective product. About 1 cup per bath or spa produces significant effect for 3 to 7 days. Oxygen baths are stimulating rather than relaxing. An energy increase is usually noticed right away. Other therapeutic benefits include body balance and detoxification, reduction of skin cancers and tumors, clearing of asthma and lung congestion, arthritis and rheumatism relief, and other conditions where increased body oxygen can prevent and control disease. Add $1/2$ cup sea salt and $1/2$ cup baking soda for extra benefits.

In most applications, especially those where anti-infective and antifungal properties are needed, we have found it more beneficial to **use H_2O_2 in an alternating series**, (usually 10 days of use, and then 10 days of rest, or 3 weeks of use, and 3 weeks of rest, in more serious cases)

About Anti-Oxidants, Free Radicals & Free Radical Scavengers

"Very few people reach their maximum potential life span. The die prematurely of wide variety of diseases - the vast majority of which are free radical diseases."

Anti-oxidants are a health byword of the nineties. They protect against the free radical attacks that are the forerunners of premature aging, heart attacks, cancer, and the opportunistic diseases such as AIDS, Candidiasis, Chronic Fatigue Syndrome, etc., that assault lowered immune defenses. Anti-oxidants "scavenge" free radicals, neutralize their damage and render them harmless.

Free radicals play a key role in the deterioration of the body. They are highly active compounds produced when fat molecules react with oxygen. They are part of normal metabolic breakdown, but also increasingly present in air pollutants, tobacco smoke, rancid foods and hydro-carbons. They are, therefore a constant presence that can be quite harmful to the body cells. After years of free radical assaults and and oxidation in cell membranes, cells become irreplaceably lost from major organs, such as the lungs, liver, kidneys and brain. This cell loss is seen as a primary cause of the deterioration effects of aging. Cells of the nervous system are particularly vulnerable to attack often resulting in senile dementia and Alzheimer's disease.

Free radical damage is linked to many degenerative diseases. Heart disease, atherosclerosis, arthritis, cancer, and immune deficiency. Damage to connective tissue results in loss of skin tone and elasticity. Wrinkling and aging skin texture occur primarily on parts of the body exposed to environmental free radical sources. A high fat diet is known to depress the body's inherent anti-oxidant enzyme response.

THE MOST POTENT ANTI-OXIDANTS

The body's own protection against free radical attack is a complex system of enzymes and nutrients that keep them in check. Some are produced internally. Others are supplied by the diet. A poor diet, inadequate exercise, illness and emotional stress result in a reduction of inherent, system anti-oxidants.

✤ **Pycnogenol** - a concentrated, highly active bioflovonoid extract from pine bark, grapeseed and other fruits. Fifty times stronger than vitamin E, 20 times stronger than vitamin C, it is one of the few dietary anti-oxidants that readily crosses the blood-brain barrier to directly protect brain cells and aid memory.

✤ **CoQ 10** - an essential catalyst co-enzyme for cellular energy in the body. The body's ability to assimilate food source CoQ10 declines with age. Supplementation provides wide ranging therapeutic benefits. See *About Enzymes & Enzyme Therapy*, pg. 29.

✤ **Germanium** - should be used only as *organic* sesquioxide. A potent adaptogen that detoxifies, blocks free radicals and increases production of natural killer cells. An interferon stimulus for immune strength and healing.

✤ **Ginkgo Biloba** - used therapeutically to combat the effects of aging. Protects the cells against damage from free radicals. Reduces blood cell clumping which leads to congestive heart disease.

✤ **Glutathione Peroxidase** - an anti-oxidant enzyme that scavenges and neutralizes cell-damaging free radicals by turning them into stable oxygen and H_2O_2, and then into oxygen and water. See *About Enzymes & Enzyme Therapy*, pg. 29.

✤ **SOD, Super-Oxide Dismutase** - an anti-oxidant enzyme that works with catalase to scavenge and neutralize free radicals. See *About Enzymes & Enzyme Therapy*, pg. 29.

✤ **Astragalus** - a strong immune enhancer and body tonic. Aids adrenal function. Vasodilating properties lower blood pressure, increase metabolism and improve circulation.

✤ **GLA, Gamma Linoleic Acid** - obtained from evening primrose oil, black currant oil and borage seed oil. A source of energy for the cells, electrical insulation for nerve fibers, a precursor of prostaglandins which regulate hormone and metabolic functions.

✤ **Shiitake mushrooms** (called oyster mushrooms when fresh) - produce a virus which stimulates interferon in the body for stronger immune function. Promote vitality and longevity. Used in Oriental medicine to prevent high blood pressure and heart disease, and to reduce cholesterol.

✤ **Reishi mushrooms** (ganoderma) - a tonic that increases vitality, enhances immunity and prolongs a healthy life. Helps reduce the side effects of chemotherapy for cancer.

✤ **Tyrosine, an amino acid formed from phenylalnine** - a growth hormone stimulant that helps to build the body's natural store of adrenalin and thyroid hormones. Rapidly metabolized throughout the body. A source of quick energy, especially for the brain.

✤ **Methionine** - a free radical de-activator and "lipotropic" that keeps fats from accumulating in the liver and arteries. Protective against chemical allergic reactions.

✤ **DiMethyl-Glycine** (once commonly known as B15) - an energy stimulant, used chiefly by athletes for endurance and stamina. Sublingual forms are most absorbable. For best results, take before sustained exercise. *Note: Too much DMG disrupts the metabolic chain and causes fatigue. The proper dose produces energy, overdoses do not.*

✤ **L-Glutathione** - an amino acid that works with cysteine and glutamine as a glucose tolerance factor and anti-oxidant to neutralize radiation toxicity and inhibit free radicals. Cleans the blood from the effects of chemotherapy, x-rays and liver toxicity.

✤ **Cysteine** - works with vitamins C, E, and selenium to protect against radiation toxicity, cancer carcinogens, and free radical damage to skin and arteries. Stimulates white cell activity in the immune system. Aids in body uptake of iron. *Note: Take vitamin C in a 3:1 ratio to cysteine for best results.*

✤ **Octacosanol** - a wheat germ derivative, used therapeutically to counteract fatigue and increase oxygen utilization during exercise and athletic sports.

✤ **Egg lipids, egg yolk lecithin** - a powerful, therapeutic source of choline and phosphatides. Used in the treatment of AIDS and other immune-deficient diseases. Must be refrigerated and taken immediately upon mixing with water to retain potency.

✤ **Wheat Germ Oil** - extracted from the embryo of the wheat berry. Rich in B vitamins, proteins, vitamin E, and iron. Goes rancid quickly. Refrigerate after opening. One tablespoon provides the anti-oxidant equivalent of an oxygen tent for 30 minutes.

See *Glossary of Healing Foods & Neutraceuticals*, pg. 64, and individual nutrient sections for complete information about these anti-oxidants.

THE MAIN ANTIOXIDANTS IN FOODS:

✤ **Selenium** - a component of glutathione. Protects the body from free radical damage and heavy metal toxicity. **Sources:** bran, brewer's yeast, broccoli, cabbage, celery, corn, cucumbers, garlic, mushrooms, onions, wheat germ, whole grains.

HOW FREE RADICALS WORK

Food + oxygen

metabolism

Energy + free radicals

Only 95-98% of free radicals formed in the body are efficiently consumed to provide energy - leaving 2 to 5% to participate in other, non-

Free radicals + cell structures

Oxidative cell damage

✤ **Vitamin E** - a fat soluble anti-oxidant and immune stimulant whose activty is increased by selenium. Neutralizes free radicals against the effects of aging. An effective anti-coagulant and vaso-dilator against blood clots and heart disease. **Sources:** almonds, walnuts, apricots, corn, safflower and peanut oil, peanut butter, wheat germ.

✤ **Beta-carotene** - a vitamin A precurser, converting to A in the liver as the body needs it. A powerful anti-infective and anti-oxidant for immune health, protection against environmental pollutants, slowing the aging process, and allergy control. **Sources:** cantaloupe, carrots, kale, mango, nectarine, papaya, prunes, spinach, squash, sweet potatoes, sea vegetables.

✤ **Vitamin C** - a primary factor for prevention of free radical damage, immune strength and health maintenance. Protects against viral and bacterial infections. Safeguards against radiation, heavy metal toxicity, environmental pollutants and early aging. Essential to formation of new collagen tissue. Supports adrenal and iron insuffiency, especially when the body is under stress. **Sources:** broccoli, brussels sprouts, grapefruit, kale, kiwi, oranges, potatoes, strawberries.

Note: The cancer-fighting potential of vitamins A, C, E, the trace mineral selenium, and beta carotene is enhanced when these anti-oxidant nutrients are taken together.

Life is the art of drawing without an eraser.

About Natural Stimulants & Energizers

The most common reason for taking stimulants is fatigue, both mental and physical. Stimulants increase the action or function of a system or metabolic process. They can create a sense of well-being, exhilaration, and self-confidence. They relieve fatigue and drowsiness. The downside to many stimulants is tolerance, dependency, lethargy, irritableness, nervousness, and restlessness. There may be difficulty in concentrating and after-effect headaches. Increasing the strength of a stimulant can increase the toxicity and/or dependency potential. Taken too often, even natural stimulants can drive a body system to exhaustion.

In combatting fatigue of all kinds, natural energizers have great advantages over chemically processed stimulants. They have more broad based activity so that they don't exhaust a paticular organ or body system. They can be strong or gentle for individual needs. In general, they are nutrient supportive rather than depleting. Specific natural remedies for fatigue can be classed under central nervous system stimulants, metabolic enhancers, and adaptogens.

➡ **Central Nervous System** (CNS) stimulants act by affecting the cerebral cortex and the medulla of the brain. Most contain either natural caffeine, naturally-occurring ephedrine, or certain free-form amino acids. In general, these substances promote alertness, energy, and a more rapid, clearer flow of thought. They also act as respiratory stimulants

➡ **Metabolic Enhancers** improve the performance of existing biochemical pathways by providing catalysts and co-factors for system support. They do not stress or deplete the body. Examples of these substances include co-enzyme factors like B vitamins, fat mobilizers like Carnitine, electron transporters such as CoQ 10, lactic acid limiters like inosine and gamma oryzonal, and tissue oxygenators like DiMethyl-Glycine (B$_{15}$).

➡ **Adaptogens** are regulators that help the body to handle stress, and maintain vitality. They are rich sources of important strengthening nutrients such as germanium, and steroid-like compounds which can provide concentrated body support. They increase the body's overall immune function with broad spectrum activity, rather than specific action. They promote recovery from illness and may be used synergistically with other tonic herbs to build strength. They are particularly beneficial in restoring the endocrine, nervous, digestive, muscle, and hepatic systems. They are usually for long term revitalization rather than immediate energy.

The following chart offers a quick look at natural stimulants and what they do. See *Glossary of Healing Foods & Neutraceuticals*, pg. 65, and individual nutrient sections for complete information about their properties, activity and benefits.

CENTRAL NERVOUS SYSTEM STIMULANTS

➡ **Coffee and caffeine** - America's most popular stimulant. See *About Caffeine*, pg. 82.

➡ **Guarana** - a rich, natural source of rainforest guaranine, for long, slow endurance energy without coffee's heated hydrocarbons that pose health problems.

➡ **Kola Nut** - a rich, natural source of caffeine from Africa, without heated hydrocarbons. Allays hunger, combats fatigue.

➡ **L-Phenylalanine** - a tyrosine precurser that works with B$_6$ as an antidepressant and mood elevator on the central nervous system. Successful in treating manic, post-amphetamine, and schizophrenic depression. Aids in learning and memory retention. A thyroid stimulant that helps curb the appetite by increasing the body's production of CCK. See *Amino Acids*, pg. 23.

➡ **Glutamine** - converts readily into 6-carbon glucose, and is therefore one of the best nutrients and energy sources for the brain. Rapidly improves memory retention, recall, sustained concentration, and alertness. Improves mental performance in cases of retardation, senility, and schizophrenia. Increases libido and helps overcome impotence. See *Amino Acids*, pg. 23.

➡ **Tyrosine** - helps build adrenalin and thyroid stores. Rapidly metabolized as an anti-oxidant throughout the body, and effective as a source of quick energy, especially for the brain. A safe therapy for depression, hypertension, in controlling drug abuse and aiding drug withdrawal. Increases libido and low sex drive. A growth hormone stimulant. See *Amino Acids*, pg. 23.

➡ **Yerba Maté** - a South American stimulant and rejuvenating herb that contains no caffeine. Naturally lifts fatigue and provides broad range nutrition to body cells. Rich in vitamins, C, B, (particularly pantothenic acid), A and E, with measureable amounts of chlorophyll, calcium, potassium, iron, magnesium and manganese. Protects against the effects of stress. Helpful in opening respiratory passages to overcome allergy symptoms. In addition to its inherent benefits, yerba maté is a catalyst substance that increases the healing effectiveness of other herbs.

➡ **Ephedra** - a long lasting CNS stimulant that calms the mind as it stimulates the body. Contains ephedrine and pseudo-ephedrine. Acts as an energy tonic to strengthen and restore body vitality. (Excellent for mental energy during a long test or meditation.) A strong, natural bronchodilator and decongestant for respiratory problems. Used in many weight loss formulas for its ability to increase metabolism. It is a cardiac stimulant and should be used with caution by anyone with high blood pressure.

➡ **Ginkgo Biloba** - a primary brain and mental energy stimulant. Increases both peripheral and cerebral circulation through vasodilation. An excellent choice as a stimulant for older people who suffer from poor memory and other aging-related CNS problems. Causes an increase in acetyl-choline levels, and therefore the ability to better transmit body electrical impulses. Best results are achieved from the extract.

➡ **Damiana** - a mild aphrodisiac, synergistic with other energy herbs in stimulating libido. A specific in a combination to treat frigidity in women and impotence in men. A mild anti-depressant tonic for the central nervous and hormonal systems.

➡ **Yohimbe** - a hormone stimulant, particularly effective in the production of testosterone. A strong aphrodisiac affecting both the male impotence and female frigidity. An effective bodybuilding and athletic formula herb where more testosterone production is desired. *Note:* Avoid if there is high blood pressure or heart arrythmia.

Note: Even when there is no dependency, most central nervous system stimulants should be for short-term use. Long term use can result in a net loss of energy and strength to the system. Most stimulants should also be avoided during pregnancy.

METABOLIC ENHANCERS

➡ **Ginger** - a warming circulatory stimulant and body cleansing herb, with effectiveness for cramping, indigestion, nausea, coughs, sinisitis, and sore throat. A catalyst in all formulas where circulation to the extremities is needed, (as in arthritis); for respiratory and lung/chest clearing combinations; in digestive system stimulants and alkalizers for clearing gas; as an aid in promoting menstrual regularity and relief from cramping and sluggishness; for all kinds of nausea, motion sickness and morning sickness; as a direct compress with cayenne to stimulate venous circulation. *Secondary uses:* as a catalyst in nervine and sedative formulas; as a gargle and part of a sore throat syrup; as a diaphoretic where sweating is needed for removing toxic wastes; as a stimulant to the kidneys for extra filtering activity;

➡ **Capsicum** - increases thermogenesis for weight loss, especially when combined with caffeine herbs or ephedra. Gives the system a little cardiovascular lift by increasing circulation. Works chiefly as a catalyst to enhance the performance of other herbs in a formula.

➡ **Bee Pollen** - a highly nutritive, tonic substance rightly known as a "superfood". Completely balanced for vitamins, minerals, proteins, carbohydrates, fats, and all essential amino acids. Use only unsprayed pollen for therapeutic applications. A full-spectrum building and rejuvenative substance, particularly for the extra nutritional and energy needs of athletes and those recuperating from illness. See *About Bee Pollen & Royal Jelly,* pg. 90.

➡ **Royal Jelly** - supplies key nutrients for energy, mental alertness and a general feeling of well-being. Enhances immunity and deep cellular health. One of the world's richest sources of pantothenic acid, which is known to combat stress, fatigue and insomnia. See *About Bee Pollen & Royal Jelly,* pg. 90.

➡ **Green Tea** - rich in flavonoids that have anti-oxidant and anti-allergen activity. It has a long history as a beneficial fasting tea, providing energy support and clearer thinking during cleansing. Contain polyphenols (not tannins as commonly believed) that act as anti-oxidants, yet do not interfere with iron or protein absorption. As with other anti-oxidants from plants, such as beta carotene and vitamin C, the green tea substances work at the molecular level, combatting free radical damage to protect against degenerative diseases. See *About Black & Green Teas,* pg. 84.

➡ **Rosemary** - an anti-oxidant herb and strong brain and memory stimulant. A circulatory toning agent, and effective nervine for stress, tension and depression.

➡ **Oats** - a long term metabolic stimulant that balances body chemistry, making easier for those trying to quit smoking or recover from addictions. A nerve and gland restorative. Use as an extract for best results.
➡ **CoQ 10** - an essential catalyst co-enzyme for cellular energy in the body. The body's ability to assimilate food source CoQ 10 declines with age. Supplementation provides wide ranging therapeutic benefits. See *About Enzymes & Enzyme Therapy*, pg. 29 .
➡ **DMG - DiMethyl-Glycine** - once commonly known as B15 - a powerful anti-oxidant and energy stimulant. Used successfully to improve Down's Syndrome and mental retardation cases, and to curb craving in alcohol addiction. DMG is a highly reputed energizer and stimulant whose effects can be attributed to its conversion to glycine. See *Amino Acids*, pg. 23.

ADAPTOGENS

➡ **Germanium** - should be used only as *organic* sesquioxide. A potent adaptogen that detoxifies, blocks free radicals and increases production of natural killer cells. An interferon stimulus for immune strength and healing. See *About Minerals & Trace Minerals*, pg. 20.
➡ **Panax Ginseng,** (Red, White and American Ginsengs) - the most effective adaptogen of all tonic herbs. Beneficial to total health and capable of stimulating both long and short term energy. Ginseng has measurable amounts of germanium, provides energy to all body systems, promotes regeneration from stress and fatigue, and rebuilds foundation strength. A central nervous system stimulant that also enhances improved sleep. Very nourishing to male reproductive and circulatory systems. Red Ginseng is particularly benificial for men since it promotes testosterone production. White and American Ginsengs are useful as stimulants for brain and memory centers for women as well as men. Ginseng benefits are cumulative in the body. Taking this herb for several months to a year is far more effective than short term doses.
➡ **Siberian Ginseng,** (Eleuthero) - a long-term tonic that supports the adrenal glands.
➡ **Schizandra** - synergistic with eleuthero for anti-stress, weight loss and sports endurance formulas. Works to support sugar regulation, and liver function and strength. Helps correct skin problems through better digestion of fatty foods.
➡ **Astragalus** - a superior tonic and strong immune enhancing herb. Provides therapeutic support for recovery from illness or surgery, (especially from chemotherapy and radiation.). Nourishes exhausted adrenals to combat fatigue. Also effective in normalizing the nervous, hormonal and immune systems.
➡ **Suma** - an ancient herb with modern results for overcoming fatigue, and hormonal imbalance. Used to rebuild the system from the ravages of cancer and diabetes.
➡ **Gotu Kola** - a brain and nervous system restorative. Wound-healing capabilities.
➡ **Fo-Ti,** (Ho-Shou-Wu)- a flavonoid-rich herb with particular success in longevity formulas. A cardiovascular strengthener, increasing blood flow to the heart.
➡ **Tienchi** - a Japanese ginseng-type herb. Used as a cardiac and blood tonic - particularly for athletes. Helps dissolve blood clots and circulatory obstructions.
➡ **Burdock** - a highly nutritional, hormone balancing herb; antibacterial, antifungal and antitumor. strong liver purifying and hormone balancing herb, with particular value for skin, arthritic, and glandular problems. A specific in all blood cleansing and detoxification combinations. An important anti-inflammatory and anti-infective herb.
➡ **Reishi** - an adaptogen mushroom for blood sugar regulation, deep immune support, anti-cancer and anti-oxidant properties, liver regeneration activity, and radiation protection. Helps strengthen those recovering from long-term illness. Excellent for children.

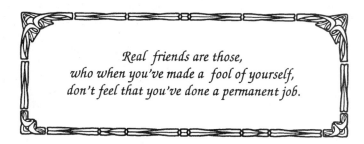

*Real friends are those,
who when you've made a fool of yourself,
don't feel that you've done a permanent job.*

Exercise - A Key To Maintaining Health

Exercise is an integral part of health. It's not just for athletes anymore. The Center for Disease Control says that a sedentary lifestyle has the effect on heart disease risk of smoking a pack of cigarettes a day! We all know that exercise speeds results in weight loss and heart recovery, but regular exercise helps any healing program. It strengthens the whole body - muscles, nerves, blood, glands, lungs, heart, brain, mind and mood. It increases metabolic rate, tissue oxygen uptake, respiratory and circulatory vigor. **Even if you didn't reduce your calorie intake, but added exercise, you would still lose weight and increase body tone.** Every exercise helps. Choose those that work for you conveniently and easily. Every series of stretches and exercises you do tones, elasticizes, shapes and contours your skin, connective tissue and muscles. **Aerobic exercise** is the best for whole body tone; the key to long-term weight and stress control, reduced cholesterol, and a stronger heart. It also stimulates antibody production, enhancing immune response. Aerobic exercise is easy, and as available as your front door.

▨ **A daily walk,** breathing deeply, for even a mile a day ($1/2$ mile out, $1/2$ mile back) makes a big difference in lung capacity and tissue oxygen. A thirty minute walk is almost a necessity for long term health. Deep exhalations release metabolic waste along with CO_2, and deep inhalations flood the system with fresh oxygen. The circulatory system is cleansed, heart strength and muscle tone are improved. Sunlight on the body adds natural Vitamin D for skin and bone health. You notice the difference from a fitness walk.

▨ **Dancing** is another great aerobic exercise. Legs and lungs show rapid improvement, not to mention the fun you have. Any kind of dancing is a good workout, and the breathlessness felt afterward is the best sign of aerobic benefit.

▨ **Swimming** works all parts of the body at once, so noticeable toning improvements come quickly with regular swimming. Just fifteen to twenty steady laps, three or four times a week, and a more streamlined body is yours.

▨ **Aerobic exercise classes** are easily available. They are held every day, everywhere, at low prices, with good music and spirit-raising group energy. Workout clothes look great on both men and women. They are comfortable, permit deep breathing, and make you feel good about your body even when you are not exercising.

↤ Whatever exercise program you choose for yourself, make **rest** a part of it. Work out harder one day, go easy the next; or exercise for several days and take two days off. It's better for body balance, and will increase energy levels when you exercise the next time. After a regular program is started, exercising **four days a week** will increase fitness level; exercising **three days a week** will maintain fitness level; exercising **two days a week** will decrease a high fitness level. But any amount of exercise is better than nothing at all.

If your schedule is so busy that you hardly have time to breathe, let alone exercise, but still want the benefits of bodywork, there is an **all-in-one aerobic exercise.** It has gotten resounding enthusiasm and response rates for aerobic activity and muscle tone - **all in one minute.** The exercise sounds very easy, but is actually very difficult, and that is why it works so well. You will be breathless (the sign of an effective aerobic workout) before you know it.

Simply lie flat on your back on a rug or carpet. Rise to a full standing position any way you can, and lie down flat on your back again. That's the whole exercise. Stand and lie down, stand and lie down - **for one minute.** Typical repetitions for most people with average body tone are six to ten in 60 seconds. Record time for an athlete in top competitive condition is about 20-24 times in a minute. Be very easy on yourself. Repeat only as many times as you feel comfortable and work up gradually. It is worth a try because it exercises muscles, lung capacity and circulatory system so well, but don't overdo it.

The body is an amazing entity. It can be streamlined, toned and maintained, no matter what age or shape you are in, with very little effort.

The FIT Rule is Frequency, at least three times a week; Intensity, enough to strengthen your heart; and Time, at least fifteen minutes per workout not including warm-ups.
The secret is continuity.

Eating For Energy & Performance

Body building is 85% nutrition. A regular long-term, very nutritious diet is the basis for high performance; not protein or even carbo-loading before an event. The major body systems involved in energy production are the liver, thyroid, and adrenal glands. Maximum anabolic effect can be achieved through food and herbal sources. Complex carbohydrates such as those from whole grains, pastas, vegetables, rice, beans and fruits, are the key to strength and endurance for both the athlete and the casual body builder. They improve performance, promote storage of muscle fuel, and are easily absorbed without excess fats.

Sixty-five to seventy-five percent of a high performance diet should be in clean-burning complex carbohydrates. Twenty to twenty-five percent should be in high grade proteins from whole grains, nuts, beans, raw dairy products, tofu and other soy foods, yogurt, kefir, eggs, and some occasional poultry, fish, and seafood. Vegetable protein is best for mineral absorption and bone density. About 10-15% should be in energy-producing fats and oils necessary for glycogen storage. The best fats are unrefined and mono-or polyunsaturated oils, a little pure butter, nuts, low fat cheeses, and whole grain snacks. The remaining fuel should be liquid nutrients; fruit juices for their natural sugars, mineral waters and electrolyte replacement drinks for lost potassium, magnesium and sodium, and plenty of pure water. When the body senses lack of water, it will naturally start to retain fluid. Waste and body impurities will not be filtered out properly, and the liver will not metabolize stored fats for energy. Six to eight glass of water a day are a must, even if you don't feel thirsty. It often takes the sensory system time to catch up with actual body needs.

Eating junk foods pays the penalty of poor performance. Athletic excellence cannot be achieved by just adding anabolic steroids to an inferior diet. The only effective action is optimal nutrition.

Exercise is an integral part of good nutrition. We have all experienced the fact that exercise eases hunger. You are thirsty after a workout as the body calls for replacement of water and lost electrolytes, but not hungry. One of the reasons rapid results are achieved in a body streamlining program is this phenomenon. Not only do muscles become toned, heart and lungs become stronger, and fats lost, but the body doesn't call for calorie replacement right away. Its own glycogens lift blood sugar levels and provide a feeling of well being. **Exercise becomes a nutrient in itself.**

Effective Diets For Sports Nutrition, Energy and Performance
Three separate diets are included on page 99 for different levels of exercise, fitness and training

➤ The first is a high vitality, active life style diet, targeted for people who lack consistent daily energy and tire easily, and those who need more endurance and strength for hard jobs or long hours. It is also for weekend sports enthusiasts who wish to accomplish more than their present level of nutrition allows.

➤ The second is a moderate aerobic diet, for people who work out 3 to 4 times a week. It emphasizes complex carbohydrates for smooth muscle use, and moderate fat and protein amounts. Complex carbohydrates also produce glycogen for the body, resulting in increased energy and endurance.

➤ The third is a training diet, concentrating more on energy for competitive sports participation, and long range stamina. For the serious athlete, and for those who are consciously body building for higher workout achievement, this diet is a good foundation for significantly improved performance. Research shows that adjusting the diet before competition can increase endurance 200% or more - well worth consideration. Athletes' nutritional needs are considerably greater than those of the average person. Recommended daily allowances are far too low for high performance needs, and have no application for competition. Consult with a good sports nutritionist, or knowledgable people at a health food store or gym to determine individual specific supplement requirements. The important consideration is not body *weight*, but body *composition*.

Each of the three diets can be useful to the serious, performing athlete. Competitive training and a training diet alone cannot insure success. Rest time, and building energy and endurance reserves are also necessary to tune the body for maximum efficiency. When not in competition or pre-event training, extra high nutrient amounts are not needed, and can be hard for the body to handle. A less concentrated diet is better for base maintenance tone, and can be easily increased for competitive performance.

Note: The FOOD EXCHANGE LIST on the next page may be used along with the DAILY DIET CHART for more choices and adjustment to individual needs.

FOOD EXCHANGE LIST

Any food listed in a specific category may be exchanged one-for-one with any other food in the category. Portion amounts are given for a man weighing 170 pounds, and a woman weighing 130 pounds.

❧ GRAINS, BREADS & CEREALS: One serving is approximately one cup of cooked grains, such as brown rice, millet, barley, bulgur, kashi, cous cous, corn. oats, and whole grain pasta;
or one cup of dry cereals, such as bran flakes, Oatios, or Grapenuts;
or three slices of whole grain bread, or twelve small wholegrain crackers;
or three six inch corn tortillas, or two rice cakes;
or two chapatis or whole wheat pita breads.

❧ VEGETABLES:
Group A: One serving is as much as you want of lettuce (all kinds), Chinese greens and peas, raw spinach and carrots, celery, cucumbers, endive, sea vegetables, watercress, radishes, green onions and chives.
Group B: One serving is approximately two cups of cabbage or alfalfa sprouts;
or one and a half cups cooked bell peppers and mushrooms;
or one cup cooked asparagus, cauliflower, chard, sauerkraut, eggplant, zucchini or summer squash;
or $3/4$ cup cooked broccoli, green beans; onions or mung bean sprouts;
or $1/2$ cup vegetable juice cocktail, cooked brussels sprouts, or 8-10 water chestnuts.
Group C: One serving is approx. $1 1/2$ cups cooked carrots, one cup cooked beets, potatoes, or leeks;
or $1/2$ cup cooked peas, corn,artichokes, winter squash or yams, or one cup fresh carrot or vegetable juice.

❧ FRUITS: One serving is approximately one apple, nectarine,mango, pineapple, peach or orange;
or 4 apricots, medjool dates or figs;
or $1/2$ honeydew or cantaloupe;
or one and a half cups strawberries or other berries, cherries or grapes.

❧ DAIRY FOODS: One serving is approx. one cup of whole milk, or full fat yogurt, for 3mg. of fat;
or one cup of low fat milk, buttermilk or yogurt, for 2gm. of fat, or $1/3$ cup of non-fat dry milk powder;
or one cup of skim milk or non-fat yogurt, for less than 1gm. of fat;
or one ounce of low fat hard cheese, such as Swiss or cheddar.

❧ POULTRY, FISH & SEAFOOD: One serving is approx. 4oz. of white fish, or fresh salmon, skinned for 3gm. of fat;
or four ounces of chicken or turkey, white meat, no skin for 4gm. of fat;
or one cup of tuna or salmon, water packed for 3gm. of fat;
or one cup of shrimp, scallops, oysters, clams or crab for 3 to 4gm. of fat.

Avoid all red meats. They are high in saturated fat and cholesterol, and unsound as a use of planetary resources. These include all beef, carved, ground, corned or smoked, veal, lamb, pork, sausage, ham, bacon, and wild game.

❧ HIGH PROTEIN MEAT & DAIRY SUBSTITUTES: One serving is approx. one block of tofu, or one egg;
or $1/2$ cup low fat or dry cottage cheese, or $1/3$ cup ricotta, parmesan or mozzarella;
or $1/2$ cup cooked beans or brown rice.

❧ FATS & OILS: One serving is approx. one teaspoon of butter, margerine or shortening for 5gm. of fat;
or one tablespoon of salad dressing or mayonnaise for 5gm. of fat;
or 2 teaspoons of polyunsaturated or monounsaturated vegetable oil for 5gm. of fat.

The following foods are very high in fat and the amounts listed are equivalent to one fat serving on the diet chart. Use sparingly as part of a high fitness diet.
 - two tablespoons of light cream, half and half, or sour cream; 1 tablespoon of heavy cream;
 - ten almonds, cashews or peanuts; twenty pistachios or spanish peanuts; four walnut or pecan halves;
 - $1/8$ avocado, or $1/4$ cup sunflower, sesame, or pumpkin seeds.

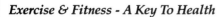

CHART FOR FOOD AMOUNTS BY SPECIFIC FITNESS DIET
Servings should be scaled up or down to fit your individual weight and type of active diet.

Daily Diet for Men			Daily Diet for Women Approx. 130 pounds		
High Energy, Active Life Diet Calories 2800 Protein 17% Carbos 70% Fat 13%	**Moderate Aerobic Diet** Calories 3250 Protein 20% Carbos 65% Fat 15%	**Training & Competition Diet** Calories 3950 Protein 23% Carbos 65% Fat 12%	**High Energy, Active Life Diet** Calories 2000 Protein 17% Carbos 70% Fat 13%	**Moderate Aerobic Diet** Calories 2200 Protein 20% Carbos 65% Fat 15%	**Training & Competition Diet** Calories 2750 Protein 23% Carbos 65% Fat 12%
6 whole grain servings	7 whole grain servings	8 whole grain servings	4 whole grain servings	4 whole grain servings	6 whole grain servings
Group A vegetables - all you want	Group A vegetables - all you want	Group A vegetables - all you want	Group A vegetables - all you want	Group A vegetables - all you want	Group A vegetables - all you want
Group B vegetables - 6 servings	Group B vegetables - 6 servings	Group B vegetables - 7 servings	Group B vegetables - 4 servings	Group B vegetables - 4 servings	Group B vegetables - 6 servings
Group C vegetables - 6 servings	Group C vegetables - 6 servings	Group C vegetables - 8 servings	Group C vegetables - 3 servings	Group C vegetables - 4 servings	Group C vegetables - 5 servings
5 fruit servings	5 fruit servings	6 fruit servings	3 fruit servings	4 fruit servings	4 fruit servings
3 dairy servings	4 dairy servings	4 dairy servings	2 dairy servings	3 dairy servings	3 dairy servings
2 poultry or seafood servings	4 poultry or seafood servings	5 poultry or seafood servings	1 poultry or seafood servings	1 poultry or seafood servings	3 poultry or seafood servings
5 fat servings	5 fat servings	6 fat servings	3 fat servings	3 fat servings	3 fat servings

**For complete sports, training and optimal energy diets,
see "Cooking for Healthy Healing" 2nd Edition by Linda Rector-Page.**

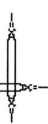

Supplements For Training, Bodybuilding & Performance

Nutritional supplements are excellent for both the serious and casual athlete. They can help build muscle tissue, maintain low body fat, and improve strength and endurance when the body is under the stress of a workout series. Clearly vitamin and mineral deficiencies result in energy loss. Supplements optimize recuperation time between workouts, are a proven adjunct to fitness and muscle growth, and speed healing from sports-related injuries.

How you take training supplements is as important as *what* you take. Your program will be more productive if you balance supplementation between workout days and rest days. Muscle growth occurs on the "off" days, as the body uses the exercise you have been giving it. In general, increased enhancement can be obtained by taking **vitamins, minerals, and glandulars** on "off" days. **Proteins, amino acids, anabolics and herbs** work best taken on "on" days, before the exercise or workout.

The following schedule contains effective products in each supplementation area:

MINERALS: You need minerals to run - for bone density, speed and endurance; anabolic enhancers
- ➡Potassium/magnesium/bromelain - relieves muscle fatigue/lactic acid buildup.
- ➡Cal/mag/zinc with boron - to prevent muscle cramping and maintain bone integrity.
- ➡Strength Systems BORON LIQUID (10mil.) - for lean muscle.
- ➡Chromium picolinate, 200mg. - for sugar regulation and glucose energy use.
- ➡Zinc picolinate, 30-50mg. daily for athletes - for immunity, healing of epithelial injuries.
- ➡MEZOTRACE - sea bottom mineral and trace mineral complex.

VITAMINS: Anti-stress factors for muscles, nerves and heart.
- ➡B Complex, 100mg. or more - for nerve health, muscle cramping, carbohydrate metabolism.
- ➡Vitamin C, 3000mg. daily w/bioflavonoids and Rutin for connective tissue strength. Take about 5 minutes before exercise to help put the vitamin into resistant areas.
- ➡Bioflavonoids - anti-oxidants to strengthen cell membrabes and prevent swelling and bruising.
- ➡Dibencozide - active co-enzyme of B_{12} for athlete's absorbability needs.
- ➡Lewis Labs BREWER'S YEAST - chromium fortified, to simulate protein synthesis.

ANTI-OXIDANTS: To increase oxygen use in blood, tissues and brain.
- ➡Vitamin E, 400IU with Selenium - for circulatory health, and protection against free radicals.
- ➡Co Q 10 - a catalyst co-emzyme factor to produce and release energy.
- ➡B_{15}- DiMethylglycine - to boost oxygen delivery; see Muscle Masters SMILAX + DMG.
- ➡Octocosonal - increases circulation and reduces muscle oxygen requirements.
- ➡Country Life ENERGIX VIALS.
- ➡Strength Systems ANTI-OXIDANT COMPOUND - for cell membrane protection; AMMONIA SCAVENGERS - between meals for free radical damage.

RAW GLANDULARS: Growth gland and hormone stimulation
- ➡Pituitary, 200mg. - the master gland, for upper body development.
- ➡Adrenal, 500mg.; see Country Life ADRENAL w/ TYROSINE - for adrenal support and cortex production.
- ➡Liver, 400mg. - for fat metabolism and detox. activity. Strength Systems LIVER TABS and Enzymatic Therapy LIQUID LIVER w/ SIBERIAN GINSENG for additional blood support.
- ➡Orchic - liquid extract best, approx 6 to 10x strength, or 1000mg. - for male testosterone support

TESTOSTERONE SUPPORT: part of a natural anabolic program for increased male performance
- ➡Source Naturals YOHIMBE 1000mg. capsules, Strength Systems YOHIMBE extract 1000mg.
- ➡Smilax, liquid - strength stamina and energy.
- ➡Muira Pauma Bark.

FREE FORM AMINO ACIDS: Hormone activators to increase body structure and strength.
- ➡Arginine/Ornithine/Lysine, 750mg. - to help burn fats for energy, natural growth stimulant; see Source Naturals SUPER AMINO NIGHT CAPS.
- ➡Carnitine, 500mg. - to strengthen heart and circulatory system during long exercise bouts.
- ➡Inosine, 1000mg. - to reduce workout stress and kick in glycogen use for extra edge performance.
- ➡Branched Chain Complex, BCAAs - for ATP energy conversion, endurance improvement; see Unipro BCAA's and Strength Systems 1500.
- ➡Strength Systems CHROMAX 1000 - for fat loss and energy (the serious athlete).
- ➡Full-1spectrum anabolics - natural steroid alternatives for body growth.
- ➡Pre-digested amino acids - easily absorbed for better performance, especially in women. Take before a workout. See Strength Systems LIQUID AMINOS.

➡Strength Systems WOMEN'S FITNESS PAKS - 22 day cycle and 8 day menstrual cycle.

ENZYMES: To process fuel nutrients for most efficient body use.
➡Pancreatin, 1400mg. - to metabolize fats, oils and carbohydrates correctly.
➡Bromelain/Papain, 500mg. - for muscle and ligament repair and strength.
➡Proteolytic Enzymes - break down scar tissue build-up and shortens recovery time after injury.

LIPIDS: Liver cleansers to metabolize fats and help form strong red blood cells.
➡Choline/Methionine/Inositol - a basic liver lipid.
➡Methionine/Lysine/Ornithine - with extra fat metabolizing agents .

FAT BURNERS: Metabolize blood and body fats, and enhance muscle growth
➡Strength Systems MCT (medium chain triglycerides).
➡Strength Systems FAT BURNERS CAPSULES.

PROTEIN/AMINO DRINKS: Daily mainstays for muscle building, weight gain, energy and endurance
➡Nature's Plus SPIRUTEIN - a maintenance drink with added body cleansers.
➡Joe Weider VEGETABLE PROTEIN POWDER - an energy drink for vegetarians.
➡Twin Lab AMINO FUEL - effective twice daily for endurance energy.
➡Twin Lab GAINERS FUEL 1000 - for maximum weight gain.
➡Strength Systems HEAVYWEIGHT BULK-UP - a competition level muscle builder.
➡Strength Systems RIGHT STUFF - for all around athletic improvement.
➡Strength Systems 100% EGG PROTEIN - highest quality egg protein.
➡Champion 900 - low fat weight gainer.

SPORTS BARS: Rich sources of various nutrients, especially carbohydrates, protein and fiber
➡Power Foods POWER BARS.
➡Strength Systems BULK UP BARS.
➡Nature's plus SPIRUTEIN ENERGY BARS.
➡Nature's Plus SOURCE OF LIFE ENERGY BARS.

SPORTSDRINKS/ELECTROLYTE REPLACEMENTS: Excellent after exertion to replace body minerals
➡Twin Lab ULTRA FUEL or Endurance QUICK FIX.
➡Alacer MIRACLE WATER .
➡Knudsens RECHARGE.
➡Twin Lab ULTRA FUEL.
➡Strength Systems CARBO COOLERS.

RECOVERY ACCELERATION
➡Strength Systems FIRST AID CAPSULES - anti-inflammatory and muscle tissue repair.

STIMULANTS: For quick, temporary, energy.
➡Excel slow release ginseng/ephedra formulas.

See *Natural Energizers & Stimulants*, page 93 for additional information.

A WORD ABOUT STEROIDS

As the standards of excellence rise in sports and competition, the use of steroids is increasing. Steroid enhancement has now spread beyond the professional and Olympic arenas to dedicated weight lifters, body builders and team players at all levels. Anabolic steroids are synthetically altered to stimulate the body's growth-enhancing activity. These substances accelerate protein breakdown into amino acids to increase muscle growth and reduce recovery time. However, science has not been able to make these substances without the risk of very serious side effects.

The dangers of synthetic steroids far outweigh any advantages.

Steroid use leads to wholesale destruction of glandular tissue, stunted growth from bone closure in males, testicle shrinkage, high cholesterol, low sperm counts with sterility noticeable after only a few months of use, enlargement and tenderness of the pectorals, weakening of connective tissue, jaundice from liver malfunction, heart enlargement, circulation impairment, and adverse side effects of hostile personality behavior and facial changes.

Free form amino acids, and naturally-occurring amino acids and proteins from herb and food sources, can act as steroid alternatives to help build the body to competitive levels without these destructive consequences. "Natural steroids" help release growth hormone, promote ammonia and acid detoxification, stimulate immunity, and encourage liver regeneration. They maximize potential, promote fast recuperation, increase stamina, and support peak performance.

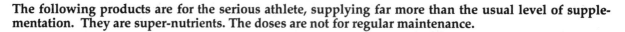

The following products are for the serious athlete, supplying far more than the usual level of supplementation. They are super-nutrients. The doses are not for regular maintenance.

- **ANABOLICS, MEGABOLICS, ULTRABOLICS, AMINOBOLICS, etc., 4-6, or 1-2 packs daily -** the mainstay of a dedicated athlete's program. They improve power, strength, endurance, build muscle tissue and stimulate growth hormone. See Strength Systems METAGRO 2, or AMINO 1000.
- **TESTOSTERONE SUPPORT -** important for male athletes and strength body builders - See Strength Systems SMILAX PLUS liquid, and ORCHIC TEST extract, 10x strength equal to 1000mg.
- **BRANCHED CHAIN AMINOS, (isoleucine, leucine, valine), 2-4 daily -** take before a workout - for endurance sports to preserve muscle mass, good ATP conversion and rebuild damaged muscles.
- **TYROSINE/ARGININE/TRYPTOPHAN/GLYCINE/ORNITHINE, needed in multigram doses for desired effect, -** to stimulate GH release; see Strength Systems NGS OCTANE.
- **GAMMA ORYZONAL (GO), 500-1500mg. daily -** a natural steroid alternative to increase testosterone secretion; for maximum weight gain and calorie use, with noticeable gain in lean muscle mass and reduction of body fat in 3-4 weeks. See also Muscle Masters TRANSFERULIC ACID 250mg.
- **BETA SITOSTEROL, 2-4 daily -** to keep blood fats and cholesterol low, and circulation clear.
- **INOSINE, 500-1500mg. daily -** to increase endurance, energy and ATP build up, take 30 minutes before working out.
- **DIBENCOZIDE B$_{12}$ -** the most active form of B$_{12}$ as a steroid alternative.
- **CHROMIUM PICOLINATE, 250mg. daily -** enhances muscle growth.
- **CoQ 10, 30-60mg. daily -** for enhanced flow of oxygen to the cells.

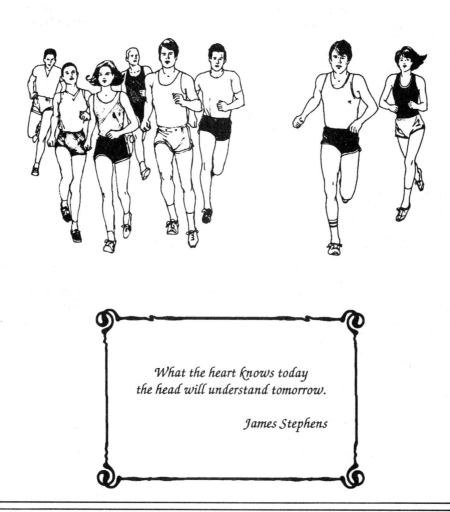

> *What the heart knows today*
> *the head will understand tomorrow.*
>
> *James Stephens*

HERBS FOR A WINNING BODY

Herbs act as concentrated food nutrients for body building. They offer extra strength for energy and endurance. They work best when taken on exercise days; in the morning with a good protein drink, or 30 minutes before exertion.

The following products are effective for both serious training and casual exercise.

◘ **Aerobic Support** - Siberian Ginseng, Ginkgo Biloba, Spirulina, Chlorella, American and Chinese Panax Ginseng, Rosemary, Chaparral, Pine Bark.

◘ **Anti-oxidants** - Ginkgo Biloba, Chlorella, Spirulina, Rosemary, Barley Green, Chaparral.

◘ **Stimulants** - Guarana Nut, Kola Nut, Ephedra, Ginkgo Biloba, Damiana, Green Tea, Coffee, Yerba Maté.

◘ **Increased Circulation** - Cayenne, Ginger, Ginkgo Biloba.

◘ **Stamina and Endurance** - Siberian Ginseng, Smilax (Sarsaparilla), Wild Yam, Schizandra, Spirulina, American and Chinese Panax Ginseng, Fo-Ti, Country Life ENERGIX vials.

◘ **Metabolic Enhancers** - Licorice Rt., Bee Pollen, Royal Jelly, American and Chinese Panax Ginseng, Green Tea.

◘ **Energy Releasers** - Siberian Ginseng, American and Chinese Panax Ginseng, Damiana, Wild Oats.

◘ **Workout Recovery And Nerve Strength** - Smilax, Vegex Yeast Paste Extract (1 teasp. in a cup of hot water at night as a source of absorbable B vitamins.)

About Herbal Steroids

Although there are no magic bullets for energy, endurance and healing of sports injuries, there are plant-derived steroids called phytosterols that do have growth activity similar to that of free form amino acids and anabolic steroids. Much testing still needs to be done on the herbs for anabolic effectiveness, especially on possible steroid strengths in normal herbal dosage form. Nevertheless, they may still be used with confidence in body building and endurance formulas. The most well-known of these herbs are:

Damiana, a mild aphrodisiac and nerve stimulant.

Sarsaparilla Root, *Smilax,* - an extract of sarsaparilla bark and root. Coaxes the body to produce greater amounts of the anabolic hormones, testosterone, cortisone, and progesterone. A blood purifying herb for nitrogen-based waste products such as uric acid. Speeds recovery time after workouts.

Saw Palmetto Berry, a urethral toning herb that increases blood flow to the sexual organs.

Siberian and Panax Ginsengs - adaptogens for over-all body balance and energy.

Wild Yam, an anti-spasmodic that prevents cramping. Contains disogenin, a progesterone precursor.

Yohimbe, a testosterone precurser for body building, and potent aphrodisiac for both male and female.

Crystal Star Herbal Nutrition Body Building Combinations:

● **MINERAL FORMULAS -** for strong body building blocks, better nutrient absorption, bone density, and endurance - MINERAL SOURCE COMPLEX™ extract, MINERAL SPECTRUM, POTASSIUM SOURCE™ and CALCIUM SOURCE™ capsules.

● **GLANDULAR FORMULAS -** for gland and hormone stimulation and growth - ADR-ACTIVE™ cap--sules, SUPER LICORICE™ extract, FEEL GREAT™ caps and tea.

● **ENERGY FORMULAS -** concentrated herbs for both immediate energy and extra endurance - SUPER MAN'S ENERGY™ extract, SUPERMAX™, ZING™, HIGH PERFORMANCE™ and GINSENG SUPER 6 ENERGY™ capsules, HIGH ENERGY™ and RAINFOREST ENERGY™ tea and caps.

● **METABOLIC ENHANCERS -** adaptogens for fat metabolism and cell production - SIBERIAN GIN--SENG extract, RECOVERY TONIC™ extract, MALE PERFORMANCE™ capsules, and GINSENG 6 RESTORATIVE SUPER™ tea and caps.

● **DRINK MIXES -** building, rejuvenating drinks with natural source amino acids, proteins, chlorophyll, enzymes, electrolytes and vitamins - ENERGY GREEN™ and SYSTEM STRENGTH™.

See *SPORTS INJURIES* in this book for more information.

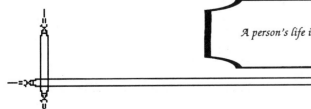

A person's life is dyed the color of his imagination.

BODY WORK FOR BODY BUILDING

➤ Stretch out before and after a workout to keep cramping down and muscles loose. Get some morning sunlight on the body every day possible for optimal absorption of nutrient fuel.

➤ Besides your major sport or activity, supplement and strengthen it with auxiliary exercise such as dancing, bicycling, jogging, and walking, and and cross training such as swimming or aerobics. This will balance muscle use and keep heart and lungs strong. Unless you are a serious, competitive athlete, make body tone your goal.

➤ *No pain does not mean no gain.* Your exercise doesn't have to hurt to be good. Once you work up to a good aerobic level and routine, you don't need to push yourself ever harder to benefit.

➤ Recuperation time is essential for optimum growth and strength. Muscles do not grow during exercise. They grow during rest periods. Alternate muscle workouts, and your training days with rest days. Move joints in their full range of motion during weight training for optimum flexibility.

➤ Weight training is beneficial for both sexes. Women do not get a bulky, masculine physique from lifting weights. They have relatively low levels of testosterone, which influences their type of muscle development.

➤ Deep breathing is important. Muscles and tissues must have enough oxygen for endurance and stamina. Breathe *in* during exertion, *out* as you relax for the next rep.

➤ Don't forget the importance of water. Good hydration is necessary for high performance, blood circulation, cardiovascular activity and overheating. Take a good electrolyte replacement drink after a workout or anytime during the day.

Fitness & Exercise Choices

Aerobic Dancing - 300-700 calories per hour
  Calisthenics - 360 calories per hour
    Cross Country Skiing - 350-1,400 calories per hour
      Cycling - 200-850 calories per hour
        Jumping Rope - 480-1,000 calories per hour
          Racquet Ball or Tennis - 350-1,000 calories per hour
            Rowing - 180-1,120 calories per hour
              Running - 400-1,300 calories per hour
                Stretching - 60-120 calories per hour
                  Swimming - 380-850 calories per hour
                    Walking - 240-430 calories per hour
                      Water Aerobics - 180-880 calories per hour
                        Weight Training - 260-480 calories per hour

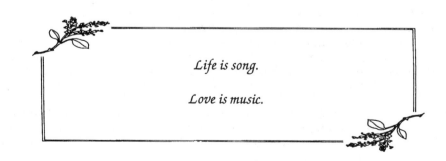

Life is song.

Love is music.

Having A Healthy Baby

PREGNANCY ✦ CHILDBIRTH ✦ LACTATION

A woman's body changes so dramatically during pregnancy and childbearing that her normal daily needs change. The body takes care of some of this need through cravings. During this one time of life, the body is so sensitive to its needs, that cravings are usually good for you. We know that every single thing the mother does or takes in affects the child. Good nutrition for a child begins *before* it is born - if possible before it is even conceived. Poor nutrition affects the fertility of both men and women, and the abscence of certain nutrients during the early months of pregnancy can result in birth defects. New research shows that adult risk for heart disease, cancer, and diabetes can be traced to poor eating habits of the parents as well as genetic proneness. The nutritional suggestions here will help build a healthy baby with a minimum of discomfort and excess fatty weight gain that can't be lost after birth.

Optimal Eating For Two
Promise yourself that at least during these few months of pregnancy and nursing, your diet and lifestyle will be as healthy as you can make it. A highly nutritious diet will help pregnancy be more of a pleasure, with less discomfort or risk of complications.
The basic rule is to satisfy your hunger with high quality unrefined foods. Most experts currently recommend 60 to 80 grams of protein daily during pregnancy, with a 10 gram increase every trimester.

✔ Eat a high vegetable protein diet, with plenty of whole grains, seeds and sprouts, with fish or seafood at least twice a week. Protein is easy to get even if you are a vegetarian. It's in almost every food, from peanut butter to bread to beans to cheese. Have a fresh fruit or green salad every day. Eat plenty of soluble fiber foods like whole grain cereals and vegetables for regularity. Eat complex carbohydrate foods like broccoli and brown rice for strength.
✔ **Drink plenty of healthy fluids** - pure water, mineral water, and juices throughout the day to keep the system free and flowing. Carrot juice at least twice a week is ideal. Include pineapple and apple juice.
✔ Eat **folacin rich foods**, such as fresh spinach and asparagus for healthy cell growth.
✔Eat **carotene foods**, such as carrots, squashes, tomatoes, yams, and broccoli for disease resistance.
✔Eat **zinc rich foods**, such as pumpkin and sesame seeds for good body formation.
✔Eat **vitamin C foods**, such as broccoli and bell peppers and fruits for connective tissue.
✔Eat **bioflavonoid-rich foods**, such as citrus fruits and berries for capillary integrity.
✔Eat **alkalizing foods**, such as miso soup and brown rice to combat and neutralize toxemia.
✔Eat **mineral-rich foods**, such as sea vegies, leafy greens, whole grains for baby building blocks. Especially include silicon-rich foods for bone, cartilage and connective tissue growth, and for collagen and elastin formation; brown rice, oats, green grasses and green drinks.
✔ Have a good protein drink several times a week for optimal growth and energy. The following is a proven example: Mix $1/2$ cup raw milk, $1/2$ cup yogurt, the juice of one orange, 2 TBS. brewer's yeast, 2 TBS. wheat germ, 2 teasp. molasses, 1 teasp. vanilla, and a pinch cinnamon.
✔ Eat small frequent meals instead of large meals.

There are several important things to avoid during pregnancy and nursing, for the greatest health to the baby.
✘ Don't diet. Low calories often mean low birth weight. Metabolism becomes deranged during dieting, and the baby receives abnormal nutrition that can impair brain and nerve development. Even if you feel you are gaining too much, a healthy diet is full of nutritious calories (not empty calories), that you will be able to lose easily after nursing. Until then, you are still eating for two.
✘ Don't restrict food variety. Eat a wide range of healthy foods to assure the baby access to all nutrients. Avoid cabbages, onions, and garlic. They upset body balance during pregnancy. Avoid red meats. Most are full of nitrates, and other chemicals the baby can't eliminate.

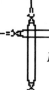

✘ Don't fast - even for short periods where fasting would normally be advisable, such as constipation, or to overcome a cold. Food energy and nutrient content will be diminished.

✘ Avoid all processed, refined, preserved and colored foods. Refrain from alcohol, caffeine and tobacco.

✘ Avoid X-rays, chemical solvents, chlorofluorocarbons such as hair sprays, and even cat litter. Your system may be able to handle these things without undue damage; the baby's can't. Even during nursing, toxic concentrations occur easily.

✘ Don't smoke. The chance of low birth weight and miscarriage is twice as likely if you smoke. Smoker's infants have a mortality rate 30% higher than non-smoker's. Nursing babies take in small amounts of nicotine with breast milk, and become prone to chronic respiratory infections.

ABOUT BREAST FEEDING

Unless there is a major health or physical problem, mother's breast milk should be the only food for the baby during the first six months of life. Despite all the claims made for fortified formulas, nothing can take its place for the baby's health and ongoing well-being. The first thick, waxy colustrum is extremely high in protein, fats (which are needed for brain and nervous system development), and protective antibodies. A child's immune system is not fully established at birth, and the antibodies are critical, both for fighting early infections and in creating solid, balanced, immune defenses that will prevent the development of allergies. The baby who is not breastfed loses nature's "jump start" on immunity. He/she faces life with health disadvantages that can last a lifetime.

Breastfed babies have a lower instance of colic and other digestive disturbances than bottle-fed babies. This is attributed to *Bifidobacteria*, the beneficial micro-organisms that make up 99% of a healthy baby's intestinal flora. Their growth is intensified by mother's milk. They are extremely important for protection against *salmonella* food poisoning and other intestinal pathogens. Bifidobacteria also produce lactic and acetic acids that inhibit the growth of yeasts and toxic amines from amino acids.

If there is simply no way to breast feed the baby, goat's milk is a better alternative than chemically made formulas, or cow's milk, both of which result in a higher risk of allergy development.

OTHER NUTRITIONAL WATCHWORDS:

✔**During Labor:** Take no solid food. Drink fresh water, have carrot juice, or suck on ice chips.

✔**During Lactation:** Promote milk quality and richness with almond milk, brewer's yeast, green drinks and green foods, avocados, carrot juice, soy milk and soy foods, goat's milk and unsulphured molasses.

✔**During Weaning:** Papaya juice will help slow down milk flow.

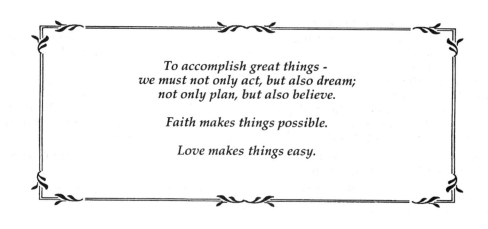

*To accomplish great things -
we must not only act, but also dream;
not only plan, but also believe.*

Faith makes things possible.

Love makes things easy.

Healthy Prenatal Supplements

Illness, body imbalance, and also regular maintenance supplementation need to be treated differently from the usual approach, even if the method is holistically oriented. The mother's body is very delicately tuned and sensitive at this time, and imbalances can occur easily.

☺ Mega-doses of anything are not good for the baby's system. Dosage of all medication or supplementation should almost universally be less than normal to allow for the infant's tiny systemic capacity. Dosage should be about half of normal. Ideal supplementation should be from food-source complexes for best absorbability.

☠ **All drugs should be avoided during pregnancy and nursing;** including alcohol, tobacco, caffeine, MSG, Saccharin, X-rays, aspirin, Valium, Librium, Tetracycline, and harsh diuretics.

☠ **Especially stay away from recreational drugs;** including cocaine, PCP, marijuana, methamphetamines, Quaaludes, heroin, LSD and other psychedelics. Even the amino acid L-Phenylalanine can adversely affect the nervous system of the unborn child.

✦ Take a good <u>prenatal</u> multi-vitamin and mineral supplement, such as Rainbow Light PRE-NATAL; especially starting six to eight weeks before the expected birth. Clinical testing has shown that mother's who took nutritional supplementation during pregnancy were far less likely to have babies with neural tube and other defects.

✦ Take a natural mineral complex (not just calcium) supplement such as MEZOTRACE SEA MINERALS for good body building blocks. In fact, **recent studies have shown that betacarotene, 10,000mg. *with* vitamin C, 500mg., niacin 50mg., and liquid herbal iron are better for skeletal, cellular and connecting tissue development than calcium supplements.**

✦ Take extra folic acid, 800mcg. daily to prevent neural tube defects. **Timing is essential. Supplemental folic acid after the first three months of fetal development cannot correct spinal cord damage.**

✦ Take Bioflavonoids 1000mg. daily, such as Crystal Star BIOFLAVONOID, FIBER & C SUPPORT™ DRINK for capillary integrity and to strengthen vein structure. Vitamin C and bioflavonoids also help prevent miscarriage. Recent tests show that over 50% of women who habitually miscarry have low levels of vitamin C and bioflavonoids.

✦ Take vitamin B$_6$ - 50mg. for bloating, leg cramps and nerve strength, as well as to prevent proneness to glucose intolerance and seizures in the baby.

✦Take kelp tablets, 4-6 daily, or Crystal Star IODINE SOURCE™ capsules, for natural potassium and iodine. Too little of these minerals mean mental retardation and poor physical development.

✦ Take natural vitamin E 200-400IU, or wheat germ oil capsules, to help prevent miscarriage and reduce baby's oxygen requirement, lessening the chances of asphyxiation during labor.

✦ Take zinc 10-15mg. daily, (or get it from your pre-natal multi-mineral). Deficiencies often result in poor brain formation, learning problems, low immunity, sub-normal growth and allergies in the baby.

✦ Some new research is showing that low doses of carnitine during the last trimester can help protect the baby from SIDS.

OTHER SUPPLEMENTATION WATCHWORDS:

✔ **During the last trimester:** Rub vitamin E or wheat germ oil on the stomach and around the vaginal opening every night to make stretching easier and skin more elastic. Begin to take extra minerals as labor approaches for an easier birth.

✔ **During Labor:** Take vitamin E and calcium/magnesium to relieve pain and aid dilation.

✔ **During Nursing:** Nutritional supplements that were used during pregnancy, such as iron, calcium, B vitaminsor a prenatal multiple, should be continued during nursing. Indeed, they may be increased for more optimum nutrition if the mother has not recovered normal strength. Breast milk is a filtered food supply that prevents the baby from overdosing on higher potencies.

☺ Take essential fatty acids, such as Omega 3 flax oils, or GLA from borage seed or evening primrose oil, for baby's brain development.

☺ Calcium lactate is beneficial with calcium ascorbate vitamin C for collagen development.

☺ Apply vitamin E oil to alleviate breast crusting.

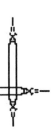

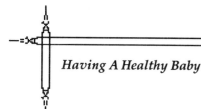

Herbs For A Healthy Pregnancy

Herbs have been used successfully for centuries to ease the hormone imbalances and discomforts of stretching, bloating, nausea and pain experienced during pregnancy, without impairing the development or health of the baby. Herbs are concentrated mineral rich foods that are perfect for the extra growth requirements of pregnancy and childbirth. The developing child's body is very small and delicate. Ideal supplementation should be from food source complexes for best absorbability. Herbs are identified and accepted by the body's enzyme activity as whole food nutrients, lessening the risk of toxemia or overdose, yet providing gentle, quickly absorbed nutrition to both mother and baby.

Herbs are good and easy for you; good and gentle for the baby.
Remember that early pregnancy and later pregnancy must be considered separately with herbal medicinals. If there is any question, always use the gentlest herbs.

DURING PREGNANCY:
* Take two daily cups of red raspberry tea, or Crystal Star MOTHERING TEA™, a red raspberry blend. Both are safe, high in iron and other minerals, strengthening to the uterus and birth canal, effective against birth defects, long labor and afterbirth pain, and elasticizing for a quicker return to normal.
* Take kelp tablets, the SEA VEGETABLE SUPREME food sprinkle on page 85, or Crystal Star IODINE SOURCE™ CAPS against birth defects.

During the last trimester, take Crystal Star PRE-NATAL HERBS for gentle, absorbable minerals and toning agents to elasticize tissue and ease delivery. Other formulas providing herbal minerals include Crystal Star IRON SOURCE™, CALCIUM SOURCE™, or MINERAL SPECTRUM™ CAPSULES, and SILICA SOURCE™ or MINERAL COMPLEX EXTRACTS.

Five weeks before the expected birth date, take Crystal Star FIVE WEEK FORMULA™ capsules to aid in hemorrhage control and correct presentation of the fetus.

DURING LABOR:
* Take Medicine Wheel LABOR EASE drops, or Crystal Star CRAMP BARK COMBO™ EXTRACT to ease contraction pain. Fifteen to 20 drops should be put into water and taken in small sips as needed during labor. Take BACK TO RELIEF™ capsules for afterbirth pain.
* For false labor, drink 4 to 6 cups catnip/blue cohosh tea to renormalize. If there is bleeding, take 2 capsules <u>each</u> cayenne and bayberry, and get to a hospital or call your midwife.

DURING NURSING:
* Add 2 TBS. brewer's yeast to your diet, along with red raspberry, marshmallow root, or Crystal Star MOTHERING TEA™ to promote and enrich milk.
* Take Vitex, (Chaste Tree Berries extract) to promote of an abundant supply of mother's milk.
* Fennel, alfalfa, red raspberrry leaf, cumin, or fenugreek teas help keep the baby colic free.
* For infant jaundice, use Hyland's BILIOUSNESS tabs.

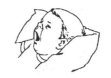

DURING WEANING:
* Take parsley/sage tea to help dry up milk.

PREVENTING SIDS - Sudden Infant Death Syndrome: If the baby has a weak system, or poor tissue or lung development (signs that it is a candidate for this condition) give a weak ascorbate vitamin C, or Ester C with bioflavonoids solution in water daily. Routinely feeding babies iron-fortified weaning foods to prevent anemia may increase the risk of SIDS, according to the British Medical Journal. New evidence indicates that infant pillows filled with foam polystyrene beads cause the baby to inhale toxic gases and suffocate.

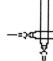

✔ HERBS TO USE DURING PREGNANCY

We suggest using the following herbs in the gentlest way during pregnancy - as hot, relaxing teas.

🌿 **Red Raspberry Leaf** - the quintessential herb for pregnancy. Raspberry is an all around uterine tonic. It is anti-abortive to prevent miscarriage, antiseptic to help prevent infection, astringent to tighten tissue, rich in calcium, magnesium and iron to help prevent cramps and anemia. It is hemostatic to prevent excess bleeding during and after labor, and facilitates the birth process by stimulating contractions.

🌿 **Nettles** - a mineral-rich, nutritive herb, with vitamin K to guard against excessve bleeding. It improves kidney function and helps prevent hemorrhoids.

🌿 **Peppermint** - may be used after the first trimester to help digestion, soothe the stomach and overcome nausea. An over-all body strengthener and cleanser. Contains highly absorbable amounts of vitamin A, C, silica, potassium and iron.

🌿 **Ginger Rt.** - excellent for morning sickness; has lots of necessary minerals.

🌿 **Bilberry** - a strong but gentle astringent, rich in bioflavonoids to fortify vein and capillary support. A hematonic for kidney function and a mild diuretic for bloating.

🌿 **Burdock Rt.** - mineral-rich, hormone balancing. Helps prevent water retention and baby jaundice.

🌿 **Yellow Dock** - improves iron assimilation; helps prevent infant jaundice.

🌿 **Dong Quai Rt.** - a blood nourisher, rather than a hormone stimulant. Use in moderation.

🌿 **Echinacea Lf.** - an immune system stimulant to help prevent colds, flu and infections.

🌿 **Chamomile** - relaxes for quality sleep, and helps digestive and bowel problems.

🌿 **Vitex** - a fertility stimulant to normalize hormone balance. Discontinue after pregnancy is realized.

🌿 **False Unicorn, Black and Blue Cohosh** - for final weeks of pregnancy only, to ease and/or induce labor.

🌿 **Wild Yam** - for general pregnancy pain, nausea or cramping; lessens miscarriage.

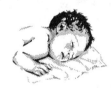

☠ HERBS TO AVOID DURING PREGNANCY

✗ **Aloe Vera** - can be too laxative. We have found George's ALOE VERA JUICE to be gentle.

✗ **Angelica** - an emmenagogue that causes uterine contractions.

✗ **Barberry** - too strong laxative.

✗ **Buchu** - too strong diuretic.

✗ **Buckthorn** - too laxative.

✗ **Cascara Sagrada** - too strong a laxative; can cause cramping and stomach griping.

✗ **Coffee** - too strong a caffeine and heated hydrocarbon source - irritates the uterus. In extremely sensitive individuals who take in excessive amounts, may cause miscarriage or premature birth.

✗ **Comfrey** - alkaloid content (carcinogen) cannot be regulated or controlled for an absolutely safe source.

✗ **Ephedra, Ma Huang** - too strong antihistamine if used in extract or capsule form. We have found it to be gentle enough as a tea to relieve bronchial and chest congestion.

✗ **Goldenseal** - can cause uterine contractions.

✗ **Horseradish** - too strong.

✗ **Juniper** - a too strong, vasodilating diuretic.

✗ **Lovage** - an emmenagogue that causes uterine contractions.

✗ **Male Fern** - too strong vermifuge.

✗ **Mistletoe** - an emmenagogue that causes uterine contractions.

✗ **Mugwort and Wormwood** - stimulates uterine contractions - can be toxic in large doses.

✗ **Pennyroyal** - stimulates oxytocin that can cause abortion. May be used in the final weeks of pregnancy.

✗ **Rhubarb Rt.** - too strong laxative.

✗ **Rue** - stimulates oxytocin production that can cause abortion.

✗ **Shepherds Purse** - too astringent. May be used after birth to control post-partum bleeding.

✗ **Tansy** - an emmenagogue that causes uterine contractions.

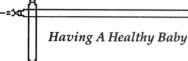

✗ **Yarrow -** a strong astringent and mild abortifacient.
✗ **Senna -** too strong laxative.
✗ **Mandrake -** an irritating, mildly toxic laxative.
✗ **Wild Ginger -** an emmenagogue that causes uterine contractions.

Bodywork For Two

➤ Get daily mild exercise during pregnancy. Take a brisk walk for fresh air, circulation, and oxygen.
➤ Sunbathe every morning for a half an hour if possible for natural vitamin D, calcium absorption and bone growth.
➤ Consciously set aside a stress-free relaxation time each day. Play your favorite restful music. The baby will know, and thrive on it.
➤ If you practice reflexology, do not press the acupressure point just above the ankle on the inside of the leg. It can start contractions.
➤ Rub cocoa butter, vitamin E oil or wheat germ oil on the stomach and around the vaginal opening every night to make stretching easier and the skin more elastic.
➤ Get plenty of rest and adequate sleep. The body energy turns inward during sleep for repair, restoration and fetal growth.

Special Problems During Pregnancy

Illness and body imbalances during pregnancy need to be treated slightly differently than a usual approach. Dosage of any medication, natural or allopathic, should be less than normal to allow for the infant's tiny systemic capacity. The mother's body is very delicately balance and sensitive at this time, and problems can occur easily.

The following schedule contains effective natural products that may be used without harm.

✦ **AFTERBIRTH PAIN -** take Crystal Star MOTHERING TEA™ or BACK TO RELIEF™ capsules, especially after a long labor, to tone and elasticize uterus and abdomen for quicker return to normal. For post-partum tearing use a sitz bath with 1 part uva ursi, 1 part yerba mansa rt., and 1 part cach comfrey leaf and root. Simmer 15 minutes, strain, add 1 tsp. salt, pour into a large shallow container; cool a little. Sit in the bath 15-20 minutes 2x daily.

✦ **ANEMIA -** Take a non-constipating, absorbable herbal iron, such as Floradix LIQUID IRON, yellow dock tea, or Crystal Star IRON SOURCE™ CAPSULES. Have a good green drink often, such as apple/alfalfa sprout/parsley juice, Green Foods GREEN MAGMA, Crystal Star ENERGY GREEN™ DRINK or Chlorella. Add vitamin C and E to your diet, and eat plenty of dark leafy greens.

✦ **BREASTS - for infected breasts:** 500mg. Vitamin C every 3 hours, 400IU vitamin E, and Beta-carotene 10,000IU daily. Get plenty of chlorophyll from green salads, green drinks, or green supplements such as CHLORELLA, Crystal Star ENERGY GREEN™ DRINK or Green Foods GREEN MAGMA.
  for caked or crusted breasts, simmer elder flowers in oil and rub on breasts. Wheat germ oil, almond oil and cocoa butter are also effective.
  for engorged breasts during nursing, apply ice bags to the breasts to relieve pain.

✦ **CONSTIPATION -** use a simple soluble fiber laxative, such as Yerba Prima COLON CLEANSE, or Crystal Star CHO-LO FIBER TONE™, or a gentle herbal laxative such as HEerbaltone. Add additional fiber fruits such as prunes and apples to your diet.

✦ **FALSE LABOR -** Catnip tea or red raspberry tea will help. See *MISCARRIAGE* page in this book.

✦ **GAS & HEARTBURN -** This is usually caused by an enzyme imbalance. Take papaya or bromelain chewables or papaya juice with a pinch of ginger, or comfrey/pepsin tablets. Or take Crystal Star PRE-MEAL ENZ™ extract drops *in water.*

✦ **HEMORRHOIDS -** Take cascara sagrada or stone root capsules as needed, or bilberry extract, or Crystal Star HEMR-EASE™ capsules. (May also use these herbs effectively mixed with cocoa butter as a suppository.)

✦ **INSOMNIA -** take a liquid or herbal calcium supplement, such as Crystal Star CALCIUM SOURCE™ capsules, or extract, *with* chamomile tea.

✦ **LABOR - For nausea during labor:** fresh ginger tea; miso broth; Alacer Emergen-C with a little salt added. **For labor pain:** crampbark extract; lobelia, scullcap, St. John's wort extract in water; for nerve pain, apply St. John's Wort oil to temples and wrists; rosemary/ginger compresses. **For post-partum bleeding:** shepherd's purse or nettles tea. **For sleep during long labor:** use scullcap tincture. (Scullcap may be used throughout labor for relaxation.) Hydrate with cool drinks frequently during labor even if there is nausea.

✦ **MORNING SICKNESS -** use homeopathic IPECAC and NAT. MUR, add vitamin B$_6$ 50mg. 2x daily, sip mint tea whenever queasy, and see *MORNING SICKNESS* program in this book.

✦ **MISCARRIAGE - for prevention and hemorrhage control -** drink raspberry tea every hour with $1/4$ teasp. ascorbate vit. C powder added, <u>and</u> take drops of hawthorne <u>or</u> lobelia extract every hour. See the *MISCARRIAGE PREVENTION* program in this book for complete information.

✦ **POST-PARTUM SWELLING & DEPRESSION -** use homeopathic ARNICA. Make a post-partum cordial with 4 slices dong quai rt., $1/2$ oz. false unicorn rt., 1 handful nettles, $1/2$ oz. St. John's Wort extract, 1 handful motherwort, $1/2$ oz. hawthorne berries, and 2 inch-long slices fresh ginger. Steep herbs in 1 pint of brandy for 2 weeks, shaking daily. Strain and add a little honey if desired. Take 1 teasp. daily as a tonic dose. Cordials and teas are more effective than capsules for post-partum healing.

✦ **STRETCH MARKS -** Apply wheat germ, avocado, sesame oil, vitamin E, or A D & E oil. Take vitamin C 500mg. 3 to 4 times daily for collagen development. See *STRETCH MARKS* program in this book.

✦ **SWOLLEN ANKLES -** use bilberry extract in water.

✦ **TOXEMIA, Eclampsia -** (Toxemia is caused by malnutrition. The liver malfunctions, becomes diseased and simply cannot handle the increasing load of the progressing pregnancy. There is a marked reduction in blood flow to the placenta, kidneys and other organs. Severe cases can be fatal, resulting in liver and brain hemorrhage, convulsions and coma. Toxemia is indicated by extreme swelling, accompanied by high blood pressure, headaches, nausea and vomiting.)
Take several green drinks such as apple/alfalfa sprout/parsley or Green Foods GREEN MAGMA for a "chlorophyll cleanout". Add vitamin C 500mg. every 3 to 4 hours, 10,000IU Beta-carotene, bilberry extract in water, and B Complex 50mg. daily. Apply PSI PROGEST CREAM as directed. Enzymatic Therapy MUCOPLEX and DGL have also been helpful, as has iodine therapy via daily kelp tablets.

✦ **UTERINE HEMORRHAGING -** Take bayberry and cayenne capsules, and get to professional help immediately. Take bilberry extract daily with strengthening herbal flavonoids for tissue integrity. Use angelica tea for uterine contraction.

✦ **VARICOSE VEINS -** Take vitamin C 500mg. with bioflavonoids and rutin, 4 daily; or bilberry extract 2x daily in water; or butcher's broom tea daily (also helpful for leg cramps during pregnancy). Drink and apply Crystal Star VARI-TONE TEA™ directly to swollen veins.

The future of American excellence, in a globalized economy without a cold war, will rest with people who can think and act with informed grace across ethnic, cultural and language lines.

The first step in achieving this excellence lies in acknowledging that we are not one big world family, or ever likely to be; but that the differences among our races, nationalities, cultures, creeds and histories are at least as profound and as durable as the similarities. America has the only chance in the world to value these different structures for their own sake, and to navigate that difference into a synergistic strength.

Unless unusually or chronically ill, a child is born with a well-developed, powerful immune system. He or she often needs only the subtle body-strengthening forces that nutritious foods, herbs or homeopathic remedies supply, rather than the highly focused medications of allopathic medicine which can have such drastic side effects on a small body. The undeniable ecological, sociological and diet deterioration in America during the last fifty years has had a marked effect on children's health. Declining educational performance, learning disabilities, mental disorders, drug and alcohol abuse, hypoglycemia, allergies, chronic illness, delinquency and violent behavior are all evidence of declining immunity and general health.

You can get a lot of help from the kids themselves in a natural health program. Kids don't want to be sick, they aren't stupid, they don't like going to the doctor any more than you do. They often recognize natural foods and therapies that are good for them. Children are naturally immune to disease. A nutritious diet and natural supplements help keep them that way.

Diet Help For Childhood Diseases

Two complete diet programs are included; a short liquid cleansing fast for rapid toxin elimination, and a raw foods purification diet for body cleansing during the beginning and acute stages of a diseases. There are also suggestions for an optimal whole foods maintenance diet for disease prevention.

Diet is the most important way to keep a child's immunity and defense mechanisms working. Germs and viruses are everywhere. They are not the major factor in causing disease; the body environment must be suitable for them to flourish. Well-nourished children are usually strong enough to deal with infection in a successful way. They either do not catch the "bugs" that are going around, contract only a mild case, or develop strong healthy reactions that are short in duration, and will get the problem over and done with quickly. It is this difference in resistance and inherent immunity that is the key factor in understanding children's diseases.

A wholesome diet can easily restore a child's natural vitality. Even children who have eaten a junk food diet for years quickly respond to fresh fruits, vegetables, whole grains, and low fats and sugars. We have noted great improvement in only a month's time. Their hair and skin take on new luster, they fill out if they are too skinny, and lose weight if they are fat. They sleep more soundly and regularly. Their attention spans markedly increase, and many learning and behavior problems diminish.

Keep it simple. Let them help prepare their own food, even though they might get in the way and you feel like its more trouble than its worth. They will have a better understanding of good food, and are more likely to eat things they have had a hand in fixing. Keep only good nutritious foods in the house. Children may be exposed to junk foods and poor foods at school or friend's houses, but you can build a good, natural foundation diet at home. For the time that they are at home, they should be able to choose only from nutritious choices.

Diet and nutritional therapy for most common childhood diseases, including measles, mumps, chicken pox, strep throat and whooping cough, is fairly simple and basic. A short liquid elimination fast, followed by a fresh light foods diet in the acute stages.

A Short Liquid Elimination Fast:

This liquid diet may last for 24 hours up to 72 hours, depending on the state of the child and the severity of the disease.

☺ Start the child on cleansing liquids as soon as the disease is diagnosed to clean out harmful bacteria and infection. Give fruit juices such as apple, pineapple, grape, cranberry and citrus juices are helpful, or give Crystal Star FIRST AID TEA FOR KIDS™. The juice of two lemons in a glass of water with a little honey may be taken once or twice a day to flush the kidneys and alkalize.

☺ Alternate fruit juices throughout the day with fresh carrot juice, bottled mineral water, and clear soups. A potassium broth or green drink (pages 53, 54ff) should be taken at least

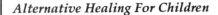

once a day. Encourage the child to drink as many healthy cleansing liquids as she/he wants. No dairy products should be given.

Supplements for the Child's Liquid Fast:

⚘ Herb teas may be taken throughout the fast. Make them about half the strength as that for an adult. Children respond to herb teas quickly, and they like them more than you might think. Just add a little honey if the herbs are bitter. We have found the following teas effective for most childhood diseases; elder flowers with peppermint to induce perspiration; catnip/chamomile/rosemary tea to break out a rash; mullein/lobelia or scullcap as relaxants; catnip, fennel and peppermint for upset stomachs.

⚘ Crystal Star COFEX TEA™ for sore throats, X-PECT-T™ to help bring up mucous, CHILL CARE™ TEA for warming against chills, and ECHINACEA EXTRACT drops in water every 3 to 4 hours to keep the lymph glands clear and able to process infective toxins.

⚘ Acidlphilus liquid, such as Natren LIFE START, Solaray BABY LIFE, or DR. DOPHILUS powder are excellent for children to keep friendly bacteria in the G.I. tract, especially if they are taking antibiotics. Use one quarter teasp. at a time in a glass of water or juice three to four times daily.

Bodywork for the Child's Liquid Fast:

⚘ A gentle enema with catnip tea is very effective for clearing the colon of impacted wastes. These hinder the body in its effort to rid itself of diseased bacteria.

⚘ Oatmeal baths help neutralize acids and rash coming out on the skin. Hydrotherapy baths (pg. 49ff.) to induce cleansing perspiration are effective. Use calendula or comfrey tea. A soothing body rub with calendula oil, Tiger Balm or tea tree oil will often loosen congestion after an herbal bath.

⚘ Ginger/cayenne compresses applied to affected and sore areas will stimulate circulation and defense mechanisms, to rid the body more quickly of infection.

⚘ Herbal steam inhalations, such as eucalyptus or tea tree oil, or Crystal Star RSPR TEA™ in a vaporizer will help to keep lungs mucous free and improve oxygen uptake.

⚘ Golden seal, myrrh, yellow dock, black walnut, yarrow, or Crystal Star THERADERM™ TEA, may be patted onto sores, scabs and lesions with cotton balls to help heal and soothe.

❦

A Raw Foods Purification Diet For Children's Diseases:
This diet may be used for initial, acute and chronic symptoms when a liquid fast is not desired, or following a liquid fast when the acute stage has passed. The body will continue cleansing, and the addition of solid foods will start to rebuild strength. Dairy products, except for yogurt should be avoided. This diet should last about three days depending on the strength and condition of the child.

On rising: give citrus juice with a teaspoon of acidophilus liquid, or $1/4$ teasp. acidophilus powder; <u>or</u> a glass of lemon juice and water with honey.

Breakfast: offer fresh fruits, such as apples, pineapple, papaya or oranges. Add some vanilla yogurt or soymilk if desired.

Mid-morning: Give a green drink, a potassium broth, (page 53) or fresh carrot juice. Add $1/4$ teasp. ascorbate vitamin C or Ester C crystals.

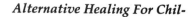

Lunch: give some fresh raw crunchy vegies with a little yogurt dip;
or a fresh vegie salad with lemon/oil or yogurt dressing.

Mid-afternoon: offer a refreshing herb tea, such as licorice or peppermint tea, or Crystal Star LICO-RICE MINTS™, or FIRST AID TEA FOR KIDS™ to keep stomach settled and calm tension,
or another green drink with $1/4$ teasp. vitamin C added.

Dinner: have a fresh salad, with avocados, carrots, kiwi, romaine and other high vitamin A foods;
and/or a cup of miso soup or other clear broth soup.

Before bed: offer a relaxing herb tea, such as chamomile or scullcap tea, or Crystal Star GOOD NIGHT TEA™. Add $1/4$ teasp. ascorbate vitamin C or Ester C crystals; **or** a cup of VEGEX yeast broth for strength and B vitamins.

Supplements for the Raw Food Children's Diet

⚕ Give a vitamin/mineral drink such as NutriTech EARTHSHAKE or Nature's Plus SPIRUTEIN (lots of flavors), or 1 teasp. liquid multi-vitamin in juice, such as Floradix CHILDREN'S MULTI-VITAMIN/MINERAL.

⚕ Continue with your acidolphilus choice. Add vitamin A & D in drops if desired, and ascorbate vitamin C or Ester C crystals in juice as outlined above.

⚕ Continue with the therapeutic herbal teas you found effective in the liquid fast, especially Crystal Star FIRST AID TEA FOR KIDS™.

⚕ Use a mild herbal laxative in half dosage if necessary, to keep the child eliminating regularly.

⚕ Use garlic oil drops or open garlic capsules into juice or water for natural anti-biotic activity; or give Crystal Star ANTI-BIO™ CAPS or EXTRACT in half dosage.

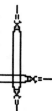

Bodywork Aids for the Raw Foods Children's Diet

⚕ Continue with herbal baths, washes and compresses to neutralize and cleanse toxins coming out through the skin.

⚕ Give a soothing massage before bed.

⚕ Get some early morning sunlight on the body every day possible for regenerating vitamin D.

❀ *When the crisis has passed, and the child is on the mend with a clean system, start them on an optimal nutrition diet for prevention of further problems, and increased general health and energy.*

An Optimal Whole Foods Diet For Children
The best health and disease prevention diet for children is high in whole grains and green vegies for minerals, vegetable proteins for growth, and complex carbohydrates for energy. It is low in fats, pasteurized dairy foods and sugars, (sugars inhibit release of growth hormones), and avoids fried foods. It is also very easy on you, the parent. Once children are taught and shown the foods that will give them health and energy they can make a lot of these simply prepared foods on their own. Make sure you tell and graphically show your child what junk and synthetic foods are. We find over and over

again that because of TV advertising and peer pressure, kids often really don't know what wholesome food is, and think they are eating the right way.

Vitamins and minerals are important for a child's physical, emotional and mental growth, and for a healthy immune system. A child's normal immune defenses are strong. If s/he is eating well, with lots of green vegies, and few sugars, refined foods or dairy products, s/he may not need extra supplementation. However, because of depleted soils and sprayed produce, many vitamins, minerals and trace minerals are no longer sufficiently present in our foods, so supplementation is often needed for good body building blocks, and to enable children to think, learn and grow at optimum levels. The most common deficiencies are calcium, iron, B₁, and vitamins A, B Complex and C.

Supplements for the Optimal Children's Diet

If your child needs more nutrition than s/he is receiving from diet, daily supplementation might include:

❧ Acidophilus, in liquid or powder; give in juice 2 to 3x daily for good digestion and assimilation.

❧ Vitamin C, or Ester C in chewable or powder form with bioflavonoids; give in juice, 1/4 teasp. at a time 2 to 3x daily. If chewable wafers are chosen, use 100mg., 250mg., or 500mg. potency according to age and weight of the child, and give 3 to 4x daily.

❧ Give a sugar-free multi-vitamin and mineral supplement daily, in either liquid or chewable tablet form. Some good choices are from Floradix, Rainbow Light, Solaray and Mezotrace.

❧ Give a protein drink each morning if the child's energy or school performance level is poor, or if a weak system is constantly leading to chronic illness. (The body must have protein to heal.) Good choices are from Nature's Plus SPIRUTEIN, and NutriTech EARTHSHAKE.

Bodywork for the Optimal Children's Diet:

❧ *Exercise is the key to health, growth and body oxygen. Don't let your kid be a couch potato, or a computer junkie. Encourage outdoor sports and activity every day possible, and make sure s/he is taking P. E. classes in school. Exercise for kids is one of the best 'nutrients' for both body and mind.*

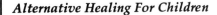

Herbal Remedies For Children

A child's body responds very well to herbal medicines. Unless unusually or chronically ill, a child is born with well-developed, powerful immune system, and this inherent resistance ability is a key factor in understanding children's diseases. They often only require the subtle, body strengthening forces that herbs or homeopathic medicines supply. The more highly focused medications of allopathic medicine can have drastic side effects on a small body. We have found that children will drink herbal teas, take herbal drops and syrups, and dissolve homeopathic medicines in the mouth much more readily than you might think. The remedies and methods listed in the following section are building, strengthening and non-traumatic to a child's system. Check suggested dosage amounts according to child's age on page 15. Conditions not listed below have their own specific page in the "AILMENTS" section of this book.

☺ **ACUTE BRONCHITIS** - Give thyme, mullein or plantain tea every 3-4 hours. Chamomile and honey tea will help curb bronchial inflammation. B & T COUGH & BRONCHIAL SYRUP.

☺ **CHEST CONGESTION** - Herbal steam inhalations with eucalyptus oil, tea tree oil, or Crystal Star RSPR™ TEA will help keep lungs mucous free and improve oxygen uptake. Hydrotherapy baths with calendula flowers or strong comfrey tea infusions will induce cleansing perspiration and neutralize body acids. Peppermint and raspberry tea are effective. Apply a soothing chest rub with TIGER BALM, WHITE FLOWER or calendula oil to loosen congestion after a bath.

☺ **COLIC** - Usually a lack of B Complex, magnesium,, calcium or potassium; sometimes mother's milk is acid from stress or tension. Give Solaray BABY LIFE for mineral and/or B Complex deficiency, or B Complex dilute liquid in water about once a week. Give Hyland's COLIC or BILIOUSNESS tabs.

Give papaya juice or apple juice. Give Natren LIFE START 1/4 teasp. in water or juice 2-3x daily, or Solaray BIFIDO-BACTERIA for infants. Give small doses of papaya enzymes. Give the baby an early morning sunbath whenever possible for vitamin D. Give a catnip enema once a week, or as needed for instant gas release.

☺ **CONSTIPATION** - Soak raisins in senna tea and feed to child for almost instant relief. Give weak licorice or mullein tea, molasses in water, or one teaspoon psyllium husk in aloe vera juice 2 times daily. A gentle catnip enema will effectively clear the colon of impacted waste, and allow the body to rid itself of diseased bacteria.

☺ **CRADLE CAP** - Massage in vitamin E or jojoba oil gently for 5 minutes. Leave on for 30 minutes, then brush scalp with soft baby brush and shampoo with TEA TREE oil or aloe vera shampoo. Repeat twice weekly. Often this is a biotin deficiency. Take biotin lozenges - 1000mcg. while nursing; the baby will receive the necessary amount through breast milk.

☺ **CUTS, BURNS & BRUISES** - Apply TEA TREE OIL, CALENDULA OINTMENT, B & T CALI-FLORA GEL, or ALOE VERA GEL every 2 or 3 hours, then apply vitamin E oil at bedtime. Apply B & T ARNIFLORA GEL for bruises and swelling.

☺ **DIAPER & SKIN RASH** - Mix comfrey, golden seal and arrowroot powders with aloe vera gel and apply to rash. Or use calendula ointment, liquid lecithin, or slippery elm powder. Dab on mineral water, or rub on vitamin A, D & E oil, or TEA TREE CREAM. Expose the child's bottom to sunlight for 20 minutes every day possible for vitamin D nutrients. Wash diapers in water with a teasp. of tea tree oil. An oatmeal bath will neutralize acids coming out through the skin.

☺ **DIARRHEA** - Give carob powder in apple juice every three hours, and offer several apples every day. Give slippery elm mixed with a little skim milk, or peppermint tea twice daily. Feed plenty of brown rice and yogurt for B Complex vitamins and friendly intestinal flora. Red raspberry, chamomile, thyme teas, and Crystal Star FIRST AID TEA FOR KIDS™ are also helpful.

☺ **EARACHE** - Use mullein essence or garlic oil ear drops directly in the ear. Or mix vegetable glycerin and witch hazel, dip in cotton balls and insert in ear to draw out infection. Give lobelia extract drops in water or juice for pain. See *EAR INFECTION* page for more information.

☺ **FEVER** - Catnip tea and catnip enemas will help a moderate fever. The diet should be liquids only - juices, herb teas, such as peppermint and red raspberry, water and broth for at least 24 hours til the fever breaks. A fever is usually a body cleansing and healing process - *a result of the problem, a part of the cure.* If the fever is sudden onset use ACONITE 30x, a homeopathic remedy. If there is nausea with the fever, use Hyland's FERRUM PHOS. See the *FEVER* page in this book for more information. See a doctor if fever is very high.

☺ **GAS & FLATULANCE** - Soak anise seed, dill seed, carraway seed or chamomile in water or juice and strain off. Give tablespoons of liquid every 3 to 4 hours until digestion rebalances.

☺ **INDIGESTION** - Give chamomile, fennel or catnip tea, or a little ground ginger and cinnamon in water. Use soy milk or goat's milk instead of cow's milk for digestibility. Give a teaspoon of acidophilus liquid before meals to build healthy flora.

☺ **INSECT BITES & STINGS** - Apply B & T SSSSTING STOP CREAM for pain and itch. (May also be used as a repellent). Or apply TEA TREE OIL. Give vitamin C 100-500mg. chewables every 4-5 hours to neutralize poison. Use vitamin B₁ as a natural insect repellent, 100mg. 2x daily.

☺ **JAUNDICE** - Give Hyland's BILIOUSNESS TABS. Prick a 100IU vitamin E oil capsule and squirt in mouth. Give a little lemon water with maple syrup.

☺ **MUMPS** - Give 10 drops mullein/lobelia tincture in water every few hours. Give Crystal Star ANTI-BIO™ DROPS in water every few hours to clear the lymph glands. Offer juices and liquids with a pinch of ginger powder in each drink for stomach cleansing. Take ginger or vinegar/sea salt baths. Make sure the child gets plenty of rest and sleep. Catnip, fenugreek, and scullcap teas are all effective.

☺ **PARASITES & WORMS** - Give raisins soaked in senna tea to cleanse the intestines. Use a garlic enema, or insert a garlic clove in the rectum at night. Give chlorophyll liquid, wormwood tea or herbal pumpkin tablets.

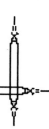

☺ **SORE THROAT -** Give Crystal Star COFEX™ TEA as a throat coat at night for almost immediate relief. Give pineapple juice 2-3x daily as an anti-viral. Use N.F. Factors HERBALSEPTIC or Nutrition resources NUTRI-BIOTIC GRAPEFRUIT SEED EXTRACT SPRAY to numb the throat. Mild zinc lozenges and licorice sticks or tea are also effective.

☺ **TEETHING -** Rub gums with honey, a little peppermint oil, or a few drops of lobelia tincture. Give weak catnip, fennel or peppermint tea to soothe irritation. Add a few daily drops of A, D & E oil to food.

☺ **THRUSH FUNGAL INFECTION -** Give Natren LIFE START, or DR. DOPHILUS powder daily, vitamin C 100mg. or Ester C chewable, and vitamin A 10,000IU. Thrush is often caused by widespread antibiotic use. Give garlic extract drops in water, or squirt a pricked garlic oil cap in the mouth. Give acidophilus liquid by mouth, and use as a suppository in the rectum.

☺ **WHOOPING COUGH -** Give Crystal Star ANTI-SPZ™ and ANTI-BIO™ capsules, lobelia or valerian/wildlettuce tincture or Nature's Way ANTSP EXTRACT to control involuntary coughing. Add 10,000IU vitamin A, and 2 cups of weak red clover, peach bark or ephedra tea daily. Apply hot ginger/garlic compresses to the chest, and use a eucalyptus steam at night. Give a liquid diet during acute stage with plenty of juices, broths and pure water.

☺ **WEAK SYSTEM -** Add a mineral supplement in liquid or chewable form, such as Floradix MULTIPLE, or Mezotrace MULTI-MINERAL COMPLEX chewable. A good general homeopathic remedy is Hyland's BIOPLASMA. Give apple and carrot juices. Include a chewable vitamin C wafer every day as a preventive against disease exposure.

✚ **First Aid tips for Kids -** Always keep tea tree oil and "RESCUE REMEDY" homeopathic drops on hand. They can handle most minor childhood emergencies naturally and effectively.

TEA TREE OIL - For infections that need antiseptic or antifungal activity - including mouth, teeth, gums, throat, ringworm, fungus, etc. Effective on stings, bites, burns, sunburns, cuts, and scrapes.

RESCUE REMEDY - For respiratory problems, coughing, gas, stomach, constipation and digestive upset. A rebalancing calmative for emotional stress and anxiety.

KIDS KIT from Hylands Homeopathic - A first aid kit with gentle all-purpose remedies.

FIRST AID TEA FOR KIDS™ - Crystal Star's gentle, all-purpose tea that addresses many childhood problems. A cleansing, detoxifying, body-balancing blend that may be taken as needed for infant jaundice and teething pain; for a fever in hot water to induce a cleansing sweat; for stomache aches, diarrhea and a generally over-acid condition, when the child is whiny and sickly.

Bifido-bacteria provides better protection and healthier intestinal flora for infants and children than regular acidophilus.

❀ To help prevent contagious disease after exposure, give 1 cayenne capsule 3x a day, 2 chewable vitamin C 500mg. wafers 3x a day, and a cup of roasted dandelion root tea daily - for 3 or 4 days.

❀ A watchword for kids: Aspirin has been linked to Reyes Syndome, a rare but sometimes deadly disease that can afflict children after bouts of flu or chickenpox.

❀ Another watchword: Infants under 12 months have little protective intestinal bacteria to fight botulism, which sometimes appears in contaminated honey. The best defense seem to be eavoidance of honey until after 1 year old.

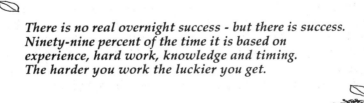

There is no real overnight success - but there is success.
Ninety-nine percent of the time it is based on
experience, hard work, knowledge and timing.
The harder you work the luckier you get.

Healthy Pets

NATURAL HEALING FOR ANIMALS

Cats and dogs usually need more nutrition than is found in most commercial animal foods. Most pet foods are derived from low quality ingredients rejected for human consumption. Pet foods that are advertised as "Complete and Balanced" are usually based on uncertain minimum nutrition requirements designed only for adequate health, not optimal health. Many vitamins and minerals are lost or lacking through non-standardized "mixmaster" processing that relies heavily on chemical additives to make the food palatable, and the shelf life long. Veterinarians today are seeing many premature and chronic health problems that seem to stem from substandard, poor quality, processed foods.

In general, animals thrive on the healthy foods and balanced diet that is good for people. Whole grains, a little meat, and lots of fresh water every day are basic. And just like people, animals need fresh greens, to keep immunity strong and their systems clean and regular. Unfortunately, also just like people, busy schedules and fast feeding make it difficult to insure that your animals are getting all the nutrition they need. Herbs, homeopathic medicines and high quality natural supplements can help maintain and restore pet health.

❤ DIET FOR A HEALTHY PET:
Most pets need some fresh vegetables every day. Greens keep their systems clean and healthy. Mix them with a little fish, raw liver and kidney, chicken, low ash canned or dry food. Most animals like cucumbers, green peppers, carrots, green onions, parsley, celery and tomato juice.

♠ Add whole grains every day for fiber and complex carbohydrates, either from a high quality kibble, or stale bread, crackers or cereal from the kitchen.

♠ Give them some dairy foods several times a week. Most animals like cheese, yogurt, kefir, cottage cheese, goat's milk and sour cream.

♠ A little fruit is good occasionally to loosen up a clogged system, but give sparingly. Most animals like raisins, coconut, cantaloupe and apples.

♠ Have fresh water available all day long. Most animals need lots of liquids every day.

♠ A good sample meal for general health can be made up all at once and divided between feedings. Mix lightly: 1 small can fish or poultry, or about 6 to 8 oz. soy protein, 3 teasp. brewer's yeast, 1 raw egg, 1 cup chopped vegetables, a little broth or water to moisten. THEY'LL LOVE IT.

♠ Avoid junk foods and refined foods for your pets. They are even worse for their smaller, simpler systems than they are for you.

Cats and dogs have slightly different diet needs. If you are mixing your own food for your animal's diet, the following knowledge is good to have.

🐈 Key foods for cats, to provide sustained energy, fiber, B vitamins, minerals, trace minerals and fatty acids; with the correct proportions of proteins and carbohydrates: liver, bone meal, sea vegetables, whole grains, rice and vegetables. Add some wheat or corn germ, bran, vegetable oil and leafy greens at least three times a week.

🐕 Key foods for dogs need to be easily digestible, and based on high quality proteins and whole grains. Dog foods should be low in saturated fat. Contrary to popular advertising, dog's do not need meat as an essential part of their diet. Their quality protein can come from eggs, soy foods and low fat dairy products, as well as occasional fish or poultry.

Notes: Don't give your dog table scraps. The animal won't get the nutritional balance it needs. Avoid heavy spices and bones. They are harmful to a dog's digestive system.

Both puppies and kittens need twice the nutrients and calories as adult animals.
Pregnant and nursing females need more protein, vitamins and minerals.
Older animals need very digestible foods, and less vitamins, minerals, proteins and sodium.

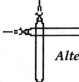

❤ SUPPLEMENTS FOR A HEALTHY PET

Food source supplements are wonderful for animals. Wheat germ oil, spirulina, kelp, brewer's yeast, bran and lecithin are all good for keeping animals as well as people in tip top condition.

Crystal Star has two very successful food and herbal supplement for animals.

HEALTHY LIFE ANIMAL MIX™ is a delicious food sprinkle packed with nutrients for a shiny coat and eyes, for healthy gums and teeth, for good temperament, regularity, immune strength and freedom from fleas and ticks. HEALTHY LIFE™ gives animals the valuable benefits of concentrated greens to keep the blood strong, the body regular and the breath and stomach sweet. It is rich in beta carotene for natural immune strength. HEALTHY LIFE™ is high in anti-oxidants such as vitamin C and E to help control arthritis and dysplasia symptoms, and help prevent damage from rancid fats or poor quality foods. It is full of natural enzymes for easier digestion and regularity. All kinds of animals love it, from hamsters to horses. Some of them (including our own) won't eat without it!

SYSTEM STRENGTH™ drink is an advanced healing combination for animals as well as people. It is a complete food-source mineral supplement, for basic body building blocks, to balance the acid/alkaline system, regulate body fluid osmosis and electrical activity in the nervous system, and to aid in digestion and regularity. SYSTEM STRENGTH™ is a rich chlorophyll and green-vitamin source, with large amounts of plant beta-carotene, B vitamins, choline, essential fatty acids with GLA, DGLA and linoleic acid, and octacosanol for tissue oxygenation. It is a vigorous source of usable proteins and amino acids. It has almost twice the amount of protein as a comparable amount of wheat germ. It is an exceptional source of alkalizing enzymes for good assimilation and digestion, and for all cell functions.
We have found it to be rapidly restorative for animal systems, even when severely ill or injured. Even very sick animals seem to know instinctively that it is good for them, and will eagerly take it as a broth from an eye dropper if they can't eat any other way.
(See ingredients and dosage listing for both of the above combinations in the back of this book.)

Homeopathic remedies are also wonderful for animals, both in liquid and tablet form. They are effective, gentle, non-toxic, and free of side effects. They heal without harming.

Keep TEA TREE OIL, *food grade 1%* H_2O_2, (1 oz. 3% solution in 1 qt. water) and RESCUE REMEDY extract on hand for your pets. These natural medicinals can handle many minor emergencies, and even some major problems. All are effective and non-toxic, and can be used externally as well as internally.

❤ BODYWORK FOR A HEALTHY PET

➤ Brush and comb your animals often. It keeps their coats shiny, circulation stimulated, and they like the attention.

➤ Avoid commercial, chemical-impregnated flea collars. They often have DDT or a nerve gas in them that is potentially toxic to pet, owner and environment. Use a mild shampoo with essential herbal oils for your pet. The oils interfere with the insect's ability to sense the moisture, heat and breath of the animal.

➤ Sprinkle cedar shavings around your animal's sleeping place to keep insects away and to make the area smell nice.

➤ Give your pet plenty of fresh air, exercise and water.

➤ Use Nature's Miracle liquid for accident clean-up. It is all natural, non-toxic, and it works.

❤ Give your pets lots of love and affection. It is always the best medicine for health and happiness. They need it as much as you do.

Nutritional Healing For Animals

ARTHRITIS:
- ☞ Avoid refined and preserved foods, especially white flour and sugar.
- ☞ Reduce red meat and canned foods. Add green and raw foods.
- ☞ Make a comfrey/flaxseed or alfalfa tea, and add to animal's drinking water.
- ☞ Give 2 teasp. cod liver oil 100-200IU vitamin E daily, 6 to 8 alfalfa tablets, and $1/4$ teasp. sodium ascorbate, Ester C powder, or vitamin C crystals daily.
- ☞ H_2O_2 1% solution in water - 1 teasp. daily for 1 month.
- ☞ Give Biogenetics BIOGUARD PLUS for PETS as directed.
- ☞ Give Crystal Star AR-EASE™ FOOD SPRINKLE FOR ANIMALS
- ☞ Shark cartilage, give continually until no evidence of the problem.
- ☞ Give Crystal Star HEALTHY LIFE ANIMAL MIX™ 2 teasp. daily; or sprinkle on SYSTEM STRENGTH™ broth mix, $1/2$ teasp. once daily.

BAD BREATH:
- ☞ Feed more fresh raw foods, less canned processed foods. Snip fresh parsley into food at each meal.
- ☞ Sprinkle a little spirulina powder or liquid chlorophyll on food.
- ☞ Give Dr. Goodpet GOOD BREATH homeopathic remedy.

BLADDER INFECTION/INCONTINENCE:
- ☞ Give vitamin C 250mg. 2 to 3 times daily, B Complex 10 to 20mg. once daily.
- ☞ Put the animal on a liquid diet for 24 hours with vegetable juices and broths - no solid foods. Offer lots of fresh water.
- ☞ Give magnesium tablets, 100mg. daily for a week.

CANCERS/LEUKEMIA/MALIGNANT TUMORS:
- ☞ Give vitamin C as sodium ascorbate powder, $1/4$ teasp. twice daily for larger animals, and cats with leukemia, or Alacer EMERGEN-C in water. As tumor starts to shrink, decrease vitamin C to a small daily pinch.
- ☞ Give Crystal Star SYSTEM STRENGTH™ broth 2 to 3x daily, $1/4$ cup or as much as animal will take.
- ☞ Shark cartilege, give continually until no evidence of the problem.
- ☞ Apply Crystal Star GINSENG SKIN REPAIR GEL™ to tumorous areas.
- ☞ Give vitamin E 200IU daily, and apply vitamin E oil locally if there is a tumor or malignancy.
- ☞ Give 1 teasp. cod liver oil, or Beta Carotene 10,000IU daily.
- ☞ Give dilute 1% food grade H_2O_2, 2 to 3 teasp. daily to both dogs and cats.
- ☞ Dilute a goldenseal/echinacea extract to $1/2$ strength. Give $1/4$ teasp. daily.
- ☞ Aloe Vera juice, 2 to 3 teasp. daily; apply gel if tumor is visible.
- ☞ Give BIOGUARD PLUS from Biogenetics as directed.

COAT & SKIN HEALTH:
- ☞ Add lecithin granules or Crystal Star HEALTHY LIFE MIX™ to food daily.
- Add 2 teasp. cod liver oil to food daily.
- Give vitamin E 100IU daily. Apply E oil or jojoba oil to affected skin areas.
- Add 1 teasp. Spirulina or kelp powder to food daily.
- Give Dr. Goodpet SCRATCH-FREE to curb itching and dry hot spots.

CONSTIPATION:
- ☞ Add more greens and veggies to the diet; decrease canned food.
- ☞ Add Crystal Star HEALTHY LIFE MIX™ for soluble food fiber.
- ☞ Mix a little garlic powder with 1 TB. olive oil and add to food.
- ☞ Exercise the animal more often. Let it outside more often for relief.
- ☞ Aloe vera juice, 2 to 3 teasp. daily.

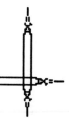

🐈 CUTS & WOUNDS:

☞ Apply a goldenseal/myrrh solution, or comfrey salve.

☞ Give vitamin C crystals (as sodium ascorbate if possible) $1/4$ to $1/2$ teasp. in a cup of water. Apply directly, and give internally throughout the day.

☞ Apply vitamin E oil. Give vitamin E 100IU daily.

☞ Apply calendula ointment.

☞ Apply Nutrition Resource NUTRI-BIOTIC GRAPEFRUIT SEED SPRAY as needed.

☞ Apply aloe vera gel and give desiccated liver tabs or powder in food daily.

🐈 DEHYDRATION:

☞ This is a major emergency for cats. Check for dehydration by pulling up the scruff of the neck. If skin is slow to return, animal is dehydrated. Take to a vet as soon as possible.

☞ Make a comfrey tea, or Crystal Star SYSTEM STRENGTH™ broth immediately. Force feed if necessary about 2 oz. an hour. Mix a little bran, tomato juice, ssame oil. Feed each hour til improvement.

☞ Try to feed green veggies; especially celery, lettuce and carrots for electrolyte replacement. Once the crisis has passed, add kelp, spirulina or a green drink to the diet.

☞ Check for worms, often a cause of dehydration.

☞ Give the animal lots of love and attention. Dehydration is often caused by depression. The animal simply curls up and will not eat or drink anything. RESCUE REMEDY is excellent in this case.

🐈 DIARRHEA:

☞ Diarrhea is often caused by spoiled food, non-food items, worms or harmful bacteria. Put the animal on a short 24 hour liquid diet with vegetable juices, broths, and lots of water.

☞ Give yogurt or acidolphilus liquid at every feeding until diarrhea ends.

☞ Give brewer's yeast and 1 teasp. carob powder at every feeding.

☞ Sprinkle crushed activated charcoal tablets on food.

☞ Aloe vera juice, 2 to 3 teasp. daily.

☞ Use Dr. Goodpet DIAR-RELIEF homeopathic remedy, or Crystal Star DIAR-EX™ extract in water.

🐈 DISTEMPER:

☞ If the problem is acute, put the animal on a short liquid diet with vegetable juices, broths, and plenty of fresh water.

☞ Give vitamin C crystals (sodium ascorbate if possible), $1/4$ teasp. mixed in a cup of water, divided throughout the day, in an eye dropper if necessary. If there is severe vomiting and loss of fluids, give some vitamin C liquid every hour. Give Dr. Goodpet CALM STRESS homeopathic remedy to calm vomiting.

☞ Add $1/2$ dropperful B complex liquid and 1 teasp. bonemeal to food daily.

☞ Give a dilute (1 drop extract in 2 teasp. water) goldenseal/myrrh, or echinacea solution. Or give echinacea tea to flush and neutralize toxins.

☞ Give yogurt or acidophilus liquid to rebuild friendly flora and immunity.

☞ Give fresh garlic, or a garlic/honey mixture daily. Give raw liver or liver tablets several times a week.

☞ Add brown rice and bran to daily food for B vitamins and system tone.

🐈 ECZEMA:

☞ Give zinc 25mg. internally, and apply zinc ointment to infected areas.

☞ Mix cottage cheese, corn oil, vitamin E oil, and brewer's yeast. Give 1 TB. daily. Or give 1 teasp. cod liver oil mixed with 1 TB. garlic powder daily.

☞ Give 1 to 2 teasp. wheat germ daily. Apply locally to sores.

☞ Reduce meat and canned foods. Add fresh veggies and greens to the diet.

🐈 EYE & EAR INFECTION:

☞ Add betacarotene 10,000IU, 1 teasp. cod liver oil, and vitamin E 100IU to the diet. Cod liver oil and E oil may also be applied locally.

☞ Give goat's milk daily in food, and apply with cotton balls to the eye.

☞ Use Dr. Goodpet EYE-C homeopathic remedy for eyes, EAR RELIEF for ears.
☞ Give homeopathic Nat. Mur in early stages; Silicea in later stages to arrest cataract development.
☞ Apply an eyebright herb tea or Crystal Star EYEBRIGHT HERBAL™ TEA to infected area.

FLEAS/TICKS/MITES: *Be sure to give floppy-eared pets a weekly ear inspection for mites and ticks.*
☞ Give fresh garlic, or mix 1/2 teasp. garlic powder and 1 teasp. brewer's yeast and sprinkle on food.
☞ Have your dog swim in the ocean, or give him a seaweed bath.
☞ String eucalyptus buds around animal's neck. Put rosemary and bay leaves, or cedar and citronella oils around sleeping area. Or grind these herbs into a powder and sprinkle on pet and sleeping area.
☞ Put eucalyptus, pennyroyal, and citronella oils on pets collar.
☞ Rub rosemary, myrrh oil, or tea tree oil directly on animal's coat between shampoos to drive off insects and leave a nice scent. Stuff a pillow with rosemary, pennyroyal, eucalyptus and mint leaves, and place on animal's bed.
☞ Sprinkle Crystal Star HEALTHY LIFE MIX™, Dr. Goodpet FLEA RELIEF homeopathic remedy, or brewer's yeast on food daily.
☞ Give 1/2 of a 100mg. vitamin B1 tablet daily to ward off insects.
☞ Apply tea tree oil directly on the insect to kill it. As an alternative to chemical dips, add a few tea tree oil drops to pet's regular shampoo. Leave on 3 to 5 minutes before rinsing.
☞ Apply jojoba oil on the bitten place to heal it faster.

GAS & FLATULENCE:
☞ Give alfalfa tabs, spirulina, or dilute chlorophyll liquid at each feeding.
☞ Sprinkle a pinch of ginger powder on food at each feeding.
☞ Give comfrey, chamomile or peppermint tea daily.

GUM & TOOTH PROBLEMS:
☞ Apply a dilute goldenseal/myrrh or propolis solution to gums.
☞ Give and apply dilute chlorophyll liquid solution.
☞ Give a natural fresh foods diet, adding crunchy raw vegies and whole grains.
☞ Apply vitamin E oil, tea tree oil, or calendula oil to gums.
☞ Vitamin C - a weak solution of ascorbate crystals in water may be rubbed on the gums.

HIP DYSPLASIA & LAMENESS (SEE ALSO ARTHRITIS):
☞ Mix 1 teasp. sodium ascorbate, or Ester-C crystals in water and give throughout the day, every day.
☞ Mix 1 teasp. bonemeal powder in one cup tomato juice, with 1 teasp. bran and 1/2 teasp. sesame oil. Give daily.
☞ Give BIOGUARD PLUS for PETS from Biogenetics as directed.
☞ Shark cartilege, give continually until no evidence of the problem.
☞ Mix 2 teasp. cod liver oil, 1 teasp. bonemeal, 1 TB. lecithin. Give daily.

INTESTINAL & STOMACH PROBLEMS:
☞ Put animal on a short liquid fast for 24 hours, with water, broth and green juices to clear intestines. Then feed yogurt or liquid acidophilus and fresh foods for 2-3 days. Give comfrey tea in the water bowl.
☞ Give Crystal Star HEALTHY LIFE MIX™ with 1/2 teasp. extra garlic powder daily.
☞ Garlic, mullein/myrrh combination, or echinacea or black walnut extract diluted in water, or mugwort tea.

MANGE & FUNGAL INFECTION:
☞ Put drops of tea tree oil in the animals shampoo and use every 2 or 3 days.
☞ Apply Pau de Arco salve, zinc ointment, fresh lemon juice to relieve area.
☞ Add bonemeal powder to food to ease tension and curb frantic licking.
☞ Use Dr. Goodpet CALM STRESS homeopathic remedy.
☞ Apply dilute echinacea tincture, or golden seal/echinacea/myrrh water solution to affected areas daily. Also sprinkle on food.

☞ Apply Nutrition Resource NUTRI-BIOTIC GRAPEFRUIT SEED spray to infected areas several times daily.

☞ Give 1 teasp. lecithin granules daily. Mix 2 teasp. cod liver oil with 1 TB. brewer's yeast and 2 teasp. desiccated liver powder. Give daily.

🐕 OVERWEIGHT:

☞ Reduce canned and saturated fat foods. Increase fresh foods, whole grains and organ meats.

☞ Give Crystal Star HEALTHY LIFE MIX™ for fiber without calories.

☞ Add more exercise to the animal's life.

🐄 PREGNANCY & BIRTH:

☞ Give red raspberry tea daily during the last half of gestation for easier birth.

☞ Give daily spirulina tabs or powder for extra protein.

☞ Give desiccated liver tabs, extra bonemeal, and cod liver oil daily.

☞ Give extra vitamin C 100mg. chewable, and vitamin E 100IU daily.

🐕 RESPIRATORY INFECTIONS & IMMUNE STRENGTH:

☞ Put animal on a short liquid diet for 24 hours to cleanse the system, with vegetable juices, broths and water. Offer comfrey tea to flush toxins faster.

☞ Give Crystal Star HEALTHY LIFE MIX™ for immune strength; COFEX TEA™ for dry hacking cough.

☞ Give Crystal Star SYSTEM STRENGTH™ broth 2 to 3 times daily, about $1/4$ cup, or as much as the animal will take.

☞ Add 1 teasp. bee pollen, vitamin E 100IU, and $1/4$ teasp. vitamin C (as sodium ascorbate if possible) dissolved in a cup of water to diet.

☞ Add dilute 1% food grade hydrogen peroxide to the diet for oxygen therapy.

☞ Add 2 to 4 garlic tablets and 6 alfalfa tablets to the daily diet.

☞ Give BIOGUARD PLUS from Biogenetics as directed.

🐕 WORMS & PARASITES:

☞ Build up parasite immunity with Crystal Star HEALTHY LIFE MIX™, as directed daily.

☞ Put the animal on a short 24 hour liquid fast with water only to weaken the parasites. Then give Crystal Star VERMEX™ CAPS as directed *with* charcoal tabs in water or an electuary for 3 to 7 days. Repeat process in a week to kill newly hatched eggs.

☞ Mix $1/2$ teasp. garlic powder and a pinch of cloves; sprinkle on food daily until worms are gone.

☞ Give spirulina for a month after worming to rebuild immune strength.

☞ Garlic, mullein/myrrh blend; echinacea or black walnut extract diluted in water, or mugwort tea.

Note: Acupuncture has been a very successful alternative treatment for animals - especially in cases of arthritis, hip dysplasia, asthma, epilepsy, cervical-disk displacements and chronic infections.

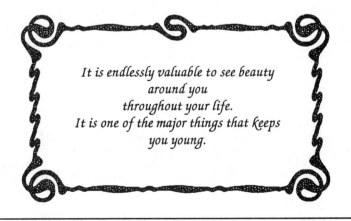

It is endlessly valuable to see beauty around you throughout your life. It is one of the major things that keeps you young.

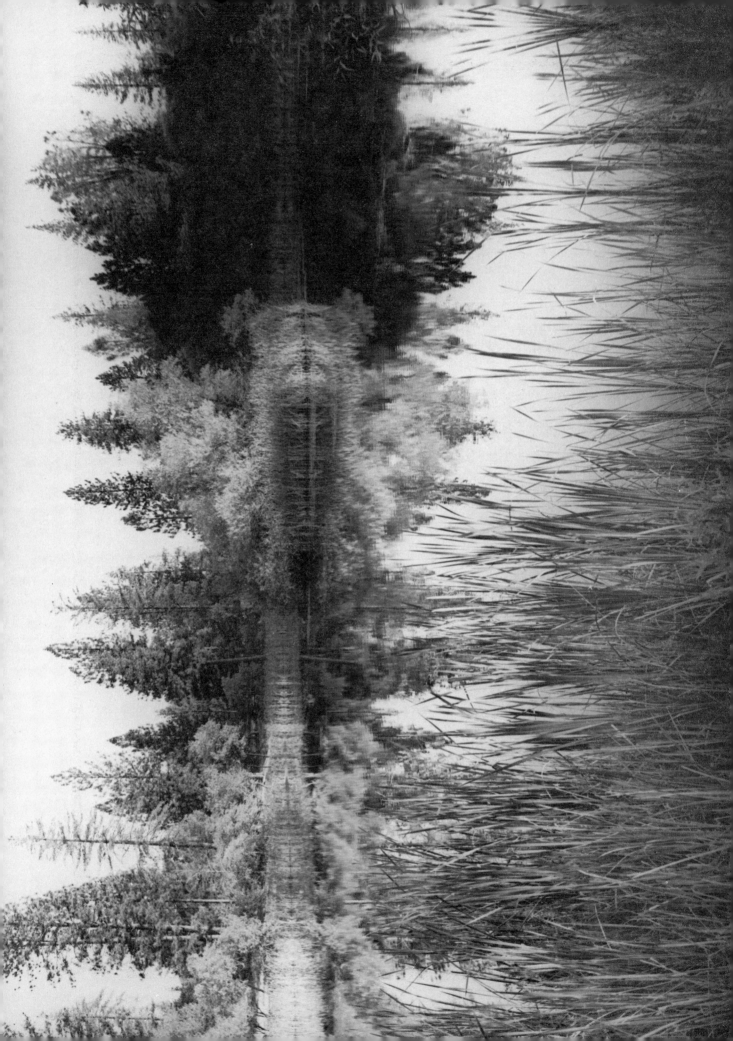

AILMENTS
IN ALPHABETICAL ORDER

Each ailment page consists of a four point program:
FOOD THERAPY, VITAMIN/MINERAL THERAPY, HERBAL THERAPY & BODYWORK

These programs can be addressed in several ways, according to the individual person's needs. A mixture of remedies may be employed in each area, or just one or two areas may be used. Pick the suggestions that you feel instinctively strong about. They are invariably the best for you, and will be the easiest to incorporate into your lifestyle.

All the recommended remedies have been found effective, but every person has a different body and is a different individual. Healing and response seem to accelerate when a person picks out his own areas of natural therapy.

✳ Bold print entries indicate the most successful, or most often used therapeutics.

✳ Where a method has also proven effective for children, a small child's face ☺ appears at the end of the recommendation.

✳ Where a method has proven particularly successful for women, a female symbol ♀ appears at the end of the recommendation.

✳ Where a method has proven particularly successful for men, a male symbol ♂ appears at the end of the recommendation.

☛ Refer to the Glossary of Healing Foods, pg. 64 for more information about any recommended food in the ailments programs.

☛ All recommended doses are daily unless otherwise specified. Dosage listed is for the major time of healing, and is not to be considered as maintenance or long term.

☛ The traditional rule of thumb for natural healing is one month for every year you have had the problem.

124

ABSCESSES

Boils ✧ Carbuncles ✧ Supperating Sores ✧ Dental Abscesses

Pus accumulation that forms due to infection, anywhere in the body - both externally and internally. Recurrent attacks of boils and abscesses indicate a depressed iummune system.

FOOD THERAPY

☙ Go on a short 1 to 3 day fresh juice diet (pg. 42ff.), followed by a fresh foods cleansing diet for 2 weeks to remove toxins.

☙ Simmer flax and fenugreek together til soft. Mash pulp. Apply to abscess as a compress.

☙ Mix fresh grated garlic with lemon juice and apply.

☙ Eat yogurt, kefir, acidophilus for friendly intestinal flora.

☙ Drink 6 to 8 glasses of pure water daily.

VITAMINS/MINERALS

Add acidophilus to the diet if taking high dose courses of antibiotics for abscess infections.

▶ Liquid chlorophyll - apply locally. Take internally, 3 teasp. daily.

▶ Take DR. DOPHILUS 3x daily.
with
▶ Garlic caps, 2 caps 3x daily.

▶ Apply and take internally Nutrition Resource NUTRIBIOTIC GRAPEFRUIT SEED extract spray and capsules as needed.

▶ Beta-carotene A 100,000IU daily for one week.
with
▶ Vit. E 400IU 2x daily or Zinc 50-75mg. daily.
and
▶ Vit. C ascorbate powder 3 to 5 grams daily, with zinc 50mg. 2x daily for 1 week.

▶ For dental abscesses: homeopathic remedies have been very successful.
✚ *Belladonna* for throbbing and redness.
✚ *Bryonia* for acute inflammation.
✚ *Pyrogenium* for undrained pus.
✚ *Silicea* to increase pus drainage after it has started.
✚ *Mercurius* for excess salivation and foul breath.

HERBAL THERAPY

☙ Echinacea extract 3x daily under the tongue.
Apply Echinacea salve or cream, or Echinacea tincture drops.

☙ Propolis tincture - apply directly and take internally, twice daily.

☙ Crystal Star ANTI-BIO™ caps - 6 daily for 3 days, then 4 daily for one week.
with
ANTI-FLAM™ CAPS and ANTI-FLAM™ CAPS and CLEANSING & PURIFYING TEA™ for one week.

☙ Take burdock rt. tea 3 to 4 cups daily.

☙ Black walnut extract. Take internally. Apply directly.

☙ Effective topical applications:
♦ Aloe vera gel.
♦ Tea tree oil.
♦ Calendula gel and tea.
♦ Body Essential SILICA GEL.

☙ For dental abscesses:
♦ Sage tea mouthwashes several times daily, especially for "dry socket" abscesses.

BODYWORK

▶ Take a catnip enema every other day for 1 week to clean out toxins.

▶ Apply a hot epsom salts compress, (2 TBS. salts to 1 cup hot water) to bring boil to a head.

▶ Apply a St. John's wort, or fresh burdock root poultice.

▶ Apply Nature's Herbs BLACK OINTMENT.

▶ Expose the area to early morning sunlight for 15 minutes a day.

▶ Apply Country Comfort COMFREY-ALOE CREAM.

▶ Apply a green or white clay compress several times daily to bring to a head.

Common Symptoms: Inflammation and infection of the skin layers; supperation with white, rather than clear drainage; weeping pus-filled sores, often accompanied by chills and fever.
Common Causes: Toxicity of the system; acid condition allowing a staph infection; viral infection.

ACIDITY ▣ ACIDOSIS
Restoring Acid/Alkaline Body Balance

Over-acidity in the body tissues is one of the basic causes of many arthritic and rheumatic diseases. Balanced body chemistry is vital to immune maintenance and disease correction.

FOOD THERAPY

A healthy body usually keeps large alkaline reserves to meet the demands of too many acid-producing foods. When these are depleted beyond a 3:1 ratio health can be seriously threatened.

🍃 Go on a short 24 hour (pg. 44) liquid fast to cleanse acid wastes. Then eat a diet of 80% alkalizing foods, including vegetable salads, sprouts, figs, apples, goat's milk, vegetable and fruit (particularly citrus) juices, soups and broths, green drinks, ume plums, etc. Acid-forming foods should be no more than 20%. Acid-forming foods include meats, poultry and eggs, fish and seafoods, lentils and peanuts, cheeses, most grains and nuts.

🍃 **Drink a daily 8oz. glass mix of tomato juice, wheat germ, brewer's yeast and lecithin. ♂**
or
🍃 **Drink 1-2 glasses of cranberry juice daily. ♀**

🍃 **Take Crystal Star SYSTEM STRENGTH™ or ENERGY GREEN™ drink mix daily.**

🍃 Eat smaller meals. Chew slowly.

VITAMINS/MINERALS

▶ Take ascorbate vitamin C crystals with bioflavonoids - 3000mg. daily for 4 weeks.

▶ HCl tabs after meals.
or
▶ High potency digestive enzymes at meals.

▶ B Complex 100mg. with extra pantothenic acid 500mg. 2 daily.

▶ Future Biotics VITAL K, 2 teasp. daily.

▶ Living Source FOOD SENSITIVITY SYSTEM daily.
or
Nutrapathic PURE & REGULAR.

HERBAL THERAPY

🍃 Crystal Star FIBER & HERBS COLON CLEANSE™ CAPS to clean out acid waste.
and
POTASSIUM SOURCE™ caps for balance, 2 daily.

🍃 Take 2 ginger caps with each meal.
and
🍃 Use ginger compresses on the kidneys to increase elimination of toxins.

🍃 Effective teas:
- ✦ Catnip ☺
- ✦ Chamomile ♀
- ✦ Fennel seed
- ✦ Wisdom of the Ancients YERBA MATÉ tea.

BODYWORK

▶ Mild exercise every day for body oxygen.

▶ Have a little wine before dinner to relax and reduce body acid.

▶ Avoid yeasted breads, pasteurized dairy, red meats, processed sugars until condition clears.

▶ Crystal Star ALKALIZING ENZYME™ BODY WRAP for almost immediate change in body pH.

▶ Reflexology point:

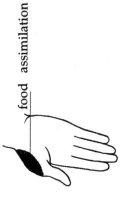

food assimilation

Common Symptoms: Frequent skin eruptions; arthritic/rheumatoid symptoms; burning, foul-smelling stools, anal itching; chronic poor digestion; acid stomach and ulcers; bad breath and body odor; alternating constipation and diarrhea; insomnia; water retention; frequent migraine headaches.
Common Causes: Mental stress and tension; kidney, liver or adrenal malfunction; poor diet with excess acid-forming foods, such as caffeine, fried foods, tobacco, or sweets. Acidosis is often related to or caused by arthritis, diabetes or borderline diabetes. Refer to those pages in this book.

ACNE ■ PIMPLES ■ BLEMISHES

Inflammation, resulting in pustules and scarring red spots, from trapped oil in sebaceous glands that harbor infective bacteria. Blackheads occur when this sebaceous oil combines with unreleased wastes and plugs the pore. Whiteheads occur when scales below the surface of the skin become filled with sebaceous oil. This conditon is more severe, because the white-heads can spread under the skin, rupture and spread the inflammation. It is a clear fact of our modern poor diet that adult acne is now more prevalent that teenage acne.

FOOD THERAPY

➤ Go on a short 1-3 day liquid cleanse (pg. 43) to clean out acid wastes. Use apple, carrot, pineap-ple and papaya juices.
   Then eat lots of fresh foods. Have a salad every day. Add of-ten to the diet: whole grains, green veggies, brown rice, fish, sprouts, low fat dairy, apples.
   Limit wheat germ, shellfish, kelp cheese, citrus, eggs and iodized salt - these foods have iodine lev-els that increase oil secretions. Drink 6-8 glasses of bottled water daily.

➤ Avoid red meats, white flour or sugar, soft drinks, caffeine, fried foods, candy, pasteurized dairy, and any foods with food addi-tives.

➤ Eliminate junk foods!

➤ Rub on lemon juice or aloe vera gel at night. Wash in the morning.

➤ Rub face with insides of papaya and cucumber skins to neutralize acid wastes.

➤ For acne scars: Place fresh - pineapple directly on the scars.

VITAMINS/MINERALS

For adult acne, do not take mega-doses of vi-tamins. They often aggravate the problem with too much iodine and vitamin E which stimulate the sebaceous glands to produce too much oil.
Add acidophilus to the diet if taking long courses of anti-biotics for acne.

◆ Mix 1/4 teasp. vitamin C crystals with 1 TB. acidophilus liquid and take 4 x daily.

◆ Pancreatin, 1 to 3 after meals to digest oils.
   with
   1 TB. Omega 3 Flax oil daily, or Wakunaga KYO-GREEN daily.
   (If there is scarring, add brome-lain 500mg. 2x daily.)

◆ For adult acne:
   ✦ Enzymatic Therapy DERMA-CLEAR program; ACNE-ZYME capsules, cream, soap, cleanser.
   ✦ Zinc 50-100mg daily.

◆ Alta Health SIL-X tabs, 3 daily.

◆ Beta carotene 25,000IU 2x daily with vitamin D 1000IU daily.

◆ B Complex 100mg. daily if acne is stress-caused (around the chin).

◆ HERPANACINE capsules.

HERBAL THERAPY

❧ Relieve inflammation and in-fection first with Crystal Star ANTI-BIO™ caps or extract, 4 x daily for 1 week.
   then take

❧ High potency royal jelly 2 teasp. daily.♀
   with

❧ Crystal Star BEAUTIFUL SKIN TEA™. Drink & apply with cot-ton balls.
   or

❧ Crystal Star BEAUTIFUL SKIN GEL™ w. propolis and royal jel-ly as directed.

❧ Apply a golden seal and myrrh solution.
   or
   Propolis tincture directly to sores.♂

❧ Evening primrose oil 4-6 daily,
   with
   Siberian ginseng or licorice tea daily.

❧ Apply tea tree oil to sores 3x daily.

❧ Use tea tree or calendula soap.

BODYWORK

▶ Apply H2O2 OXYGEL to affect-ed areas for one month. Do not squeeze. Both whiteheads and blackheads will come to the sur-face and be eliminated.

▶ Wash face and affected areas with a mild hypo-allergenic cleanser. Exfoliate with a gentle, alkalizing scrub.

▶ Steam face with Swiss Kriss Herbs; or with lavender (may also pat on lavender water), or eucalyptus and thyme.

▶ Get some early morning sun on the face every day possible. Get fresh air and exercise daily, and plenty of rest to eliminate toxins.

▶ Apply 2-3 Nutrition Resource NUTRI-BIOTIC liquid concen-trate drops directly and massage in.

▶ Apply white clay and let dry several times daily to bring to a head.

▶ Use only water-based cosmetics.

Common Symptoms: Inflamed and infected pustules on the face, chest and back. Often itching and scarring.
Common Causes: Gland (particularly pituitary), and hormone (particularly male) imbalance during high growth years, and before menstruation; high fat diet, especially saturated fats and fried foods; poor digestion of fats; essential fatty acid deficiency; excess sugar; (a rise in blood sugar is multiplied by 5 when it gets to the skin. Sugar-saturated skin is susceptible to acne infection); poor liver function; poor elimination/ constipation; heredity; some oral contraceptives; allergies and allergy-causing cosmetics; stress; lack of green veggies.

ADRENAL GLAND HEALTH

Small glands resting on top of the kidneys, the adrenals are comprised of two parts: the cortex, responsible for cortisone production, and the medulla, which secretes adrenaline. The cortex helps maintain body balance, regulates carbohydrate and sugar metabolism (balancing dysfunction that results in hypoglycemia or diabetes), and produces certain sex hormones. The medulla produces epinephrine (adrenaline) and norepinephrine to speed up metabolism to cope with stress. During stressful periods the adrenals increase metabolism to ward off negative effects. Adrenal function is impaired by long term cortico-steroid drug use, because these drugs cause the adrenals to shrink in size.

See following page for a discussion of ADDISON'S DISEASE and CUSHING'S SYNDROME

BODYWORK

➤ Massage therapy is effective in improving adrenal function. Most therapists will use muscle testing to determine the degree and indications of the dysfunction and then work to clear the adrenal pathways.

➤ Reflexology point:

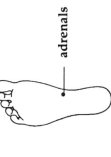

— adrenals

➤ Moderate exercise, such as a daily walk benefits adrenal health.

➤ Adrenal glands position in the body atop the kidneys:

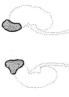

HERBAL THERAPY

❧ Crystal Star ADR-ACTIVE™ capsules or ADRN™ extract, 2x daily with BODY REBUILDER caps to stimulate hormone rebalance.

❧ High potency Premier One or YS ROYAL JELLY, 2 teasp. daily. (highest source of natural pantothenic acid available).

❧ Siberian ginseng capsules or extract 2x daily. ♂

or

Siberian ginseng/astragalus capsules, 4 daily. ♂

❧ ATOMODINE 1-2 drops daily. ♀

❧ Effective teas:
   ◆ Licorice rt.
   ◆ Hawthorne
   ◆ Gotu kola

❧ Effective extracts:
   ◆ Echinacea rt.
   ◆ Astragalus rt.
   ◆ Milk thistle seed

VITAMINS/MINERALS

▶ Adrenal complex glandular, such as Country Life ADRENAL with TYROSINE. ♂

▶ Enzymatic Therapy LIQUID LIVER w. SIBERIAN GINSENG. ♂

▶ Pantothenic acid 500-2000mg. daily.

   with

   B Complex 100mg.
   and

   Tyrosine 500mg. daily.

▶ American Biologics SUB-ADRENE, 5 drops daily.

▶ Ascorbate vitamin C 3000mg. or Ester C 1500mg. daily.

▶ High potency digestive enzymes, such as Rainbow Light DOUBLE STRENGTH ALL-ZYME, to stimulate adrenal cortex production.

▶ Co Q10 30mg. 2x daily as an antioxidant.

FOOD THERAPY

❧ The importance of good diet is essential to adrenal health. Eat small, instead of large meals, low in sugar and fats. Eat lots of fresh foods, cold water fish, brown rice, legumes and whole grains.

❧ Add more high potassium foods such as potatoes, fish, and avocados to the diet. (Intake should be about 3 to 5 grams daily.) Cut down on high sodium foods.

❧ See **Diet For Hypoglycemia** in this book for more specifics.

❧ Take 2 teasp. each daily in fruit juice:
   ◆ Brewer's yeast
   ◆ Wheat germ

❧ Make a mix of flax seed/bran/broth/honey. Take some each morning to feed adrenals.

❧ Avoid hard liquor, tobacco and excess caffeine.
   Avoid fats, fried foods, red meats and highly processed foods.

Common Symptoms: Lack of energy and alertness; a sense of being "driven" and anxious, followed by great fatigue, weakness and lethargy; poor memory, low blood pressure and poor circulation; moodiness and irritability; sugar dysfunctions (hypoglycemia and diabetes); low immunity; brittle nails, dry skin; food cravings, especially for sugar.
Common Causes: Continued stress; poor diet with too much sugar and refined carbohydrates; over use of alcohol and nicotine, or recreational drugs; too much caffeine; vitamin B and C deficiencies.

ADDISON'S DISEASE

A lifelong disease resulting from an underactive adrenal cortex. Continual, severe adrenal exhaustion - characterized by unhealthy weight loss, nausea, low blood sugar, low blood pressure, and lethargy. The ability to cope under stress is greatly impaired. There is usually discoloration and brownish pigmentation of the skin, particularly on the knees, elbows, scars, skinfolds and palms. These areas, the mouth and skin freckles become abnormally dark. The hair darkens, and dark striations appear on the nails. Body hair decreases. Circulation is reduced and the person always feels cold.

☞ Good diet is critical in overcoming Addison's Disease. Alcohol, caffeine, tobacco, and highly processed foods must be avoided.

☞ Take Enzymatic Therapy ADRENAL CORTEX CONCENTRATE, with PITUITARY and ADRENAL CONCENTRATES to stimulate yet balance ACTH output, and feed adrenals.

☞ Take brewer's yeast, such as Lewis Labs, 2TBS. daily, with extra B Complex 100mg. and pantothenic acid 1000mg.

☞ Royal Jelly, 60,000 to 100,000mg. or more, 2x daily,

☞ Licorice extract, taken under the tongue or in water, 2x daily.

CUSHING'S SYNDROME

A rare, dysfunctional disease caused by overactive adrenal cortex. It is an opportunistic condition, allowed by immune suppression, and sometimes brought on by overdose of cortico-steroid drugs, (particularly those used for rheumatoid arthritis). It is also a metabolic disease that causes the formation of kidney stones. It is characterized by obesity in the stomach, face and buttocks, but severe thinness in the limbs. There is muscle wasting and weakness, poor wound healing, thinning of the skin leading to stretch marks and bruising. Peptic ulcers, high blood pressure, mental instability, and diabetes also accompany Cushing's. The face may get acne-like sores and the eyelids are often swollen. Particularly in women, there is scalp balding, yet excess body and facial hair, and a variety of menstrual disorders. Because of its rarity, our experience has been limited with this disease. The following protocols have been found helpful:

☞ A vegetarian diet should be followed, low in fat, sodium and sugar. Add high potassium foods daily.

☞ Add green drinks, such as chlorella with germanium and protein for healing.

☞ Take supplemental potassium in large doses - particularly herbal potassium drinks, such as Future Biotics VITAL K 2 TBS. daily, or Enzymatic Therapy HERBAL K.

❦

➤ **ADRENAL HEALTH SELF-TEST:** This common diagnostic test is performed by many chiropractors, massage therapists and naturopaths. Home blood pressure testing kits make this test an easy way to monitor your own adrenal health.

1) Lie down and rest for 5 minutes. Take a blood pressure reading.
2) Stand up and immediately take another blood pressure reading. If your blood pressure is *lower* after you stand up, your adrenals are probably functioning poorly. The amount of drop in blood pressure is usually in ratio to the amount of adrenal dysfunction.

Stimulation and nourishment of the adrenals will improve immune resistance, and aid in the healing of arthritis, bronchitis, hypoglycemia, diabetes, allergies, exhaustion, fatigue, and the hormone imbalances found in P.M.S. and menopause.

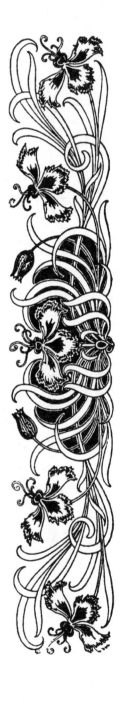

AGE SPOTS ■ LIVER SPOTS

An external sign of harmful waste accumulation, particularly in the liver; a result of free radical damage in skin cells. Lipofuscin is the age-related pigment that seems to actually appear as the age spots. It can oxidize, and thus cause the look of brown spots. Eliminating the cause (see below) is essential to eliminating the spots.

FOOD THERAPY

☙ Go on a short liquid diet (pg. 43) to clear the liver of toxins. Age spots are often the visible sign that the liver is throwing off metabolic wastes through the skin.

☙ Then drink carrot/beet/cucumber juice once a week for the next month to keep the liver clean.

☙ Then, follow the liver cleansing program in this book. Include lots of fresh foods and green salads. Avoid acid forming foods such as red meat, caffeine, etc.

☙ Avoid rancid nuts and oils.

☙ Take 2 TBS. brewer's yeast daily, or Bio-Strath LIQUID YEAST as directed.

☙ Take a glass of lemon juice and water daily, and apply lemon juice to spots.

VITAMINS/MINERALS

► Apply PSI PRO-GEST CREAM several times daily for 3 months.

► Anti-oxidants are the key to preventing the accumulation of lipofuscin, particularly vitamin E 400IU with selenium 100mcg., 2x daily, and CoQ 10 10mg. 3x daily.

► Ascorbate vitamin C crystals with bioflavonoids, 1/4 teasp. in water 4x daily.
with
► Beta carotene A 100,000IU and vitamin D 1000IU daily to clear the liver.

► Am. Biologics OXY-5000 FORTE.

► Take vitamin E 400IU; prick oil capsules and apply to spots. ♂

► Rainbow Light DETOX-ZYME 3-4 daily.

► High Omega 3 fish or flax oil 3 x daily.

► B Complex 100mg. 2x daily.

► Evening primrose oil 2-4 daily.

HERBAL THERAPY

❧ Biotec AGELESS BEAUTY 4 daily to metabolize rancid fats in the liver and destroy free radicals. ♀

❧ High potency royal jelly, 2 teasp. daily. ♀
or
Take 1 dropperful Superior BEE SECRETION daily.

❧ Crystal Star LIV-ALIVE™ capsules and LIV-ALIVE™ tea.
with
HERBAL ENZYMES™ capsules as a liver digestive stimulant.
and
GINSENG SKIN REPAIR GEL™ (with natural UV sunscreen protection.)

❧ Apply Dong Quai extract to spots. Take Dong Quai/Ginseng capsules 3 to 4 daily. ♀

❧ Effective teas: Take both internally and apply to spots.
  ✦ Rosehips
  ✦ Licorice rt.
  ✦ Chamomile
  ✦ Dandelion root

BODYWORK

► Avoid excess sun exposure. Get plenty of fresh air and some exercise at least three times a week.

► Reflexology: press point on stomach just above the navel. Stroke downward in the area of the liver under the right breast.

► Rub on Care Plus H2O2 OXY-GEL every night for 1 to 3 months til spots clear.

► Reflexology point:

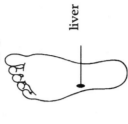

liver

► Sunscreens help prevent age spots from darkening.

Common Symptoms: Brown mottled spots on the hands, neck and face.
Common Causes: Hormonal imbalances; excessive sun exposure, especially with a thinned ozone layer; liver malfunction and exhaustion; long term use of hair colors and permanents; certain birth control pills; lack of exercise; too much exposure to the sun; poor assimilation and digestion, especially of saturated or rancid fats.

AGING & LONGEVITY

Slowing The Aging Process - Living Longer In Health

The *quality* of our lives is what matters. Disease and aging are two different things. Disease and aging are largely genetically controlled, disease is usually the result of individual diet, lifestyle and environment. We can slow the aging process by maintaining the best internal environment possible to prevent disease. We know that the lifespan of the individual can be increased. The human body is designed for rejuvenation at any age, because youth is not a chronological age. It is a state of good health and optimistic spirit. **Don't Worry. Be Happy.** Research shows that a pessimistic outlook on life depresses both personality and immune response. An optimistic, well-rounded, loving life needs friends and family. Regular contact is important for you and for them. Doing for and giving to others at this stage of life when there is finally the time to do it graciously makes a world of difference to the quality of life. Enjoy a regular sex life. (Endocrine activity keeps you young.) There is nothing like love and emotional involvement to keep life interesting and worthwhile. Age is not the enemy; illness is.

FOOD THERAPY

Healthy longevity can be greatly enhanced and extended through some simple dietary watchwords. Diet must improve to stay youthful. It must be optimally nourishing as the years pass.

ꙮ Nutritional quality, not quantity is the key. Fewer calories are needed for good body function as metabolism slows. Optimum body weight should be about 10 to 15 pounds less than in one's 20's or 30's. **Consciously eat smaller meals with less volume of food.**

ꙮ Keep dietary fats and oils low - 2 to 3 TBS. a day from unsaturated vegetable sources. Avoid fried foods, red meats and highly processed foods.

ꙮ Promote an alkaline system with plenty of fresh vegetables, whole grains, green drinks and miso.

ꙮ Have ocean foods several times a week for thyroid and metabolic balance.

ꙮ Eat cultured foods; yogurt, kefir and tofu products, sauerkraut, a glass or two of wine in the evening, etc, to promote better nutrient assimilation.

ꙮ Drink *plenty* of bottled water or mineral water daily. Drink alcohol in moderation. Alcohol tolerance decreases as the nervous system changes with age.

VITAMINS/MINERALS

Get plenty of food source vitamins and minerals for body building blocks and healthy cell regeneration. Food grown supplements, such as Living Source, or New Chapter are easily assimilated.

▶ Anti-oxidants are key to anti-aging:
   ✦ CoQ 10, 10mg, 3x daily
   ✦ Pycnogenol 50mg. daily
   ✦ Germanium 60mg. 2x daily
   ✦ Vitamin E 400IU with Selenium
   ✦ Beta-or Marine Carotene 25,000IU
   ✦ Ester C with bioflavonoids
   ✦ Glutathione, 50mg. for enhanced T-cell function.
   ✦ Am. Biologics OXY-5000 FORTE.

▶ Take an occasional "oxygen bath" with 1/2 cup 35% food grade H_2O_2 in spa or bath.

▶ Digestive/assimilation enhancers:
   ✦ Schiff ENZYMALL
   ✦ Solaray SUPER DIGESTAWAY

▶ Broad spectrum supplements:
   ✦ NutriTech ALL 1 vitamin drink. ♂
   ✦ Biotec BIOGUARD, 3 daily.
   ✦ Co. Life LIFESPAN 2000.
   ✦ Mezotrace SEA MINERALS COMPLEX 2 daily w/ extra vit. D

▶ Ener-B internasal B12 every other day

▶ Body Essentials SILICA gel internally.

HERBAL THERAPY

Herbal source nutrients insure gland balance and help stimulate immune response. Gentle herbal tonics and nutrients keep the system clear and immunity strong.

☙ Herbal immune enhancers:
   ✦ Sun CHLORELLA tabs or drink.
   ✦ Crystal Star SYSTEM STRENGTH™ drink mix.
   ✦ Crystal Star GINSENG SIX DEFENSE RESTORATIVE TEA.
   ✦ Bee pollen, and/or propolis.

☙ Herbal gland/cell revitalizers:
   ✦ Efamol Evening Primrose oil caps 2-4 daily. ♀
   ✦ YS royal jelly 2 teasp. daily.
   ✦ Dong Quai/Damiana caps or extract for women. ♀
   ✦ Siberian Ginseng tea or caps daily for men. ♂
   ✦ Enzymatic Therapy LIQUID LIVER w. SIB. GINSENG. ♂
   ✦ Wisdom of the Ancients YERBA MATÉ tea.
   ✦ Crystal Star GREEN TEA CLEANSER™ for free radical prevention.
   ✦ Body Essentials SILICA GEL, 1 TB. 3x daily in 3 oz. liquid.

☙ Brain nutrients:
   ✦ Ginkgo Biloba 2 daily
   ✦ Gotu Kola
   ✦ Dr. Chang's LONG LIFE TEA

BODYWORK

Regular exercise prolongs fitness at any age. Exercise helps maintain stamina, strength, agility, circulation and joint mobility. Exercise is a nutrient in itself.

▶ Do deep breathing and mild stretching exercises every morning - outdoors if possible, to oxygenate the tissues, limber the body, and help clear it of the previous night's waste and metabolic eliminations. Stretches at night before bed help insure muscle relaxation and better rest. Remember that it is normal to sleep less as metabolism slows.

▶ Take a walk every day, especially after your largest meal, for better circulation, energy, strength, stress reduction and enzyme function.

▶ Maintain your desired weight. Ten to 30 pounds of extra weight can take two years off your life. Thirty to 50 pounds takes off four years, and over fifty pounds takes off eight years. Consciously undereat to keep slim. Extra weight ages you sexually, physically and mentally.

▶ Don't smoke. In addition to its other well-documented hazards, smoking uses up tissue oxygen, which feeds the brain and helps prevent disease.

Common Symptoms: Memory loss or impairment; loss of sex drive; low immunity; a decrease in lean body mass; lower metabolic rate; decreasing physical activity; poor digestion, assimilation and elimination; arthritic and joint stiffness; weakened respiratory capacity; poor skin, organ and muscle tone; thyroid decrease; multiple drug regimens.

AIDS ■ ACQUIRED IMMUNE DEFICIENCY

AIDS and related syndromes are the result of immune system breakdown. The body becomes unable to defend itself against infection or disease. AIDS and several other immune-deficient conditions are caused by HIV (human immunodeficiency virus). They include an acute mononucleosis-like syndrome, an asymptomatic state as a carrier of HIV, an AIDS related complex (ARC), and "full blown" AIDS syndrome. The weakened immune system is also susceptible to a broad spectrum of other "opportunistic" diseases, and eventually becomes overwhelmed by them. The most common of these are *pneumocystis carinii*, a pneumonia infection, *Kaposi's sarcoma*, a connective tissue cancer, *Epstein-Barr Virus (EBV)*, *Cytomegalovirus (CMV)* an EBV-associated infection, *candidiasis*, *herpes simplex virus*, *tuberculosis* and *salmonella*, a parasitic infection.

FOOD THERAPY

There is usually a great deal of toxicity, fatigue and malabsorption in AIDS and related conditions. A liquid fast is therefore not recommended as being too harsh for an already weakened system.

☙ The diet should, however, have the highest possible nutrition. A modified macrobiotic diet is ideal for high resistance and immune strength. Intestinal chemistry and pH environment must be changed to optimize disease protection. See diet recommendations on the following pages.

☙ Take a potent protein/vitamin/mineral drink, such as NutriTech ALL 1 for increased strength and energy.

☙ Take 3-4 glasses of fresh carrot juice daily, or 300,000IU beta or marine carotene to stimulate effective T-cell activity.

☙ Take a potassium broth (pg. 53) every day for ongoing detoxification. A good juicer is really necessary.

☙ **Other diet watchwords:**
♣ All produce should be fresh and organically grown when possible.
♣ No fried foods of any kind. Avoid concentrated sweeteners, and highly processed foods of all kinds.
♣ Flush the body with 6 to 8 glasses of mild herb teas and bottled water daily. Add 1/2 teasp. ascorbate vitamin C to each daily drink for optimum results.

VITAMINS/MINERALS

Because such vigorous treatment is necessary, supplementation is recommended at all stages of healing to change intestinal environment, strengthen immunity, allow nutrient assimilation and increase tissue oxygen.

▶ Purifying supplements:
♣ Egg yolk lecithin. Active lipids help make cell walls virally resistant.
♣ Care Plus H2O2 OXY GEL rubbed on the feet, or 3% liquid, 1TB. in 8oz. water taken internally.
♣ Am. Biologics DIOXYCHLOR.
♣ Ester C powder w. bioflavonoids, 10-30 g. daily - injection or orally.

▶ Rebuilding supplements:
♣ Enzymatic Therapy RAW THYMUS sublingual.
♣ Carnitine 500mg. 2x daily.
♣ Ener-B internasal B12 daily.
♣ Natra-Bio THYMUS EXTRACT.

▶ Effective anti-oxidants:
♣ Germanium 150mg. sublingual 6 daily with astragalus caps 4 daily.
♣ CoQ 10, 30 mg. 3 x daily.
♣ Quercetin w. Bromelain 500mg. 3x daily.
♣ Pycnogenol 50mg. 2x daily.
♣ Vitamin E 1000IU daily, with selenium as selenomethionine.
♣ Glutathione 50mg. for HIV positive

▶ Effective enzymes:
♣ Rainbow Light DETOX-ZYME
♣ Biogenetics BIOGUARD S.O.D.
♣ Acidophilus complex with bifidus - refrigerated, highest potency, 3 teasp. daily with biotin 1000mcg.

HERBAL THERAPY

❦ Aloe vera juice 3 glasses daily to curb virus spread, with garlic extract caps 8 daily.

❦ Ecomer SHARK LIVER OIL or Cartilade Technologies SHARK CARTILAGE, 740mg.

❦ Crystal Star DETOX™ capsules, ANTI-VI™ tea or extract, HERBAL DEFENSE TEAM™ caps or extract as directed.
with
LIV-ALIVE™ caps or extract.
and
ADRACTIVE™ caps or extract, HEARTSEASE/ANEMI-GIZE™ caps for stronger blood and energy.

❦ Sun CHLORELLA, starting with low dosage, gradually increasing. Enzymatic Therapy LIQUID LIVER w. SIBERIAN GINSENG.

❦ Health Concerns POWER MUSH-ROOMS as directed.

❦ Effective anti-viral herbs:
♦ Echinacea/pau de arco extract 3x daily.
♦ St John's wort extract proven effective against retro viruses.

❦ Effective immuno-modulators:
♦ Siberian ginseng extract
♦ Garlic/rosehips/chaparral caps
♦ Astragalus extract or capsules
♦ Reishi mushroom capsules

BODYWORK

It is absolutely necessary to detoxify the liver for holistic healing to be effective. See LIVER CLEANSING pages in this book.

▶ Reflexology point:

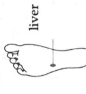

liver

▶ Avoid anal intercourse.
→ Avoid needle-injected and all pleasure drugs.
→ Practice safe sex.
→ Make sure all blood transfusion plasma has been tested for HIV virus.

▶ Take a colonic once a week until recovery is well underway to remove infected feces from the intestinal tract.

▶ Get fresh air and sunlight on the body every day. Get mild exercise daily, and plenty of rest. Do deep breathing exercises every morning and evening, especially when recovering from pneumocystis

▶ See Overheating Therapy, pg. 38.

▶ See Hydrotherapy, pg. 49.

The Holistic Approach To AIDS

More and more people with this tragic disease are turning to alternative therapies and taking responsibility for their own research and treatment. This kind of direct action enables things to move very fast, and we are getting a clearer understanding of treatment and response. A much more positive picture is emerging. Indeed there are enough success stories just in the last eighteen months from the people themselves, and the holistic practitioners working with them, to indicate that holistic therapies are showing more promise than ever. AIDS, ARC, and other immune deficiency diseases are no longer seen to be inevitably fatal as they once were. Holistic programs are frequently causing symptoms to abate and gradually disappear. The advance of the virus itself has been slowed in many instances, and improved longevity and quality of life are observed even in full-blown AIDS cases. As more people with these diseases see their own progress, return to work, and pick up their lives, more expertise is coming into the field via holistic physicians, homeopaths, naturopaths, chiropractors, therapists, nutritional counselors and others.

California cities have become the leaders in shattering the numerous myths about AIDS, and in natural and unorthodox treatment efforts. They are a mecca for dedicated people with the latest knowledge and successful therapies. Seek them out if you are HIV positive and need help. We are seeing improvement, energy return, and diminishment of symptoms every day.

The following schedule is an updated listing of holistic therapies we are aware of that have achieved measureable success with AIDS and its attendant conditions. Doses are generally quite high when beginning these therapies. They may be reduced as improvement is observed. Treatments may be used together or separately as desired by each individual, along with the recommendations of a competent professional with personal case knowledge.

❖ **Ascorbate vitamin C crystals - use calcium ascorbate, or a mixed mineral ascorbate *with bioflavonoids*; to flush and detoxify the tissues. Take orally 10-20 teasp. daily for 2 to 3 weeks, then reduce to 10 grams twice a week. Mega-doses may be resumed as necessary. Intravenous dose - 100-150 grams daily for 2-3 weeks, reducing to 30 grams every week for maintenance.**

❖ Vitamin E - 1000IU daily, with selenium as sodium selenite drops or selenomethionine, and beta or marine carotene 100,000IU as an anti-infective.

❖ **Raw thymus extract - 1 tablet 3 x daily or $1/2$ dropperful 3 x daily - $1/2$ dropperful 2 x daily to strengthen immunity.**

❖ Echinacea extract/pau de arco extract - $1/2$ dropperful 3x daily, and/or reishi and shiitake mushrooms, to stimulate production of interferon, interleukin and lymphocytes; or 4-6 cups daily of the following immune restorative tea: prince ginseng roots, dry shiitake mushrooms and soaking water, echinacea angustifolia root, schizandra berries, astragalus, ma huang, pau de arco bark, St. John's wort. Steep 30 minutes. (See Crystal Star GINSENG 6 DEFENSE RESTORATIVE™ TEA.)

❖ Acidophilus culture complex with bifidus - refrigerated, highest potency, 3 teasp. daily with biotin 1000mcg.

❖ Fresh vegetable juices - a good juicer such as Champion or Vitamix is critical to juice potency. Take carrot/beet/cucumber juice 1-3 x daily with garlic extract and flax oil added, to detoxify the liver. Chew 1 to 3 DGL tablets during the day to neutralize released acids.

❖ Aged aloe vera juice - 2-3 glasses daily; found to block the virus spread from cell to cell.

❖ Egg lipids from egg yolk lecithin - highest potency, such as Jarrow Corp., or Source Naturals EGGS ACT liquid.

❖ **Potent anti-oxidants - such as CoQ 10 30mg., Germanium 100-150mg., Pycnogenol 50mg. 4x daily, DMG sublingual (di-methyl-glycine), Glutathione 50mg. 2x daily, and Octacosonal 1000mg. to overcome the side effects and nerve damage from AZT, and to strengthen white blood cell and T-cell activity. Take with Solaray QUERCETIN PLUS with bromelain 500mg. 3x daily for respiratory improvement, and digestive enzymes, such as Rainbow Light DETOX-ZYME.**

❖ Carnitine - 500mg. daily for 3 days. Rest for 7 days, then take 1000mg. for 3 days. Rest for 7 days. Take with high omega 3 flax oils, 3-6 x daily, or evening primrose oil 500mg, 3 x daily.

❖ **Vitamin B complex - 100-200mg. 3 x daily, with extra pantothenic acid 250mg. and zinc picolinate 30-60mg.**

❖ Hydrogen peroxide, food grade oxy gel or 3% solution - by injection with a qualified practitioner or orally 1 TB. in 8oz. of water, 3-4 x daily, or rubbed on the feet morning and evening. Alternate use, one week on and one week off for best results.

❖ Germanium - highest potency 200mg. 6x daily, or 150mg sublingually, 4x daily, with astragalus capsules, 4 daily.

❖ Sun CHLORELLA - 15-20 tablets or 2 packets of granules daily for immune building.

❖ Ecomer SHARK LIVER OIL or Cartilade Technologies SHARK CARTILAGE 740mg. - 1 cap for every 12 pounds of body weight for 3 weeks before meals then 4-6 caps daily - increases leukocytes and white blood cell activity to fight infection.

❖ St. John's wort extract or Crystal Star ANTI-VI™ EXTRACT (50% St. John's Wort/50% Lomatium) 3 x daily.

❖ **Propolis extract with KYO-Green garlic extract.**

❖ Overheating therapy has been effective for inhibiting growth of the invading virus. Hydrotherapy has been effective in re-stimulating circulation.

❖ Curcuma combinations are effective as anti-cancer formulas against Kaposi's Sarcoma and other tumors.

Common Early Symptoms: It can take from 2 to 5 years or longer after infection for symptoms to appear - extreme fatigue; loss of appetite and weight; inability to heal even minor ailments; night sweats; enlarged liver and/or spleen; skin disorders; constant respiratory infections; malabsorption with bowel inflammation and chronic diarrhea.

Common Causes: Sex with an HIV positive person; drug abuse and sharing infected needles; infected blood transfusions. Immune deficiency susceptibility because of an unhealthy lifestyle: poor nutrition on a wide scale; toxic pleasure drug use; anal intercourse with bowel permeability; widespread antibiotic use; smoking; stress; inadequate sleep and exercise. *It is also becoming widely known that HIV is not the only culprit in the AIDS connection. Syphilis is usually massively present in AIDS victims, as are parasites and other viruses that are now thought to set the stage for AIDS and related conditions.*

Note: It is relatively easy to transfer HIV virus through anal intercourse, more difficult through vaginal or oral sex. Enzymes in the saliva, friendly flora in the intestinal tract, and HCl in the stomach produce a hostile environment that destroys the virulence of HIV. There is no such protection in the colon. Suppression of the immune system is believed to occur when the HIV virus slips through the intestinal wall and into the bloodstream. Normal immune response is to attack the virus with macrophages that then die and are removed through the lymphatic system. These toxic wastes are finally dumped into the colon on its last leg of clearance from the body. but in an unprotected colon without friendly bacteria or good defensive pH environment, new HIV viruses hatch from the dead macrophages, and multiply in the feces all over again, repeating the same cycle. The immune system cannot detect the virus in the colon and does not marshal its forces until the infection is in the bloodstream; often too late if immune defenses are exhausted.

Diet Defense Against AIDS & Related Complexes

A high resistance, immune-building diet is primary to success in overcoming AIDS and related conditions. It is a major disease, and treatment must be approached with vigorous commitment. The intestinal environment must be changed to create a hostile site for the pathogenic bacteria (this protocol is also effective against candida albicans and some types of cancer). The following liquid and fresh foods diet is for the ill person who needs drastic measures - a great deal of concentrated defense strength in a short time. It represents the first "crash course" stages of the change from cooked to living foods. It has been successful in the reversal of HIV positive to HIV negative, and in symptom recession of full-blown AIDS cases. Optimal diet improvement also helps prevent the other attendant diseases associated with immune deficiency. The space in this book only allows for an abbreviated form of this diet. The complete program with supporting recipes, may be found in "COOKING FOR HEALTHY HEALING" by Linda Rector-Page. See also the BLOOD CLEANSING DIET for immune deficient diseases in this book (pg. 48).

This is a modified, enhanced macrobiotic diet, emphasizing more raw than cooked foods, and mixing in acidophilus powder with foods that *are* cooked to convert them to living nourishment with friendly flora. As with other immune depressing viral diseases, the pathogenic HIV bacteria live on dead and waste matter. For several months at least, the diet should be vegetarian, low in dairy, yeasted breads and saturated fats. Meats, fried foods, dairy products except yogurt and kefir, coffee, alcohol, salt, sugars and all refined foods must be eliminated. Of course, all drugs should be excluded, (even prescription drugs if possible). The ultra purity of this diet controls the multiple allergies and sensitivities that occur in immune deficiency, yet still supplies the needs of a body that is suffering primary nutrient deprivation. For most people, this way of eating is a radical change, with major limitations, but the health improvement for AIDS is excellent.

The following is a suggested daily outline:

On rising: take 2-3 TBS. cranberry concentrate in 8 oz. of water with $1/2$ teasp. ascorbate vitamin C crystals with bioflavonoids;
or cut up $1/2$ a lemon (with skin) and blend in the blender with 1 teasp. honey and 1 cup distilled water. Strain.
Add $1/2$ teasp. Natren LIFE START II lactobacillus complex or Alta Health CANGEST powder to either of these drinks.

Take a brisk walk for exercise and morning sunlight.

Breakfast: have a glass of fresh carrot juice with 1 t.easp. Bragg's LIQUID AMINOS, **and** whole grain muffins or rice cakes with kefir cheese;
or a cup of soy milk or plain yogurt mixed in the blender with a cup of fresh fruit, sesame seeds, walnuts;

or oatmeal, amaranth or buckwheat pancakes with yogurt and fresh fruit;

and 1/2 teasp. Natren LIFE START II lactobacillus or Alta Health CANGEST powder mixed in 8 oz. aloe vera juice;

Midmorning: take a weekly colonic. On non-colonic days, take a potassium broth or essence with 1 TB. Bragg's LIQUID AMINOS and 1/2 teasp ascorbate vitamin C crystals *with bioflavonoids added;*

and have another fresh carrot juice, or pau de arco tea, with 1/2 teasp. Natren LIFE START II powder added.

Lunch: have a fresh green salad with lemon/flax oil dressing, with plenty of tofu, avocado, nuts, seeds and alfalfa sprouts;

or an open-faced sandwich on rice cakes, or a chapati with fresh vegies and soy or yogurt cheese;

or a cup of miso soup with rice noodles or brown rice;

or some steamed vegies and tofu with millet or brown rice;

and take a cup of pau de arco tea or aloe vera juice with 1/2 teasp. ascorbate vit. C and 1/2 teasp. Natren LIFE START II powder added.

Midafternoon: have another carrot juice with Bragg's LIQUID AMINOS and 1/2 teasp. Natren LIFE START II added;

and a green drink such as Sun CHLORELLA, Green Foods GREEN ESSENCE, or Crystal Star ENERGY GREEN, with 1/2 teasp. ascorbate vitamin C crystals added.

Dinner: have a baked potato with Bragg's LIQUID AMINOS, soy cheese or kefir cheese and a green salad;

and another potassium broth or black bean or lentil soup with 1/2 teasp. Natren LIFE START II added;

or black bean or lentil soup and a tofu and vegie casserole with yogurt and soy cheese;

or a fresh spinach or artichoke pasta with steamed vegies and lemon/flax oil dressing;

or a Chinese steam stir-fry with shiitake mushrooms, brown rice and vegetables.

Sprinkle 1/2 teasp. Natren LIFE START II or Alta Health CANGEST powder over any cooked food at this meal.

Before Bed: take a glass of aloe vera juice with 1/2 teasp ascorbate vit. C crystals and 1/2 teasp. Natren LIFE START II;

and a fresh carrot or papaya juice, or alkalizing drink such as Crystal Star SYSTEM STRENGTH™.

☛Unsweetened mild herb teas and bottled water are recommended throughout the day for additional toxin cleansing and alkalizing.

☛One half teasp. ascorbate vitamin C powder with bioflavonoids may be added to any drink throughout the day to bowel tolerance for optimum results.

The goal for overcoming HIV infection is staying strong. Strength greatly reduces the chances of succumbing to full-blown AIDS or to another infection. It allows you to survive while research for a virus-inhibiting compound goes on. In some cases, a strong person can even develop resistance to the virus effects indefinitely.

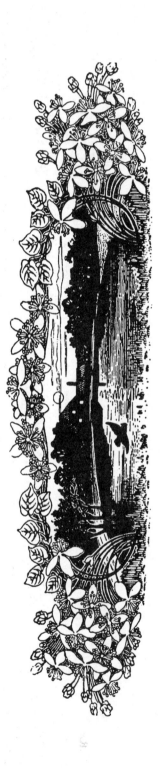

ALCOHOL ABUSE

As with other addictive practices, alcohol abuse is both brought on and marked by stress and depression - a lack of confidence about one's self, or reason for one's life. As fatuous as it may seem, contentment, or purposely making a major life style change is sometimes the best medicine for changing body chemistry - and thus curbing the craving for alcohol effects.

FOOD THERAPY

🍃 Go on a short juice fast (pg. 42 or 43) to clean out alcohol residues. Then follow the HYPOGLYCEMIA DIET in this book for 3 months. Take an extra daily protein drink, such as Nature's Plus SPIRUTEIN or Nutri Tech ALL 1 to balance body chemistry, replace electrolytes, and add strength quickly. Add 1TB. flax seed oil during withdrawal stage.

🍃 Add plenty of mineral-rich foods to your diet for a solid nutritional foundation. (See COOKING FOR HEALTHY HEALING by Linda Rector-Page.)

🍃 The continuing diet should be high in magnesium foods. Include wheat germ, bran, brewer's yeast, whole grains and cereals, brown rice, green leafy vegetables, potatoes, miso, low fat dairy, eggs and fish.

🍃 Avoid refined and fried foods, sugary or heavily spiced foods and caffeine. They aggravate alcohol craving.

🍃 Cleanse the liver. No alcohol detox program will work without liver regeneration See LIVER DETOX program in this book.

🍃 Take a Vegex broth every night for B vitamins and to curb craving.

VITAMINS/MINERALS

▶ Vitamin C is a key: Take up to 10,000mg. (or to bowel tolerance), ascorbate vitamin C crystals with bioflavonoids - ¼ teasp. at a time in juice throughout the day for at least one month to change body chemistry.

▶ Mega-vitamin therapy is effective: To curb alcohol craving, take either of the following combinations daily with meals for a month:
2 Glutamine 500mg.
2 Cysteine 500mg.
2 B Complex 100mg.
3 Ascorbate Vit. C 1000mg.
2 Niacinamide 500mg.
2 Zinc 50mg. ♂

or

3 Solaray CHROMIACIN
2 Twin Lab GABA Plus
3 Glutamine 500mg.
2 Magnesium 400mg. ♀

To calm nerves and withdrawal effects:
▶ 2 daily - raw brain glandular with taurine 500mg. and zinc 30mg. ♂

▶ B15 DMG, 125mg. with B6 200mg. and carnitine 500mg. daily.

or

▶ DLPA 750mg. with tyrosine 500mg. and 500mg. magnesium. ♀

HERBAL THERAPY

🌿 Crystal Star WITHDRAWAL SUPPORT™ CAPS as directed for several months.

with

🌿 Evening primrose oil caps 2-4 daily. ♀

🌿 Spirulina 500mg., or Sun CHLORELLA granules or Crystal Star ENERGY GREEN™ drink daily.

with

🌿 Rainbow Light DETOX-ZYME 3 daily. ♂

🌿 Crystal Star LIV-ALIVE™ caps or extract for detoxification, ADR-ACTIVE™ caps and HIGH ENERGY TEA™ for energy support.

🌿 4 chaparral caps and/or 2 cups Angelica tea during craving times.

🌿 Effective extracts - capsule or lquid:
♦ Passion flower
♦ Silymarin (milk thistle) for detoxification
♦ Scullcap
♣ Hops to decrease desire
♦ Valerian/wild lettuce

🌿 Medicine Wheel SERENE EXTRACT to calm nerves.

🌿 Massage Care Plus OXYGEL into head and neck once a day.

BODYWORK

▶ Acupuncture and massage therapy realignment are successful in curbing craving for alcohol.

▶ Improved fitness and system oxygen are important. Get fresh air, sunlight and exercise every day.

▶ Foot reflexology:

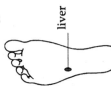
liver

▶ Although it seems to state the obvious, avoid the places, people and circumstances that sharpen your desire to escape through alcohol. This usually means major life change and may seem impossible. But it almost always starts the road to lasting success and is often the only way.

Initial withdrawal symptoms include high anxiety, rapid pulse with tremors, hot flashes and drenching perspiration, dehydration, insomnia, and hallucinations.
Liver detoxification shortens withdrawal time significantly.

Common Symptoms: Alcohol dependence, and using alcohol for daily calories instead of food; short term memory loss; liver degeneration and disease; nervousness and poor coordination; high LDL cholesterol and blood sugar; immune depression; poor enzyme production leading to poor fat and protein metabolism, and especially to mineral deficiency; anger; lack of emotional control, aggressive/compulsive behavior toward friends and family members.
Common Causes: Excessive intake of alcohol influenced by inherited, socio-psychological and physiological factors; hypoglycemia; poor diet, with too much refined, sugary food and too little fresh, high mineral foods; unrelieved daily stress, tension and emotional depression.

ALCOHOL TOXICITY ■ HANGOVER

There are effective natural means of reducing alcohol's damage to your body and brain. The real idea is to reduce alcohol consumption below the toxicity level.

FOOD THERAPY

☙ Eat vitamin B-rich and high fiber foods to give stability and soak up blood alcohol.

☙ No sugar or "hair of the dog". Both may *seem* to make you feel better, but really drag out a hangover.

☙ Effective tonics:
◆ Brewer's yeast, raw egg, orange juice, cayenne. Drink all at once - straight down.
◆ Tomato juice, mixed green and yellow onions, celery, parsley, hot pepper sauce, basil, water, fennel seeds, rosemary leaves, Bragg's LIQUID AMINOS. Drink - straight down.
◆ **Revitalizing Tonic** on page 60 in this book.
◆ Knudsen's **VERY VEGGIE** juice, V-8 juice or the **vegetable juice on pg. 55.**

☙ Crystal Star BIOFLAV., FIBER & C SUPPORT™ drink. Excellent results within a half hour.

☙ Electrolyte replacement drink, such as Knudsen's RECHARGE or mineral water.

VITAMINS/MINERALS

▷ *Before you drink, to minimize toxicity to the brain:*
✦ Vitamin C powder or Alacer ENERGEN-C with bioflavs. 1/2 teasp. in water *with* 2 vitamin B Complex capsules.

or

✦ Cysteine 500mg. *with* 2 evening primrose oil caps before drinking *and* before retiring.
✦ B15 DMG sublingual *with* Ener B internasal B12 before drinking.

▷ *Anti-oxidant and enzyme therapy together are effective after the fact.*
✦ Am. Biologics INFLA-ZYME FORTE tablets, 2-4 between meals.
✦ Glutamine 500mg. with vitamin E 400IU with selenium 2x daily to reduce oxygen loss.
✦ Biotec CELL GUARD with SOD 6 tablets.

▷ Healing vitamin blend: 1 each
✦ Flax seed oil 3x daily
✦ Vitamin B1 thiamine 500mg.
✦ B2 riboflavin 100mg. 1 daily
✦ B6 250mg. daily
✦ Emulsified A 25,000IU, 2 daily

▷ Homeopathic *Nux Vomica* at night before retiring after drinking.

HERBAL THERAPY

☙ *Before you drink, to minimize toxicity:*
✦ Crystal Star ASPIR-SOURCE™ capsules before drinking, *with a* GINSENG 6 SUPER ENERGY™ capsule. ♀
✦ GINSENG 6 DEFENSE RESTORATIVE™ tea,

and/or

✦ Jade Medicine SAGES GINSENG tablets.
✦ Siberian ginseng extract as needed.

☙ *Nervines and enzyme therapy together are effective after the fact.*
✦ Cayenne/ginger capsules to settle stomach and relieve headache.
✦ Scullcap tea to soothe nerves and oxygenate the brain.
✦ Angelica tea to relieve a headache caused by poor vascular activity.
✦ Milk thistle seed extract for liver support.
✦ Crystal Star WITHDRAWAL SUPPORT™ caps.

☙ *Take a quick liver tonic if you think you have alcohol poisoning:*
Steep for 20 minutes - hibiscus, cloves, allspice, and the juice of 2 lemons in white grape or orange juice. Drink slowly.

BODYWORK

▶ Apply cold compresses to the head *before and after* a long hot shower, to wash toxins off combing out through the skin. (You won't believe what a difference this makes.) Or, take alternating hot and cool showers to stimulate circulation and eliminate blood alcohol.

▶ Take a whirlpool spa or sauna for 20 minutes.

▶ Get outside in the fresh air as soon as possible - the more oxygen in the lungs and tissues, the better.

▶ Rub Care Plus OXYGEL on the feet, or take a teaspoonful of 3% dilute solution in a glass of water to oxygenate the blood and brain.

▶ A hangover should be gone by five o'clock the next day. If it isn't, you probably have alcohol poisoning. Take an enema (catnip, chlorophyll, coffee), or if the case is severe, get your stomach pumped at an urgent care center.

Common Symptoms: Sensitivity to light, headache, eyeache, bad taste in the mouth; weakness; debility; shakiness; dull mind and senses; lethargy.
Common Causes: Alcohol poisoning from too much alcohol; liver exhaustion and consequent malfunction.

ALLERGIES ■ CHEMICAL & CONTAMINANT

As allergic reactions multiply in America, we find ourselves pinpointing and treating them ever more specifically. Chemical allergies are caused particularly by petro-chemicals that the body stores in the fatty tissues in an attempt to remove them as alien substances from its delicate functions and balance. An allergic reaction occurs after a second exposure to an irritant, as the body's inflammatory response is alerted and histamines are produced. Repeated chemical exposures set off rampant free radical reactions in the body, which can tolerate only a certain level of contaminates before toxic overload results and an allergic reaction sets in.

FOOD THERAPY

🍃 Go on a short 3 to 7 day liquid diet (pg. 43) to begin toxin release. Have one each of the following daily:
◆ a glass of fresh carrot juice
◆ a potassium broth (pg. 53)
◆ 2 cups miso soup

🍃 Then, eat organically grown foods as much as possible. Avoid canned foods. Avoid caffeine, which inhibits liver filtering function, and foods sprayed with colorants, waxes or ripening agents.

🍃 Have a bowl of high fiber cereal every morning. Eat plenty of fruits, vegetables and whole grains for fiber protection.

🍃 Take 2 TB. each daily in food:
♣ Brewer's yeast
♣ Wheat germ
♣ Lecithin granules

🍃 Drink only bottled water.

🍃 Crystal Star ENERGY GREEN™ or SYSTEM STRENGTH™ drinks for detoxification and blood building.

🍃 Eat legumes and sea vegetables to excrete lead.

VITAMINS/MINERALS

A good supplement program can reinforce the body against chemical assault, and help keep immune response intact.

▶ Anti-oxidants are the key:
✦ Ascorbate vitamin C with bioflavonoids - 3-5000mg. daily.
✦ Vitamin E 400IU w/ selenium.
✦ CoQ10 - 30mg. 2x daily.
✦ Beta/marine carotene 150,000IU.
✦ Glutathione 50mg. 3 daily.
✦ Solaray yeast free selenium.

▶ Take a food grown multi-vitamin/mineral daily.

▶ Enzymatic Therapy ADRENAL GLANDULAR COMPLEX.
with
Enzymatic Therapy raw THYMUS COMPLEX as directed.

▶ Biotec CELL GUARD, or Biogenetics BIOGUARD, S.O.D. w/ catalase, 6 daily.

▶ Vital Health FORMULA 1 oral chelation with EDTA, 2 packets daily. ♂

▶ B complex 100mg. daily with extra B6 200mg. and zinc 50mg. daily.

HERBAL THERAPY

🌿 Crystal Star DETOX CAPSULES with GREEN TEA CLEANSER™ or CLEANSING & PURIFYING TEA for 6 weeks.
then
LIV-ALIVE™ tea or LIV-ALIVE™ capsules for 1 month to restore liver function. (Add FIBER & HERBS COLON CLEANSE™ capsules if desired.)

🌿 Blood detoxification herbs:
◆ Garlic oil caps, 2-4 daily.
◆ Sun CHLORELLA or Green Foods GREEN MAGMA.
◆ Liquid chlorophyll 1 teasp. every 4 hours.
◆ Aloe vera juice with herbs, 1 glass every 4 hours.
◆ Pau d' arco tea every 4 hours.

🌿 NutriBiotic GRAPEFRUIT SEED EXTRACT CAPSULES.

🌿 4 Evening primrose oil caps *with* 2 cysteine caps 500mg. daily.

🌿 Effective capsules:
◆ Astragalus ♂
◆ Kelp 10 tabs daily, or Crystal Star IODINE THERAPY caps 4 daily. ♀
◆ Siberian ginseng *extract* caps. ♂

BODYWORK

▶ Use Coca's Pulse Test or muscle testing to identify allergens. (See page 347 in the appendix section.)

▶ Foot reflexology:

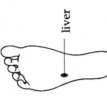

liver

▶ See page 91 about free radical scavengers and anti-oxidants for more information.

▶ Avoid antacids; they interfere with enzyme production, and the ability of the body to carry off chemical residues.

▶ Avoid as much as possible: smoking and secondary smoke, pesticides and fungicides, phosphorus fertilizers, fluorescent lights, aluminum cookware and deodorants, electric blankets; microwave ovens, and non-filtered computer screens.

Common symptoms: Always feeling "low energy" and "under the weather" regardless of how much sleep one gets; abnormal metabolism; skin rashes; chronic respiratory inflammation; ringing in the ears; nausea; diarrhea; headaches; low immune response.
Common Causes: Repeated exposure and sensitivity to toxic chemicals and environmental pollutants.

ALLERGIES ◼ ENVIRONMENTAL & SEASONAL
Allergic Rhinitis ✧ Hayfever

Allergic rhinitis seems to result from two main areas - allergies to environmental pollutants, such as asbestos, smoke and fumes, and allergies to seasonal conditions, such as dust, pollen or spores. This type of allergic reaction often occurs when the body has an excess accumulation of mucous, which then harbors environmental irritants. Most drugstore medications only relieve or mask symptoms. They also have a rebound effect - the more you use them, the more you need them. Cortico-steroid drugs for this type of allergy, taken over a long period of time, do not cure, and often make the situation worse by depressing immune defenses, and impeding allergen elimination.

FOOD THERAPY

Diet change and cleansing of the internal environment is the single most beneficial thing you can do to control allergic rhinitis reactions.

🍃 Begin with a short three to seven day cleansing diet (Pg. 42) to rid the body of excess mucous build-up, release allergens from the body, and pave the way for diet and nutritional changes to have optimum effect.
◆ Then start a diet with non-mucous-forming foods: fresh vegetables and fruits, whole grains, cultured foods such as yogurt, raw dairy, and seafoods.
◆ For a complete diet to overcome allergies, see COOKING FOR HEALTHY HEALING, by Linda Rector Page.

🍃 Avoid all refined and preserved foods, sugars, caffeine, dairy products and fatty, mucous-forming foods during healing.

🍃 Lemon water in the morning, and a green drink, such as CHLORELLA or Crystal Star ENERGY GREEN™, during the day will flush excess mucous and support clean body energy.
or
🍃 Crystal Star BIOFLAV., FIBER and C SUPPORT™ drink mix daily.

VITAMINS/MINERALS

Natural supplements help reinforce the body's defenses against allergens, and build resistance to further attacks.

▶ CoQ10, 30mg. 3x daily, with high Omega 3 flax oils 3 x daily.

▶ Ascorbate Vitamin C or Ester C powder *with bioflavonoids* $1/4$-$1/2$ teasp. every 3 hours to flush and detoxify tissues; then reduce to 5000mg. daily.
with

▶ Quercetin 1000-2000mg. daily with bromelain 500mg.

▶ High potency royal jelly 2 teasp. daily. ♂

▶ B complex 100mg. with extra pantothenic acid 500mg. and B6 100mg. 2x daily after meals, morning and evening. (Or use as a preventive measure before high risk seasons.)

▶ Alta Health CANGEST or Professional Nutrition DOCTOR DOPHILUS.

▶ Raw thymus and adrenal 3 x daily.

▶ Germanium SL 150mg. 3x daily; with B12 SL 500mcg. 3x daily

HERBAL THERAPY

Homeopathic and herbal remedies help even acute attacks without side effects.

🌿 Crystal Star ALRG™ and/or ANTI-HST™ caps, or ALRG-HST™ extract with ADR-ACTIVE™ caps.

🌿 Natra-Bio BIOALLERS oral homeopathic liquid, 3x daily. (When buying, specify for type of allergen.)
with
Crystal Star RESPIRATOR TEA™.

🌿 Effective homeopathic remedies:
◆ Hyland's HAYFEVER tabs
◆ BioForce POLLINOSAN tabs
◆ BioForce SINUSAN tabs

🌿 Effective preventive herbs:
◆ Crystal Star ADR-ACTIVE™ capsules or ADRN™ extract.
◆ Twin Lab PROPOLIS tincture.
◆ Unsprayed Bee Pollen granules.
◆ Garlic tabs 6 daily.
◆ Evening primrose oil 4-6 daily.
◆ Crystal Star ALLR-HST™ TEA with ephedra extract.

🌿 Effective extracts: 10 drops 3x daily.
◆ Butcher's broom as an anti-flam.
◆ Bilberry
◆ Ginkgo Biloba leaf to inactivate biochemical substances.
◆ Lobelia
◆ Echinacea root - tonic dose

BODYWORK

Exercise is important to increase oxygen uptake in the lungs and tissues. Mental relaxation is also a key, since stress and tension aggravate allergies.

▶ Take a daily walk with deep breathing exercises.

▶ Relax. Stress and tension aggravate allergies.

▶ Take some *fresh* grated horseradish in a spoon with lemon juice. Hang over a sink to release great quantities of excess mucous *fast*.

▶ Use Coca's Pulse Test or muscle testing to identify allergens. (See page 347 in the appendix.)

▶ Stop smoking and avoid secondary smoke. It magnifies allergies reactions.

▶ Acupressure points:
During an attack, press tip of nose hard as needed for relief.
or
Press hollow above the center of upper lip as needed.

Common Symptoms: Runny, watery, itchy nose and eyes; sneezing and coughing attacks; sore, irritated throat; chronic lung, bronchial and sinus infections; skin itching and rashes; asthma; frontal headaches; insomnia; menstrual disorders; hypoglycemia; learning disabilities.
Common Causes: Pollen, spore, mold and other airborne allergens reacting with excess mucous and waste accumulation in the body; adrenal exhaustion; free radical damage lowering anti-histine levels and liver function; stress; hypoglycemia; candida albicans yeast overgrowth; EFA deficiency.

ALLERGIES ◼ FOOD SENSITIVITY & INTOLERANCE

Food allergy - an antibody response to a certain food. Food intolerance - an enzyme deficiency to digest a certain food. Both can occur with either foods or food additives. This type of sensitivity is the fastest growing allergy group as people are more and longer exposed to chemically altered, enzyme-depleted, processed foods that the human body is not equipped to handle. When the body consumes these foods its own enzyme capacity must assume all digestive responsibilities. This capacity eventually weakens, total food assimilation does not occur, and large amounts of undigested fats and proteins are left that the immune system treats as potentially toxic are not eliminated. It releases prostaglandins, leukotrienes, and histamines into the bloodstream to counteract the perceived threat, and food intolerances occur. Food allergies have become extremely widespread. As the body's toxic burden increases it becomes increasingly less able to tolerate even small doses of an allergen. Common ones include intolerance to wheat, dairy products, fruits, sugar, yeast, mushrooms, eggs, coffee, corn and greens. Although some of these foods are healthy in themselves, they are often heavily sprayed or treated, and in the case of animal products, secondarily affected by antibiotics and

FOOD THERAPY

🍃 Go on a short 24 hour liquid diet (pg. 44) to clear the system of allergens. Then follow a diet emphasizing fresh, organic produce and grains.

🍃 Include manganese-rich foods: buckwheat, nuts, legumes, blueberries.

🍃 Eat cultured foods to add friendly flora to the G.I. tract for digestion.

🍃 Avoid common food allergens: mushrooms, pasteurized dairy foods, wheat, chocolate, eggs, yeast, sugar, corn, nightshades such as potatoes, tomatoes, eggplant, nuts, etc. Foods commonly sprayed with heavy sulfites or pesticides: lettuce, apples, carrots, cole slaw, citrus, peanuts, cane, green beans should also be avoided.

🍃 Take 2TB. apple cider vinegar with honey at each meal to acidify saliva.

🍃 Crystal Star BIOFLAVONOID, FIBER & C SUPPORT™ drink daily.

🍃 See "COOKING FOR HEALTHY HEALING" by Linda Rector-Page for a complete diet program to overcome food allergies.

🍃 Try a food rotation diet to eliminate suspect allergen foods.

VITAMINS/MINERALS

▶ Quercetin Plus w. bromelain 3 daily.

▶ Ester C up to 5000mg. daily with bioflavonoids

   and/or

   CoQ 10, 30mg. 2x daily to help the liver produce anti-histimines.

▶ Alta Health manganese with B₁₂ sublingual.

▶ A full spectrum digestive enzyme such as Rainbow Light DOUBLE STRENGTH ALL-ZYME ♂ or Alta Health CANGEST. ♂ and Betaine HCl with meals, or Dr. DOPHILUS ¼ teasp. in liquid before meals. ☺

▶ Rainbow Light FOOD SENSITIVITY capsules with meals. ♀

▶ Liquid chlorophyll 1 teasp. 3x daily before meals.

   with

   Enzymatic Therapy LIQUID LIVER capsules as directed.

▶ For lactose intolerance
   ✚ Lactaid drops or tablets.
   ✚ Nature's Plus SAY YES TO DAIRY.

HERBAL THERAPY

🌿 Y.S. bee pollen/royal jelly/honey combination, 2 teasp. daily . ♂

🌿 Crystal Star ANTI-HST™ capsules or ALRG-HST™ extract to help normalize anti-histamine production.

🌿 Nature's Works SWEDISH BITTERS, or Crystal Star BITTERS & LEMON CLEANSE™ extract.

🌿 George's aloe vera juice daily. ♂

🌿 Effective capsules:
   ◆ Reishi mushroom.
   ◆ Golden seal root

🌿 Crystal Star HERBAL ENZYMES after meals. ♂

🌿 Natra Bio homeopathic:
   ◆ FOOD ALLERGY - GRAIN.
   ◆ FOOD ALLERGY -DAIRY.

🌿 Crystal Star CANDID-EX™ capsules if the allergy is related to gluten or wheat foods. (Also see CANDIDA ALBICANS page in this book.)

🌿 Omega 3 flax seed oil with meals.

BODYWORK

▶ Many childhood allergies are the result of feeding babies meats and pasteurized dairy foods before 10-12 months. Babies do not have the proper enzymes before this time to digest these. Feed mother's milk, soy milk, or goat's milk for at least 8 months to avoid food allergies.

▶ Use Coca's Pulse Test or muscle testing to identify allergens. (See page 347 in the appendix.)

▶ Use a garlic/catnip enema to cleanse the digestive tract, and balance colon pH.

▶ Reflexology point:

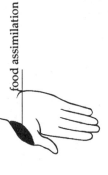

food assimilation

Common Symptoms: The inability to eat normal amounts of a food; cyclical headaches; hypoglycemia; hyperactivity in children; excessively swollen stomach, nausea or tiredness after eating palpitations, sweating, mental fuzziness after eating.
Common Causes: Eating chemically altered, sprayed, injected or processed foods that the body cannot handle; overconsumption of too few foods; food additives such as nitrites and sulfites; stress; poor diet; alkalosis with low gastric pH and enzyme deficiency; insufficient sleep; emotional trauma; chronic infections; eating a particular allergen food.

ALZHEIMERS DISEASE

Senility ✧ Cerebral Atherosclerosis ✧ Memory Deterioration ✧ Lack Of Alertness

The growing number of people living into their 70's, 80's, and 90's is creating an expanding population of people who suffer from significant loss of brain function. The medical community is reporting that Alzheimer's disease is now a common condition that increases strongly with age. But many of those diagnosed are really victims of too many drugs or other cerebral dysfunctions called "senility". Natural therapies have been successful in slowing the deterioration of brain function.

FOOD THERAPY

A highly nutritious diet is showing without question to be a deterrent of onset.

☙ Follow the Hypoglycemia Diet in this book. Eat organically grown foods as much as possible, with emphasis on vegetable protein-rich brain foods: eggs, soy foods, sea vegetables, whole grains, seeds, fresh vegetables, etc. The diet should be low in fats, salt, meat, and dairy, with plenty of fiber.

☙ Eat plenty of B vitamin foods, such as brown rice and other whole grains, brewer's yeast, molasses, liver, fish and wheat germ. (They block aluminum toxicity and protect the brain.)

☙ Eat tryptophan-rich foods, such as poultry, low fat dairy products and avocados. There is almost always tryptophan deficiency in Alzheimer's disease.

☙ Make up a mix of the following ingredients and take 1-2 TBS. each morning with cereal or juice: ♂
Lecithin granules
Brewer's yeast
Wheat germ oil
Oat or rice bran
Blackstrap molasses
Canola oil

☙ Drink only bottled water for good blood circulation and brain health.

VITAMINS/MINERALS

▶ Niacin therapy 250-500mg. 3 x daily.
with
Omega 3 fish or flax oils 3 x daily.

▶ Ester C w/ bioflavonoids, up to 3000mg. daily.
with
PC 55 - phosphatidyl choline 3x daily, or choline 1-5 grams daily.
with
B Complex 100mg., pantothenic acid 1000mg. *and* pancreatin for uptake, to block aluminum apsorption.

▶ ENER-B vit. B12 inter-nasal gel every 2-3 days, and/or folic acid 400mcg.

▶ Effective anti-oxidants:
✤ Vitamin E 800IU w. selenium daily.
✤ Beta carotene, 25-50,000IU daily.
✤ CoQ 10, 30mg. 2x daily.
✤ Solaray TRI-O₂ 2 daily.

▶ Golden Pride ORAL CHELATION THERAPY, 1 cap 2x daily, *and*
A liquid potassium 2 teasp. daily. ♂

▶ Cal/Mag/Zinc 4 daily to lower blood aluminum.
with
Evening primrose oil 500mg. 4 daily.

▶ Glutamine and/or glycine 500mg.

HERBAL THERAPY

☙ Crystal Star MENTAL CLARITY™ capsules. (Do not take if there is blood pressure imbalance.)
or
CREATIVI-TEA™ 2 x daily. ♀

☙ Ginkgo biloba liquid extract or capsules 2, 3 x daily.
with
Garlic, 4 capsules daily.

☙ YS royal jelly 2-3 teasp. daily. ♀

☙ Ginseng/gotu kola caps 2 daily.
or
Siberian ginseng extract drops. ♂

☙ Crystal Star GINSENG 6 SUPER TEA™ or CAPSULES.

☙ Crystal Star POTASSIUM SOURCE caps 4 daily with rosemary tea. ♀

☙ Brain nutrients:
♦ Ginkgo biloba 2 daily
♦ Gotu kola
♦ Bilberry extract
♦ Dr. Chang's LONG LIFE TEA
♦ Wisdom of the Ancients YERBA MATÉ tea.

BODYWORK

Beware of fluoridated water. It increases absorption of aluminum from deodorants, pots and pans, etc. by over 600%.

▶ Get daily mild exercise and/or use hot and cold hydrotherapy for brain and circulation stimulation.

▶ Decrease prescription diuretics if possible. They leach potassium and nutrients needed by the brain.

▶ Avoid aluminum and alum containing products: cookware, deodorants, dandruff shampoos, anti-diarrhea compounds, canned foods, salt, buffered aspirin and analgesics, antacids, refined and fast foods, relishes, pickles, tobacco, etc. Read labels!

▶ Reflexology pressure points for the brain:
↣ Squeeze all around the hand and fingers.
↣ Pinch the end of each toe. Hold for 5 seconds.

▶ Have silver amalgam dental fillings removed. They can cause mercury toxicity that releases into the brain, and affects brain health.

Common Symptoms: Loss of ability to think clearly and remember past or present facts, names, places, etc.; loss of touch with reality; confusion and impaired judgement; difficulty in completing thoughts or following directions; personality and behavioral change.
Common Causes: Poor or obstructed circulation; arteriosclerosis; anemia from long or excessive drug use; decrease in hormone output; lack of exercise, and body/brain oxygen; lack of enough pure water; fluid accumulation in the brain; thyroid malfunction; aluminum toxicity from a wide variety of aluminum-containing products; mercury toxicity from silver-amalgam dental fillings; inherited predisposition to mental illness; emotional shock and loss, such as the death of a spouse.

ANEMIA

Hemolytic ✧ Iron-Deficiency ✧ Pernicious Anemia ✧ Thalassemia ✧ Sickle Cell

Hemolytic: vitamin B12 and/or folic acid deficiency causing red blood cells to be destroyed more quickly than they are replaced. **Iron-Deficiency:** caused by a lack of iron, or poor absorption of iron. **Thalassemia:** an inherited defect, usually affecting people of Mediterranean origin. **Sickle Cell:** an inherited abnormal hemoglobin defect among blacks. **Pernicious:** an auto-immune disease caused by a deficiency of vitamin B12, due to poor intake or absorption; common among elderly people.

FOOD THERAPY

Food and herbal iron sources are best for absorbability.

▲ Eat iron-rich foods: liver, organ meats, figs, seafood, molasses, beets, brown rice, whole grains, poultry, eggs, grapes, raisins, yams, almonds.

▲ Eat manganese-rich foods, such as whole grains, greens, legumes, nuts, pineapples and eggs for iron uptake.

▲ Eat cultured foods, such as yogurt, kefir, and soyfoods for friendly bacteria and B12 formation.

▲ Eat potassium rich foods, such as broccoli, bananas, sunflowerseeds, vegetables, whole grains, and dried fruits; or take a potassium broth until red blood count improves (pg. 53).

▲ Eat vit. C rich foods, such as citrus fruits, cruciferous vegetables, tomatoes green pepper, for iron absorption.

▲ Avoid oxalic acid-forming foods: sodas, caffeine, chocolate, red meat, etc.

▲ Make a mix of the following and take 2TBS. daily in food:
   ♣ Brewer's yeast
   ♣ Wheat germ
   ♣ Sesame seeds
   ♣ Dried, crushed sea vegetables

▲ Take a protein drink (pg. 63) or a green drink (pg. 54) every morning.

VITAMINS/MINERALS

▶ ENER-B Vit. B12 internasal gel every 2 days.

with

Betaine HCl or Alta Health MANGANESE at meals for best uptake.

▶ Sun Chlorella 15-20 tabs daily.

▶ B Complex 100mg. with extra pantothenic acid and B6.

▶ Vitamin E 800IU with CoQ10 30mg. - especially for thalassemia.

▶ **Absorbable iron sources:**
   ✦ Enzymatic Therapy LIQUID LIVER w. SIB. GINSENG 2 x daily. ♂
   ✦ Strength Systems DESICCATED LIVER 3 daily, or desiccated liver tabs 6 daily.♂
   ✦ Floradix liquid iron 2x daily.
   and

▶ Take your choice of iron with vitamin C for best absorption.

▶ KAL folic acid w/ B12 and zinc 50mg. to regain menstrual periods.

▶ For sickle-cell anemia: take folic acid 800mcg., vitamin B6 100mg. 2x daily, zinc 50mg. daily, and vitamin E 400IU 2x daily.

HERBAL THERAPY

❧ Crystal Star HEARTSEASE/ANEMI-GIZE™ capsules, and IRON SOURCE™ capsules or extract 3x daily til blood count improves.
   or
ENERGY GREEN DRINK™ mix daily.

   and

Extra bee pollen 1000mg. daily.

❧ Spirulina 6 tabs daily, with Bee Pollen tablets 6 daily.

❧ Effective teas:
   ◆ Yellow dock
   ◆ Pau de arco
   ◆ Dandelion root and leaf

❧ Effective capsules:
   ◆ Beet root
   ◆ Fo-Ti
   ◆ Kelp (espec. during pregnancy)
   ◆ Crystal Star POTASSIUM SOURCE™ capsules as a source of B12.

❧ Effective extracts:
   ◆ Siberian ginseng ♂
   ◆ Dong quai/ damiana ♀
   ◆ Ginseng Co. CYCLONE CIDER

BODYWORK

▶ Get some mild exercise daily to enhance oxygen uptake. Get morning sunlight every day possible for vit. D.

▶ Avoid pesticides, sprays and fluorescent lighting that cause mineral leaching from the body.

▶ Poor food combining accounts for an amazing amount of iron deficiency. Get a good food combining chart, or see "COOKING FOR HEALTHY HEALING" by Linda Rector-Page.

Common Symptoms: Overall weakness; dizziness and fainting; heart palpitations; breathlessness; lack of libido; gastro-intestinal bleeding; ulcers; slow healing; fatigue; pallor; violent mood swings; irritability; spots before the eyes. Secondary signs of deficient iron include apathy, brittle nails, poor appetite, hair loss, pale skin and lips, headaches, and poor memory.
Common Causes: Recurring infections and diseases indicating low immunity and mineral deficiency; B12 and folic acid deficiency; pregnancy; poor diet or poor food assimilation; candida albicans, lupus, or other auto-immune condition; parasites; excessive menstruation; lack of green vegetables; alcoholism.

APPENDICITIS

Chronic

Appendicitis is an inflammation of the appendix, a small 2 inch tube opening into the beginning of the large intestine. It is usually caused by blockage from a small, hard lump of fecal matter, which in turn results from a fiber-deficient diet. The blockage stops the natural flow of fluids, unfriendly bacteria swarm in and inflamation results. The suggestions on this page are for chronic, recurring appendicitis. If there is danger of appendix rupture, you need emergency treatment. **DON'T DELAY!**

FOOD THERAPY

🥬 Go on a short vegetable juice diet (pg. 43) to clear and clean the intestine. Take one potassium drink (pg. 53) daily during this fast.

🥬 **Make sure the diet is high in soluble fiber to help prevent attacks.**

🥬 Then, eat sweet fruits for a day to encourage healing.

🥬 Then, resume a mild foods simple diet and include a glass of carrot juice daily for 2 weeks.

🥬 Avoid refined and fried foods on a continuing basis.

🥬 Take no solid food or laxatives during an appendicitis flare-up.

VITAMINS/MINERALS

▶ Beta carotene 25,000IU 4x daily, with
Liquid chlorophyll in water 3 x daily.

▶ **Dr. DOPHILUS** lactobacillus compound powder $1/4$ teasp. in water 4 x daily.
or
DDS powder for gentle, friendly bacteria and enhanced peristalsis.

▶ Ester C or ascorbate vit. C crystals $1/4$ teasp. in water 4 x daily.

▶ Vit. E 400IU 2 x daily.

▶ Living Source STRESS MANAGEMENT COMPLEX multivitamin daily.
and
Rainbow Light ULTRA-ZYME tablets at meals.

▶ Zinc picolinate 30mg. daily.

HERBAL THERAPY

🌿 **Crystal Star MIN-ZYME-MINOS™ drink mix for alkalinity and better food absorption.**

🌿 Crystal Star ANTI-BIO™ capsules or extract every 2 hours to reduce infection and inflammation.

🌿 Effective teas:
  ◆ **Alfalfa**
  ◆ **Buckthorn**
  ◆ **Slippery Elm**
  ◆ **Agrimony**

🌿 Solaray REFRESH capsules or Yerba Prima COLON CARE SYSTEM after an attack for 6 days to clean the colon of infection.

🌿 Echinacea extract 4 x daily under the tongue.

BODYWORK

➤ Do not take high colonics or enemas during an attack.

➤ Keep the colon clean. Constipation is usually the cause of an attack. Use a mild catnip enema. ☺

➤ Use alternating hot and cold cayenne/ginger compresses on affected area and along spine.

➤ Reflexology point:

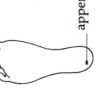

appendix

➤ Position of appendix in the body:

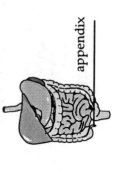

appendix

Common Symptoms: Intense, recurring sharp pain on the lower right side at the waist.

Common Causes: Poor diet, lacking in fiber and roughage; too many antibiotics; too many laxatives resulting in lack of peristalsis and friendly bowel flora.

ARTERIOSCLEROSIS ■ ATHEROSCLEROSIS

Both arteriosclerosis and atherosclerosis block the flow of blood from the arteries to the heart, and damage the circulatory system. Atherosclerotic plaque is largely composed of cholesterol. Its first signs begin underneath the inner wall of the artery suggesting that a vitamin B6 deficiency and a diet high in animal fats is the cause rather than cholesterol as previously thought. Arteriosclerosic plaque is the build-up of calcium on the inside of the artery walls. Both conditions are not only preventable, but reversible. Love and affection, both given and taken, really reduces heart and arterial problems.

FOOD THERAPY

ಈ Follow the **HEALTHY HEART DIET** in this book. As a rule, vegetarians have healthier hearts and arteries.

ಈ Avoid saturated fatty foods, such as red meats, full-fat dairy products, fried foods and refined, low fiber foods.

ಈ Eat plenty of high fiber whole grains, particularly in the form of cereals, rather than bread or pasta, and lots of fresh greens.

ಈ Eat foods rich in anti-oxidant vitamins C, E and Beta-carotene.

ಈ Take one cup daily of the following mix:
♠ 2 teasp. wheat germ, 2 teasp. honey, 1 TB. lecithin, in 1 cup fenugreek tea.

ಈ Eat smaller meals, especially at night.
♠ Have a little wine at dinner for digestion and relaxation.

ಈ Crystal Star BIOFLAVONOID, FIBER & C SUPPORT™ drink or wafers daily, as a tonic to address the causes of arteriosclerosis.

ಈ Reduce coffee consumption to 1 cup daily.

VITAMINS/MINERALS

▶ Golden Pride ORAL CHELATION THERAPY, 1 cap 2x daily. ♂
and
Carnitine 500mg. daily.

▶ Alta Health SIL-X silica tabs on a regular basis for prevention.

▶ Phosphatidyl choline daily.
with
✦ Chromium picolinate 2 daily,
✦ Garlic oil extract caps 6 daily,
✦ Vitamin E 400IU w. selenium daily.

▶ Vitamin B6, 100mg. 3x daily
with
Beta carotene 25,000IU 2 x daily.
and
Ester C 3-5000mg. daily with bioflavonoids and rutin.

▶ Effective anti-oxidants:
✦ Co. Life Pycnogenol, 1 to 2 daily.
✦ Country Life B15 DMG sublingual
✦ Germanium 100mg. 2x daily.
✦ CoQ 10, 10mg. 2x daily.

▶ Niacin 500mg. 2 x daily
with
Zinc 50mg. daily to raise HDL levels.

▶ High potency, 1400mg. pancreatin with meals as a fat/oil digestant. ♂

▶ Future Biotics VITAL K liquid. ♂

HERBAL THERAPY

🌿 Crystal Star HEARTSEASE/ HAWTHORNE™ capsules or HAWTHORNE extract 2 x daily.
and/or
HEARTSEASE CIRCU-CLEANSE TEA™, a blood purifying tea w. butcher's broom. ♀

🌿 Ginkgo Biloba extract under the tongue 2-3x daily.
with

🌿 Sun Chlorella tabs 15-20 tabs or 1 packet daily.
or

🌿 Solaray ALFAJUICE capsules as diected.

🌿 Ginseng Co. CYCLONE CIDER liquid drops, or Ginseng/cayenne caps daily. ♂

🌿 High omega 3 flax oil 3 x daily.

🌿 Body Essentials SILICA GEL 1 TB. 3x daily for 1 month in 3oz. liquid.

🌿 Evening primrose oil caps, 4-6 daily for 1 month, then 3-4 daily.

🌿 George's ALOE VERA JUICE, 1 8oz. glass daily with a pinch of ginger powder added to each glass.

🌿 Butcher's broom or astragalus tea for a limited time to increase circula-

BODYWORK

▶ Stop smoking. Keep your weight down. Relax. The stress and tension from stressful life styles can cause big artery problems.

▶ Take a brisk walk daily. Then use a dry skin brush over the body to stimulate circulation.
or
Take an alternating hot and cold shower to increase blood flow.

Common Symptoms: Poor circulation with cold hands and feet, and leg cramps; mild heart attacks; mental and respiratory deterioration; blurred vision; high blood pressure.
Common Causes: Too much saturated fat and refined food in the diet; vitamin B6 deficiency; smoking; obesity; stress; lack of aerobic exercise; too much caffeine and alcohol; excess salt.

ARTHRITIS

As the country's number one crippling disease, there are two major categories of arthritis, unified by two major symptoms - skeletal pain and joint malfunction. **Osteoarthritis**, the most common type, affects 40 million Americans - 80% of the people over 50. It is a "wear and tear" disease affecting weight-bearing joints by forming calcified deposits in them, and the bones by a breakdown in the buffer cartilage that protect bone ends. **Rheumatoid arthritis** is a systemic disease, with chronic inflammation of the joints, muscles, ligaments and tendons. Arthritis is not a simple disease in any form, affecting not only the bones and joints, but also the blood vessels, kidneys, skin, eyes and brain.

FOOD THERAPY

🍃 Diet change is the single most beneficial thing you can do to control both arthritis. See the following pages for a brief cleansing/control diet. See COOKING FOR HEALTHY HEALING by Linda Rector-Page for a complete diet with corresponding recipes.

🍃 A good, alkalizing diet can prevent or neutralize arthritis even in longstanding cases. Start a healing program with a short juice fast to clear out toxic wastes. (pg. 42ff.) Then follow an 80% raw foods diet for two months. A modified macrobiotic diet can be particularly helpful on a long term basis. (page 52)

🍃 Foods to add to your diet: Artichokes, cabbages, basic cereal grains, such as rice, oats and corn, cold water fish, fresh fruits and vegetables, leafy greens, garlic, onions, olive oil, sweet potatoes, squashes, eggs and parsley.

🍃 Foods to avoid: refined foods, saturated fatty foods from meat and dairy products, wheat pastries and other high gluten foods that are also high in sugar, cholesterol and fat. Nightshade family foods such as peppers, eggplant, tomatoes and potatoes; caffeine, colas, chocolate and highly spiced foods.

VITAMINS/MINERALS

▶ Quercetin Plus w/Bromelain, 2 daily.
or
▶ Bio-genetics BIOGUARD PLUS with Betaine HCl at meals.
and/or
Apply Body Essentials SILICA GEL to joints. Take internally as directed.

▶ Pantothenic acid therapy sources:
✦ YS royal jelly 2 teasp. daily.
✦ Enzymatic Therapy ADRENAL COMPLEX.

▶ DLPA 750mg. or GABA as needed.

▶ Solaray SL Germanium 150mg. daily, with Cysteine 500mg. 2x daily, and CoQ 10 30mg. 2x daily.

▶ Ester C 500mg. with bioflavonoids, up to 10 daily for collagen synthesis.

▶ CAL/MAG CITRATE w. boron and vitamin D for uptake, with pycnogenol 50mg. 3 x daily. ♀

▶ Am. Biologics INFLAZYME FORTE for pain and stiffness. ♂

▶ Country Life LIGA-TEND as needed; with B Complex 100mg. daily. ♀

▶ Omega 3 FLAX OIL 3x daily. Expect pain diminishment in 2 to 4 months.

HERBAL THERAPY

🌿 Crystal Star AR EASE caps and/ or tea, or GREEN TEA CLEANSER and 4 each LIV-ALIVE™ and ADRN-ALIVE™ capsules daily.

🌿 Ginkgo biloba extract daily.
with
Cartilade SHARK CARTILAGE 3 daily.

🌿 Yerba maté tea to stimulate the body's own cortisone.

🌿 Effective capsules:
✦ Yucca 4 daily.
✦ Devil's claw rt. 4 daily.
✦ Turmeric 4 daily.
✦ Alfalfa 10 daily.
✦ Green tea extract caps 6 daily, and cayenne/ginger compresses.

🌿 Strength Systems FIRST AID caps for green-lipped muscle therapy.

🌿 Evening primrose oil 4 daily. ♀

🌿 Aloe vera juice 1 glass daily. ♂ and apply aloe vera gel daily.

🌿 Sun CHLORELLA 2 packets or 20 tabs daily.

🌿 Crystal Star ALKALIZING ENZYME™ herbal wrap.

BODYWORK

Note: High doses of aspirin for arthritic pain can cause tinnitus and gastritis.

▶ Massage therapy, hot and cold hydrotherapy, epsom salts baths, chiropractic adjustments and overheating therapy are all effective. See page 49ff.

▶ Apply H2O2 Care Plus OXYGEL to affected areas every 24 hours. And/or take an energy/oxygen bath (pg. 49).

▶ Effective local applications:
→ PSI PRO-GEST cream
→ Chinese WHITE FLOWER oil.
→ B & T TRIFLORA gel.
→ Silica gel around joints.
→ Cajeput/wintergreen oil rubs
→ Bioforce ARNICA LOTION (Dilute 1 part to 5 parts water).

▶ Avoid tobacco smoke. Tobacco is a nightshade plant. *Note:* Motrin is also a nightshade derivative. It *is* an antiinflammatory, but should not be used by nightshade-sensitive people.

▶ To relieve pain, press the highest spot of the muscle between thumb and index finger. Press in the webbing between the two fingers, closer toward the bone that attaches to the index finger. Press into the web muscle, angling the pressure toward the bone of the index finger. Press for 10 seconds at a time.

Common Symptoms - Rheumatoid Arthritis: Inflammation and swelling of the joints; pain affecting the whole body; destruction of cartilage tissue due to poor calcium assimilation; digestive problems; great fatigue; anemia; ulcerative colitis; chronic lung and bronchial congestion; neurological depression; liver malfunction.
Common Symptoms - Osteoarthritis: Stiffness, pain, joint immobility; bone deterioration; inorganic sediment in the joints; pain and swelling in joints and spine during damp weather.
Common Causes Of Both Osteoarthritis & Rheumatoid Arthritis: Calcium depletion; osteoporosis; gland and hormone imbalance; prolonged use of aspirin or cortico-steroid drugs, that eventually impair the body's own healing powers; poor diet, lacking in fresh vegetables and high in acid and mucous-forming foods; food allergens; auto-toxemia from poor bowel movements and constipation; inability to relax; resentments and a negative attitude toward life that lock up the body's healing ability.

Cleansing Diets For Arthritis Control

The following brief diet programs for arthritis may be used for several weeks to help detoxify the body and flush out inorganic mineral deposits. Small and subtle dietary changes are not successful in reversing arthritic conditions. Vigorous diet therapy is necessary. For permanent results, the diet must be changed to non-mucous and non- sediment-forming foods. See COOKING FOR HEALTHY HEALING, by Linda Rector-Page for more explicit information and recipes.

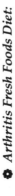

❖ Arthritis Liquid Cleansing Diet:

On rising: take a glass of lemon juice and water; **or** a glass of fresh grapefruit juice.

Breakfast: take a glass of potassium broth or essence (pg. 53); **or** a glass of carrot / beet / cucumber juice.

Mid-morning: have apple or black cherry juice; **or** a green drink, such as Sun CHLORELLA, a drink from page 54ff, or Crystal Star ENERGY GREEN™ drink.

Lunch: have a cup of miso soup with sea vegies snipped on top, **and** a glass of fresh carrot juice.

Mid-afternoon: have another green drink, a cup of Crystal Star GREEN TEA CLEANSER™; **or** an herbal tea, such as alfalfa/mint, or Crystal Star AR-EASE™ TEA.

Dinner: have a glass of cranberry / apple, or papaya juice, or another glass of black cherry juice.

Before bed: take a glass of celery juice, or a cup of VEGEX yeast extract broth; **or** a cup of miso soup.

❖ Arthritis Fresh Foods Diet:

On rising: take a glass of lemon juice and water, or grapefruit juice; **or** a glass of apple cider vinegar in water with honey.

Breakfast: have a glass of cranberry, grape or papaya juice, or Crystal Star BIOFLAVONOID, FIBER & C SUPPORT™ DRINK or WAFERS; **and** some fresh fruits, especially cherries, bananas, oranges and strawberries.
And have 2 teasp. daily of the following mix. Two **each**: sunflower seeds, lecithin granules, brewer's yeast, wheat germ. Mix into yogurt, or sprinkle on fresh fruit or greens.

Mid-morning: take a glass of potassium broth (pg. 53) or essence; **and/or** more fresh fruit with yogurt; **or** a green drink such as Crystal Star GREEN TEA CLEANSER™, or Sun CHLO-RELLA or Green Foods GREEN MAGMA with 1 teasp. Bragg's LIQUID AMINOS™ added.

Lunch: have a large dark green leafy salad with lemon/oil dressing; **and/or** a hot vegie broth or onion soup; **and/or** some marinated tofu or tempeh in tamari sauce.

Mid-afternoon: have a cup of miso soup with sea vegies on top; **or** a green drink, alfalfa / mint tea, or Crystal Star LICORICE MINTS TEA.

Dinner: have a Chinese greens salad with sesame or poppy seed dressing; **or** a large dinner salad with soy cheese, nuts, tamari dressing, and a cup of black bean or vegie broth or miso soup; **or** some quick steamed vegetables and brown rice for absorbable B vitamins.

Before bed: have a cranberry or apple juice, or black cherry juice; **or** a cup of VEGEX yeast extract broth; and/ or celery juice.
✓Make sure you are drinking 6 to 8 glasses of bottled mineral water daily to keep inorganic wastes releasing quickly from the body.

Supplements for the Fresh Foods Diet: As the body starts to rebuild with a stronger, more alkaline system, supplements may be added to speed this process along.

✦ Ascorbate Vitamin C powder and bioflavonoids in juice ($^{1}/_{4}$ teasp. four times daily) for interstitial tissue and collagen development.
✦ High Omega 3 flax oil 3 teasp. daily. Add Rainbow Light ALL-ZYME caps or Alta Health CANGEST caps, for assimilation, and alfalfa tabs, 6 to 10 daily to help alkalize the system.
✦ Take Crystal Star AR EASE™ caps as directed, and/ or Quercetin Plus with Bromelain 500mg. daily to aid the release of inorganic calcium and mineral deposits.
✦ Use DLPA 750 - 1000mg. daily, germanium 100mg., or highest potency Bio-genetics BIO-GUARD PLUS™ for pain relief.
✦ Niacinamide 500mg. daily to help joint pain, flexibility and circulation.

ASTHMA

Asthma affects about 3 per cent of the U.S. population, but is most common in children under the age of ten, with a 2:1 ratio of boys to girls. Extrinsic or atopic asthma is an allergy related condition, due to antigen-antibody stimulation by foods or food additives coupled with poor digestive/assimilation elements. Intrinsic or bronchial asthma, is due to chemical toxicity, hypersensitivity of the airways to cold air, bronchial infection and emotional stress. Both types can appear at the same time.

FOOD THERAPY

❧ Go on a short mucous cleansing liquid diet (pg. 42) for a week. Then follow a non-mucous-forming, low salt diet for the next 3 months. (See next page for a brief version), or "COOKING FOR HEALTH HEALING" by Linda Rector-Page for a complete version of this diet.)

❧ Maintain a vegetarian diet as much as possible.

❧ During an attack - eat only fresh raw foods. Include fresh apple or carrot juice daily.

❧ Make a syrup of pressed garlic juice, cayenne, and honey. Take 1 teasp. daily as a liver cleansing bile stimulant for fatty-acid metabolism.

❧ Avoid all foods with sulfites and MSG. Avoid mucous-forming foods, such as pasteurized dairy products, meats except fish and seafoods, high gluten breads, and sugars. Avoid refined and preserved foods, fried and fatty foods, and caffeine. Reduce salt and heavy starches.

❧ Mix fresh grated horseradish and lemon juice. Take a spoonful and hang over a sink to expel mucous in large quantities.

VITAMINS/MINERALS

▶ Ester C or ascorbate vit. C powder w/bioflavs. & rutin 5000mg. daily.
with
Beta-carotene100,000IU.
or

▶ Quercetin Plus 1000-2000mg. daily, with
Bromelain 500mg, vit. C 3000mg. and magnesium 500mg. daily.

▶ Pantothenic acid therapy sources:
✦ High potency royal jelly or bee pollen, 2 teasp. daily.
✦ Pantothenic acid caps 1000mg. daily with PABA 500mg.
✦ B Complex 150mg. daily with extra B6 100mg. ♂

▶ Raw Adrenal complex and/or Raw Thymus glandular 2 x daily.

▶ Bioforce ASTHMASAN drops. ♂

▶ Alta Health MANGANESE w. B12 2 daily, or Ener-B internasal B12 esp. for sulfite-induced asthma.

▶ Use food grade H2O2, 3% dilute solution in 8oz. water in a vaporizer at night for relief and tissue oxygen.

▶ Reishi mushroom capsules.

▶ Pancreatin, 450mg, before each meal to digest clogging fats and oils, and/or HCl, 1 tablet after each meal.

HERBAL THERAPY

❧ Crystal Star ASTH-AID™ tea and capsules to clear the chest, and ANTI-HST™ or ALRG-HST™ extract to produce antihistamines.
with
ADR-ACTIVE™ capsules or extract.

❧ Crystal Star ANTI-SPAZ™ capsules as needed every hour to control spasmodic wheezing. ☺
with
X-PECT-T™ tea for mucous release.

❧ For acute attacks: Lobelia extract under the tongue as needed. ☺

❧ Two teas for chronic asthma:
① 1 pt. ginger rt, 1 pt. ephedra, 1 pt. schizandra berries.
② 1 part each: bupleurum, fenugreek seed, gotu kola.

❧ Therapeutic teas:
◆ Green tea
◆ Ephedra
◆ Nettles
◆ Gotu kola
◆ Scullcap
◆ Pau de arco

❧ Effective extracts under the tongue:
◆ Ginkgo biloba extract.
◆ Heritage ATOMODINE dilute for iodine therapy.
◆ Lobelia as a chest muscle relaxant

BODYWORK

▶ Use eucalyptus oil in a vaporizer at night and/or a catnip/garlic enema twice a week. ☺

▶ Apply an onion poultice to the chest.

▶ Biofeedback is effective for asthma.

▶ Avoid tobacco smoke.

▶ Massage and gently scratch the lung meridian from top of shoulder to end of thumb to clear chest of mucous. Massage between the shoulder blades.

▶ Do deep breathing exercises to increase lung capacity and chest muscles outdoors if air quality is acceptable. Before aerobic exercise, deplete the body of chemicals that induce asthma attacks by starting with a short warm up. Then take a walk, bicycle ride, or other exercise, exhaling strongly to expel toxins.

▶ Reflexology point:

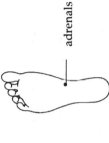

adrenals

Common Symptoms: Difficult breathing; choking; wheezing; coughing; difficulty in exhaling.
Common Causes: Food allergies, particularly to additives or preservatives, excess sugar, pasteurized dairy products, meats, wheat; adrenal exhaustion and imbalance; hypoglycemia; poor circulation; environmental pollutants; emotional stress.

Liquid Mucous Cleansing Diet For Asthma & Respiratory Disease

Follow for three to five days at a time as needed for mucous release.

A program to overcome asthma and other chronic respiratory problems is usually more successful when begun with a short mucous elimination diet. This allows the body to rid itself first of toxins and mucous accumulations causing congestion before an attempt to change eating habits. Then avoid pasteurized dairy products, heavy starches and refined foods that are inherently a breeding ground for continued congestion. All respiratory problems will benefit from this way of eating. The first stage, a high vitamin C liquid diet, should be followed for 3 - 5 days. It often produces symptomatic relief from respiratory problems in 24 to 48 hours.

On rising: take a glass of cranberry, apple or grapefruit juice; **or** lemon juice in hot water with 1 teasp. honey; **or** a glass of cider vinegar, hot water and honey.

Breakfast: take a hot potassium broth or essence (page 53), or Crystal Star SYSTEM STRENGTH™ DRINK with 1 teasp. liquid chlorophyll, Sun CHLORELLA or Green Foods GREEN MAGMA.
Add 2 or 3 garlic capsules and $1/4$ to $1/2$ teasp. ascorbate vitamin C or Ester C powder with bioflavonoids in water.

Mid-morning: have a glass of fresh carrot juice; **and/or** a cup of comfrey/fenugreek tea, or Crystal Star RESPIRATOR TEA™ or ASTH-AID TEA™.

Lunch: have a hot vegetable, miso or onion broth, or Crystal Star SYSTEM STRENGTH™ DRINK;
Add 2-3 more garlic capsules and $1/4$ to $1/2$ teasp. ascorbate vitamin C or Ester C powder with bioflavonoids in water.

Mid-afternoon: have a cleansing herb tea, such as alfalfa/mint or Crystal Star GREEN TEA CLEANSER™; **or** another green drink such as Sun CHLORELLA, or Crystal Star ENERGY GREEN™.

Dinner: have a hot vegie broth, potassium essence, or miso soup with sea vegies snipped on top; **or** another glass of carrot juice.
Take 2-3 more garlic capsules, and $1/4$ to $1/2$ teasp. ascorbate vitamin C or Ester C powder in water.

Before bed: take another hot water, lemon and honey drink; **or** hot apple or cranberry juice.

❧ Salts should be kept low during this diet, but a little Bragg's LIQUID AMINOS can be added to any broth or juice for flavor.
❧ Drink six to eight glasses of bottled water or mineral water each day for best cleansing results.
❧ If you have a cold, include even more liquids than described above, such as hot broths, mineral water, fruit and vegetable juices, or a little brandy with lemon.

Supplements for the Mucous Cleansing Diet

♣ Add 1 teasp. acidophilus liquid, or $1/4$ to $1/2$ teasp. acidophilus powder to any broth or juice.

♣ Ascorbate vitamin C or Ester C powder may be taken thoughout the day in juice or water, to bowel tolerance for tissue flushing and detoxification. Take up to 10,000mg. daily for the first three days, then 5,000mg. daily til the end of the *liquid* fast.

♣ Try to stay away from cortisone compounds that eventually weaken the immune system, and from over-the-counter drugs that often simply drive the congestion deeper into the lungs and tissues.

See "COOKING FOR HEALTHY HEALING" by Linda Rector Page for the complete diet.

148

ATHLETE'S FOOT ◼ FUNGAL SKIN INFECTIONS

Athlete's foot and other fungal infections thrive in dampness and warmth. Make sure that any concurrently occurring fungal infections (such as athlete's foot and "jock itch") are treated simultaneously, so that infection is not continually passed from one area to another.

FOOD THERAPY

❧ Avoid acid forming foods such as red meats, caffeine and fried foods.

❧ Eat plenty of cultured foods such as yogurt, tofu and kefir to keep the body alkaline and nutrients absorbed.

❧ Add lots of fresh fruits and vegetables to the diet during healing.

❧ Drink 6-8 glasses of water daily to keep elimination system free and flowing.

❧ Apply a honey/garlic poultice to the area to impede bacterial growth.

❧ Dab cider vinegar between the toes 3 or 4 x daily. Wipe inside of shoes with vinegar.

VITAMINS/MINERALS

▶ Apply a few drops of Nutrition Resource NUTRIBIOTIC GRAPE-FRUIT SEED SPRAY or CREAM and massage in.

▶ Zinc 50mg. 2 x daily.
with
Alta Health MANGANESE & B12 daily.

▶ Vit. E 400IU 2 x daily. Also apply to sore area.

▶ Acidophilus powder ½ teasp. 3 x daily. Also dissolve in water and apply to area directly.
and
take 4-6 garlic extract capsules daily to destroy fungus.

▶ Lysine 1000mg. daily.

▶ Crush or open the following and mix together in a bowl.
B2 500mg., niacin 1000mg., pantothenic acid 500mg.
Add 2 teasp. sesame oil and 2 teasp. brewer's yeast. Apply to area at night. Put on an old sock to cover and leave on overnight.

HERBAL THERAPY

❧ Apply echinacea cream.

❧ Apply black walnut tincture. ♀

❧ Apply tea tree oil as needed.

❧ Evening primrose oil caps 4 daily for 2 weeks for fungal peeling.

❧ Mix powders of whey and slippery elm with water. Apply.

❧ Dust feet with myrrh/golden seal powder.

❧ Apply aloe vera gel.

❧ Apply witch hazel freely.

❧ Open a capsule of Crystal Star's anti-fungal WHITES OUT #2™. Make a solution with water. Dab twice daily onto affected areas.
or
Open a WHITES OUT™ #2 capsule and apply directly to toes.

❧ Apply lomatium extract to area, or Crystal Star ANTI-VI™ extract.

❧ Apply Crystal Star FUNGEX™ gel.

BODYWORK

▶ Keep feet well aired and dry. Keep shoes well-aired and change socks daily. Go barefoot as much as possible where appropriate. Expose feet to natural sunlight every day to inhibit fungal growth.

▶ Open garlic capsules and apply the powder between the toes every morning and night.

▶ Use castile or tea tree oil soap.

▶ Apply N.F. HERBAL-SEPTIC liquid daily to affected area. ☺

▶ Apply Care Plus OXYGEL H2O2, to affected area.

Common Symptoms: Burning, itching skin infection between the toes; area will be dry, scaly, cracked, bleeding and tender, with weeping bacterial odor.
Common Causes: Tight or non-porous shoes, so that perspiration cannot evaporate; infection from fungus micro-organisms in locker rooms and showers; yeast overgrowth; prolonged anti-biotic use that lowers immune defenses, and allows unfriendly bacteria to thrive and take hold.

BACK ACHE ◼ CHRONIC LOWER BACK PAIN

Lumbago ◇ Herniated Disc ◇ Scoliosis

The spine is the major seat of human nerve structure, and as such manifests many of the body's emotional, psychological and physical stresses. Causes for back conditions can be as wide-ranging as a slipped disc and family financial problems. In addition to diet improvement and supplementation, a good massage therapist who treats more than just the physical problem, is often the best answer.

FOOD THERAPY

🍃 Uric acid aggravates back pain. Avoid red meats, pasteurized dairy and caffeine.

🍃 The diet should be high in minerals and vegetable proteins. Vegetarians have stronger bone density.
Take a high mineral drink daily, such as Crystal Star ENERGY GREEN™ or SYSTEM STRENGTH™.
and/or
A protein drink such as Nature's Plus SPIRUTEIN or NutriTech ALL 1.

🍃 Drink 6-8 glasses of pure water daily to keep kidneys flushed and functioning well.

🍃 Take a potassium broth (pg. 53) once a week for strength and kidney cleansing.

VITAMINS/MINERALS

▶ Twin Lab CSA 250mg, 1 daily.

▶ Stress B Complex with extra B6 100mg. daily and B12 SL 2000mcg.

▶ Alta Health MANGANESE with B12 for spine cell development .

▶ DLPA as needed for chronic pain. ♀
or
▶ Country Life LIGATEND capsules.

▶ Mezotrace SEA MINERAL/TRACE MINERAL COMPLEX 3 x daily.

▶ Vit. C 3-5000mg. with bioflavonoids.
and
Emulsified A & D daily for connective tissue strength.

▶ Bromelain 500mg, 2 x daily,
with
a high magnesium CAL/MAG CITRATE formula.
and
Boron 3mg. daily for better uptake.

▶ Care Plus OXYGEL rubs every night until relief.

HERBAL THERAPY

🌿 Crystal Star SILICA SOURCE™ or MINERAL SOURCE™ COMPLEX extracts for good collagen growth.
and/or
BONZ™ caps or tea for strengthening.

🌿 Crystal Star RELAX CAPS™ or ANTI-SPAZ™ capsules for spasm control. BACK TO RELIEF™ or ANTI-FLAM™ capsules, with St. John's wort as an analgesic and anti-inflammatory.

🌿 Effective herbal compresses:
 ◆ Hops/Lobelia
 ◆ Comfrey/Lobelia
 ◆ Horsetail

🌿 Effective extracts or capsules:
 ◆ St. John's wort
 ◆ Passion flower
 ◆ Devil's claw

🌿 Alta Health SIL-X silica extract for strength and collagen building.

🌿 Nature's Way ANTSP tincture as needed.

🌿 Crystal Star BLDR-K TEA™ if kidneys are inflamed.

BODYWORK

▶ **Regular, non-jarring exercise is the most important key in treating and preventing back pain. Exercises, such as swimming, cycling, walking, rowing and cross-country skiing will build back strength gradually.**

▶ Apply wet, cayenne/ginger heat packs to spine and lower back.

▶ Massage into back:
 → B&T TRIFLORA GEL. ♀
 → Chinese WHITE FLOWER oil.
 → Cajeput/wintergreen oil.
 → MINERAL ICE GEL.
 → DMSO with ALOE GEL. ♂

▶ Get plenty of bed rest with head and legs propped up. Sleep on a firm mattress.

▶ Reflexology points:

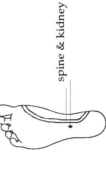

spine & kidney

150

Common Symptoms: Spinal stress and pain; inability to do even small bending or pushing actions.
Common Causes: Poor posture; improper lifting, sitting or standing; kidney/bladder problems; arthritis; slipped disc; deep-seated emotional stress; kidney malfunction; high heels; overweight; protein, calcium and other nutrient deficiency; green vegetable deficiency; osteoporosis or osteoarthritis; sleeping on a mattress that is too soft; congenitally poor spinal alignment. If you have fallen or bruised the spine or tailbone, and have persistent pain after 5 days, see a qualified massage therapist or chiropractor.

BAD BREATH & BODY ODOR

Both of these conditions are manifestations of the same problem - poor diet, poor food digestion, poor assimilation, causing rotting food and bacteria formation that the body throws off through the skin and breath.

FOOD THERAPY

❧ Start with a short 24 hour liquid diet (pg. 44) with apple juice and 1 TB. psyllium husks to cleanse the bowel.

❧ Then follow a diet with lots of crunchy fresh fruits and green vegetables. Eat high chlorophyll foods like parsley and sprouts.

❧ Eat plenty of cultured foods such as yogurt, tofu and kefir for better intestinal flora activity.

❧ Have a glass of lemon juice and water every morning.

❧ Drink 6-8 glasses of water daily to keep the kidneys clear.

❧ Add liquid chlorophyll drops to either apple or carrot juice to neutralize stomach acids and cleanse the digestive tract.

❧ Eat light, less concentrated foods.

❧ Reduce or avoid red meats and other heavy animal protein, fried foods, and heavy sweets.

❧ Eat smaller, meals, and chew well for best enzyme activity.

❧ Brush teeth and tongue after every meal.

VITAMINS/MINERALS

▶ Acidophilus 4-6 x daily.

▶ Betaine HCl before each meal, or Schiff ENZYMALL tabs w. ox bile. ♀

▶ Liquid chlorophyll, 1 teasp. in water after meals
or
take a green drink such as Green Foods GREEN MAGMA. Wakunaga KYO-GREEN, or Crystal Star ENERGY GREEN drink once a day.

▶ Chew propolis lozenges.

▶ Solaray ALFAJUICE capsules.

▶ Odorless garlic caps to control low-grade infections.

▶ Vitamin C 1000mg. with 500mg. bioflavonoids 3x daily, **with** zinc 50mg. 2 x daily.

▶ B Complex 100mg.daily.

▶ High Omega 3 fish or flax oils to improve circulation/blood fat release.

▶ **For morning breath:** Just before bedtime, floss between all teeth, then brush with baking soda rather than toothpaste. Brush your tongue but do not use mouthwash. Morning breath should be eliminated or greatly reduced.

HERBAL THERAPY

❧ Crystal Star PRE-MEAL ENZ™ before meals, or HERBAL ENZ™ at/after meals.
and/or
MEAL'S END TEA for digestion and fresh breath after eating.

❧ Effective teas:
♦ Peppermint
♦ Fenugreek/sage
♦ Rosemary ♀
♦ Alfalfa/mint

❧ Use Natureworks HERBAL BITTERS, or Crystal Star BITTERS & LEMON CLEANSE™ to boost liver function and stimulate effective digestion.

❧ Put pinches of cloves, ginger, cinnamon, nutmeg or anise in a cup of water and drink as a natural antacid.

❧ BioForce GOLDENROD extract as directed.

❧ Keep colon and bowel clean with a gentle herbal laxative such as HERBALTONE, or a fiber drink such as Crystal Star CHO-LO FIBER TONE™.

❧ Apply aloe vera gel under arms. ♀

BODYWORK

▶ Exercise to cleanse metabolic wastes being improperly expelled through skin and lungs.

▶ Take a mineral salts bath such as Para Labs BATH THERAPY at least once a week. ♀

▶ Clean teeth with myrrh gum powder, or Toms toothpaste with myrrh.

▶ Effective mouth deodorizers:
→ Coslo BREATH SPRAY.
→ TIBS essential oil breath drops.
→ Use tea tree oil mouthwash.

▶ Effective body deodorants:
→ Dab underarms/feet with vinegar.
→ Dust with a mix of 2 parts baking soda and 1 part arrowroot.

▶ Use a dry skin brush all over the body daily to remove toxins coming out through the skin. Then shower with an oatmeal/honey "scrub" soap.

▶ Wear natural fiber clothing so the skin can breathe. Wear sandals when possible.

▶ Reflexology point.

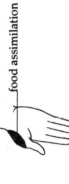

food assimilation

Common Symptoms: Bad taste in the mouth and mouth odor; foul smelling perspiration.
Common Causes: Poor diet with a green vegetable deficiency; enzyme deficiency; poor digestion, leading to indigestion; poor mouth or body hygiene; sluggish intestinal system and chronic constipation; stress and anxiety; gum disease and tooth decay; food intolerances; HCl deficiency; low grade chronic throat infection; smoking liver malfunction; post-nasal drip.

BEDWETTING

Most experts agree that barring any physical/mechanical obstruction or infection, youthful bedwetting is psychologically based. However, nutritional therapies have had such notable success in this area that we cannot help but believe that nutritional deficiencies are also a part of the problem.

FOOD THERAPY

❧ Avoid oxalic acid-forming foods, such as cooked spinach, sodas, rhubarb, caffeine, cocoa, chocolate, etc.

❧ No junk foods. Avoid refined sugars, excess salts and spicy foods as irritants.

❧ Avoid food colorings, preservatives and pasteurized cow's milk as possible allergens.

❧ Take a small glass of cranberry/apple juice each morning to clean the kidneys.

❧ No liquids before bed. Eat a little celery instead to balance organic salts.

❧ Take a spoonful of honey before bed. ☺

VITAMINS/MINERALS

▷ Hylands BEDWETTING tablets before bed. ☺

▷ Twin Lab LIQUID MINERALS.
or
Mezotrace SEA MINERAL COMPLEX chewable. ☺

▷ Country Life CAL SNACK, milk free chewable calcium. ☺

▷ Twin Lab CSA 250mg. 1 daily.

▷ Floradix LIQUID MULTI VITAMIN daily.

▷ Magnesium 100mg. daily. ☺

HERBAL THERAPY

❧ Crystal Star BLDR-K™ tea at dinner. Use half strength for children. ☺

❧ Crystal Star RELAX CAPS™ or VALERIAN and WILDLETTUCE extract in water for stress-related bedwetting.

❧ Give the child cinnamon sticks to chew on before bed.

❧ Effective teas: Use as extract drops in water if possible.
  ◆ Scullcap
  ◆ Cinnamon bark ☺
  ◆ Horsetail at dinner
  ◆ Cornsilk
  ◆ Plantain

❧ Effective tea combination: Parsley/oatstraw/juniper/uva ursi.

❧ Ginkgo biloba extract drops in water, mixed with a little honey before bed. ☺

❧ Crystal Star CALCIUM SOURCE™ capsules or extract drops in water.

BODYWORK

➤ See a good chiropractor or massage therapist if a compressed nerve or an obstruction is the suspected cause.

➤ Muscle testing (applied kinesiology) is effective here in determining what allergies may be the cause.

➤ Good circulation is a key. Good daily exercise is an answer; especially bicycle riding. ☺

➤ Leave a night light on so the child will feel free to get up at night.

➤ Give a relaxing massage before bed to ease muscles and fears. ☺ ◎

Common Symptoms: Involuntary urination during the night beyond toilet training age.
Common Causes: Inherited organ weakness; excess sugar, salt, spices or dairy in the diet; food allergies; stress, emotional anxiety and behavioral disturbances; bad dreams; allergies; hypoglycemia or diabetes; compressed nerve or congenital obstruction in the bladder area.

BLADDER INFECTIONS
Bacterial Cystitis ✧ Incontinence

Recurrent bladder infections are very common in women, because of the proximity of the bladder and the urethra to the vagina. Well over 75% of American women have at least one urinary tract infection in a ten year period - almost 30% have one at least once a year. Most also involve infection of the kidneys, making the problem progressively more serious. - with an alarming number of cases resulting in kidney failure. *Note: The active chemical in many spermicidal creams and foams, nonoxynol-9, causes recurring cystitis and yeast infections. Beware.*

FOOD THERAPY

🍃 Avoid acid and sediment-forming foods, such as caffeine, black tea, tomatoes, cooked spinach, etc. Avoid carbonated drinks, concentrated starches, fried, salty and fatty foods, sugars, pasteurized dairy and refined foods.

🍃 Add plenty of celery, watermelon, ume plum balls and green drinks (pg. 54ff) to the diet.
A yeast-free diet is best, with no baked breads.

🍃 During acute stage, take 2 TBS. cider vinegar and honey in water each morning, cottage cheese at noon, and a glass of white wine at night.

🍃 Drink a minimum of 10 glasses of distilled water and/or alkalizing juices daily to keep acid wastes flushed. Acidify the urine with cranberry juice - 2 glasses daily.

🍃 During acute period: take 4 to 6 glasses of cranberry juice daily, and carrot/beet/cucumber juice every other day to neutralize and cleanse infection.

◗ Chlorophyll liquid 3 teasp. daily or Green Foods GREEN MAGMA drink daily during healing.

VITAMINS/MINERALS

◗ Dr. DOPHILUS 2 caps 3 × daily to replace friendly flora, especially if taking anti-biotics.
(May also use 1 TB. acidophilus powder in warm water as a douche.♀)
with
Garlic caps 6 daily and zinc 30mg.

◗ Take Enzymatic Therapy HERBAL K with uva ursi caps for 10 to 14 days to disinfect. On the tenth day begin Solaray CRAN-ACTIN caps, 2 daily as directed.

◗ Ascorbate or Ester C 3-5000mg. with bioflavonoids 2000mg. daily.
with
Beta-carotene 25,000IU 4-6x daily.
or
Take together 6 time daily: Ascorbate or Ester C 1000mg, bromelain 500mg., and Lysine 1000mg.

◗ Nutrition Resource NUTRIBIOTIC GRAPEFRUIT EXTRACT caps as directed to kill infecting bacteria.

◗ Vitamin E 800mg. to help reduce interstitial cystitis scarring

◗ High Omega 3 flax oil with B6 250mg. 2x daily.

HERBAL THERAPY

🌿 Crystal Star BLDR-K™ capsules 6 daily,
or BLDR-K FLUSH™ tea. ♀
or PROSCAPS™. ♂
with
ANTI-BIO™ capsules each time if problem is severe.

🌿 Effective teas, 3 cups daily:
◆ Cornsilk ♀
◆ Plantain/oatstraw
◆ Marshmallow rt.
◆ Uva ursi/nettles/buchu
◆ Watermelon seed
◆ Dandelion/juniper bry.
◆ Horsetail tea from extract
◆ Catnip ☺

🌿 Ginkgo biloba or echinacea extract, 3x daily, with Crystal Star BLDR-K™ extract.

🌿 Bioforce BLADDER IRRITATION tincture.

🌿 Solaray CORNSILK BLEND caps.

🌿 If infections develop regularly after intercourse, rinse the vagina and labia with golden seal/echinacea tea.

🌿 Thuja as a gentle diuretic for incontinence.

BODYWORK

➤ Apply wet heat, or hot comfrey compresses across lower back and kidneys to relieve pain and ease urination.

➤ If there is accompanying hemorrhage, take 1 oz. marshmallow rt., steep in 1 pt. hot milk. Take every $\frac{1}{2}$ hr. to staunch bleeding.

➤ Take a mild catnip or chlorophyll enema to clear acid wastes.

➤ Take hot and cold sitz baths to release fluids and flush out acids.

➤ Reflexology point:

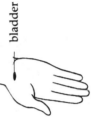

bladder

➤ Biofeedback treatment has been successful for both women and men where there is incontinence.

➤ Urinate as frequently as desired. Do not try to hold it in. Use plain white toilet paper.

Common Symptoms: Frequent, urgent, painful urination; pain in lower back and abdomen; often a fever as the body tries to throw off infection; strong odor urine; cloudy urine.
Common Causes: Overuse of antibiotics; venereal disease; stress; spermicide and contraceptives; kidney malfunction; excess acid-forming foods and food allergens; aluminum cookware, deodorants, etc.; lack of adequate fluids to keep the body flushed; poor elimination. tampons and diaphragms pinching the neck of the bladder, hampering waste elimination.

♀ BLADDER INFECTIONS ▨ INTERSTITIAL CYSTITIS ▨ URETHRITIS ♀

Chronic UTIs are often non-bacterial. Interstitial cystitis has been called "migraine of the bladder". Many of the same things that both trigger and benefit migraine headaches affect interstitial cystitis the same way. It is another of today's immune system breakdown diseases; the body will be at risk until immunity is strengthened. Attend to healing immediately, because of the great pain, and because the virus spreads rapidly in an immune deficient environment. Antibiotics do not help and may aggravate this virus. They can actually attack the bladder lining when there is no bacterial infection to attack.

FOOD THERAPY

❧ Avoid these trigger foods: aged proteins such as yogurt, pickled herring, cheeses, sauerkraut, citrus fruits, citrus juices and red wine until condition normalizes.

❧ Take green drinks (pg. 54ff) and carrot juice during acute stages, and as a preventive.

❧ Increase leafy greens and fiber foods in the diet.

❧ Take 1 TB. each daily as a preventive:
♦ Lecithin
♦ Brewer's yeast

❧ Note: cranberry juice is *not* beneficial for interstitial cystitis.

❧ Cleanse the kidneys with watermelon juice, or watermelon seed tea. Strengthen them with well-cooked beans and sea vegetables.

VITAMINS/MINERALS

▶ Vitamin C therapy: ascorbate or Ester C powder, 1/4 teasp. every hour during acute stages to help restore normal immunity.
and
Lysine 1000mg. with bromelain 500mg. 6x daily.

▶ Enzymatic Therapy ACID-A-CAL capsules 4-6 daily.

▶ Nature's Plus vitamin E 800IU daily.

▶ CoQ 10 10mg. 3x daily.
with
Emulsified A 25,000IU

▶ Sun CHLORELLA 15-20 tabs daily for 1 month.

HERBAL THERAPY

❧ Crystal Star BLDR-K™ extract and/or BLDR-K™ tea; a full course of echinacea extract or Crystal Star PAU DE ARCO/ECHINACEA extract. Take ANTI-FLAM™ caps if needed. and then HERBAL DEFENSE TEAM™ caps to help restore immunity.

❧ Omega 3 flax oil caps 3 x daily.

❧ Effective teas:
♦ Cornsilk
♦ Dandelion
♦ Uva ursi
♦ Astragalus
♦ Chaparral
♦ Watermelon seed

❧ Effective extracts:
♦ Ginkgo Biloba extract
♦ Bilberry extract as an anti-inflammatory.

❧ Solaray ALFAJUICE caps as a potent anti-oxidant and green source.

❧ Nutribiotic GRAPEFRUIT SEED EXTRACT drops in water as directed for 1 month.

BODYWORK

The active chemical in many spermicidal creams and foams, nonoxynol-9, increases the risk of all types of cystitis.

▶ Reflexology point:

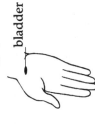

bladder

▶ Do not wear tampons if you have recurring cystitis.

▶ Sitz baths during an infection help bring cleansing circulation to the infected area. Alternate hot and cold for best re-sults. See Appendix instructions (pg. 347).

▶ Position of bladder/urethra:

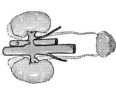

Common Symptoms: Scarred, tough, atrophied bladder, so that normal urination is impossible; pain goes away during urination, then immediately returns; breakdown of bladder tissue, even when infection is not present; cloudy urine with foul odor; systemic fever and aching.
Common Causes: Viral infection; environmental and food allergies; lowered immunity; dietary "triggers" causing acidity in the system; pelvic congestion from chronic constipation, lowered libido, or heavy, painful menstrual periods; dehydration.

BONE HEALTH & GROWTH

Breaks ◇ Brittle Bones ◇ Cartilage Regrowth

Continuing research is showing that several common medications put bone health at risk. L-thyroxine - a thyroid stimulant; cortico-steroid drugs such as hydrocortisone, cortisone and prednisone - prescribed for rheumatic conditions and respiratory diseases; phenytoin and phenobarbital - anti-seizure drugs; heparin - a blood thinner, and furosemide - a diuretic.

FOOD THERAPY

Vegetarians have denser, better formed bones, and stronger immune systems.

☙ Maintain a mineral-rich vegetable protein diet with whole grain complex carbohydrates.

☙ The liver is vital to bone marrow formation. Keep it healthy.

☙ Avoid red meats, refined foods, caffeine, and acid-forming foods.

☙ Good foods for bones:
- for calcium and silicon -
  ◆ green vegetables
  ◆ fish and seafood
  ◆ sea vegetables
  ◆ whole grains
- for boron -
  ◆ dried fruits
  ◆ nuts and seeds
  ◆ honey,
  ◆ a little wine
- for vitamin C -
  ◆ papayas
  ◆ bell peppers
  ◆ broccoli
  ◆ cantaloupe

Note: Sugar and citrus inhibit calcium absorption.

☙ Take high potency digestive enzymes or betaine HCl for mineral absorption.

VITAMINS/MINERALS

There is much more to strong bones than just getting plenty of calcium. Without the proper amounts of other minerals as well as vitamin D - you won't absorb the calcium.

▶ Alta Health SILICA/MANGANESE AM/PM complex or Body Essentials SILICA GEL internally 2x daily.
  with
  Calcium ascorbate C 3000mg. and Vit. B6 250mg. daily.

▶ A & D 25, 000IU/1,000IU daily
  with
  Mezotrace SEA MINERAL COMPLEX 2 daily, and vit. E 400IU ♂

▶ Solaray CAL/MAG CITRATE or Enzymatic Therapy OSTEO PRIME caps.

▶ ENER B vit. B12 every 3 days.

▶ Body Essentials SILICA GEL 1 TB. 3x daily for 1 month in 3oz. liquid.

▶ Effective bone knitters/healers:
  ◆ PSI PROGEST CREAM
  ◆ Twin Lab CSA capsules

▶ Collagen tablets 6 daily, or Nutrapathic CALCIUM COLLAGEN COMPLEX tablets.

HERBAL THERAPY

Absorbable minerals are key factors in bone building. Herbs are one of the best ways to get them.

Phyto-hormone herbs can be an important part of continuing bone health and formation.

❧ Effective estrogen/progesterone stimulating and balancing herbs for marrow formation:
  ◆ Dong quai/Licorice rt. ♀
  ◆ Black cohosh/sarsaparilla ♂

❧ Twin Lab propolis extract. ♂

❧ Crystal Star BONZ™ capsules or tea daily.
  and/or
  ENERGY GREEN™ or SYSTEM STRENGTH™ drink mix, and CALCIUM SOURCE™ caps or extract for balanced calcium.s. ♀

❧ Crystal Star SILICA SOURCE™ extract for collagen formation; SUPER SARSAPARILLA EXTRACT for phyto-progesterone to help lay down bone material.

❧ Solaray ALFAJUICE for active Vit. K and chlorophyll.

❧ Effective herbal bone healers:
  ◆ Nettles
  ◆ Horsetail extract

BODYWORK

▶ Aerobic exercise and light weight training are some of the best ways to build and elasticize bones, and prevent bone loss.

▶ Get some sunlight on the body every day possible for natural vitamin D.

▶ NO SMOKING. It increases bone brittleness and inhibits bone growth.

▶ Swim or walk in the ocean when possible;
  or
  take daily kelp or dulse tablets.

▶ Avoid aluminum pots and pans, deodorants and fluorescent lighting. Both leach calcium from the body.

▶ For bone breaks:
  → take homeopathic *Arnica Montana.*
  → apply *Arnica Gel* to reduce swelling.
  → apply a clay or turmeric paste poultice and cover with gauze.

Common Symptoms: Easy bone breaks; poor bone healing.
Common Causes: Mineral deficiency or poor assimilation; poor diet with too many refined foods, and too much meat protein, causing phosphorus imbalance; enzyme deficiency; heavy metal or drug toxicity; steroids or too many cortico-steroid drugs; stress; too much alcohol and/or tobacco.

BONE SPURS ◼ PLANTAR WARTS

Contrary to popular belief, bone spurs are the result of acid/alkaline imbalance in the body which favors an overly acid condition. They often accompany rheumatoid arthritis, because individuals with this disease are deficient in stomach acid and normal enzyme production.

FOOD THERAPY

❧ Make sure your diet is rich in whole foods, vegetables and fiber - low in sugars, meat, refined carbohydrates and saturated fats. Eliminate hard liquor and fried food.

❧ Drink black cherry juice daily. Take a potassium drink or green drink often to keep acid/alkaline and kidney balance good.

❧ Rub cut papaya skins on affected areas.

❧ See other diet suggestions on ARTHRITIS and GOUT pages in this book.

❧ Effective enzyme balancing foods:
♣ Miso soup
♣ Fresh vegetables
♣ Brewer's yeast
♣ Cranberry juice

VITAMINS/MINERALS

▶ Enzymatic Therapy ACID-A-CAL and/or CHERRY FRUIT capsules. ♀

▶ Vitamin C up to 5000mg. daily with extra bioflavonoids 500mg. daily, for collagen and interstitial tissue formation.

or

▶ Mix Vitamin C crystals with water to a paste. Apply to spur, and secure with tape. Leave on all day for several weeks to see improvement.

or

Apply Crystal Star VITAMIN C GEL.

▶ Cal/Mag/Zinc 4 daily. ♀

▶ Country Life LIGA-TEND for at least 1 month.

▶ Magnesium/Potassium/Bromelain capsules for enzymes. ♂

or

Quercetin Plus w/ Bromelain. ♀

▶ Take Betaine HCl to increase stomach acid for better assimilation.

HERBAL THERAPY

❦ Crystal Star AR-EASE™ capsules to dissolve crystalline deposits, *with* BITTERS & LEMON CLEANSE™ extract each morning.   and/or

ANTI-FLAM™ caps to take down inflammation.

❦ Body Essentials SILICA GEL 1 TB. 3x daily for 1 month in 3oz. liquid. Also apply topically.

❦ Effective topical applications:
◆ Propolis tincture.
◆ A mixture of wintergreen oil, witch hazel, and black walnut tincture.
◆ Tea tree oil.
◆ A paste mixture of green clay and liquid chlorophyll.

❦ Apply NatureWorks SWEDISH BITTERS extract.

❦ Take echinacea extract internally 2x daily, and apply several times daily.

or

Apply BioForce echinacea cream.

BODYWORK

➤ Apply epsom salts compresses.

➤ For plantar warts:
➤ Soak feet in the hottest water you can stand for as long as you can.
➤ Apply dandelion stem juice 3x daily. Let dry each time.

➤ Rub H₂O₂ OXYGEL directly on the wart or spur twice daily. Removal takes about 2 months.

➤ Apply DMSO for pain and to help dissolve crystalline deposits.

➤ Crystal Star ALKALIZING ENZYME BODY WRAP™ to rebalance body chemistry.

Common Symptoms: Inflammation and infection; painful spurs on heels and joints; great pain from ingrown nodules on the feet.
Common Causes: Low acid diet aggravating liver congestion and poor or irregular kidney function; insufficient stomach acid; constipation and toxemia from excess fats and refined carbohydrates; too little vegetable protein.

BRAIN HEALTH & ENERGY
More Mental Activity ✧ Less Mental Exhaustion & Burn-Out

The brain controls the entire body. It takes 50% of our blood sugar and 20% of our inhaled oxygen, yet is only 2% of our body weight. It is also our primary health maintenance organ and the seat of energy production. When it is functioning well, total body health is improved. The brain is an incredibly sensitive organ, responding quickly but only temporarily to drugs and short term stimulants. The best way to get good long term brain enhancement is to feed it and use it. Brain nutrients have a rapidly noticeable effect on increased brain performance. Good, consistent brain nourishment can straighten out even grave mental, emotional and coordination problems.

FOOD THERAPY

Brain foods are especially rich in potassium, zinc, magnesium, iron, sodium and iodine. Neurotransmitter levels can be significantly increased by a single nutritious meal.

🍃 Alcohol, tobacco and drugs depress brain function - increasing the need for neurotransmitter replenishment through brain foods.

🍃 Include frequently in the diet: Sea vegetables, fish and sea foods, sprouts, fertile eggs, wheat germ, unsaturated oils, brown rice, tofu, apples, oranges, grapefruit, wheat germ and beans.
Cold water fish are excellent as brain food because they are primarily fat and water

🍃 Drink plenty of pure water every day for brain health.

🍃 Take a protein/mineral/energy drink every morning, such as one from pg. 63, or Nature's Plus SPIRU-TEIN, or Crystal Star SYSTEM STRENGTH™ drink.

🍃 Make a mix of 2TBS. each and take 1 to 2 teasp. daily: lecithin for phospho-tides, brewer's yeast for myelin for-mation.

VITAMINS/MINERALS

Good brain work requires over 20% of the body's total energy supply. It has a large appetite for blood sugars, oxygen, vitamins, minerals, amino acids and fatty acids.

▶ Anti-oxidants are the brain key:
❖ Pycnogenol 50mg. 3x daily
❖ CoQ 10 30mg. daily
❖ Ener B vit. B12 internasal gel
❖ DMG sublingual
❖ Carnitine 500mg. daily.
❖ Germanium 150 SL 200mg. daily - esp. if there is brain cancer.

▶ Glutamine pwdr. 1/4 teasp. with Glycine pwdr. 1/4 teasp.

▶ Germanium 50-100mg. w/ Suma or Rainbow Light MIND SYSTEM caps
and
Choline 600mg. daily.

▶ B Complex 150mg. w/ extra niacin 500mg.

▶ Other good brain nutrients: ♂
❖ Vit. E with selenium. ♂
❖ Phosphatidyl choline.
❖ Future Biotics VITAL K drink.
❖ Omega 3 fish/flax oils.
❖ Magnesium 800mg.
❖ Tyrosine 500mg.
❖ Zinc Picolinate 30mg. daily.
❖ Taurine
❖ Nutrapathic BRAIN ALERT tabs.

HERBAL THERAPY

Many mineral-rich herbs provide key biochemical ingredients for effective neuro-transmission.

🌿 Crystal Star MENTAL CLARITY™ capsules, CREATIVI-TEA™, and MEDITATION™ tea.

🌿 Crystal Star RAINFOREST ENER-GY™ tea and capsules.

🌿 Ginkgo Biloba extract 3 x daily.

🌿 Effective herbal neurotransmitter stimulants:
◆ Alfalfa
◆ Cayenne
◆ Dandelion

🌿 Ginsengs are key brain nutrients:
◆ Crystal Star SUPER GINSENG 6™ tea and capsules.
◆ Crystal Star ROYAL MU tea. ♂
◆ Ginseng/Gotu Kola capsules.
◆ Ginseng/Damiana capsules. ♂

🌿 Effective herbal brain foods:
◆ Rosemary
◆ Royal jelly
◆ Kelp tabs 6 daily.
◆ Parsley/sage tea
◆ Gotu kola

🌿 Evening primrose oil 2-4 daily for good brain electrical connections. ♀

BODYWORK

▶ Get some mild aerobic exercise, such as a daily 20 minute walk for brain oxygen. Practice deep brain breathing for increased oxygen nutrient levels. (See Bragg's booklet on this subject.)

▶ Cheerfulness, optimism and relaxation assure better brain function.

▶ Tobacco, alcohol, marijuana all inhibit brain release of vasopressin, impairing memory, attention and concentration.

▶ Reflexology point: Squeeze all around hand for brain stimulation.

▶ Brain views: External and Internal:

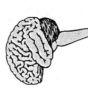

Common Symptoms: Spaciness and lack of concentration; inability to remember well or for a reasonable length of time.
Common Causes: Lack of protein, potassium or other minerals; mental burnout; overwork with no rejuvenating "down time"; stress; poor diet.

BRONCHITIS

Chronic bronchitis is a condition in which excessive mucous is secreted in the bronchi. The typical victim is forty or older, with lowered immunity from prolonged stress, fatigue or smoking. The disease usually develops slowly over a course of years, but will not go away on its own. The bronchial walls thicken and the number of mucous glands increases. The person becomes increasingly susceptible to respiratory infections, during which bronchial tissue becomes inflamed, and mucous becomes thicker and more profuse. The recent type of viral bronchitis which affects women, is very hard to treat, and lasts from three weeks to five months. Bronchitis can be incapacitating, and lead to serious, even potentially fatal lung disease.

FOOD THERAPY

Avoid cough suppressants. Coughing helps get rid of mucous.

🌿 Go on a short mucous cleansing liquid diet (pg. 42) to clear the body of mucous. Then follow a basically vegetarian, cleansing diet for several weeks. Reduce fats, dairy, salts and clogging heavy foods. See "COOKING FOR HEALTHY HEALING" by Linda Rector-Page for a complete non-mucous forming diet.

🌿 Avoid sugars, dairy foods, heavy starches and fatty foods during healing to reduce congestion. Keep the bowels clean so that the system can eliminate mucous well.

🌿 **Take plenty of cleansing soups broths, hot tonics, high vitamin C juices, vegetable juices and green drinks. (pg. 53ff.)**

🌿 Make an onion/honey syrup - *(Put 5 to 6 chopped onions and 1/2 cup honey in a pot and cook over very low heat for two hours. Strain and take 1 TB. every two hours.),* or use the onion garlic broth on page 57.

🌿 Take lemon juice in water each morning and flax seed tea each night during acute stages to alkalize the blood and cleanse the colon.

🌿 Crystal Star SYSTEM STRENGTH™ drink mix daily for 1 month.

VITAMINS/MINERALS

▶ Ester C or ascorbate vitamin C crystals with bioflavanoids 1000mg. in water, 5-10,000mg. or to bowel tolerance at first, then reducing to 3-5000mg. daily.

▶ Zinc lozenges as needed every two hours with Cysteine 500mg. for chest congestion and Alta Health SIL-X silica to relieve inflammation.

▶ Beta carotene 100,000IU with garlic caps 6 daily and bee pollen 1000mg.

▶ Effective anti-oxidants:
   ✦ Pycnogenol 50mg. 2-4x daily.
   ✦ Biogenetics BIOGUARD PLUS
   ✦ CoQ 10, 30mg. 2x daily.
   ✦ Country Life DMG SL tabs.

▶ Enzymatic Therapy ADRENAL and/or THYMUS COMPLEX. ♀

▶ **Rub food grade H2O2 Care Plus OXYGEL on chest and lung area and overcome infection. ♂** Use eucalyptus, wintergreen, mullein oils, or H2O2 in an inhaler.

▶ Standard Homeopathics HYLAVIR tabs. Rub tea tree oil on the chest. ☺

HERBAL THERAPY

🌿 Crystal Star ANTI-BIO™ capsules or extract 6x daily *with* RESISTANCE SUPPORT™ caps, 2 daily as an anti-oxidant, and X-PECT™ tea or SUPER LICORICE™ extract as expectorants.

🌿 Crystal Star FIRST AID™ CAPS, 4 at a time to relieve acute conditions.
   and
Crystal Star BRNX™ EXTRACT as needed daily.

🌿 Effective extracts, 3 to 4 x daily:
   ◆ Lobelia as an expectorant.
   ◆ Echinacea rt. extract daily.
   ◆ Licorice rt. as an expectorant.
   ◆ Reishi mushroom extract caps.

🌿 Effective teas:
   ◆ Ephedra as a bronchodilator
   ◆ Licorice rt.
   ◆ Coltsfoot
   ◆ Wild cherry
   ◆ Hyssop/horehound

🌿 Herbal expectorant tea formula: Steep in a pot with 4 cups water for 25 minutes - licorice rt., horehound, roseships, coltsfoot, lobelia, pleurisy rt., wild cherry bk. ☺

🌿 Cayenne/ginger capsules 4-6 daily. Apply cayenne/ginger compresses to the chest. (See page 49ff.)

BODYWORK

▶ Avoid smoking, secondary smoke and smog-plagued areas. Get fresh air and sunshine every day. Air pollutants help cause bronchitis.

▶ Take a hot sauna or steam bath and follow with a brisk rubdown, and chest/back percussion with a cupped hand to loosen mucous.

▶ Apply alternating hot and cold witch hazel compresses to the chest to stimulate circulation.

▶ Deep breathing exercises daily, morning & before bed to clear lungs.

▶ Avoid inhaling cold air. Cover mouth and nose with a scarf or mask so that infectious microorganisms are not sucked into the lungs, causing pneumonia.

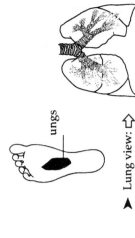

▶ Reflexology point:

lungs

▶ Lung view: ⇧

Common Symptoms: ● Acute Bronchitis: Slight fever; inflammation; headache, nausea, lung and body aches; hacking, mucous-producing cough.
● Chronic Bronchitis: Difficult breathing and shortness of breath; repeated attacks of acute bronchitis; chest congestion; mucous-producing cough and wheezing that lasts for 3 months or more; fatigue, weakness and weight loss; low grade lung infection.
Common Causes: High mucous and acid-forming diet; suppressive "cold preparations"; lack of exercise and poor circulation; smoking and smog; low immunity, stress and fatigue.

BRUISES ■ EASY BRUISING

If there is continued, excessive and frequent bruising see a physician for a clotting time blood test.

FOOD THERAPY

❧ The diet should be light, low fat, and high in minerals and trace minerals to lay a solid foundation for strong capillaries and skin.

❧ Eat vitamin K rich foods, such as alfalfa sprouts, sea vegetables, green peppers, citrus fruits and green vegetables.

❧ Avoid pasteurized dairy foods during healing.

❧ Take a green drink once a week for prevention (pg. 54ff). or Crystal Star ENERGY GREEN DRINK™ mix.

❧ Crystal Star BIOFLAVONOID, FIBER & C SUPPORT™ drink or wafers.

VITAMINS/MINERALS

▶ Apply DMSO 2 x daily for a week.

▶ Apply Enzymatic Therapy CELL-U-VAR cream daily.

▶ Ascorbate vitamin C with bioflavonoids and rutin 1000mg. every 2 hours during healing. with Emulsified vitamin A & E.

▶ Omega 3 flax oil 3 daily for 1-3 months.

▶ Take for 36-48 hours until discolortion subsides.
Bromelain 500mg. 2 x daily. ♂
or
Quercetin Plus with bromelain 4-6 daily.

▶ Homeopathic *Arnica Montana* to reduce swelling and repair blood vessels.

▶ Vitamin K, 4 daily.

▶ Apply Twin Lab POTASSIUM CHLORIDE LIQUID directly.

▶ Collagen tabs or powder daily.

HERBAL THERAPY

❦ Crystal Star SILICA SOURCE™ or bilberry extract for capillary strength and collagen formation. and/or GINSENG SKIN REPAIR™ GEL

❦ Apply Body Essentials SILICA GEL several times daily.

❦ Effective applications:
◆ **Arnica extract**
◆ Aloe vera gel
◆ **Chinese WHITE FLOWER oil**
◆ Wheat germ oil
◆ Witch hazel
◆ Tea tree oil ☺

❦ Apply PAU DE ARCO GEL frequently as needed.

❦ Solaray **TURMERIC** capsules and **ALFAJUICE** capsules 4 daily, *each.*

❦ Make strong rosemary/thyme tea. Strain and add to a hot bath. Soak 25 min. ♀

❦ Crystal Star SYSTEM STRENGTH™ drink for food source minerals and potassium.

❦ Alfalfa or kelp tabs 6-8 daily, as vitamin K sources.

BODYWORK

▶ Apply ice frequently and squeeze bruise to release blood congestion. Rub vigorously.

▶ Apply Care Plus H₂O₂ OXYGEL to bruise 3-4x daily.

▶ Apply B & T ARNIFLORA gel 3-4 x daily. ☺

▶ Effective compresses:
→ Comfrey rt. and comfrey cream
→ Onion
→ Aloe vera
→ Golden seal

▶ Do not take aspirin if bruising is frequent.

Common Symptoms: Black and blue skin discolorations.

Common Causes: Vit. K deficiency; thin capillary and vein walls; poor collagen formation; mineral-poor diet. Easy bruising is usually found in people who are overweight, or who take anti-clotting drugs. Unusual easy bruising is also an early warning sign of cancer.

BURNS
1st Degree, 2nd Degree & 3rd Degree

FOOD THERAPY

☙ Apply ice water immediately, then vinegar soaked compresses.

☙ Drink plenty of fluids, especially potassium broth (pg. 53) and green drinks (pg. 54ff). Get plenty of proteins and mineral-rich foods for fast tissue repair.

☙ For immediate relief with no blistering or irritation, dip cotton balls in strong fresh ginger juice or strong black tea and apply.

☙ Effective compresses:
   ♦ Honey
   ♦ Cold black tea
   ♦ Egg whites or raw potato for scalds.

☙ Use baking soda or cider vinegar in warm water for acid/chemical burns.

VITAMINS/MINERALS

▶ Germanium SL 150mg. 3 x daily.

▶ Apply pure vitamin E oil every 3-4 hours. Take vitamin E w. selenium 2-3x daily for a week.

▶ Take ascorbate vit. C 3-5000mg. daily. Make a solution of ascorbate crystals in water and apply.

▶ American Biologics SUB-ADRENE for cortex formation.

▶ Nutribiotic spray as needed to counteract bacterial infection.

▶ Future Biotics HERBAL K , several doses daily.

▶ Homeopathic Arnica Montana followed by Hypericum tincture.

▶ NutraPathic CALCIUM COLLAGEN tabs.

▶ B Complex 100mg. with extra niacin 250mg. for fluid loss.

▶ Beta carotene 25,000IU 4x daily, with zinc 30mg. 3 x daily.

▶ Solaray CAL/MAG w. D and potassium for fluid/potassium loss.

HERBAL THERAPY

❧ Apply Crystal Star or Califlora CALENDULA GEL.
   or
   Crystal Star RAINFOREST ENERGY™ GEL.
   with
   Crystal Star POTASSIUM SOURCE™ capsules.

❧ Apply Pau de Arco Gel frequently as needed.

❧ Effective herbal compresses:
   ♦ Comfrey leaf/wheat germ oil
   ♦ Tea tree oil.☺

❧ Make a strong anti-infection healing tea of elder blossoms, red clover, yarrow and golden seal. Strain and apply.
   or
   Comfrey, nettles, marshmallow, scullcap, red clover and apply.

❧ Alta Health SIL-X silica, Crystal Star SILICA SOURCE™ extract or horsetail tea for healing and new collagen formation.

❧ Green tea or gotu kola tea, 2 cups daily for nerve and tissue healing.

BODYWORK

Get medical help fast for anything other than a first degree or small second degree burn.

▶ Flush with cold water; then apply ice packs until pain is relieved.

▶ Apply Care Plus OXY GEL.

▶ Apply aloe vera gel and/or "aloe ice" gel frequently.

▶ Apply Body Essentials SILICA GEL frequently.

▶ If the burn is 3rd degree, treat for shock until help arrives.
   → Cayenne: 1/4 teasp. tincture, or 2 opened capsules in 1 tsp. warm water.
   → Cut away loose clothing that has not adhered to the skin.
   → Apply ice water if skin is not charred. If charred, apply cloths dipped in aloe vera gel or juice, or a fresh comfrey leaf poultice.

Common Symptoms: 1st degree - sunburn, minor blistering and pain.
2nd degree - blistering, scarring gland structure damage; hair follicles burned off.
3rd degree - extensive tissue damage; oozing, charring, severe loss of body fluids; electrolyte loss and shock.

BURSITIS
Acute & Chronic Tendonitis ✧ Tennis Elbow

Inflammatory conditions in the tendons or bursa, the sac-like membrane that contains joint protecting fluids. Both conditions can develop calcified deposits in the shoulder, elbow, hip or knee. Both can result from strain, a blow to the affected body part, or in the case of bursitis, as a secondary symptom of arthritis or rheumatism.

FOOD THERAPY	VITAMINS/MINERALS	HERBAL THERAPY	BODYWORK
✷ Avoid acid-forming foods, such as caffeine, salts, refined foods, red meats, etc.	▶ Quercetin Plus 3 daily with extra bromelain 500mg. **and** Am. Biologics INFLAZYME FORTE to reduce inflammation.	❦ Alta Health SIL-X silica for connective tissue growth, and CANGEST caps for acid/alkaline balance. **with** Source Naturals organic GERMANIUM 100mg. daily.	▶ Take a mineral or epsom salts bath once a week. Apply hot castor oil packs to affected areas.
✷ Keep the body alkaline with foods like celery, avocados, potatoes, wheat germ, sweet fruits, sprouts, greens, brewer's yeast, oats and sea vegetables.	▶ Country Life LIGA-TEND as needed, or 4 daily.	❦ Apply B&T TRI-FLORA analgesic gel, or hot comfrey/olive oil compresses. **with** Solaray TURMERIC capsules.	▶ Apply Care Plus OXY GEL to affected areas every 24 hours. ▶ Apply ice packs to inflamed area during acute stages. Apply wet warm compresses during later stages for faster healing.
✷ Keep the kidneys flushed and healthy with a green drink or carrot/beet/cucumber juice.	▶ Take DLPA 500-750mg. as needed Apply DMSO roll-on with aloe vera gel as needed for pain.		▶ Use affected area gently. Intense athletic activity is inadvisable until trauma is relieved. Regular mild aerobic and stretching exercises are recommended to keep joint system free.
✷ Add to the diet for *organic* calcium uptake: ✦ Salmon and sea foods ✦ Dark green leafies ✦ Cultured foods ✦ Broccoli and potatoes	▶ Biotec EXTRA ENERGY ENZYMES with SOD 6-10 daily, or ENER-B vit. B12 nasal gel. ▶ Enzymatic Therapy ACID-A-CAL capsules to dissolve sediment. **with** Ascorbate vit. C or Ester C with bioflavonoids and rutin 3000mg. daily for collagen formation.	❦ Crystal Star AR EASE™ caps or tea, with ANTI-FLAM™ caps or extract as needed to reduce swelling and inflammation, **with** ADR-ACTIVE™ capsules for essential cortex formation, and RELAX™ capsules for stress relief.	▶ Avoid smoking and tobacco as acid-producing habits. ▶ Reflexology point: 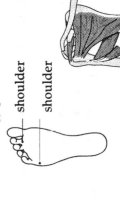 — shoulder — shoulder
✷ Crystal Star BIOFLAVONOID, FIBER & C SUPPORT™ drink as needed.	▶ Solaray BIO-ZINC or zinc picolinate daily.	❦ Apply Body Essentials SILICA GEL to joints. Take internally as directed.	
✷ Take high omega 3 flax oil 1 teasp 3 x daily. Improvement usually in 2 - 6 weeks.	▶ American Biologic A & E EMULSION w. SUB-ADREN extract. **and** Niacinamide 500mg. 2x daily for 1 week, then daily *with* DMG 125mg. daily.	❦ Use Crystal Star ALKALIZING/ ENZYME BODY WRAP™ to change body pH almost immediately.	▶ Bursa area view:
✷ See the ARTHRITIS DIET in this book for more information.			

Common Symptoms: Both tendonitis and bursitis involve inflammation and tenderness where tendons affix to bones, causing limited motion in the affected body part. The pains are usually severe and shooting with swelling and redness, especially in damp weather.
Common Causes: Poor diet causing metabolic imbalance; stress; toxemia; a direct blow to the affected area.

CALLOUSES ■ CORNS ■ BUNIONS

Bunions - thickened layers of skin on the sides of the big toe. Callouses - thickening of the skin formed on the site of continual pressure - usually on the hands or feet. Corns - thickening of the skin, hard or soft, on the feet. See also PLANTAR WARTS in this book.

FOOD THERAPY

🍃 Go on a 24 hour (pg. 44) vegetable juice liquid diet to clear out acid wastes. Then eat lots of fresh raw foods for a month. Have a green salad every day. Take a green drink or carrot/beet/cucumber juice every 3 days to flush the kidneys and rebalance the acid/alkalinity.

🍃 Avoid fats, fried foods, sugars and alcohol.
Avoid red meats, caffeine, chocolate, sodas, and other oxalic acid-forming foods.
♣ Eat a low salt diet.
♣ Eat 2-3 apples a day.

🍃 Avoid antacids. They aggravate and upset acid/alkaline imbalance. The body needs adequate HCL for proper mineral assimilation.

VITAMINS/MINERALS

▶ Enzymatic Therapy ACID-A-CAL 3x daily. ♀

▶ Betaine HCl, or Alta Health CANGEST with meals for better mineral assimilation.

▶ Apply Nutrition Resource NU-TRIBIOIC GRAPEFRUIT SEED extract spray or ointment full strength, *and* take the capsules 2x daily.

▶ Cal/mag/zinc 4 daily with B Complex 100mg. 4 daily.
and with
Ascorbate vitamin C w/ bioflavonoids 1000mg.
Also make a solution of vitamin C crystals and water and apply directly.

▶ Vitamin E 400IU daily. Apply E oil daily.

▶ Beta-carotene 50,000IU 2 x daily.

▶ Lecithin 1900mg. 3 daily for smooth skin and improved body flow.

HERBAL THERAPY

🌿 Apply tea tree oil 2-3x daily.

🌿 Apply a weak golden seal root solution.

🌿 Effective poultices:
◆ Green clay mixed w/ liquid chlorophyll. ♂
◆ Flaxseed/garlic

🌿 Mix and apply: witch hazel, wintergreen oil, and black walnut tincture.

🌿 Take 1 teasp. liquid chlorophyll in water 3 x daily with Crystal Star ECHINACEA extract.

🌿 Apply Care Plus H₂O₂ OXY-GEL or 3% solution several times daily for a month.

▶ Apply NatureWorks SWEDISH BITTERS and take 1 teasp. daily.

BODYWORK

➤ Make a footbath with 2 handfuls of comfrey root to 1 gallon warm water. Soak feet 15 minutes daily.

➤ Massage affected area with castor oil.

➤ Apply hot epsom salts compresses.

➤ Apply Body Essentials SILICA GEL directly or as a compress.

➤ Rub green papaya skins on callouses daily. ♀

➤ Apply olive oil compresses to corns.

➤ Apply raw garlic poultices to bunions.

➤ Apply DMSO for pain. ♂

Common Symptoms: Staph or strep type infection; pain and inflammation of nodules and growths on the feet.
Common Causes: Toxemia; sometimes alkalosis; kidney malfunction causing acid/alkaline imbalance; too many sweets, caffeine and saturated fats; excess sebaceous gland output causing poor skin elimination of wastes; poor calcium elimination.

CANCER

See immediately following pages for suggestions for specific cancer sites: Organ Cancer, Lung & Stomach Cancer, Prostate Cancer, Breast, Ovarian, Cervical & Uterine Cancer.
Today's statistics show that 30% of all Americans will contract some kind of cancer in their lives. New evidence indicates that 90% of all cancer is environmentally caused and therefore preventable. Diet and nutrition are by far the most important of the environmental factors. It is felt that America's enormous incidence of breast and colon cancer, (500% compared to the rest of the world), is due to poor nutrition. It is vitally important to follow a very concentrated program incorporating several aspects of natural healing. Diet, exercise, enemas, vitamin therapy and herbs all need to be coordinated for there to be remission. A concerted effort is needed for at least 6 months to a year.

FOOD THERAPY

🍃 Follow a *strict, intensive* macrobiotic diet (following page) during healing. Pay particular attention to vegetable protein and soluble fiber foods, such as brown rice, whole grains, soy foods, nuts, seeds, and sprouts. Have some miso soup, sea vegetables and 2 TBS. brewer's yeast every day.
♦ The recommended continuing diet should be high in fresh fruits, vegetables and fiber, low in meats and fat.

🍃 Fast with only fresh juices for 2 days each week.
♦ Fruit juices such as cranberry or grape the first day.
♦ Vegetable juices such as potassium broth, a green drink, or carrot juice the second.

🍃 Take a carrot/beet/cucumber juice once a week to clean the liver and kidneys.

🍃 Specific anti-cancer foods: onions, garlic, yams, cruciferous vegetables, shiitake mushrooms, green and orange vegetables, legumes, rice and potatoes, yogurt, fish, sea vegetables and seafood, apples, carrots and tomatoes.

VITAMINS/MINERALS

Recent mainstream research shows that supplements are effective in combatting the effects of chemotherapy and radiation, healing from surgery, oxygenating the tissues and detering cancerous growth:

▶ Green superfoods are a key:
✚ Biotec CELL GUARD w. SOD.
✚ Green Foods GREEN MAGMA.
✚ Sun CHLORELLA.
✚ Crystal Star ENERGY GREEN™.

▶ Anti-oxidants are anti-carcinogenic:
✚ Germanium 100mg. 2x daily.
✚ CoQ 10 30 mg. 3x daily.
✚ Beta carotene 100,000IU daily.
✚ Pycnogenol 50mg. 2x daily.
✚ Ester C w/ bioflavonoids.
✚ Vit. E w/ selenium.
✚ Biogenetics BIOGUARD PLUS.

▶ Rainbow Light DETOX-ZYME, or Alta Health CANGEST with meals.

▶ High Omega 3 flax okil - 3x daily.
with
Solaray CHROMIACIN caps daily.

▶ Future Biotics VITAL K liquid.

▶ Natren LIFE START II, $1/2$ teasp. 3 x daily for liver health.

▶ Am. Biologics CARTILADE caps.

HERBAL THERAPY

🌿 Ginseng therapy is showing outstanding results.
♦ Crystal Star GINSENG 6 DEFENSE RESTORATIVE™ TEA and SUPER GINSENG 6™ capsules.
♦ Siberian ginseng *extract* capsules or liquid daily.

🌿 Pau de arco or calendula tea 4 cups daily.

🌿 Iodine therapy w. sea vegetables:
♦ Atomodine extract
♦ Crystal Star SYSTEM STRENGTH™ drink.
♦ Kelp tabs 8-10 daily.

🌿 Crystal Star DETOX™ capsules *and* PAU DE ARCO/ ECHINACEA EXTRACT as directed. with
GREEN TEA CLEANSER™ every morning to reduce carcinogens.

🌿 Highest potency royal jelly, 2 teasp. daily.

🌿 Herbs to reduce the effects of chemotherapy and radiation:
♦ Licorice Rt.
♦ Reishi mushroom.
♦ Astragalus.
♦ Garlic 6-10 caps daily.

BODYWORK

Get aerobic exercise regularly. It is a nutrient in itself. No healing program will make it without some exercise.

▶ Avoid tobacco in all forms, synthetic hormones, particularly estrogen, X-Rays, excessive alcohol and caffeine.

▶ Take a coffee enema once a week for a month (1 cup strong brewed in a qt. of water) or chlorella implants.

▶ Get some sunlight on the body every day possible (esp. for organ cancers).

▶ Effective poultices for external growths:
→ Garlic/onion
→ Comfrey Lf.
→ Green clay
→ Crystal Star GINSENG SKIN REPAIR™ GEL.

▶ Care Plus OXYGEL rubbed on the feet daily, or on affected area, or taken at 3% dilution 1 teasp. in 8oz. water daily to increase body oxygen uptake.

Common Symptoms: Chronic constipation or diarrhea; sudden appearance or enlargement of growths; enlarged or swollen organs; internal bleeding and non-healing wounds; blood passing in the stool; unexplained chronic pain in a specific area.
Common Causes: Poor diet with too many food additives, refined and junk foods, alcohol, tobacco, etc., all of which deprive the body of oxygen use; too much fat and animal protein; lack of dietary fiber; low minerals and protein, preventing continued healthy cell and tissue formation; over-use of drugs; stress; an over-acid, mucous-filled system where vital organs cannot cleanse enough waste to maintain health.

DIET DEFENSE AGAINST CANCER

The natural healing world has concentrated on cancer problems intensely in the past few years, and has learned and realized much about how to deal with this often unnecessary killer.

❖ Cancers are opportunistic, attacking when immune defenses and bloodstream health are low.

❖ Cancerous cells seem to crave dead de-mineralized foods, and starving them out feels like any drug withdrawal. The fight against this isn't easy, but as healthy cells rebuild, the craving subsides.

❖ Cancers also seem to live and grow in the unreleased waste and mucous deposits in the body. Avoid red meats, pork, fried foods, refined carbohydrates, sugars, caffeine, preserved or artificially colored foods, heavy pesticides and spraed foods. All of these clog the system so that the vital organs cannot clean out enough of the waste to maintain health. They deprive the body of oxygen use, and provide little or no usable nutrition for building healthy cells and tissue. Avoid antacids. They interfere with enzyme production, and the body's ability to carry off heavy metal toxins.

❖ Most cancers are caused or aggravated by poor diet and nutrition. Many cancers respond well to diet improvement. Nutritional deficiencies accumulate over a long period of time - too much refined food, fats and red meats; too little fiber and fresh foods; natural vitamin and mineral imbalances. These deficiencies eventually change body chemistry. The immune system cannot defend properly when biochemistry is altered. It can't tell its own cells from invading toxic cells, and sometimes attacks everything or nothing in confusion.

❖ Love your liver! It is the main organ to keep clean and working well. It is a powerful chemical plant in the body that can keep the immune system going, healthy red blood cells forming, and oxygen in the bloodstream and tissues.

❖ Overheating therapy has been effective against cancer. See Paavo Airola's book HOW TO GET WELL.

❖ New, viable research on colon cancer is showing that plain aspirin *beneficially inhibits* substances that are involved in pathogenic cell proliferation. Other cancers are also expected to respond favorably.

❖ Regular exercise is almost a "cancer defense" in itself. It enhances oxygen use and accelerates passage of material in the colon.

❖ The primary answer to cancer seems to lie in promoting an environment where cancer and degenerative disease can't live - where inherent immunity can remain effective. These diseases do not seem to grow or take hold where oxygen and minerals (particularly potassium) are high in the vital fluids. Vegetable proteins and amino acids in the body allow the maximum use and assimilation of these two elements.

❖ Don't be discouraged, no matter how many times you have to return to a juice and raw foods diet. Many people have overcome this "incurable" disease.

🍃

Intensive Building/Balancing Macrobiotic Diet:

A macrobiotic diet is very effective against cancer and other degenerative diseases, helping to rebuild healthy blood and cells, and preventing diseased tissue from continued growth. This way of eating is non-mucous forming, low in fats that can alter body chemistry and enhance cancer potential in the cells, and high in vegetable fiber and protein. It is stimulating to the heart and circulatory system through its emphasis on oriental foods such as miso, bancha green tea, and shiitake mushrooms. It is alkalizing with umeboshi plums, sea vegetables and soy food. It is high in potassium, natural iodine, other minerals and trace elements. Its greatest benefit is that it is cleansing and strengthening at the same time, and offers a truly balanced way of eating that is easily individualized for one's environment, the seasons, and the constitution of the person using it. The strict form recommended here for an intensive healing programs should be followed for three to six months.

On rising: take a potassium broth or essence (page 53), or carrot/beet/cucumber juice;
or cranberry concentrate (2 teasp. in water) or red grape juice;
and a vitamin/mineral drink such as Nutritech ALL 1, or Crystal Star SYSTEM STRENGTH™.

Breakfast: make a mixture of 2 TBS. **each:** brewer's yeast, wheat germ, lecithin and bee pollen granules. Sprinkle some on a whole grain cereal, granola or muesli, or mix with yogurt and dried fruit;
and/or use on fresh fruit, such as strawberries or apples with kefir or kefir cheese; add a whole grain breakfast pilaf such as Kashi, bulgar or millet, with apple juice or kefir cheese topping.

Mid-morning: take a green drink (pg. 54ff.) Sun CHLORELLA, Green Foods GREEN MAGMA, Crystal Star ENERGY GREEN™ or fresh wheat grass juice. Add 1 teasp. Bragg's LIQUID AMINOS to any choice;
and/or an herb tea, such as pau de arco, Jason Winters tea, or Crystal Star CHINESE ROYAL MU, or MEDITATION™ TEA;
or a glass of fresh carrot juice, or Green Foods GREEN ESSENCE DRINK;

or a cup of miso soup with sea vegetables snipped on top. (Have 2 TBS. dry sea vegetables daily.)

Lunch: have some steamed broccoli or cauliflower with brown rice, tofu and a little soy cheese;
or an oriental stir fry with brown rice and miso sauce;
or a fresh green salad with whole grain pitas or chapatis;
or a black bean, onion or lentil soup, or a 3 bean salad;
or falafels in pita bread with some raw or steamed vegies and a tamari dressing;
or a cabbage or slaw salad with oriental sesame dressing.

Mid-afternoon: have a cup of bancha , kukicha twig tea, or roasted dandelion tea, or Crystal Star CIRCU-CLENZ™ TEA or MIN-ZYME-MINOS™ DRINK;
and some whole grain crackers with kefir cheese or a soy spread;
or crunchy raw vegies with a little gomashio (sesame salt) sprinkled on top.

Dinner: have a brown rice, millet, bulgar, or kasha casserole with tofu, or tempeh and some steamed vegetables;
or a hearty dinner salad with some sea vegies, nuts and seeds, and whole grain bread or chapatis;
or baked, broiled or steamed fish or seafood with rice and peas or other vegies;
or a baked vegie casserole with mushroom/yogurt or kefir cheese sauce;
or stuffed cabbage rolls with rice, and baked carrots with tamari and a little honey.

Before bed: have a cup of VEGEX yeast paste broth, or a relaxing herb tea, such as alfalfa/mint or red clover tea, **or** a glass of organic apple juice.

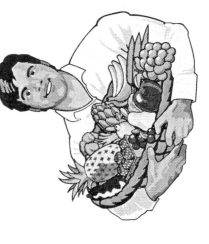

•*Note: In order for the macrobiotic balance to be set up, and work correctly with the body in this phase of healing, several foods and food types must be avoided:*
- Red meat, poultry, preserved, smoked or cured meats of all kinds, and dairy products
- Coffee, black teas,carbonated drinks, and some stimulant herb teas
- Nightshade plants, such as tomatoes, potatoes, peppers and eggplant
- Sugars, corn syrup and artificial sweeteners; and tropical and sweet fruits
- All refined, frozen, canned and processed foods
- Hot spices, white vinegar, and table salt

≈ **Supplements and Herbal Aids for the Intensive Macrobiotic Diet:**

❖ Siberian ginseng extract or tea several times daily.
❖ Take ascorbate vitamin C crystals in water 3 to 5000mg. daily, with ginkgo biloba extract drops.
❖ Mega-potency acidolphilus and Barley GREEN MAGMA to combat the effects of chemotherapy.
❖ Wheat germ oil, vitamin E 400IU with selenium,or germanium 100mg. to add tissue oxygen.
❖ Crystal Star PAU DE ARCO/ECHINACEA extract, IODINE THERAPY™ or POTASSIUM SOURC™E capsules, and high omega 3 FLAX OIL to inhibit tmor growth.

≈ **Bodywork for the Intensive Macrobiotic Diet:**

➤ Get morning sunlight and mild exercise every day possible to accelerate the passage of toxins.
➤ Overheating therapy is effective for degenerative disease. See P. Airola, "HOW TO GET WELL", for the proper technique.

See "COOKING FOR HEALTHY HEALING" by Linda Rector-Page for an initial cleansing and complete diet program for cancer control.

Specific Suggestions For Particular Cancer Sites

Cancer is not one disease, but many types of cancers. It includes a large group of malignancies which vary in development, cause, and behavior according to their location in the body. There can be more than one type of cancer in a particular organ or location. The fundamental link between all cancers is that the cells have been desensitized to normal growth constraints. The damaged cells grow uncontrolled and may move (metastasize) to other sites in the body.

❖ *Prostate (and Testicular) Cancer* is the most common cancer in males in the U.S., striking one in nine men over age seventy. It is associated with a high fat diet and rich, high cholesterol foods. A highly nutritious diet is a proven weapon against this kind of cancer. Increased risk for this type of cancer is associated with low vitamin A levels. There is frequency of urination, difficulty in starting and stopping urination, feelings of urgency or straining, and other symptoms similar to prostatitis. As the cancer outgrows the small prostate gland it often eats its way into the bladder or rectum, or even the pelvis and back causing severe damage. A monthly self-exam should be a part of your prevention plan, especially if you are over fifty.

+ **Causes:** High fat, high sugar, low fiber diet; raised testosterone levels (particularly from steroids).

+ **Major Symptoms:** Lumps in prostate and/or testicles; thickening and fluid retention in the scrotum; painful, weak, interrupted urination; persistent, unexplained back pain.

+ **Therapy:** High potency royal jelly 2 teasp. daily, evening primrose oil 4 daily, Crystal Star PAU DE ARCO/ECHINACEA extract; high fiber, low fat diet excretes hormones linked to cancer; Vitamin E *with* selenium 200mcg.; CoQ 10, 30mg. 2x daily; vitamin C 5-10,000mg. daily (best as an ascorbic acid flush - page 347); beta or marine carotene 100,000IU, cysteine 500mg. daily; regular daily exercise.

❖ *Organ Cancer - (liver, pancreas, bladder, kidney, lymphatic)*

+ **Causes:** DDT and other similar pesticides have been linked to pancreatic and all organ cancers. (Although they are banned in this country, we receive them in foods imported from other countries.); high fat, high cholesterol, high sugar, low vegetable and fresh fruit diet.

+ **Major Symptoms:** Frequent and often painful, burning urination; blood in the urine; extreme lethargy.

+ **Therapy:** : Crystal Star DETOX™ *or* LIV-ALIVE™ capsules as directed. Germanium, 200mg. 3x daily, *with* burdock tea 2 cups daily or more. (Eat fresh burdock daily if available.); Vitamin E *with* selenium 200mcg.

❖ *Breast Cancer* - Post-menopausal women have the highest risk, with 75% of all cases occurring in women over 40. Since fat cells act as the storage depots of the body, they also store environmental, chemical and food-related toxins. Those who are overweight are more prone to risk - *and* they have a much harder time overcoming the disease. Also at risk are women who have overly high, or imbalanced estrogen secretion; e.g., those who had their first period before age 12; those who did not go through menopause til after age 55; those who did not have a child before age 30; and those who did not carry a pregnancy full-term. (Vegetarian women have fewer instances of breast cancer than non-vegetarians, because they seem to process estrogen differently.) Long term synthetic estrogen and/or oral contraceptive use is also suspect as a risk factor for breast cancer.

- **About mammograms:** Radiation from X-Rays can severely harm breast tissue and cell balance - especially those from older mammography machines. Although mammograms have improved in the last 20 years both in clarity and amount of dosage, we still hear enough horror stories about swift fibroid onset to recommend that mammograms should not be done routinely or without suspected cause. When a mammogram screens the breasts of a woman under fifty, it only detects dangerous lesions about 50% of the time, because a younger women's breasts are so dense. *No study has shown that death rates from breast cancer are reduced by mammogram screening in women under 50.* Therefore, because even low-dose radiation can cause possible breast fibroids, mammograms in this age group should only be necessary if there are *abnormal findings* such as lumps or nipple infections. Even in women over fifty, where the effect of radiation is less, if there is no family breast cancer history or suspected reason for alarm, mammograms should be undertaken with care. Check out your chosen facility thoroughly. By the time a tumor has reached the size that can be detected, it has probably been growing for 10 years or more and has likely spread to other body areas. While early detection can mean less radical medical intervention, **prevention through immune enhancement and a healthy lifestyle should be the primary goal - not early detection.**

A *breast cancer prevention plan* should include: 1) A decrease in body fat through reduction of fat intake to 20% of the diet - particularly the fats from sugary foods, dairy products and alcohol. 2) An increase in anti-oxidant nutrients - beta carotene, vitamin E and C, selenium and wheat germ oil. 3) The addition of plenty of fish, sea vegetables, complex carbohydrates from whole grains, soy foods and green and orange vegetables to the diet. 4) Avoidance of unnecessary exposure to radiation. 5) Limited exposure to exogenous estrogen - from birth control pills or estrogen replacement, or meats and poultry and dairy foods that are regularly injected with synthetic estrogen. 6) A breast self-exam once a month. 7) The taking of positive, conscious steps to decrease the stress and increase the relaxation and enjoyment of life.

+ **Causes:** Hypothyroidism, especially when linked to iodine deficiency; vitamin E, C and selenium deficiency; too much refined sugar, red meat and dairy; emotional stress and tension; tinted glasses that block the full spectrum of light to the pineal gland causing deficiencies in vitamin D and other nutrients necessary for hormone balance.

+ **Major Symptoms:** Discharge from the nipple, lumps or thickening of the breast; scaly skin patches, especially around the nipple; change in breast texture or color; persistent enlargement of lymph nodes in the armpit; breast changes that are not related to regular menstrual cycle; chronic swelling and sores around the mouth, gums or jaw.

+ **Therapy:** Primary diet recommendations - reduce dietary fat to 20% or less. Add 4-6 gms. of soluble fiber daily from complex carbohydrates and fresh or dried fruits. Add cruciferous vegetables, such as broccoli and cauliflower, and green and orange vegetables daily. Use flax seed tea for fiber and cleansing. American Biologics natural vitamin E emulsion 400IU with selenium 200mcg. daily to relieve soreness and help reduce cystic nodule size; carnitine 250mg.; Prof. Services PRO-GEST cream; royal jelly 1/4 teasp. 2x daily with CoQ 10, 30mg. 2x daily; beta-carotene, particularly from marine sources 25,000IU. Vitamin C with bioflavonoids, up to 10,000mg. *daily* (best as an ascorbic acid flush - page 347). Unsaturated fatty acids such as evening primrose oil or borage seed oil; omega 3 flax oil; flax seed tea; iodine therapy with kelp, Atomodine, or Crystal Star IODINE

THERAPY™ capsules or extract. Regular exercise is a key protective factor against breast cancer.

A final word of warning - removal of the ovaries following any type of breast surgery involves hormone-related health problems, such as osteoporosis, increased cholesterol and heart attack risk. Chemotherapy does not improve a woman's chances for survival, especially if the cancer has spread to the lymph nodes.

❖ *Cervical and Uterine Cancer* - While obesity is linked to all types of cancer, overweight women are particularly likely to develop cancer of the cervix and/or uterine lining. Women past menopause, especially those who have never been pregnant, are also at risk. High blood pressure, long term oral contraceptive use, untreated severe dysplasia and synthetic estrogens have all recently been linked to cervical and uterine cancer. If localized cervical cancer is not treated, it usually spreads to underlying connective tissue, nearby lymph glands, the uterus, and the genito-urinary tract. Women can lower their risk. The current drug temoxophyd can engender endometrial and liver cancer.

Note: the Am. Cancer Society has now quietly dropped its recommendation that women have a PAP test every year - advocating it only if the woman is at high risk.

+ **Causes:** Vitamin E and A deficiency; a history of sexually transmitted diseases; early teen-age intercourse; infertility, or conversely, having more than five births; cervical dysplasia or benign fibroids aggravated by excess estrogen production from a high fat diet and lack of fiber; cancer of the penis in a sexual partner may cause cellular mutation; exposure to carcinogenic substances, such as heavy metals, asbestos, herbicide chemicals, nicotine, etc.; serious vaginal infections, such as trichomoniasis.

+ **Major Symptoms:** Bleeding between menstrual periods; painful, heavy periods; unusual vaginal discharge; bleeding during intercourse indicating presence of polyps.

+ **Therapy:** Calcium supplementation has shown results in preventing precancerous lesions from becoming cancerous. Unsaturated fatty acids therapy from evening primrose, and high omega 3 fish or flax oil; a diet rich in fresh fruits and vegetables, esp. cruciferous vegetables; keep fats low - include soy foods for protein instead of meats or dairy products; high potency royal jelly 2 teasp. daily; Beta-carotene 100,000IU daily, particularly from marine sources; Ester C 5- 10,000mg. daily, vitamin E 800IU daily with selenium 200mg., Green Foods GREEN MAGMA, Prof. Services PROGEST CREAM.

❖ *Colo-rectal and Colon Cancer* - Now the number two cause of death in the United States, 100,000 people die every year from colon cancer. Overweight men are particularly at risk. A low fat, high fiber diet can dramatically reduce the risk of developing benign polyps that often lead to colon cancer.

+ **Causes:** A diet high in fat, (especially saturated fats from red meat) and low in soluble fiber.

+ **Major Symptoms:** Persistent diarrhea, changing to persistent constipation for no apparent reason; blood in the bowel movement.

+ **Therapy:** Fiber is still the dietary key for colon cancer. Add foods such as whole grain cereals, (particularly wheat bran) sweet potatoes, baked beans, dried fruits, cruciferous vegetables, soy foods, legumes and other high fiber (but low roughage) foods to the diet. Inhibitory vitamins are A, C & E, beta carotene 100,000IU, and selenium 200mcg., taken together. Two cups of green tea, as a preventive; flax seed tea for fiber and cleansing. For precancerous colon polyps: Vitamin C, Green Foods GREEN MAGMA drink. As a preventive measure, daily low dose aspirin coupled with a high fiber diet has shown positive results.

❖ *Ovarian Cancer* - Women at risk seem to be those who have never had children, who are past menopause and overweight from a high fat diet - with a family history of cancer.

+ **Causes:** A family history of cancer; juvenile epilepsy; certain anti-inflammatory medication (alicylates, non-steroidals, cortico-steroids); thyroid disorders, alcohol-induced diabetes.

+ **Major Symptoms:** There are often no symptoms until the cancer has mestastisized.

+ **Therapy:** Unsaturated fatty acids therapy from evening primrose, and high omega 3 fish or flax oil; a diet rich in fresh fruits and vegetables, esp. cruciferous vegetables; keep fats low - include soy foods for protein instead of meats or dairy products; high potency royal jelly 2 teasp. daily; beta-carotene 00,000IU daily, particularly from marine sources; Ester C 5-10,000mg. daily, vitamin E 800IU daily with selenium 200mg., Green Foods GREEN MAGMA, Prof. Services PROGEST CREAM.

❖ *Lung Cancer* - Smoking hurts everybody and makes everyone more at risk for cancer, even unborn fetuses; continuing heavy metal, toxic chemical and radioactive exposure; exposure to toxic pesticides and herbacides; chronic lung weakness from bronchitis or T.B.

+ **Causes:** Smoking and secondary smoke; long term exposure to heavy metals, or chemicals such as those in pesticides, asbestos and radioactive materials.

+ **Major Symptoms:** Persistent cough and chest pain; blood in the sputum.

+ **Therapy:** Vitamin A *and* Beta-carotene, particularly from marine sources; vitamin E 1000IU with selenium 200mcg. B complex 150mg., green tea, or Crystal Star GREEN TEA CLEANSER™ as a preventive; H2O2 OXYGEL applied to the chest; Vit. B12 w/ folic acid; Siberian ginseng extract 4 to 6 x daily; germanium 200mg. 3x daily; reishi mushroom tea or capsules daily for interferon.

❖ *Stomach Cancer* - The elderly are particularly at risk, because of decreasing HCl production and lack of dietary fiber. As with other cancers, a high fat diet is always linked to stomach cancer. This type of cancer takes a long time to develop, sometimes as much as fifteen years.

+ **Causes:** High intake of meat proteins and nitrates - low intake of fresh fruits, vegetables and olive oil (and the vitamins C and E in them); a high fat, low fiber diet; HCl deficiency; stomach polyps.

+ **Major Symptoms:** Pernicious anemia; chronic indigestion and gastritis; pain after eating.

+ **Therapy:** Green tea, or Crystal Star GREEN TEA CLEANSER™ as therapy and as a preventive; Green Foods GREEN MAGMA, pancreatin for digestion of protein; allium vegetables such as onions, garlic, leeks, and scallions; small frequent meals - no large meals. Inhibitory vitamins are A, C & E, beta carotene, and selenium 200mcg., taken together.

CANDIDA ALBICANS ■ CANDIDIASIS

Candidiasis is a state of inner imbalance, not a germ, bug or disease. Candida albicans is a strain of yeasts commonly found in the gastro-intestinal and genito-urinary areas of the body. It is generally harmless, but when resistance and immunity are low, the yeast is able to multiply rapidly, feeding on sugars and carbohydrates in these tracts. It releases toxins into the bloodstream, and causes far-reaching problems. It is a stress-related condition, brought about because the body is severely out of balance, usually either from repeated rounds of antibiotics, birth control pills, or cortico-steroids, a nutritionally poor diet that is high in refined carbohydrates and alcohol, and a life-style short on rest.

FOOD THERAPY

The food recommendations for the initial diet are critically important in controlling candida yeast proliferation to normal levels. Candida yeasts grow on carbohydrates, preserved, processed and refined foods, molds, and gluten breads.

✿ **Do not eat the following foods for the first month to 6 weeks:** Sugar or sweeteners of any kind, gluten bread and yeasted baked goods, dairy products (except plain kefir or kefir cheese, or yogurt and yogurt cheese), smoked, dried, pickled or cured foods, mushrooms, nuts or nut butters (except almonds and almond butter), fruits, fruit juices, dried or candied fruits, (the phosphoric acid carbonated drinks, coffee, black tea, caffeine, binds up calcium and magnesium) alcohol or foods containing vinegar. Chemical foods and drugs, such as anti-biotics, steroids, cortico-steroids, and tobacco must be avoided.

This is a long, restrictive list, but for the first critical weeks, when the energy-sapping yeasts must be deprived of nutrients and killed off, it is the only way.

✿ **Acceptable foods during this first stage:** Lots of fresh and steamed vegies (especially onions, garlic, ginger root, cabbage,and broccoli), poultry, seafood, fish and sea vegetables, olive oil, eggs, mayonnaise, brown rice, amaranth, buckwheat, barley and millet, soy and vegetable pastas, tofu and tempeh, plain yogurt, rice cakes/crackers, some citrus fruit and herb teas. This is a short, limited list; but diet restriction is the most important way to stop yeast overgrowth.

✿ Try to have a green drink and/or miso soup every day.

VITAMINS/MINERALS

For best results rotate anti-yeast and anti-fungal products, so that yeast strains do not build up resistance to any one formula.

▶ Maintaining bowel flora is critical to overcoming yeast growth.
✦ DDS acidophilus.
✦ Prof. Nutr. DR. DOPHILUS in water as directed. (May also be used as a vaginal application.)
✦ Women's Health RELEAF formula.

▶ To help kill the yeasts:
✦ Pro. Spec. CAPRICIN 3x daily.
✦ Am. Biologics DIOXYCHLOR with taurine
✦ Solaray CAPRYL.
✦ NutraPathic NUTRAMUNE for 1 mo., then slowly add D-YEAST.
✦ Nutrition Resource NUTRIBIOTIC grapefruit seed extract.

▶ For allergic reactions:
✦ Bromelain 500mg. with Lysine 1000mg.
✦ Ascorbate C 3000mg. w. bioflavs.

▶ For immune support:
✦ Biotin 1000mcg. with B complex and taurine.
✦ Zinc picolinate 50mg.
✦ Ascorbate C or Ester C w. bioflavonoids - up to 5000mg. daily.
✦ Marine carotene 100,000IU or Crystal Star SYSTEM STRENGTH™ drink.
✦ Enzymatic Therapy THYMUS/LUNG and IMMUNOPLEX.

▶ For protein/nutrition:
✦ Source of Life protein drink.
✦ Full spectrum pre-digested amino acid compound.

HERBAL THERAPY

Herbs are prime agents for restoring body homeostasis.

❦ To kill the yeasts:
✦ **Pau de Arco tea 4 cups daily.**
✦ **Crystal Star PAU DE ARCO/ECHINACEA extract, CANDIDEX™ caps and CRAN PLUS™ tea.**
✦ **Black walnut extract.**
✦ **Garlic 6-10 daily.**

❦ For gland balance:
✦ Heritage ATOMODINE liquid.
✦ Crystal Star ADR-ACTIVE™.
✦ Evening primrose oil caps.
✦ Enzymatic Therapy ADRENAL COMPLEX.

❦ For bowel / digestive regulation:
✦ Sonne #7 Bentonite.
✦ Barberry tea 2 cups daily.
✦ Crystal Star CHO-LO FIBER TONE™ drink or capsules.
✦ Enzymatic Therapy IBS capsules.

❦ To build immunity:
✦ Green superfoods: Sun CHLORELLA, Living Foods SUPERFOOD, Crystal Star ENERGY GREEN™.
✦ Echinacea extract, tonic dose.
✦ Astragalus and hawthorne extr.
✦ Crys. Star. HERBAL DEFENSE™.

❦ For tissue oxygen:
✦ Germanium 30-100mg. daily.
✦ Rub Care Plus OXYGEL on abdomen. Take w. ascorbate C 2000mg.

❦ To clean the liver:
✦ Natren LIFE START II.
✦ Alta Health CANGEST caps.

BODYWORK

A positive mind and outlook are essential to overcome this body stress. Relax and have a good laugh every day.

▶ Get enough sleep. Adequate sleep and rest are primary factors in the body's ability to overcome debilitating, yeast-induced fatigue.

▶ Exercise and oxygen are keys to overcoming candida. Regular aerobic exercise is necessary for optimum body oxygen use.

▶ Soak any fungal infected areas in tea tree oil solution. (May also be used in water as a vaginal douche.) Use Grapefruit Seed Extract as a vaginal douche or enema for cleansing.

▶ Avoid antibiotics, birth control pills and cortico-steroid drugs unless absolutely necessary. They set up an easy environment in which candida can flourish.

▶ Use applied kinesiology to test for food and product sensitivities.

▶ Reflexology point:

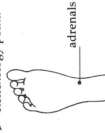

adrenals

CANDIDA ALBICANS CLEANSING DIET FOR THE FIRST TWO MONTHS OF HEALING

Diet change is the most important and effective way to rebuild strength and immunity from candida overgrowth. The initial cleansing diet here concentrates on releasing dead and diseased yeast cells from the body. This phase usually requires 2-3 months to bring about complete cleansing. It may also be used as the basis for a personal "rotation diet", in which you slowly add back individual foods during healing that caused an allergic reaction to candida. As you start to see body improvement, and symptoms decrease (usually after three to six months), start to add back some whole grains, fruits, juices, a little white wine, some fresh cheeses, nuts and beans.

Remember - sugars and refined foods will allow candida to grow again.

Note: We have been working successfully with candidiasis since 1984 and have found repeatedly that a too-rigid diet does not work over the long term, because the sufferer cannot stick to it (except in a very restricted, isolated environment), and the body becomes imbalanced the other way. In addition, we are learning that the disease itself, and the immune response to it are changing. The recommended diets in "HEALTHY HEALING" and "COOKING FOR HEALTHY HEALING" are real people diets, used by people suffering from candida who have shared their experience with us. They are being continually modified to meet changing needs and to take advantage of an ever-widening network of information.

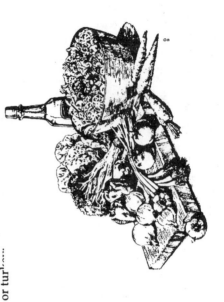

On rising: take 2 teasp. cranberry concentrate, or 2 teasp. lemon juice in water to clean the kidneys;
or a glass of water with 1 teasp. Sonne #7, and 1 teasp. raw unfiltered apple cider vinegar with 1 teasp. honey, if there is flatulence.

Breakfast: take NutriTech ALL 1 vitamin/mineral drink in water;
then take 1 or 2 poached or hard boiled eggs on rice cakes with a little butter or flax oil;
or almond butter on rice cakes or wheat free bread;
or oatmeal with 1 TB. Bragg's LIQUID AMINOS;
or amaranth or buckwheat pancakes with a little butter and vanilla.

Mid-morning: take a green drink (page 54ff.) or Sun CHLORELLA or Green Foods BARLEY GREEN, or Crystal Star ENERGY GREEN™ in water;
or a cup of pau de arco tea, or chamomile, barberry, or echinacea extract drops in a cup of water;
or a small bottle of mineral water.

Lunch: have a fresh green salad with lemon/olive or flax oil dressing;
or open face rice cake or wheat free bread sandwiches, with a little mayonnaise or butter, some vegies, seafood, chicken or tur'·····
or a vegetable or miso soup with butter and cornbread;
or steamed vegies with tofu and brown rice;
or chicken, tuna or vegetable pasta salad, with mayonnaise or lemon/ oil dressing.

Mid-afternoon: have some rice crackers, or baked corn chips, with a little kefir cheese or butter;
or some raw vegies dipped in lemon/oil dressing or spiced mayonnaise;
or a small mineral water and hard boiled or deviled egg with sesame salt or sea vegetable seasoning.

Dinner: baked, broiled or poached fish or chicken with steamed brown rice or millet with flax oil and veggies;
or a baked potato with Bragg's LIQUID AMINOS, or a little kefir cheese, or lemon oil dressing;
or an oriental stir fry with brown rice and a miso or light broth soup;
or a tofu and vegie casserole;
or a vegetarian pizza on a chapati or pita crust;
or a small omelet with vegie filling;
or a hot or cold vegetable pasta salad.

Before bed: have a cup of herb tea such as chamomile, peppermint, or Crystal Star LICORICE MINTS TEA.

✱ Note: Brewer's yeast does not cause or aggravate candida albicans yeast overgrowth. It is still one of the best immune-enhancing foods available.

◗ Supplementation should be included in the cleansing diet phase to boost body energy in the yeast reduction and killing process. See the vitamin/mineral and herbal suggestions on the preceding page. For best results choose supplements to help kill the yeasts, to balance and restore intestinal flora, to help clean the liver, for bowel regulation, glandular rebalance, and allergic reactions.
See COOKING FOR HEALTHY HEALING, by Linda Rector-Page for a complete control diet for Candida albicans - to enhance liver function for detoxification, improve digestion, create an environment for better nutrient assimilation, and build immunity to prevent recurrence.

DIAGNOSIS INFORMATION FOR CANDIDA ALBICANS OVERGROWTH

Because much of the traditional medical community has chosen not to recognize, diagnose or treat Candidiasis, the alternative professions of Naturopathy, Homeopathy, Chiropractic and Holistic medicine have seen and dealt with most of these cases over the past twelve years. Their energy and dedication have advanced the knowledge and understanding of the symptoms and treatment of Candidiasis to a great degree; better pin-pointing of symptoms and treatment, shortening of healing time, lessening of overkill, and more understanding of the large, overriding psychological aspect of the disease.

The common symptoms for Candida Albicans overgrowth occur in fairly defined stages:

+ 1st symptoms: Bowel problems; heartburn and chronic indigestion with flatulence and bloating; recurring cystitis and vaginitis; chronic fungal infections of the skin and nails; athlete's foot.

+ 2nd symptoms: Allergy/immune reactions such as asthma, hives, eczema, hayfever, skin rashes, acne; frequent and chronic headaches and muscle aches; earaches; chronic bronchitis; sensitivity to odors.

+ 3rd symptoms: Central nervous system reactions, such as extreme irritability; confusion, and a "spacey" feeling; memory lapses, and the inability to concentrate; chronic fatigue and lethargy, often followed by acute depression.

+ 4th symptoms: Gland and organ dysfunctions such as hypothyroidism, adrenal failure, and hypoglycemia; ovarian problems, including frigidity and infertility; male impotence and lack of sex drive.

☞**Ask yourself the following questions as a measure of self-diagnosis. Several "yes" answers should alert you to Candida.**

✓ Have you recently taken repeated rounds of antibiotic or cortico-steroid drugs, such as Symycin, Panmycin, Decadron, Prednisone, etc. or acne drugs for 1 month or longer?
✓ Have you been troubled by PMS, vaginitis or vaginal yeast infections, endometriosis, abdominal pains, prostatitis, or loss of sexual interest?
✓ Are you bothered by unexplained frequent headaches, muscle aches and joint pain?
✓ Do you crave sugar, bread, or alcoholic beverages?
✓ Are you frequently bothered by chronic fungal infections, such as ring worm, jock itch, nail fungus, athlete's foot? Or hives, psoriasis, eczema or chronic dermatitis?
✓ Are you over-sensitive to tobacco, perfume, insecticides, or other chemical odors?
✓ Do you have recurrent digestive problems, gas or bloating? Do you have chronic constipation alternating to diarrhea?
✓ Are you now taking, or have you previously taken birth control pills for more than 2 years? Have you been pregnant more than twice?
✓ Are you bothered by chronic fatigue, erratic vision, spots before the eyes, poor memory or continuing nervous tension?
✓ Do you feel depressed and sick all over, yet the cause cannot be found? Are the symptoms worse on damp, muggy days with joint and muscle pain?

CONTROLLING CANDIDA ALBICANS

Candida albicans is a modern opportunistic yeast strain that takes advantage of lowered immunity to overrun the body. Healthy liver function and a strong immune system are the keys to lasting prevention and control of candida overgrowth. The whole healing/rebuilding process usually takes from 3-6 months or more, and is not easy. The changes in diet, habits and life style are often radical. Some people feel better right away; others go through a rough "healing crisis". (Yeasts are living organisms - a part of the body. Killing them off is traumatic.) But most people with candida are feeling so bad anyway, that the treatment and the knowledge that they are getting better, pulls them through the hard times. Be as gentle with your body as you can. Give yourself all the time you need, at least 3 to 6 months. Of course you want to get better quickly, but multiple therapies all at once can be self-defeating, psychologically upsetting, and too traumatic on the system. Just stick to it and go at your own pace.

A comprehensive and successful program for overcoming this disease includes the following stages:

Stage 1: Kill the yeasts through diet change and supplement therapy. Avoid antibiotics, cortico-steroid drugs and birth control pills, unless there is absolute medical need.

Stage 2: Cleanse the dead yeasts and waste cells from the body with a soluble fiber cleanser or bentonite.

Stage 3: Strengthen the digestive system by enhancing its ability to assimilate nutrients. Strengthen the afflicted organs and glands, especially the liver. Restore normal metabolism, and promote friendly bacteria in the gastro-intestinal tract.

Stage 4: Rebuild the immune system. Stimulating immune well-being throughout the healing process supports faster results.

Note: Candida albicans can mimic the symptoms of over 140 different disorders. For instance, chronic fatigue syndrome (EBV), salmonella, intestinal parasite infestation and mononucleosis all have similar symptoms, but are treated very differently. Have a test for candida before starting a healing program to save time, expense, and for more rapid improvement.

Note: While Candida symptoms appear mostly in women, men and children also get yeast infections. Both sexual partners need to be treated because candida is passed back and forth during intercourse. See "THRUSH" in the Children's Ailments section, and the "FUNGAL INFECTIONS" and "ATHLETE'S FOOT" pages for more information concerning yeast overgrowth in men and children.

CARPAL TUNNEL SYNDROME

While carpal tunnel syndrome has long been as a problem for knitters and needle-workers, and those doing repetitive task jobs, such as carpenters, musicians and assembly-line workers, it is becoming a common ailment of the computer age, affecting more than one out of ten Americans who work on computer terminals. Standard medical treatment is usually cortisone shots to control swelling, or in severe cases, surgery to enlarge the carpal tunnel opening. Natural therapies can both relieve pain and act as a preventive to the development of CTS.

FOOD THERAPY

🍃 **Make sure your diet is rich in vitamin B6 foods, such as whole grains, organ meats (especially liver), green leafy vegetables, beans and legumes.**

🍃 Eat plenty of fresh foods with at least one green salad every day. Add celery for good cell salt activity, and sea vegetables or miso soup to alkalize.

🍃 Avoid caffeine, hard liquor and soft drinks. They bind magnesium. Avoid other oxalic acid-forming foods, such as cooked spinach, rhubarb and chocolate.

🍃 Take a glass of lemon juice and water each morning. Make a mix - add 2 teasp. to the daily diet:
  ◆ Lecithin granules
  ◆ Brewer's yeast
  ◆ Molasses
  ◆ Toasted wheat germ

🍃 Have a green drink (pg. 54ff.) or fresh carrot juice often.

🍃 Crystal Star BIOFLAV., FIBER & C SUPPORT DRINK™ for collagen support and tissue integrity.

VITAMINS/MINERALS

▶ Vit. B6 500mg. daily, with B Complex 100mg. for 3 months.
with
Niacin 500mg. 2 x daily to increase circulation.
and
Ascorbate vitamin C w/ bioflavonoids 3-5000mg. daily for connective tissue formation.

▶ Enzymatic Therapy LIQUID LIVER w. SIB. GINSENG.

▶ Quercetin Plus or pycnogenol, 2 daily, with bromelain 500mg.
and
Ester C with bioflavs. 550mg. 6 daily.

▶ Nutrapathic CALCIUM/COLLAGEN capsules.

▶ Effective natural pain control:
  ✚ Country Life LIGATEND. ♂
  ✚ GABA with Taurine. ♀
  ✚ DLPA 500mg. as needed.
  ✚ Twin Lab CSA as needed.

HERBAL THERAPY

🌿 Crystal Star RELAX CAPS™ for nerve restoration.
with
SILICA SOURCE™ extract for rebuilding collagen and connective tissue.
and
META-TABS™ if there is an underactive thyroid.

🌿 Evening primrose oil caps 4 daily for prostaglandin formation. ♀

🌿 Ginkgo biloba extract as needed 2-3x daily.

🌿 Solaray TURMERIC capsules for inflammation.

🌿 Effective extracts:
  ◆ Scullcap
  ◆ Passion flower
  ◆ Lobelia

🌿 Alta Health SIL-X silica 2-3x daily.

🌿 Hylands NERVE TONIC as needed. ♀

BODYWORK

Self Test for CTS: Hold out your right hand, bend your left index finger and tap the middle of your right wrist where your wrist joins your hand. If you get a tingling sensation or shooting pains down your fingers, you probably have carpal tunnel problems.

▶ Massage affected areas frequently. Apply cajeput oil or Chinese WHITE FLOWER oil.

▶ Reflexology point:

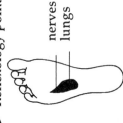

nerves
lungs

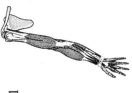

▶ Massage area with CarePlus OXY-GEL.

▶ Carpal tunnel affected area:

Common Symptoms: Poor grip; intense numbness, tingling, pain and swelling in the wrist and hand, often involving shoulder nerves as well; chronic muscular weakness and atrophy; nerve inflammation.

Common Causes: Continued stress on the wrist, hand and arm nerves from repetitive tasks; vitamin B6 deficiency, and/or birth control pills creating a B6 deficiency, leading to the disorder; underactive thyroid;too much protein; lack of magnesium; glandular imbalance during pregnancy; body electrical system "shorts" from prostaglandin imbalance.

CATARACTS ◼ CONJUNCTIVITIS

Cataracts are the leading cause of impaired vision in America, affecting over 4 million people. They appear as cloudy or opaque areas on the crystalline lens of the eye which focuses light, and block light entering the eye. Natural therapies have shown that progression can be arrested and *early* cataracts reversed. Conjunctivitis, an inflammation of the lining of the eyelid is often caused by a viral infection, and can be extremely contagious. See also EYESIGHT page in this book.

FOOD THERAPY

🍃 A preventive diet and life style are the key to eye health. Reduce intake of fats, choesterol, and salt. Add food sources of magnesium, such as seafoods, whole grains, green vegetables, molasses, nuts and eggs.

🍃 Avoid refined carbohydrates and all sugars, red meats, caffeine, and tobacco. Avoid rancid foods as sources of free radicals.

🍃 For cataracts:
Blood sugar stability is a key factor. Include green leafy vegies, sea vegetables, seafood, celery, citrus fruits, brewer's yeast, sprouts, apples and apple juice in the diet. Add legumes for sulphur-containing amino acids.

🍃 For conjunctivitis:
Apply yogurt, grated potato or apple to inflammation.

Take a potassium broth (pg. 53) often to feed the optical tissue.
and
A glass of carrot juice daily for three months.

🍃 Crystal Star BIOFLAV., FIBER & C SUPPORT™ drink. with rutin.

VITAMINS/MINERALS

▶ Golden Pride ORAL CHELATION therapy, 1 cap 2x daily. ♂

▶ Enzymatic Therapy ACID-A-CAL caps daily, with chromium picolinate 200mcg.

▶ Anti-oxidants are key preventives, especially in the de-activation of heavy metals:
✦ Vit. E w/ Selenium. ♂
✦ Ascorbate Vitamin C w. bioflavonoids 3000mg. daily.
✦ Beta carotene 150,000IU daily, with vitamin D 1000IU.
✦ Glutathione 50mg. daily.
✦ Germanium100mg. 3x daily.
✦ Pycnogenol 50mg. 2x daily. ♂

▶ Quantum SEE capsules.

▶ For cataracts: Histidine caps 2 daily *and* quercetin plus with bromelain 4-6 daily.

▶ For conjunctivitis: 1 drop castor oil in the eyes 3 x daily, and zinc 50mg. 2 x daily.

▶ B Complex 100mg. *with* extra B2 100mg. 3x and B6 100mg. 3x daily.

▶ Homeopathic SILICEA tabs.

HERBAL THERAPY

🌱 Use Crystal Star EYEBRIGHT HERBAL™ tea as an eyewash.
and
Take bilberry extract as soon as cataracts are noted to retard formation and remove chemicals
and/or
SUGAR STRATEGY HIGH™ capsules for sugar regulation.

🌱 Aloe vera juice (without ascorbic acid) drops in the eye 2 x daily.

🌱 High potency royal jelly 2 teasp. daily, with spirulina tabs 4-8 daily.

🌱 Effective teas and eyewashes for cataracts:
◆ Eyebright
◆ Rosehips
◆ Chaparral

🌱 Effective teas and/or washes for conjunctivitis:
◆ Bilberry
◆ Aloe vera juice
◆ Chamomile
◆ Chickweed

🌱 Solaray VIZION capsules.

🌱 Ginkgo biloba extract or capsules 4 x daily.

BODYWORK

▶ Do long slow neck rolls and other good eye exercises (see Bates Method book).

▶ Avoid long exposure to the sun. Get your exercise early in the day.

▶ Avoid aspirin, commercial antihistamines and cortisone as detrimental to eye health.

▶ For conjunctivitis: palm eyes to release infection and stimulate circulation.

▶ Reflexology point:

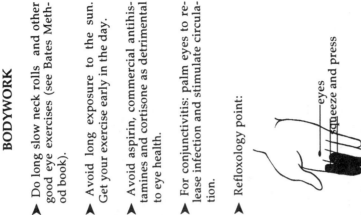

eyes — squeeze and press

Common Symptoms: ● Conjunctivitis: Inflammation of the eye and eyelid; pussy discharge; swollen, bloodshot eyes, with pain and sometimes blurred vision.
● Cataracts: Continuing lens opacity and gradual loss of vision.

Common Causes: ● Conjunctivitis: Allergic reaction from irritating fumes from chemicals, smoke or pollutants; infection from eye injury.
● Cataracts: Free radical damage from heavy metal and environmental pollutants or ultra-violet rays; too much fat, sugar, salt and cholesterol in the diet; diabetes (See Diet For Diabetes Control in this book); poor circulation and/or constipation; liver malfunction; protein deficiency with poor enzyme activity.

CELLULITE

When the body's circulation and elimination process become impaired, connective tissue loses its strength. Unmetabolized fats and wastes become trapped in the vulnerable cells just beneath the skin instead of being expelled through normal means. Over a period of time these waste materials harden and form the puckering, distorted skin effect we know as cellulite. When regular fat is squeezed the skin appears smooth - cellulitic skin will ripple like an orange peel, or have the texture of cottage cheese. Because it is unattached material, dieting and exercise alone are not able to dislodge cellulite. An effective program for cellulite release should be in four parts: 1) Stimulate the body's elimination function. 2) Increase circulation and metabolism. 3) Control excess fluid retention. 4) Re-establish connective tissue elasticity.

FOOD THERAPY

🍃 Follow a diet high in complex carbohydrates. Eat plenty of fresh unrefined foods. Reduce fats. Eat light, easily-digested foods.
   ♣ Eat only fruits and fruit juices un- til noon. Use only poly or mono-unsaturated oils.
   ♣ Avoid all fried and fatty foods.

🍃 Take Crystal Star LIV-ALIVE TEA™ or carrot/beet/cucumber juice, to clean the liver so it can metabolize fats better. Avoid heavy caffeine, carbonated drinks, and oxalic-acid-forming foods that cause liver malfunction.

🍃 Graze - eat smaller, more frequent meals, instead of 2 to 3 large ones.

🍃 See "COOKING FOR HEALTHY HEALING" by Linda Rector-Page for a complete cellulite diet.

🍃 Don't smoke. It impedes both circulation and metabolism.

VITAMINS/MINERALS

▶ Apply Natureworks SILICA GEL as directed.

▶ Solaray CENTELLA or CENTELLA VEIN caps. ♀

▶ Enzymatic Therapy CELL-U-VAR program as directed. ♀

▶ Carnitine 500mg. daily.
   with
   Bio-tec AGELESS BEAUTY tabs to dissolve and flush rancid fats and waste material.

▶ Effective liver aids to help metabolize fats:
   ♣ High potency lipotropics.
   ♣ High Omega 3 flax or fish oils.
   ♣ Rainbow Light TRIM-ZYME.
   ♣ Source Naturals SUPER AMINO NIGHT tabs.

▶ Esteem Plus 1 daily at lunch as directed.

▶ Body Essentials SILICA GEL internally 1 TB. in 3 oz. liquid and externally on problem areas.

HERBAL THERAPY

🌿 Effective herbs for cellulite:
   ◆ Bilberry caps or extract for bioflavonoids.
   ◆ Gotu kola extract to normalize connective tissue integrity.
   ◆ Bladderwrack to stimulate thyroid function and tone tissue.
   ◆ Kola nut to potentiate lipolysis.
   ◆ Butcher's broom to increase circulation.

🌿 Crystal Star CEL-LEAN™ capsules, 3 daily, before meals.
   with
   META-TABS capsules if there is a lazy thyroid.

🌿 Apply Yerba Prima VIVALO cream to trouble spots daily.

🌿 Apply Care Plus H2O2 OXYGEL gel to fatty areas. (In some cases the fat globules will release coming out through the skin in little white bumps.)

🌿 Evening Primrose oil caps 4 daily as essential fatty acids.
   with
   Crystal Star HOT SEAWEED BATH™ to stimulate circulation and potentiate lipolysis.

BODYWORK

The best approach is prevention. Maintain a slim subcutaneous fat layer by keeping the body slender and toned.

▶ Massage. Massage. From periphery towards the heart. Use a dry skin brush, loofa or ayate cloth to stimulate lymph glands.

▶ Regular aerobic exercise can help by toning tissue and maintaining underlying tissue integrity. An hour's walk every day, especially after a large meal is excellent.

▶ Crystal Star TIGHTENING & TONING BODY WRAP™, a rapid inch-loss treatment for firmer, smoother skin.
   and/or
   CEL-LEAN™ gel, tea or wafers for follow up and trouble spots.

▶ Reflexology point:

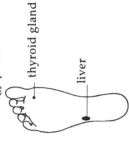

thyroid gland

liver

Common Symptoms: Lumps, bumps and "cottage cheese" around thighs, hips and love handles; trapped waste and fluid in pockets beneath the skin; tightness, heaviness in the legs; soreness and tenderness when tissue is massaged.
Common Causes: Poor quality nutrition resulting in liver exhaustion, resulting in reduced metabolism of fats - which are then often thrown off as lumpy "chicken fat". Inadequate exercise; insufficient water intake; increased/imbalanced hormonal activity; crash dieting with usual rapid regain of weight; some drugs that imbalance body processes.

CEREBRAL PALSY

Cerebral palsy is a broad term for brain-centered motor disorders which usually appear at birth or during early childhood. This type of palsy is characterized by a loss of control over voluntary muscles and abrupt, jerking, muscle contractions.

FOOD THERAPY

🍃 Eat organically grown foods as much as possible. Include plenty of leafy greens in the diet with a fresh salad every day.

🍃 Take a potassium broth every other day for 3 months (pg. 53). Go on a cleansing juice fast one day a week until symptoms improve (usually 3-4 months).

🍃 No refined foods, saturated fats, red meats, fried or fatty foods, caffeine or canned foods.

🍃 Make a mix of 2 TBS. each of the following. Take some daily.
   ♣ Brewer's yeast
   ♣ Lecithin
   ♣ Wheat germ

🍃 A modified macrobiotic diet is effective. See pg. 52 in this book, and "COOKING FOR HEALTHY HEALING" by Linda Rector-Page for a complete daily diet.

VITAMINS/MINERALS

▶ Twin Lab CSA for spinal/nerve pain and tension.

▶ B Complex 150mg. daily, **and** Lexon SUPREME B BLEND inositol cocktail powder for muscle atrophy.♂ or Twin Lab CHOLINE/INOSITOL caps. ♀

▶ Phosphatidyl choline or Egg Yolk Lecithin 6 daily. ♂

▶ Effective anti-oxidants:
   ✤ Octacosonal 1000mg. 4 daily
   ✤ Vit. E 400IU 3 x daily
   ✤ CoQ 10 30mg. daily

▶ Country Life RELAXER (GABA with Taurine) ♀

▶ Tyrosine 500mg. daily for L-Dopa formation.

▶ Magnesium 800mg. for better muscle/nerve coordination.

HERBAL THERAPY

🌿 Crystal Star RELAX CAPS™ 2-4 daily as needed for tension. and/or ANTI-SPZ™ capsules or CRAMP BARK COMBO™ extract. with

🌿 Evening primrose oil caps 6 daily.

🌿 Crystal Star SYSTEM STRENGTH™ drink for stability and alkalinity.

🌿 Effective herbal anti-oxidants:
   ✦ Rosemary
   ✦ Chaparral
   ✦ Care Plus H2O2 OXYGEL applied to affected muscle areas.

🌿 Ginkgo biloba extract *and/or* Hawthorne extract 3 to 4x daily.

🌿 An effective tea: One part each of gotu kola, bilberry, ginger, butcher's broom and lady slipper.

BODYWORK

▶ Stay away from all pesticides.

▶ Use hot and cold hydrotherapy to stimulate circulation.

▶ Continuing massage of the muscles is a key deterrent to atrophy.

▶ Reflexology point:

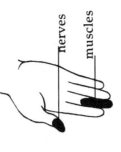
nerves
muscles

Common Symptoms: A muscle-nerve disorder with spastic and uncontrollable muscle movement; often atrophy of the muscles.
Common Causes: Hereditary through drug abuse or over-use in the mother; clogged motor control centers in different locations in the brain, malnutrition as an infant; heavy metal poisoning; nerve malfunction through deficient prostaglandin formation.

CERVICAL DYSPLASIA ▨ CERVICAL CARCINOMA
Condyloma Acuminata (Genital Warts) ◇ HPV (Human Papilloma Virus)

Pre-cancerous, abnormal tissue lesions of the cervix, both dysplasia and carcinoma, are a growing, serious problem in America. Both conditions seem to be the result of risky life-style habits and reduced immunity from poor nutrition. Early age of first intercourse, multiple sexual partners increasing sexually transmitted diseases, such as *herpes simplex type 2* and *papilloma viruses*, lower socio-economic class with its traditionally nutrient-poor diet, smoking, and oral contraceptives, are all considered to be high risk factors for this type of disease. Natural treatments deal with the causes of genital warts and require strong commitment and significant lifestyle changes, with positive outlook and good body / mind connection for immune support.

FOOD THERAPY

Nutrition intake must be optimized for there to be any permanent improvement - especially after the long courses of anti-biotics commonly given as the medical approach.

❧ Follow a cancer-preventing macrobiotic diet, pg. 52.
♦ Increase fresh fruits, vegetables (especially cruciferous, green and orange veggies), and complex carbohydrates as protective factors.

❧ Avoid red meat and poultry foods. These may have been contaminated with estrogens or other hormone treatments.

❧ Reduce dietary fat, again especially from animal foods. Reduce caffeine, hard liquor and processed foods.

❧ Add vegetable juices and/or green drinks (pg. 53-55ff.) for immune support and supplementing vitamin deficiencies.

❧ Add 2 TBS. chopped sea vegetables as a viable source of marine carotene. Add fish for omega 3 oils.

VITAMINS/MINERALS

Supplementation should concentrate on strengthening against deficiencies caused by oral contraceptives that can cause cell abnormalities, and smoking.

▶ Take daily:
♦ Marine carotene or beta-carotene 200,000IU.
♦ Folic acid 800mcg. 2x during treatment, then 1x daily.
♦ Ascorbate vitamin C 3000mg.
♦ Vitamin B₆ up to 200mg.
♦ Vit. B₁₂ SL, or ENER-B internasal gel.

▶ Increase immune support:
♦ Sun CHLORELLA or Green Foods GREEN MAGMA, two packets daily.
♦ Zinc picolinate 30mg. daily.
♦ Vitamin E400IU w. selenium 200mcg. 2x daily.

▶ Quercetin with bromelain 2 daily with Pycnogenol OPC 85 2 daily.

▶ Apply Pro. Serv. PRO-GEST CREAM or oil as directed.

HERBAL THERAPY

❦ Crystal Star ANTI-VI™ EXTRACT and/or TEA.
or
Crystal Star DETOX™ capsules for one month as a blood cleanser, followed by ANTI-VI™ or ECHINACEA 100% extract, and a course of vaginal packs.

❦ Burdock tea, 2 cups daily.

❦ Highest potency royal jelly 2 teasp. daily.

❦ Evening primrose oil capsules, 6 daily.

❦ Golden seal/chaparral suppositories (powders mixed with coca butter).

❦ Crystal Star CALCIUM SOURCE™ caps or extract to prevent pre-cancerous lesions from becoming cancerous.

BODYWORK

High-risk life style factors must be eliminated for there to be permanent improvement and prevention of further invasive lesions. Recurrence often occurs after standard surgery alone.

▶ Eliminate smoking, the use of oral contraceptives and multiple sexual partners.

▶ Surgery may be avoided by using *botanical vaginal packs*, such as Crystal Star DIRECT (special order only), grapefruit seed extract, Body Essentials SILICA GEL, or chlorella, placed against the cervix to draw out toxic wastes and slough abnormal cells. *Abstain from sexual intercourse during vag pack treatment.* See Appendix for a pack you can make yourself.

▶ Use a barrier contraceptive to prevent new contact with HPV or herpes viruses.

▶ Alternating hot and cold hydrotherapy or sitz baths will promote immune activity to the pelvic area.

Common Symptoms: Sexually transmitted disease, resulting in a class 4 Pap smear; heavy painful periods; bleeding between periods; pain during intercourse; genital warts or herpes; chronic gonorrhea or any unusual vaginal discharge; fever and the need to urinate more frequently; infertility.
Common Causes: Early age of first intercourse; frequent abortions; multiple sexual partners; *herpes simplex type 2* and *papilloma viruses*; lower socio-economic class with its traditionally nutrient-poor diet; early start/continued smoking; vit. A, Beta-carotene, C, B₆ deficiency; exposure to environmental carcinogens; long-term oral contraceptive use. Low grade bacterial infection.

CHICKEN POX

This is usually a childhood disease, lasting from seven to ten days. One bout of chicken pox provides immunity against recurrence for the rest of your life.

FOOD THERAPY

🍃 Take 2 lemons in water with a little honey every 4 hours to flush the system of toxins and clean the kidneys.

🍃 Stay on a liquid diet for the first 3 days of infection, with plenty of fruit and vegetable juices. Then have a raw foods diet, some apples, bananas, yogurt, avocados and a fresh salad daily for the rest of the week.

🍃 Avoid all dairy products except a little yogurt or kefir cheese. ☺

🍃 Dab honey or wheat germ oil on scabs to heal and prevent infection. ☺

VITAMINS/MINERALS

▶ Beta carotene 25,000IU.

▶ Ascorbate vitamin C or Ester C crystals, $\frac{1}{4}$ teasp. every 2-3 hours to bowel tolerance, to flush the tissues, relieve itching, and neutralize the viral activity. ☺

▶ Take vitamin E internally 400IU daily. Apply oil to scabs.

▶ Use Nutribiotic GRAPEFRUIT SEED EXTRACT spray to control infection and heal sores.

▶ Apply Home Health SCAR-GO
or
Enzymatic Therapy DERMA-ZYME OINTMENT to heal scars.

▶ Zinc 30mg. 2x daily for a month after disease has run its course to re-establish immunity.

▶ Raw thymus glandular to encourage the production of T-lymphocytes.

HERBAL THERAPY

🌿 Crystal Star THERA-DERM™ tea & wash. Take internally, and apply with cotton balls to lesions.
and
Apply LYSINE & LICORICE GEL to sores.

🌿 Apply B & T CALIFLORA gel as needed. ☺

🌿 Take cayenne/lobelia caps every 3 to 4 hours.

🌿 Apply a golden seal/ myrrh solution
or
A strong tea of yellow dock, burdock and golden seal every 4 hours.

🌿 Effective topicals applications:
♦ Royal jelly
♦ Comfrey salve
♦ Aloe vera gel
♦ St. John's wort salve

🌿 Apply Advanced Research PAU DE ARCO GEL frequently if sores become infected.

🌿 Apply fresh comfrey leaf compresses to sores.

BODYWORK

▶ Use a catnip enema twice during acute stage to clean out toxins. ☺

▶ Effective baths for skin itching and healing:
→ Peppermint/ginger
→ Cider vinegar/sea salt
→ Oatmeal
→ Ginger
Note: Wet compresses may be applied often with any of the above to control itching.

▶ No aspirin. It has been linked to Reye's syndrome, a rare but deadly disease that can afflict children after bouts of chicken pox or some types of flu. It also tends to aggravate sores.

▶ Apply Care Plus OXYGEL to sores.

Common Symptoms: Mild fever and headache, with small blister-type lesions all over the body that erupt, crust and leave a small scar. The blisters and scabs are highly infective. Keep the child isolated from other children, frail elderly people or those who have never had chicken pox.
Common Causes: A viral infection, usually allowed to become virulent by reduced immunity from a poor diet - too many sugars, sweets, refined carbohydrates, and mucous-forming foods; lack of green vegetables.

176

HIGH SERUM CHOLESTEROL

Low Density Lipoproteins ✧ High Triglygerides

Cholesterol is a fat-related substance in the body that is needed by the body for nerve, hormone, and cell function. Abnormal metabolism and over-indulgence in high cholesterol foods leads to serious deposits in arterial linings, and to gallstones. There are two kinds of cholesterol. HDL (high density lipo-protein, or good) cholesterol, LDL/VLDL (low density and very low density lipo-proteins, or bad) cholesterol. Triglycerides are a related type of blood fat that travels with cholesterol as lipo-proteins. High triglycerides can cause blood cells to stick together, impairing circulation and leading to heart attack or stroke.

FOOD THERAPY

Vegetarians who occasionally eat eggs and small amounts of low fat dairy are at the lowest risk for arterial or heart disease.

☙ A low fat, high fiber diet is the key to reducing cholesterol. Reducing sugar is the key to lowering triglycerides. See the Healthy Heart Diet in this book; or "COOKING FOR HEALTHY HEALING" by Linda Rector Page for a complete daily diet.

☙ Foods that lower cholesterol: olive and unsaturated oils, whole grains and soluble fiber foods, soy foods fresh fruits and vegetables, yogurt and cultured foods, wheat germ, brewer's yeast.

☙ Cholesterol in foods such as eggs is not the culprit. (Eggs are a whole food, with phosphatides to balance the cholesterol.) The prime contributor to high blood cholesterol levels is saturated fat and over-eating. Concentrate on substantially reducing animal fats, red meats, fried foods, high fat dairy foods, salt, sugar, and refined foods in your diet.

☙ Eat smaller meals, especially at night. A little wine with dinner reduces stress and raises HDLs.

VITAMINS/MINERALS

▶ If dietary means have not been successful, use niacin therapy to reduce *all blood fats and benefit nerves. (Do not use if glucose intolerant, have liver disease or a peptic ulcer.)*
   ✦ 1500mg. daily ♂
   ✦ 1000mg. daily ♀
   ✦ Bio-Resource LO-NIACIN with glycine 500mg. if sugar sensitive.
          or

▶ Niacin-bound chromium, as Solaray CHROMIACIN or CHROMEMATE to regulate sugar use.

▶ Sun CHLORELLa tabs 10-20 daily.

▶ Beta carotene 100,000IU daily.

▶ Lipotropics to enhance the liver:
   ♣ Nutrapathic FAT METABOLIZER capsules as directed.
   ♣ Solaray LIPOTROPIC 1000.
   ♣ Omega 3 flax seed or fish oil
   ♣ Vitamin E 400IU, 2x daily. ♀
   ♣ Arginine 1000mg. daily (unless you have herpes or EBV). ♂

▶ Ester C w. bioflavs. 2000mg. daily.

▶ Golden Pride ORAL CHELATION THERAPY, 1 cap 2x daily. ♂
          and
   Carnitine 500mg. daily.

HERBAL THERAPY

☙ Guggulipids 500mg. w. 25mg. guggulsterone 3x daily to reduce both LDL, VLDL, and triglyceride levels.

☙ Crystal Star CHO-LO FIBER TONE™ drink mix, 2 TBS. in water morning and evening. and/or CHOL-EX™ capsules, 3 daily for 2 months.

☙ Crystal Star HEARTSEASE/ CIRCU-CLENSE™ tea, and hawthorne extract 2 to 3x daily.

☙ Source Naturals MEGA GLA or evening primrose oil 4 daily. ♀

☙ Solaray TURMERIC extract tabs.

☙ To raise HDL's:
   ✦ Alfalfa seed powder
   ✝ Brewer's yeast

☙ To lower LDL/triglyceride levels:
   ✦ Reishi mushroom capsules
   ✦ Suma
   ✦ Ginger rt.
   ✦ American or Chinese ginseng
   ✦ Garlic 6 tabs daily. ♂

☙ Activated charcoal tablets 3 daily with meals.

BODYWORK

Accurate lipoprotein and cholesterol fractions testing is available, and is worthwhile as a means of monitoring your progress as you make life style improvements.
Ideal cholesterol levels should be from 140 to 165 mg/dl, with LDL cholesterol from 30 to 50 mg/dl, and HDL cholesterol from 80 to 90 mg/dl. (Over 244 is an ideal heart attack victim; 210 is the average American level.)
Ideal triglyceride levels should be around 200 to 240 mg/dl. Every one percent increase in blood cholesterol translates into a two percent increase in heart disease risk.

▶ Eliminate tobacco use of all kinds. Nicotine raises cholesterol levels.

▶ Reduce your body weight. Most overweight people have abnormal metabolism and biochemistry. **If your are 10 pounds overweight, your body produces an extra 100mg. of cholesterol every day.**

▶ Take a brisk daily walk or other regular aerobic exercise of your choice to enhance circulation.

▶ Practice a favorite stress reduction technique at least once a day.

Common Symptoms: Plaque formation on the artery walls; poor circulation; leg cramps and pain; high blood pressure; difficult breathing; cold hands and feet; dry skin and hair; palpitations; lethargy; dizziness; allergies and kidney trouble.
Common Causes: Stress; diet high in saturated fats, low in soluble fiber; EFA deficiency.

CHRONIC FATIGUE SYNDROME
Epstein-Barr Virus

Although some of the defining characteristics of CFS and EBV are different, they are both the result of disordered immune function which allows yeast infections, allergies, and virus activity. While protocols vary, current thinking states that chronic fatigue syndrome is due to a chronic infection from the Epstein Barr virus - a common, latent virus in humans that replicates and becomes active when normal immune response is compromised. Support and enhancement of immune system function is the key to reducing susceptibility and achieving resistance and remission. A recent survey has indicated that vitamins, minerals and other natural therapies are more helpful than prescription drugs in rebuilding immune response and overcoming these diseases. Concentration should be on system detoxification, enhancing liver function and immune support.

FOOD THERAPY

Keep the diet at least 50% fresh foods during intensive healing time.

🍃 A highly nutritious diet must be maintained. Emphasize foods that build immunity. Include often:
♣ defense foods, such as cruciferous vegetables
♣ antibody forming foods, such as onions and garlic
♣ oxygenating foods, such as wheat germ;
♣ high mineral foods, such as sea vegetables and whole grains;
♣ soluble fiber foods, such as prunes and bran;
♣ cultured foods, such as yogurt and miso;
♣ protein foods, such as seafood, fish and whole grains.

🍃 Take a protein drink every morning such as Nature's Plus ENERGY DRINK, or an alkalizing enzyme therapy drink such as Crystal Star SYSTEM STRENGTH™ drink each day for a month.

🍃 Avoid acid-forming, allergen-prone and body stressing foods like junk and fast foods. Eliminate caffeine, red wine, refined sugars, cheese and processed foods.

🍃 Immune defense cells are created in bone marrow. Keep new cell development strong with vegetable proteins, B vitamins (esp. B12 and folic acid) and oxygen.

VITAMINS/MINERALS

▶ Effective anti-oxidants:
✦ Germanium 150mg. SL
✦ CoQ 10 30mg. 3x daily.
✦ Vit. E 400IU w. selenium 200mcg.
✦ Chlorella 20 tabs daily.
✦ Pycnogenol 30mg. 3x daily.

▶ Vitamin C or Ester C crystals with bioflavonoids, 1/4 teasp. every half hour to bowel tolerance to flush the tissues and act as an anti-viral agent for 10 days. Then reduce to 3-5000mg. daily. *with* Marine carotene 100,000IU daily.

▶ Effective energizers:
✦ Country Life DMG SL tabs
✦ Ener B12 internasal gel
✦ Biotec CELL GUARD tablets.
✦ Am. Biologics DIOXYCHLOR w. taurine tablets.

▶ Raw Lymph complex, and/or Raw Thymus SL *with* Biotin 1000mcg. for immune stimulation.
with
Tyrosine 500mg. daily. ♀

▶ Magnesium 500mg. daily with Grapefruit Seed extract capsules.

▶ Natren LIFE START 2, or Dr. DOL-PHILUS as a liver detoxifier, with evening primrose oil caps, 4 daily.

▶ Bromelain 500mg. daily with Future Biotics VITAL K. ♂

HERBAL THERAPY

🌿 Ginkgo biloba extract as needed.

🌿 Crystal Star ADR ACTIVE™ caps or extract, with BODY REBUILD-ER™ caps.
and
ANTI-VI™ extract or tea.
and
LIV-ALIVE™caps or LIV-ALIVE™ tea for the first 3 months of healing.

🌿 Crystal Star SUPER LICORICE™ w. an herbal source potassium

🌿 Effective extracts:
◆ Licorice rt.
◆ Echinacea
◆ Hawthorne lf. and flwr.
◆ Siberian ginseng

🌿 Effective liver detoxifiers:
◆ Bupleurum
◆ Milk thistle extract

🌿 Immune building herbs:
◆ Schizandra bry.
◆ Astragalus
◆ Golden seal/myrrh
◆ Reishi mushroom
◆ Pau de arco

🌿 Effectiv anti-viral herbs:
◆ St. John's wort
◆ Lomatium, 10 drops 3x daily.

🌿 Anti-fungal herbs:
◆ Black walnut
◆ Garlic capusles

BODYWORK

▶ Take a daily deepbreathing walk for tissue oxygen uptake. Walk at least twenty minutes to stimulate lymphatic system and cerebral circulation.

▶ Rub Care Plus OXY GEL onto soles of the feet for nascent oxygen. Alternate daily use, one week on and one week off. Too much reactivates symptoms. A little is great; act is not.

▶ Get some early morning sunlight on the body every day possible for vitamin D.

▶ Relax. An optimistic mental attitude and frame of mind play a major role in releasing the body from stress, a big factor in lowered immunity. **Remember that immune stimulation itself has an anti-viral effect.**

▶ Stretching exercises and massage will cleanse the lymph system and enhance oxygenation. Use hot and cold alternating hydrotherapy to stimulate circulation.

▶ Avoid tobacco in all forms. Nicotine destroys immunity. It takes 3 months to rebuild immune response even after you quit.

▶ Overheating therapy is effective in controlling and overcoming Epstein-Barr Virus. See Airola "HOW TO GET WELL" for this technique.

DIAGNOSIS INFORMATION FOR CONTROLLING CHRONIC FATIGUE & EBV

As increasing mental, emotional and physical stresses occur in our environment, susceptibility to chronic viral infections has become more and more prevalent.

Natural healers and therapists have now been working with Chronic Fatigue Syndrome and EBV for several years. These problems are quite difficult to diagnose and treat because they represent a degenerative imbalance in the endocrine system, and metabolism of the entire body. A number of important things should be recognized to achieve successful and effective control over this condition:

1) Chronic fatigue syndromes act like recurring systemic viral infections. These viruses often go undetected because their symptoms mimic simple illnesses like colds, flu, or acute but less debilitating mononucleosis. Following the acute stages these viruses penetrate the nuclei of immune system T-cells where they seem to be able to survive and replicate indefinitely. Multiplication of the virus and recurring symptoms appear with a rupturing of the organism and its release into the bloodstream. This can occur at any time, but almost always arises when the person is under stress or has reduced immune response due to a simpler illness such as a cold or cough.

2) Chronic Fatigue and EBV take longer to overcome than Candida or Herpes Virus. The symptoms are similar but the viral activity is more virulent and debilitating to the immune system, and entrenchment in the glands and organs is more deep seated. It takes two to four weeks to notice consistent improvement, and three to six months or even longer to feel energetic and normal. However, most people do respond to natural therapies in three to six months. Many achieve near normal functioning in two years even though the virus may persist in the body.

3) **Symptoms are greatly reduced by aerobic exercise. Even light stretching, shiatzu exercises, or short walks are noticeably effective when they are done regularly every day.**

4) A good diet is of prime importance in keeping the body clear of toxic wastes and balancing the lymphatic system. Drink plenty of fresh liquids, and clear the bowels daily.

5) **Like Candida, Chronic Fatigue Syndrome and EBV are serious, but be gentle with yourself. Don't get so wound up in the strictness of your program that it further depresses you and takes over your life. It is clear in almost every case that people who learn to identify and manage mental, emotional and physical stress in their lives recover fastest.**

6) The outward symptoms for chronic fatigue conditons are similar to mononucleosis, AIDS, ARC, candidiasis, M.S., lupus, fibrocystis myalgia and other opportunistic disease. There are many AIDS-like symptoms, but CFS does not kill and tends to go into remission. However, like AIDS it can be passed through bodily fluids. Do not kiss on the mouth. Do not feed table scraps to pets. Wear a condom during intercourse. Do not donate your blood. When having lab testing, notify lab personnel to take precautions. It is always best to be tested for viral titers that measure your body's reaction to the virus, or elevated levels of EBV anti-bodies so that your treatment will be correct.

7) No conventional medical treatment or drugs on the market today help this condition, and most hinder immune response and recovery.

CRITERIA FOR CHRONIC FATIGUE SYNDROME

A) Persistent, debilitating fatigue in a person who has no previous history of similar symptoms, that does not resolve with bed rest, and that is severe enough to reduce and impair average daily activity below 50% percent of normal for that person for at least 6 months.
B) Other conditions with similar symptoms have been excluded through examination and testing.
C) The following symptoms should be evident on at least two occasions within a two month period: ○ Low grade fever; ○ throat infections without pus; ○ sore lymph nodes in the armpit and neck.

Common Symptoms: ●First symptoms: Recurrent sore throat; low grade fever; lymph node swelling; headache and aching muscles and joints; sleep disorders; fatigue which rest does not help; poor digestion; lethargy; classic flu or mononucleosis symptoms.
●Second symptoms: Ringing in the ears; exhaustion; chronic depression and irritability; fogginess, spaciness and muddled thinking; low grade infection and fever; moodiness; diarrhea; sharper muscle aches and weakness; vertigo.
●Third symptoms: Extreme fatigue; herpes; aching ears and eyes; weakened immune response; paranoia; chronic exhaustion; weight loss and loss of appetite; MS-like nerve disorder.

Common Causes: CFS develops from EBV and other opportunistic viruses that attack a weakened immune system, particularly if there is a history of mononucleosis and/or yeast related problems; emotional stress; environmental pollutants causing chemical sensitivities; smoking; widespread antibiotic or cortico-steroids that lower immunity; a low nutrition diet that depletes magnesium and other vitamins and minerals; low levels of cortisol, an immune-stimulating hormone that is secreted in response to stress.

POOR CIRCULATION

Sluggish circulation can stem from many body conditions, and is itself one of the first signs of serious disorder. High blood pressure, arterioscleriosis, varicose veins, Reynaud's disease, phlebitis, and heart disease are all connected with circulatory system health. Investigate further if your condition does not improve.

FOOD THERAPY

🍃 Keep the colon clear and your cholesterol down with a high fiber diet; at least 60% fresh foods.

🍃 Make the following drink; take some daily for almost immediate improvement:
1/2 cup tomato juice,
1/2 cup lemon juice,
6 teasp. wheat germ oil
1 teasp. brewer's yeast.

🍃 Avoid red meats, fried and fatty foods, excess caffeine and salts, refined foods, and sugar.

🍃 Citrus fruits, juices and dried fruits have good bioflavonoid content to strengthen vein and tissue walls.

🍃 See the Healthy Heart Diet in this book, or "COOKING FOR HEALTHY HEALING" by Linda Rector-Page for a complete circulatory improvement diet.

🍃 Eat smaller meals more often. Avoid large or heavy meals.

VITAMINS/MINERALS

▶ Carnitine 500mg. 2x daily.
with
Vitamin B₁₂ SL, or Ener-B B₁₂ internasal gel every 3 days.
and
Golden Pride ORAL CHELATION therapy, 1 cap 2x daily. ♂

▶ Niacin therapy: 250mg. 3-4x daily, with PABA 500mg. 2 x daily.
or
Solaray CHROMIACIN capsules 2 x daily. ♂

▶ Key anti-oxidants:
♣ Pycnogenol 50mg. 2x daily.
♣ Germanium 100mg. 2x daily.
♣ CoQ 10 30mg. daily.
♣ Solaray TRI O2 capsules.

▶ High Omega 3 flax or fish oils 3x daily. ♀

▶ Vit. E w/ Selenium 400IU daily.
and
Ester C with bioflavonoids 500mg., 2 tabs 3x daily.

▶ B Complex 100mg. with extra B6 250mg. 2x daily.

▶ FutureBiotics VITAL K 3 teasp. daily.

HERBAL THERAPY

🌿 Ginkgo biloba extract 2-3x daily or as needed, especially for cold hands and feet.

🌿 Butcher's broom caps or tea as a naural blood thinner. (Use on a temporary basis.)

🌿 Crystal Star HEARTSEASE/ HAWTHORNE™ capsules and hawthorne or ginkgo biloba extract; ♀ or a few drops of Crystal Star RECOVERY TONIC™ in water. ♂
and/or
HEARTSEASE/CIRCU-CLIENSE™ tea daily.

🌿 Effective herbal stimulants:
♦ Cayenne/ginger caps 4 daily.
♦ Siberian ginseng extract ♂
♦ Bilberry extract daily. ♂

🌿 Effective teas:
♦ Crystal Star MEDITATION™
♦ Crystal Star ROYAL MU™
♦ Kukicha twig or Crystal Star GREEN TEA CLEANSER™
♦ Pau de Arco

🌿 Ginseng Co. CYCLONE CIDER as needed.

🌿 For Reynaud's Syndrome, use Solaray GINK-ALERT caps.

BODYWORK

▶ Apply alternating hot and cold cayenne/ginger compresses to areas in need of stimulation. Or wrap feet in towels soaked in cayenne/ginger solution.

▶ Use a dry skin brush over the body before your daily shower.

▶ See a chiropractor or massage therapist for a structure workout to clear any obstructions and open energy pathways.

▶ Take a brisk aerobic walk every day to get your blood moving.

▶ Aromatherapy:
→ Juniper essential oil
→ Cajeput oil
→ Sage oil

▶ Apply Crystal Star CELLEAN™ gel as directed.

▶ Biofeedback has been notably successful for cold hands and feet.

Common Symptoms: Cold hands and feet; poor memory; migraine headaches; numbness; ringing in the ears and hearing loss; dizziness when standing quickly; shortness of breath; high triglyceride and cholesterol levels; varicose veins.
Common Causes: Cholesterol plaque on artery walls; constipation; lack of exercise; toxic or obstructed system.

CIRRHOSIS of the LIVER

Cirrhosis, or scarring, of the liver tissue is a serious, degenerative condition, preventing the liver from its proper function. Usually a consequence of excess alcohol consumption, it is also almost always a part of other severe liver infections, such as hepatitis, EBV, and AIDS related syndromes. If the diet is also low in nutrition, the liver becomes exhausted, and even more serious debilitation results.

FOOD THERAPY

A continuing optimum nutrition diet is the key to liver regeneration.

- Take a carrot/beet/cucumber juice daily for 1 week, then every other day for a week, the every 2 days, then every 3 days, etc. for a month to detoxify the liver.
  Then take a glass of lemon juice and water each morning, and follow a diet for Hypoglycemia. (See HYPOGLYCEMIA pages in this book, or "COOKING FOR HEALTHY HEALING" by Linda Rector-Page.)

- Include two glasses of carrot juice daily for at least a month during healing. Eat plenty of fresh fruits and vegetables. Particularly eat vegetable protein, such as sprouts whole grains, tofu, wheat germ, and brewer's yeast.

- Avoid all alcohol, fried, salty or fatty foods, caffeine, refined sugar and tobacco.

- Add 2 teasp. each to the daily diet:
  ◆ Lecithin
  ◆ Brewer's yeast
  ◆ Wheat germ oil

VITAMINS/MINERALS

- **Carnitine 500mg. 2x daily.**

- **Choline 600mg., or choline/inositol daily to prevent fat accumulation in the liver.**

- Enzymatic Therapy LIVA-TOX.

- Natren LIFE START II, 3 x daily to clean and restore liver tissue.
  with
  Beta-carotene 100,000IU daily
  and
  Ascorbate vit. C crystals 5000mg. daily or to bowel tolerance.

- Effective anti-oxidants:
  ◆ Vit. E 400IU with selenium 100mg. 2 x daily.
  ◆ B15 sublingual, 1 daily.
  ◆ Nature's Plus Germanium w. Suma 1 daily.
  ◆ CoQ10 50mg. 3x daily.

- Branched-Chain Aminos to heal scarring and inflammation, and to promote weight loss, 2 tablets before meals.

- Effective lipotropics:
  ◆ Solaray LIPOTROPIC 1000.
  ◆ Methionine 2 x daily.
  ◆ Lecithin capsules 2 daily.

HERBAL THERAPY

- ❦ Crystal Star LIV-ALIVE™ caps, or extract, and/or LIV-ALIVE™ tea (3 cups daily for 3 weeks, then 1 cup daily for a month.)
  or
  GREEN TEA CLEANSER™ daily for 3 to 6 months.

- ❦ Effective teas:
  ◆ Oregon grape root
  ◆ Dandelion root
  ◆ Hyssop

- ❦ Milk thistle capsules or extract 3 x daily.

- ❦ Sun CHLORELLA or Green Foods GREEN MAGMA granules, 1 packet daily.

- ❦ Make the following tea mix. Take 1 cup daily: bilberry, ginkgo biloba lf., ginger rt.

- ❦ George's ALOE VERA JUICE, 1 glass daily, with garlic capsules 4 daily.

- ❦ Crystal Star GINSENG 6 DEFENSE RESTORATIVE™ tea to help heal internal scarring.

BODYWORK

▶ Take a coffee enema once a week for a month to flush out and stimulate liver activity. (1 cup strong brewed in a quart of water), or chlorella or spirulina implants.

▶ Drink 6-8 glasses of pure water daily. Take an early morning sunbath whenever possible.

▶ Reflexology point:

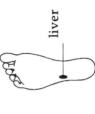

liver

▶ Liver area:

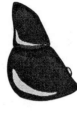

Common Symptoms: Sluggish, reduced energy; constipation alternating to diarrhea; often jaundice; skin itching/irritation; rings under the eyes. Severe symptoms include anemia and large bruise patches.
Common Causes: Liver toxicity from excess alcohol and/or drugs; excess refined foods and sugars; long term malnutrition.

COLDS ▦ UPPER RESPIRATORY INFECTION

Cough ◇ Sore Throat

A "cold" is usually an attempt by the body to cleanse itself of wastes, toxins and bacterial overgrowth that have built up to the point where natural immunity cannot handle or overcome them. The glands are always affected, and as the endocrine system is on a 6 day cycle, a normal "cold" usually runs for about a week as the body works through all its detoxification processes. Natural remedies are effective in speeding recovery and reducing discomfort. **See following pages for what to do for FLU.**

FOOD THERAPY

ᴥ If you have a cold:
Go on a liquid diet during the acute stage, with green drinks or potassium broth (pg. 53ff) to clean out infection and mucous.
Then eat light meals when fever and acute stage has passed - esp. fresh and steamed vegetables, fresh fruits and juices, and cultured foods for friendly intestinal flora.
Drink six to eight glasses of liquids daily to flush the kidneys.

ᴥ Take 2 TBS. cider vinegar, and 2 teasp. honey in water each morning. and
2 TBS. each lemon juice and honey with 1 teasp. fresh grated ginger at night.

ᴥ Crystal Star BIOFLAV., FIBER & C SUPPORT™ drink for nasal congestion - clears in 15 to 20 minutes.

ᴥ To release quantities of mucous all at once, take fresh grated horseradish in a spoon with lemon juice, and hang over the sink.

ᴥ To prevent a cold:
Keep immune response strong with a optimum nutrition, esp. during high risk seasons, plenty of rest and regular exercise.

VITAMINS/MINERALS

▶ **Ester C or ascorbic acid crystals -** 1/4 teasp. every half hour to bowel tolerance to flush the body and neutralize toxins. Use as a preventive as well, to decrease the length and severity and to boost immunity.

▶ **Low dose zinc lozenges** dissolved under the tongue to kill harmful throat bacteria.
with
CoQ 10mg. 3x daily.

▶ **Quercetin Plus 3x daily** for inflammation.

▶ Preventive supplements:
✦ Beta carotene 25,000IU 4x daily.
✦ Zinc 30mg. daily. ♂
✦ Garlic oil caps 6 daily.
✦ Vitamin E 400IU w. selenium.
✦ Acidophilus liq. 3 tsp. daily. ☺

▶ Nutribiotic **GRAPEFRUIT SEED EXTRACT** spray or gargle (3 drops in 5oz. water) to release mucous and phlegm and clear sinuses.

▶ Effective homeopathic remedies:
✦ Nu-Age COUGH
✦ Boiron OSCILLOCOCCINUM ☺
✦ **Eupatorium Perfoliatum** ☺
✦ Hylands C-PLUS ☺

▶ H₂O₂ nasal spray (make with several drops of 3% solution in 5 oz. water) to reduce congestion and clear sinuses.

HERBAL THERAPY

❦ During acute phase:
◆ Crystal Star FIRST AID CAPS™ every hour during acute stages to promote sweating and eliminate toxins. (Use as a preventive in initial stage.)
◆ Zand INSURE HERBAL extract and capsules and HERBAL LOZENGES every 2 hours.

❦ Crystal Star ANTI-BIO™ capsules and extract to flush the lymph glands as directed for 6 days.
with
COLD SEASON DEFENSE™ caps. and/or
CHILL CARE™ tea to warm, CO-FEX™ TEA as a throat coat. ☺

❦ Other effective teas:
◆ Horehound
◆ Coltsfoot
◆ Pau de arco

❦ Effective capsules:
◆ Cayenne/ginger
◆ Echinacea/golden seal
◆ Ephedra - a natural antihistamine to relieve post-nasal drip and phlegm without drowsiness.

❦ During recovery phase:
◆ Zand ASTRAGALUS extract.
◆ Crystal Star HERBAL DEFENSE TEAM™ extract or caps.

❦ Effective expectorants:
◆ Zand DECONGEST extract
◆ Crystal Star X-PECT-T™ ☺

BODYWORK

▶ Rest is important. Adequate sleep is necessary. Vigorous exercise stresses an already stressed body too much for continuing recovery.

▶ Open all channels of elimination with hot baths or showers, hot broths and tonics, (pg. 57ff.) brandy and lemon, and catnip enemas.

▶ Apply hot ginger compresses to the chest.

▶ Use eucalyptus steams or in a vaporizer to open sinus passages and quiet a cough.

▶ See a massage therapist to open up blocked body meridians.

▶ Avoid drug store cold remedies. They halt the body cleansing and balancing processes, and generally make the cold last longer.

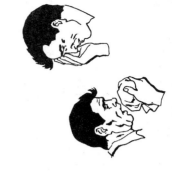

A WORD ABOUT THE CHRONIC COLD

Unfortunately, the common cold is quite common - a miserable condition indeed. There seem to be almost as many cold remedies as there are colds. As we have said, a cold is usually a cleansing condition, and sometimes it is just better to let this happen so your body can start fresh, with a stronger immune system. But it is hard to work, sleep, and be around other people with your misery and cold symptoms.

With this in mind, we have developed a quick cold check that has been successful at minimizing misery while your body gets on with its job of cleaning house.

1) Take a brisk daily walk to rev up the immune system, and get you out of the house into fresh air. A walk puts cleansing oxygen into the lungs, and stops you from feeling sorry for yourself. It works wonders!

2) Take plenty of ascorbate vitamin C or Ester C, preferably in powder form with juice, spread throughout the day. Take Zinc lozenges as needed, and other supplements of your choice.

3) No smoking or alcohol (other than a little brandy and lemon). They suppress immunity. Avoid refined flours, sugar, and pasteurized dairy foods. They increase production of thick mucous.

4) Eat lightly but with good nutrition. During an infection, nutrient absorption is less efficient. A vegetarian diet is the best at this time so the body won't have to work so hard at digestion.

5) Drink plenty of liquids; 6-8 glasses daily of fresh fruit and vegetable juices, herb teas, and water. These will help flush toxins through and out of the system.

6) Keep warm. Don't worry about a fever unless it is prolonged or very high. (See fevers as cleansers and healers) Take a long hot bath, spa or sauna. Lots of toxins can pass out though the skin. Increase room humidity so the mucous membranes will remain active against the virus or bacteria.

7) Stay relaxed. Let the body concentrate its energy on overcoming the cold. Go to bed early, and get plenty of sleep. Most regeneration of virus-damaged cells occurs between midnight and 4 a.m.

8) Think positively about becoming well. Optimism is often a self-fulfilling prophecy. ✣

DO YOU HAVE A COLD or THE FLU? HERE ARE THE DIFFERENCES.

Colds and flu are distinct and separate upper respiratory infections, triggered by different viruses. (Outdoor environment - drafts, wetness, temperature changes, etc. do not cause either of these illnesses.) The flu is more serious, because it can spread to the lungs, and cause severe bronchitis or pneumonia. In the beginning stages the symptoms can be very similar. Both colds and flu begin when viruses - (that, unlike bacteria, cannot reproduce outside the cells) - penetrate the body's protective barriers. Nose, eyes and mouth are usually the sites of invasion from cold viruses. The most likely target for the flu virus is the respiratory tract. Colds and flu respond to different treatments. The following symptomatic chart can help identify your particular condition and allow you to deal with it better.

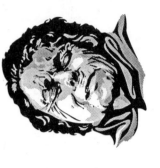

A Cold Profile Looks Like This:
✚ Slow onset.
✚ No prostration.
✚ Rarely accompanied by fever and headache.
✚ Localized symptoms such as hoarseness, listlessness, runny nose and sneezing.
✚ Mild fatigue and weakness as a result of body cleansing.
✚ Mild to moderate chest discomfort, usually with a hacking cough.
✚ Sore or burning throat common.

A Flu Profile Looks Like This:
❖ Swift and severe onset.
❖ Early and prominent prostration with flushed, hot, moist skin.
❖ Usually accompanied by high (102°-104°) fever, headache and sore eyes.
❖ General symptoms like chills, depression and body aches.
❖ Extreme fatigue, sometimes lasting 2-3 weeks.
❖ Acute chest discomfort, with severe hacking cough.
❖ Sore throat occasionally.

FLU ▦ VIRAL RESPIRATORY INFECTION

Flu infections are longer and stronger than colds. Flu treatment programs work best in a series of stages for complete recovery. ACUTE, or infective stage, either viral or bacterial, and including aches, chills, prostration, fever, sore throat, etc. This phase should be used for 2 to 4 days. RECUPERATION, or healing stage, to replenish the body's natural resistance. This phase should be followed for one to two weeks. MAINTENANCE, or immune support stage, to be used for two to three weeks, especially in high risk seasons. **See previous page for diagnosis information.**

FOOD THERAPY

ઍ During the acute stage: take only liquid nutrients - plenty of hot, steamy chicken soup, hot tonics and broths to stimulate mucous release (pg. 56ff). Plenty of vegetable juices and green drinks (pg. 54ff) to alkalize and rebuild the blood and immune system.

ઍ During the recuperation stage: follow a vegetarian, light "green" diet. Have a salad every day, cultured foods like yogurt and kefir for friendly flora replacement, and steamed vegetables with brown rice for strength. Crystal Star ENERGY GREEN™ drink mix to return body vitality and rebuild healthy blood. ♂

ઍ During maintenance and all stages: Avoid all refined foods, sugars, and pasteurized dairy foods. They increase mucous clogging and allow a place for the virus to live. Avoid alcohol and tobacco as immune suppressors. Avoid caffeine foods. They inhibit iron and zinc absorption. Crystal Star SYSTEM STRENGTH™ drink to alkalize the body and add concentrated food source minerals.

ઍ If you just can't seem to "get over it", make up 1 gallon of Crystal Star CLEANSING & FASTING™ tea, and take 5 to 6 cups daily *with* 12 to 15 FIBER & HERBS COLON CLEANSE™ capsules daily until the virus is removed.

VITAMINS/MINERALS

▶ Homeopathic remedies are excellent against the flu, because they can be so specific as to symptom.
✦ Boiron OSCILLOCOCCINUM
✦ B&T Alpha CF
✦ **BioForce INFLUAFORCE**
✦ Hylands remedies specific to individual symptoms of the flu. ☺

▶ During acute stage: Ester C or ascorbic acid crystals: $1/4$ teasp. every half hour to bowel tolerance to flush the body and neutralize toxins.
and

▶ Zinc lozenges dissolved under the tongue to deactivate virus activity in the throat, or zinc capsules 30mg.
or
Nutribiotic **GRAPEFRUIT SEED EXTRACT** spray.

▶ Effective anti-infective/antioxidants:
✦ Germanium 100mg.
✦ Beta carotene 100,000IU
✦ Food grade 3% H_2O_2 (1TB. in 8oz. water)
✦ Vitamin E 800IU daily.

▶ Effective maintenance:
✦ Raw Thymus tincture to build cell immunity.
✦ Professional Nutrition DR. DO-PHILUS in papaya juice. ☺
✦ CoQ 10, 10mg. 3 x daily.
✦ Iron with C 2 daily.
✦ Pantothenic acid for adrenal support.

HERBAL THERAPY

❦ During acute stage: Crystal Star ANTI-VI™ extract as needed several times daily, or ANTI-BIO™ extract or capsules every 2 hours til improvement is noticed.
with
CLEANSING & PURIFYING TEA™ or GREEN TEA CLEANSER™. ☺

❦ Crystal Star FIRST AID CAPS™ to raise body temperature and reduce virus multiplication.

❦ Ephedra tea to inhibit flu virus and induce sweating.

❦ Effective anti-viral extracts:
✦ **Echinacea angustifolia**
✦ St John's Wort
✦ Lomatium
✦ Osha Root ☺

❦ Effective recovery herbs:
✦ Calendula tea 4 cups daily.
✦ Astragalus capsules or extract
✦ Wisdom of the Ancients SYM-FRE tea.

❦ For maintenance and immune strength: Sun chlorella tabs or granules, Wakunaga KYOGREEN, or Green Foods GREEN MAGMA.

❦ Cayenne/bayberry capsules - to normalize gland activity.

BODYWORK

➤ During the acute stage: Get plenty of bed rest, so the body can concentrate on overcoming the virus.

➤ Gargle with a few drops of tea tree oil in water for sore throat.

➤ Use overheating therapy to overcome a flu virus. Take a hot sauna, spa, or bath to raise body temperature and increase circulation. Heat deactivates viruses.

➤ To begin the maintenance phase: Have a complete massage therapy treatment to cleanse remaining pockets of toxins, and clear body meridians. Plus it makes you feel so good again!

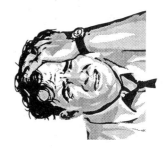

COLD SORES ■ CANKER SORES ■ FEVER BLISTERS ■ HERPES SIMPLEX

These mouth sores are quite common and indicate recurrent body chemistry imbalance, sometimes coupled with a hypothyroid condition. They are usually the result of a herpes simplex virus 1 infection, occurring after a fever, illness, body stress, and consequent reduced immunity. They can also be caused by food sensitivities, nutrient deficiencies, or hormone imbalance, such as before menses.

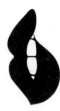

BODYWORK

➤ Apply Nutrition Resource NUTRIBIOTIC GRAPEFRUIT SEED EXTRACT SPRAY to sore as needed.

➤ Effective rinses to alter body and mouth pH:
→ Golden seal solution
→ Aloe vera juice
→ Echinacea solution
→ Golden seal/myrrh solution. Swish in mouth every 1/2 hour.

➤ Effective topical applications:
→ Care Plus OXYGEL
→ Crystal Star LYSINE/LICORICE GEL™
→ Black walnut tincture
→ Tea tree oil
→ Comfrey/aloe salve
→ Red raspberry tincture
→ B & T SSSTING STOP

➤ Apply ice packs frequently. Follow with vitamin E oil.

➤ Relax more. Get plenty of sleep and rest.

HERBAL THERAPY

❧ Take aloe vera juice internally. Apply aloe vera gel frequently.

❧ Crystal Star HRPS™ capsules 4-6 daily, to alkalize and heal.
and/or
THERA-DERM™ tea. Apply to sores. Drink 2 cups daily.

❧ Licorice extract - apply directly, take internally.

❧ Crystal Star RELAX CAPS™ as needed to calm the tension often causing sores. ♀

❧ Apply St. John's wort salve. Take St. John's wort capsules or Crystal Star ANTI-VI™ extract as anti-virals.

❧ Burdock tea 2 cups daily to balance hormones. ♀

❧ White Oak extract as an astringent. ♂

❧ Propolis lozenges - apply propolis extract directly, and take under the tongue.

VITAMINS/MINERALS

▶ Ascorbate vitamin C crystals with bioflavonoids: Take 1/4 teasp. every 2-3 hours in juice. Make a strong solution in water and apply directly to sores every half hour until they subside.

▶ Take Lysine 1000mg. daily. Apply LYSINE CREAM at first signs of blisters.

▶ Quercetin Plus w. Bromelain 500mg. 2x daily.

▶ Liquid chlorophyll 3 teasp. daily before meals.

▶ Pro. Nutrition DR. DOPHILUS, or Natren LIFE START II, 1/4 teasp. 3 to 4x daily in water. ☺

▶ Dr. Diamond HERPANACINE capsules as directed 2x daily.

▶ B Complex 100mg. daily w/ extra B6 250mg., with zinc lozenges 2 to 3 daily.

▶ Effective homeopathic remedies:
✚ Hylands *Hylavir* ☺
✚ *Natrum Muriaticum*

FOOD THERAPY

🍃 Add more cultured foods to your diet for prevention: yogurt, kefir, sauerkraut, etc.

🍃 Avoid high arginine foods, such as coffee, peanut butter, nuts, seeds, corn, etc.

🍃 Keep the diet alkaline: eliminate red meats, caffeine, refined and fried foods, sugars, sweet fruits, etc.

🍃 Eat a mineral-rich diet: plenty of salads, lots of raw and cooked vegetables, whole grains. Baked potatoes and steamed broccoli are especially good.

🍃 For prevention, take 2 TBS. brewer's yeast every day. Drink a fresh carrot juice once a week.

🍃 Crystal Star SYSTEM STRENGTH™ drink toalkalize the body for prevention.
and/or
BIOFLV., FIBER & C SUPPORT drink for concentrated food flavonoids.

Common Symptoms: Contagious herpes simplex virus sores on the face and mouth - beginning with a small sore bump, and turning into a very sore, often pussy blister. Lips and inside of the mouth are usually also sore.
Common Causes: Herpes simplex virus 1; B Complex deficiency; premenstrual tension and consequent hormone imbalance; gluten sensitivity; over-acid diet; recurring virus infection; emotional stress.

COLITIS ■ SPASTIC COLON ▩ IBS (Irritable Bowel Syndrome)

Enteritis ✧ Ileitis

A chronically inflamed colon is often a result of food allergies or sensitivities - usually to wheat, cheese, corn or eggs. Colon membranes become irritated, and the body forms pouchy pockets in reaction. In severe cases ulcerous lesions line the sides of the colon.

FOOD THERAPY

🍃 Go on a mono diet for 2 days with fresh apples and apple juice.
Then eat a low fat, mild diet with plenty of soluble fiber, but low roughage. Include fresh fruits, green leafy salads with olive oil and lemon dressing, whole grain cereal, such as oatmeal, brown rice, steamed vegetables (esp. potatoes and cabbage), fruit fiber from prunes, apples and raisins.
Foods should be mildly cooked, never fried.

🍃 Gentle fiber foods include apple pectin, rice bran, and gum guggul.

🍃 Eat cultured foods, such as yogurt and kefir for friendly intestinal flora.

🍃 Avoid nuts, seeds, dairy foods and citrus fruits while healing. Spicy foods and caffeine are also irritants.

🍃 Have a glass of fresh carrot juice 3x a week. Keep the body hydrated with plenty of water.

VITAMINS/MINERALS

Liquid and chewable supplements are best for colitis irritation.

▶ Effective enzymes:
   ✦ Chewable papaya enzymes
   ✦ Alta Health CANGEST powder or tablets.
   ✦ Solaray SUPER DIGEST-AWAY capsules.

▶ Enzymatic Therapy chewable DGL tabs before meals.
and IBS capsules (enteric-coated peppermint oil) between meals.
with
   Royal Jelly 2 teasp. daily.

▶ High omega 3 flax seed oil 3 teasp. daily.

▶ Country Life BROMELAIN with 2000gdu. activity. ♂

▶ Chlorophyll liquid 3 teasp. daily in water before meals.
with
   Schiff emulsified vit. A 50,000IU daily.

▶ Nature's Life liquid PHOSPHORUS FREE CAL/MAG. ♂

▶ Homeopathic *Silicea* tablets.

HERBAL THERAPY

🌿 Yerba Prima or George's ALOE VERA JUICE with HERBS morning and evening.

🌿 Peppermint oil drops in water 2 x daily.

🌿 Crystal Star BWL-TONE™ capsules with GREEN TEA CLEANSER™ 2 cups daily.
and/or
CHO-LO FIBER TONE™ drink mix, 1 heaping teasp. in water morning and evening.

🌿 Effective anti-spasmodics:
   ✦ Crystal Star RELAX CAPS™ and/or ANTI-SPZ™ capsules.
   ✦ Chamomile tea
   ✦ Valerian/wild lettuce

🌿 Effective teas:
   ✦ Slippery elm
   ✦ Pau de arco
   ✦ Rosemary

🌿 Alfalfa tablets 6-10 daily, with bee pollen 2 teasp. daily.

🌿 Sonné bentonite liquid, 1 teasp. morning and evening to clean out wastes.

BODYWORK

If there is appendicitis-like sharp pain, seek medical help immediately.

▶ Effective gentle enemas to rid the colon of fermenting wastes and relieve pain:
   ↪ Peppermint tea
   ↪ White oak bark
   ↪ Slippery elm
   ↪ Chamomile
   ↪ Lobelia

▶ Apply warm ginger compresses to spine and stomach.

▶ Acupressure help:
Stroke the abdomen up across and down.

▶ Consciously practice relaxation techniques to reduce stress.

▶ Avoid antacids. They often do more harm than good by neutralizing the body's HCl needed for good assimilation of food.

▶ Many elimination channel problems mimic IBS. A physical exam can help pinpoint the problem.

▶ Eat smaller, more frequent meals. No large meals.

Common Symptoms: Abdominal cramps and pain; recurrent constipation, usually alternating with bloody diarrhea; rectal hemorrhoids, fistulas and abcsesses; rectal abscesses and inflammation; blood and mucous in the stool; dehydration and mineral loss.
Common Causes: Excess refined foods and sweets; lack of dietary fiber; food allergies; Candida albicans; vitamin K deficiency; anemia and electrolyte imbalance; emotional stress, depression and anxiety; too many antibiotics.

CONSTIPATION ▦ COLON & BOWEL HEALTH ▦ WASTE MANAGEMENT

The colon and bowel are the depository for all waste material after food nutrients have been extracted and processed to the bloodstream. It is hardly any wonder that up to 90% of all diseases generate from an unclean colon. Decaying food ferments, forms gases, as well as 2nd and 3rd generation toxins, and the colon becomes a breeding ground for putrefactive bacteria, viruses, parasites, yeasts, molds, etc. Ideally, one should eliminate as often as a meal is taken in. Bowel transit time should be approx. 12 hours. To promote healthy bowel function, include plenty of fiber and liquids in your diet, exercise regularly and establish a regular daily time for elimination.

FOOD THERAPY

➤ **Start with a short easy colon cleansing juice fast (pg. 43) to rid the bowel of current wastes.**
Then, follow a mild food, low fat, largely vegetarian diet, with plenty of high fiber fruits, whole grains, cereals, salad greens, and cultured foods like yogurt and kefir to establish friendly intestinal flora. **Take plenty of liquids daily; at least 6-8 glasses of juice or water.**

➤ **Good colon health foods:**
♣ Flax seed, Bran, Whey, Brewer's Yeast, Yogurt, Acidophilus, Greens.

➤ Avoid all refined foods, saturated fats, fried foods, and caffeine.

➤ To restore peristaltic action, mix equal parts of flax seed and oat bran in water. Let sit overnight. Take 2 TBS. in the morning

➤ Aloe vera juice with herbs 8oz. daily in the morning.

➤ Chew food well, and eat smaller meals. No large heavy meals.

➤ Crystal Star BIOFLAV., FIBER & C SUPPORT™ drink for 3 gms. fiber in every serving.

VITAMINS/MINERALS

Avoid drugstore antibiotics, antacids, and milk of magnesia. They kill friendly intestinal flora.

▶ Prevent constipation by adding some of these supplements to the diet:
♦ Acidophilus liquid
♦ Garlic capsules
♦ Brewer's yeast
♦ Omega 3 flax seed oil

▶ Take a good food *food source* multiple vitamin to control initial gas and stomach rumbling as the additional dietary fiber combines with the minerals in the G.I. tract.

▶ Crystal Star BWL-TONE™ caps or Enzymatic Therapy IBS if there is bowel irritation.

▶ Apple pectin or HCl tablets at meals. ♂

▶ Chlorophyll liquid 3 teasp. daily before meals.
or
Sun CHLORELLA or Green Foods GREEN MAGMA.

▶ Laci LeBeau SUPER DIETER'S tea for temporary relief.

▶ Alta Health CANGEST for better assimilation and liver activity.

HERBAL THERAPY

❦ Crystal Star FIBER & HERBS COLON CLEANSE™ capsules 2, 3x daily.
and/or
LAXA-TEA to flush wastes gently and quickly the first few days.

❦ Planetary Formulas TRIPHALA to promote a firm, healthy odor-free stool.

❦ Psyllium husks and/or Sonné liquid bentonite or Crystal Star CHO-LO FIBER TONE™ drink in water, to gather up colon waste and flush it out. *Note: If there is a history of sluggish colon activity, wait 1½ hours after taking before eating.*

❦ Milk thistle seed extract to enhance bile output and soften stool.

❦ Effective herbal laxatives:
♦ Senna leaf and pods ♀
♦ Cascara sagrada to increase peristalsis and normalize evacuation.
♦ **HERBALTONE caps** ♀
♦ Solaray REFRESH
♦ **YERBA MATE tea, 2 TBS. in 2 CUPS water 2x daily.**
♦ Flax seed tea
♦ Fennel/ginger caps 4 at a time to also freshen breath.

BODYWORK

The protective level of fiber in the diet can be easily measured:
→ *the stool should be light enough to float.*
→ *bowel movements should be regular, daily and effortless.*
→ *the stool should be almost odorless, signalling increased transit time in the bowel.*
→ *there should be no gas or flatulence.*

▶ Take a colonic irrigation to start your program. A grapefruit seed extract colonic is extremely effective, especially if there is colon toxicity along with constipation. (Dilute to 15 to 20 drops per gallon of water.) Take a catnip enema once a week to keep cleansing well. (See page 49ff.) *Note: Enemas may be given to children and infants. Use smaller amounts according to size and age. Allow water to enter very slowly, and allow them to expel when they wish.*

▶ Take a brisk walk daily.

▶ Stroke and press each of the reflexology points for 3-5 minutes:

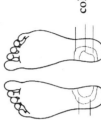

colon points

Common Symptoms: Infrequent bowel movements; flatulence and gas; fatigue, nausea and depression; nervous irritability; coated tongue; headaches; bad breath and body odor; mental dullness; sallow skin.
Common Causes: Poor diet, drugs, travel and stress all affect bowel regularity; too many refined carbohydrates; deficient fiber; autotoxemia from too much red meat, pasteurized dairy, fried foods, caffeine and alcohol; overeating; overuse of drugs and laxatives; hypothyroidism; lack of exercise.

INFORMATION & DIET SUGGESTIONS FOR COLON HEALTH

Most poor health conditions that we endure extend from poor elimination in one way or another. Elements causing constipation and colon toxicity come from three basic areas:
1) Non-food chemicals in our food and pollutants in the environment, ranging from relatively harmless to very dangerous. The body can tolerate a certain level of contamination. When that individual level is reached, and immune defenses are low, toxic overload causes illness. A strong system can metabolize and excrete many of these toxins, but when the body is weak or constipated, they are stored as unusable substances. As more and different chemicals enter the body they tend to interreact with those that are already there, forming mutant, second generation chemicals far more harmful than the originals. Evidence in recent years has shown that most bowel cancer is caused by environmental agents.
2) Over-accumulation of body wastes and metabolic byproducts that are not excreted properly. These wastes can also become a breeding ground for parasite infestation. A new nationwide survey has revealed that one in every six people studied have one or more parasites living somewhere in the body.
3) Slowed elimination time, allowing waste materials to ferment, become rancid, and then recirculate through the body as toxic substances.
These and other factors result in sluggish organ and glandular functions, poor digestion and assimilation, lowered immunity, faulty circulation, and tissue degeneration.

✱ The key to avoiding bowel problems is often nutritional. A high fiber, unrefined foods diet is important to both cure and prevention of waste elimination problems. Diet improvement can also correct the diseases these problems cause. Even a gentle and gradual improvement from low fiber, low residue foods will help almost immediately. In fact, graduated change is often better than a sudden, drastic about-face, especially when the colon, bowel or bladder are painful and inflamed. Constipation is usually a chronic problem, and while body cleansing progress can be felt fairly quickly with a diet change, it takes from three to six months to rebuild bowel and colon elasticity with good systolic/diastolic action. There is no easy route, but the rewards of a regular, energetic life are worth it.

After the initial cleansing juice diet, the second part of a good colon health program is rebuilding healthy tissue and body energy. This stage may be used for 1 - 2 months for best results. It emphasizes high fiber through fresh vegetables and fruits, cultured foods for increased assimilation and enzyme production, and alkalizing foods to prevent irritation while healing. During this diet avoid refined foods, saturated fats or oils, fried foods, meats, caffeine or other acid or mucous forming foods, such as pasteurized dairy products, during this diet.

On rising: take a glass of George's or Yerba Prima aloe vera juice with herbs;
or Sonne's LIQUID BENTONITE, with 1 teasp. liquid acidophilus added; **or** Crystal Star CHO-LO FIBER TONE™ capsules, or drink mix in apple or orange juice.

Breakfast: Soak a mix of dried prunes, figs and raisins the night before; take 2 to 4 TBS. with 1 TB. blackstrap molasses, **or** mix with yogurt;
or make a mix of oat bran, raisins, and pumpkin seeds, and mix with yogurt or apple juice, or a light vegie broth. Add 2 teasp. brewer's yeast or Lewis Labs FIBER YEAST;
and have some oatmeal or a whole grain cereal, granola or muesli with yogurt or apple juice;
or have a bowl of mixed fresh fruits with apple juice or yogurt.

Mid-morning: take a green drink (page 54ff), Sun CHLORELLA, Green Foods GREEN ESSENCE, or Crystal Star ENERGY GREEN™ drink;
or pau de arco, green tea or Crystal Star GREEN TEA CLEANSER™ to alkalize the system.
or a fresh carrot juice;

Lunch: have a fresh green salad every day with lemon/oil dressing, or yogurt cheese or kefir cheese;
or steamed vegies and a baked potato with soy or kefir cheese;
or a fresh fruit salad with a little yogurt or raw cottage cheese topping.

Mid-afternoon: have another fresh carrot juice, or Crystal Star SYSTEM STRENTH™ drink;
and/or green tea or slippery elm tea, or Wisdom of the Ancients YERBAMATE TEA.
and/or some raw crunchy vegies with a vegetable or kefir cheese dip, or soy spread.

Dinner: have a large dinner salad with black bean or lentil soup;
or an oriental stir fry and miso soup with sea vegetables snipped on top;
or a steamed or baked vegetable casserole with a yogurt or soy cheese sauce;
or a vegetable or whole grain pasta with a light lemon or yogurt sauce.

Before bed: have some apple or papaya juice;
or another glass of aloe vera juice with herbs;
or Crystal Star CHO-LO FIBER TONE™ drink or capsules, Crystal Star BIOFLAV., FIBER & C SUPPORT™ drink for 3gms. fiber in every serving.

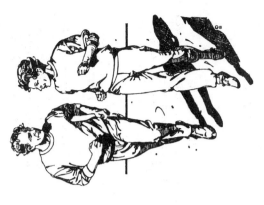

188

COUGH

Chronic ◇ Dry & Hacking ◇ Smokers

This type of cough is not the result of infection per se, but evidence of continuing throat irritation from smoking, environmental pollens, etc., or chemical pollutants. It should be regarded as a sign of reduced immunity, and treated both topically, and as part of an immune-stimulating program.

FOOD THERAPY

❧ Take 2 TBS. honey and 2 TBS. lemon juice in water or cider vinegar to stop the tickle.

❧ Drink cleansing fruit juices. Eat high vitamin C foods, such as sprouts, green peppers, broccoli, and cherries.

❧ Take a cup of hot black tea with the juice of 1 lemon and 1 teasp. honey.

❧ Take a cup of hot water with 2 TBS. brandy and 2 TBS. lemon juice.

❧ Avoid pasteurized dairy products during acute stages.

VITAMINS/MINERALS

▶ Enzymatic Therapy ORAL-ZYME lozenges, or other low dose (10-30mg.) lozenge under the tongue til dissolved.

▶ Ricola lozenges / pearls.

▶ Ascorbate vitamin C or Ester C powder: $1/4$ teasp. every half hour to bowel tolerance. with

Beta-carotene 25,000IU 2x daily.

▶ Propolis tincture or lozenges.♂

▶ Effective homeopathic remedies:
✤ BioForce *Biotussin* drops and tablets.
✤ Nu-Age *Cough.*
✤ Hylands cough syrup. ☺
✤ B&T cough syrup. ☺
✤ Standard Homeopathic *Hy-lavir* tablets. ☺
✤ Bioforce *Santasapina* or *Dros-inula* cough liquids.

▶ Garlic capsules 4 to 6 daily.

HERBAL THERAPY

❧ Crystal Star COFEX TEA™, especially at night. Usually works within 24 hours. ☺
and/or
X-PECT™ TEA as an expectorant.

❧ Crystal Star SUPER LICO-RICE™ extract drops.

❧ Horehound, licorice, and wild cherry drops, syrups, or teas.

❧ Effective teas or steams:
◆ Eucalyptus
◆ Peppermint
◆ Slippery Elm

❧ Propolis extract under the tongue or lozenges as desired.

❧ Crystal Star ANTI-SPZ™ capsules, 4 at a time as needed.

❧ Natures Way ANTSP tincture.

❧ Sage or rose hips tea with lemon juice, honey, and fresh ginger root.

❧ Clove tea for spasmodic coughing or hiccups.

BODYWORK

▶ Eliminated smoking and secondary smoke from your environment.

▶ Effective gargles:
➤ Tea tree oil drops in water.
➤ Slippery elm tea
➤ Aloe vera juice

▶ Steam eucalyptus or tincture of benzoin in a vaporizer at night.

▶ Effective lozenges:
➤ Zand HERBAL INSURE
➤ BioForce *Santasapina*

▶ Avoid commercial cough syrups, and drugstore over-the-counter medicines. They often make the problem worse by suppression, which forces the infection deeper into the tissues.

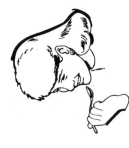

Common Symptoms: Hacking, dry or chronic coughing with no phlegm or mucous eliminated; chronic rough smoker's-throat cough from constant irritation.

Common Causes: Low grade chronic infection of throat and sinuses; mucous-forming diet; allergies; smoking irritation.

CROHN'S DISEASE
Regional Enteritis

Crohn's disease is chronic inflammation of the digestive tract, with painful ulcers that form in one or more sections, or all along its length. When the ulcers heal they leave thick scar tissue that narrows the tract and adversely affects elimination. Although a direct cause has not been defined, poor assimilation of nutrients is always involved, and accompanying ulcerous bleeding often causes anemia. A strictly followed, highly nutritious, mild foods diet has proven to be an effective non-toxic alternative to cortico-steroid drugs.

FOOD THERAPY

❧ Diet improvement is the key:
1) Start with an alkalizing liquid diet for 3 days:
  ❦ Carrot and apple juice
  ❦ Grape juice
  ❦ Pineapple green drinks.
2) Then add mild fruits and vegetables for a week:
  ❦ Carrots, potatoes, yams, apples, papayas, bananas, etc.
3) Add steamed and raw vegetables, brans, cultured foods for 2 weeks:
  ❦ Yogurt, kefir, miso, etc.
  ❦ Salads, broccoli, cabbage
  ❦ Oat bran, rice bran, etc.
4) Finally add rice, whole grains, wheat germ, tofu, fish, and seafood for healing protein.
5) The continuing diet should be high in complex carbohydrates and soluble fiber, and low in saturated fats.

❧ Avoid nuts, seeds, and citrus while healing. Eliminate red and fatty meats, saturated fats and fried foods. Increase high fiber and fresh foods.

❧ Drink only bottled water. Over treated tap water can often cause inflammatory bowel diseases.

❧ Effective green drinks:
  ❦ Crystal Star ENERGY GREEN™
  ❦ Green Foods GREEN MAGMA
  ❦ Sun CHLORELLA

VITAMINS/MINERALS

Avoid commercial antacids. They eventually make the inflammation worse by causing the stomach to produce more acids.

▶ Take 1 teasp. chlorophyll liquid in water 3 x daily.

▶ Enzymatic Therapy IBS capsules, LIQUID LIVER w. Siber. Ginseng, and/or
DGL tablets as needed.

▶ Ascorbate vit. C w. bioflavonoids powder, $1/4$ teasp. 4 to 6x daily.

▶ Zinc picolinate 15-30mg. daily.
with
Vit. E 1000IU daily.
and
Magnesium 200mg. 3x daily. ♂

▶ Dr. DOPHILUS powder $1/4$ teasp. 3x daily.

▶ Chewable bromelain 40mg. or papaya enzymes after meals. ♂

▶ Lewis Labs FIBER YEAST each morning. ♀

HERBAL THERAPY

❧ Crystal Star BWL TONE™ caps and/or GREEN TEA CLEANSER™ for 3 months.
with
George's aloe vera juice 4 glasses daily to gently aid bowel recovery.

❧ Evening primrose oil caps 500mg. 2 x daily. ♀
and
Wisdom of the Ancients YERBA-MATE tea.

❧ Crystal Star CHO-LO FIBER TONE™ drink or Sonné liquid bentonite to gently clean out toxins.

❧ Bee pollen 2 teasp. daily.

❧ Effective herbal anti-oxidants to scavenge the free radicals involved in Crohn's disease attacks.
  ◆ Garlic capsules 4-6 daily.
  ◆ Spirulina
  ◆ Pau de Arco
  ◆ Fenugreek

❧ Effective herbal flavonoids:
  ◆ Hawthorne
  ◆ Bilberry
  ◆ Rosehips

BODYWORK

▶ Peppermint tea enemas once a week for the first month of healing.

▶ Apply hot, wet ginger compresses to stomach and lower back.

▶ Consciously work to reduce stress in your life.

▶ Reflexology points:

stomach & colon area

▶ Crohn's disease region:

Common Symptoms: Inflammation and soreness along the entire G.I. tract; bouts of diarrhea with a low grade fever; abdominal distention, tenderness and pain from food residue and gas; abnormal weight loss and depression.

Common Causes: Low dietary fiber, with excess refined sugar and acid-forming foods, leading to a severely inflammatory condition which forms deep ulcers along the entire length of the digestive tract from rectum to mouth; multiple food intolerances, particularly to wheat and dairy; emotional, acid-causing stress; zinc deficiency.

CUTS ▨ SCRAPES ▨ WOUNDS

FOOD THERAPY

🍃 Place ice packs on the area immediately to stop bleeding and reduce trauma.

🍃 Apply wheat germ oil directly.

🍃 Squeeze a fresh lemon on the area to clean and disinfect.

🍃 Eat plenty of fresh greens every day for faster healing.

VITAMINS/MINERALS

▶ Apply Vit. E oil. Take 400IU daily internally.

▶ Nutribiotic GRAPEFRUIT SEED EXTRACT spray to counteract infection.

▶ Apply Amer. Biologics DIOX-YCHLOR directly.

▶ Ester C w/ bioflavs. and rutin, 3-5 grams daily. Apply a weak solution directly to cut. with Pantothenic acid 500mg. for collagen/protein formation.

▶ Zinc picolinate 50mg, 2 x daily.

▶ Nature's Plus GERMANIUM PLUS 25mg. daily for a month if wound is slow healing.

▶ Vit. K 100mg. 3 × daily for clotting ability. ♀ with Cal/mag/zinc 4 daily for faster healing. ♂

▶ Apply propolis extract. Take 1/2 dropperful 2x daily.

▶ Enzymatic Therapy DERMA-ZYME ointment for slow healing cuts.

HERBAL THERAPY

❧ Apply aloe vera gel as needed.

❧ Apply yarrow compresses to aid clotting ability.

❧ Apply Deva FIRST AID drops, or Bach Flower RESCUE REMEDY drops.

❧ Crystal Star ANTI-BIO™ capsules or extract to overcome infection and inflammation.

❧ Propolis lozenges - apply propolis extract directly, and take under the tongue.

❧ Apply royal jelly as needed. Take 2 teasp. daily internally.

❧ Apply Country Comfort GOLDEN SEAL/MYRRH salve, or COMFREY/ALOE salve.

❧ Apply a mix of St. John's wort/cayenne and marshmallow rt.

❧ Apply cranesbill powder directly to sore.

❧ Gotu Kola capsules, 4 daily for connective tissue and nerve healing.

❧ Apply cayenne tincture to stop bleeding, and take drops internally as needed for shock.

BODYWORK

▶ Apply Pau de Arco Gel frequently as needed.

▶ Apply Crystal Star GINSENG SKIN REPAIR™ gel with germanium and vitamin C.

▶ Apply Arnica cream as needed.

▶ Apply a green clay poultice to reduce swelling.

▶ Clean with H₂O₂ and apply tea tree oil drops every 2 to 3 hours.

▶ Apply DMSO for bruising. Apply morning and evening for 2-3 days for best results.

▶ Apply alternating hot and cold witch hazel compresses.

▶ Prick open and apply a vitamin A&D capsule.

▶ Apply B & T califlora, or other good calendula gel. Dilute Crystal Star 25% CALENDULA gel to clean out cut, then apply homeopathic *Hypericum* tincture. *Note: After a deep cut do not apply calendula gel right away. It heals so fast that the outside closes up before the inside has been healed. Apply after the inside begins to heal.*

CYSTS ▣ POLYPS ▣ BENIGN TUMORS ▣ LIPOMAS ▣ WENS

Benign growths of varying size - found both internally on the intestinal, urethral, genital passage linings, and externally anywhere on the skin. They often arise from an excessive growth of fat cells. They are responsive to the body's growth-regulating mechanisms and quite receptive to natural therapies. They can be annoying, unsightly, and in some cases lead to cancer.

FOOD THERAPY

☙ Go on a short 1 to 3 day liquid diet for to set up a healing environment, stimulate the liver and clean the blood. Then follow with a fresh foods diet for the rest of the week.

☙ Avoid red meats, caffeine, pasteurized dairy products and acid-forming foods.

☙ Eliminate saturated fats (mostly animal fats), fried foods, chocolate, margarine, shortening and other refined fats.

☙ Add more fish, seafoods, sea vegetables and unsaturated oils, such as flax and sunflower oil to the diet.

VITAMINS/MINERALS

▶ Beta carotene 25,000IU every 4 hours for a month.
with
Natures Plus Vit. E 800IU daily.

▶ Shark cartilage capsules and Carnitine 500mg. daily, especially for lipomas and wens.
with
High omega 3 fish or flax oils 3 x daily to control fat metabolism.

▶ Ascorbate C crystals with bioflavonoids $1/4$ teasp. 4x daily for a month.

▶ Organic germanium 25-50mg. daily,
with
Sun CHLORELLA 1 packet daily in water.

▶ Folic acid 400mcg. daily to correct cell formation.
with

▶ Vit. B6 250mg. 2x daily until condition clears. ♀

▶ Zinc picolinate 50mg. 2x daily for a month. Then a maintenance dose of 30mg. daily. ♂

HERBAL THERAPY

❧ Echinacea or milk thistle extract 4x daily to clear lymph nodes and regulate liver function.
and/or

❧ Crystal Star ANTI-BIO™ extract as an anti-infective.

❧ Apply tea tree oil for 4 to 6 weeks.

❧ Pau de arco tea 4 cups daily for a month.
with
Comfrey compresses on the affected area.

❧ Chaparral caps 6 daily, or extract 4x daily for 1-2 months.

❧ Evening primrose oil 500mg. 6 daily, with Nature's Plus Vit. E 800IU. ♀

❧ Apply Nutrition Resource GRAPEFRUIT SEED EXTRACT directly, 2x daily, esp. if the growth is increasing in size.

❧ Propolis lozenges - apply propolis extract directly, *and* take under the tongue.

BODYWORK

▶ NO smoking. Nicotine aggravates gland imbalances that allow these deposits to form.

▶ Massage into affected area daily, Care Plus H2O2 OXYGEL for 3 weeks, for noticeable reduction without pain.

▶ Apply Advanced Research PAU DE ARCO GEL frequently as needed.

▶ Scrub skin with a loofa or dry skin brush regularly to keep sebaceous glands unblocked.

▶ Apply liquid garlic directly with a cotton swab.

▶ Apply Crystal Star GINSENG SKIN REPAIR GEL™ with germanium and vitamin C for several weeks.

Common Symptoms: A lump or bulge seen or felt under the skin; in the case of vaginal cysts, there is often bleeding during intercourse; where there are colon, ladder or cervical polyps there is often rectal, urinal or vaginal bleeding; wens usually form over nerve ganglia.
Common Causes: Internal toxicity and infection; diet contains excess acid or mucous forming foods; poor assimilation/digestion of fats; for sebaceous cysts, gland outflow blocked with sebum deposits; accumulation of dead skin cells, local cosmetic irritants.

DANDRUFF ▨ SEBORRHEIC DERMATITIS

Dandruff appears as dry, flaky particles of skin in the hair. It can result from a variety of conditions, both physical and emotional, appearing when skin cells turn over at a faster rate than normal and break away in large flakes into the hair. It tends to occur more in the winter and fall months. While dandruff appears to be a dry skin condition, it is actually the opposite - too much oil is being produced, clogging sebaceous glands.

FOOD THERAPY

ꝛ Make sure the diet is low in sugars, starches and animal fats. Eliminate fried foods. They clog the body so it cannot eliminate wastes properly. Avoid dairy products, refined sugars and flours, chocolate, nuts and shellfish. These are traditional allergens that are sometimes involved with dandruff. Eliminate refined sugars. They deplete the body of B vitamins.

ꝛ Add sulphur-rich foods to the diet: Lettuce, oats, green pepper, onions, cucumber, eggs, fish, cabbage, wheat germ.

ꝛ Eat lots of green salads, steamed vegetables, and whole grains to nourish the glands.

ꝛ Make a mix and take 2 TBS. daily in food:
   ♣ Lecithin
   ♣ Brewer's yeast
   ♣ Wheat germ

ꝛ Eat plenty of cultured products like yogurt and kefir to encourage healthy intestinal flora and better digestion.

VITAMINS/MINERALS

▶ B Complex 100mg. daily with extra B6 100mg., and folic acid 400mcg.
      and
PABA 1000mg.
      and
Niacin 500mg. for increased circulation.

▶ Schiff emulsified A & D
      with
Lecithin caps or choline/inositol caps, 2 daily.

▶ Zinc picolinate 50mg. 2x daily. ♂
      with
Beta carotene 25,000IU 4x daily.

▶ Omega 3 flax oils 3x daily.

▶ Evening primrose oil caps 4-6 daily.
      or
Rainbow Light ORGANIC EFA VIT. A caps. ♀

▶ Biotin 600mcg. daily. ♂

▶ Vit. E w/ selenium 400IU daily.

HERBAL THERAPY

ꝛ Alta Health SIL-X silica capsules for 1 month.

ꝛ Effective herb minerals:
   ✦ Crystal Star MINERAL SPECTRUM™ capsules.
   ✦ Crystal Star SYSTEM STRENGTH™ drink mix.
   ✦ Crystal Star SILICA SOURCE™ extract.
   ✦ Kelp tabs 8 daily.

ꝛ Effective mineral rinses:
   ✦ Rosemary/yarrow
   ✦ Nettles
   ✦ Chaparral

ꝛ Steep bay leaves in olive oil until fragrant. Rub on scalp before shampoo. Leave on 30 minutes and shampoo out.

ꝛ Massage jojoba or rosemary oil into scalp. Leave on 1 hour. Shampoo out.

ꝛ Steep cider vinegar and peppermint oil drops in 1 cup water. Rinse hair.

BODYWORK

Avoid over-the-counter commercial ointments that often do more harm than good by clogging sebaceous glands.

➤ Use jojoba, aloe vera or biotin shampoos.

➤ Get some regular circulation-stimulating exercise daily.

➤ **Add drops of tea tree oil to hair rinse, and use daily. Or use tea tree oil shampoo.**

➤ Massage head with both hands and all the fingers at once, for 5 minutes every day to stimulate scalp circulation and slough dead skin cells.

➤ Add a few drops Nutrition Resource NUTRIBIOTIC GRAPEFRUIT SEED EXTRACT to shampoo, and use daily.

➤ **Rinse the hair with cider vinegar and water after every wash to keep sebum deposits from clogging pores. Or try a shampoo specifically designed to remove build-up.**

Common Symptoms: Scaling flakes on scalp and eyebrows; redness, and itching, burning scalp.
Common Causes: Sebaceous gland malfunction; too much alcohol, saturated fat, sugar and starch in the diet; essential fatty acid deficiency; lack of green vegetables; excessively strong or harsh hair dyes.

DEPRESSION
Anxiety ✧ Paranoia

The mental and emotional state that we call depression can stem from as wide a range of causes as there are individuals. In general, there seem to be five broad spectrum origins for depression. 1) Great loss, as of a spouse or child, and the inability to mourn or express grief. 2) Bottled-up anger and aggression turned inward. 3) Behavior, often learned as a child, that gets desired attention or controls relationships. 4) Biochemical imbalance characterized by amino acid and other nutrient deficiencies. 5) Drug-induced depression.

FOOD THERAPY

Food and nutrition are key factors in the brain's behavior and well-being. Poor diet is often the cause of depression, especially in teenagers and the elderly.

☙ Sufficient protein (about 15% of total calorie intake) minimizes depression. Eat plenty of fresh vegetables and whole grains. Include fish, sea foods and legumes for protein. Keep tissue oxygen high for red blood cell formation. (See the HEALTHY HEART DIET in this book.) Make sure there is good soluble fiber in your diet.

☙ Have a glass of carrot juice 2 to 3x a week with a pinch of sage and 1 teasp. Bragg's LIQUID AMINOS.

☙ Make a mix of 1/4 cup each and take 2 TBS. daily:
♣ Lecithin granules
♣ Brewer's yeast
♣ Wheat germ
♣ Pumpkin seeds

☙ Eliminate all preserved, refined and junk foods. Avoid sweets, alcohol and drugs.

☙ Drink bottled water. Several studies indicate that treated water can cause neurotransmitter imbalances.

VITAMINS/MINERALS

▶ Relief from depression:
♣ DLPA 750mg, as needed.
♣ Tyrosine 500mg, with B6 100mg, 2 to 3x daily.
♣ Country Life RELAXER caps.
♣ Natrol SAF capsules. ♀
♣ GABA caps with glycine.

▶ Magnesium 500mg, 2x daily. and/or Solaray CHROMIACIN. ♂

▶ Country Life Maxi-B Complex with taurine daily, *and MOOD FACTORS capsules as needed.* ♂

▶ Enzymatic Therapy THYROID/ TYROSINE capsules ♀, with Vit. B12 internasal or sublingual

▶ Brain oxygenators:
♣ Germanium w/suma.
♣ CoQ 10 10mg, 3x daily.
♣ Biotec EXTRA ENERGY ENZYMES 6 daily.
♣ Glutamine 1000mg.
♣ Wheat germ oil capsules.

▶ Vitamin C with bioflavonoids is a natural tranquilizer and helps withdrawal from drugs and chemical dependencies.

HERBAL THERAPY

☙ Ginkgo Biloba extract drops as needed.

☙ Bach Flower RESCUE REMEDY and sage tea as needed.

☙ Crystal Star DEPRESSEX™ extract for mental calm, RELAX CAPS™ for nerve repair.

☙ Crystal Star CREATIVI-TEA™. Steep 1 oz. tea in brandy for 3 days. Add cherry juice and steep for 24 hours. Take 3 TBS. daily.

☙ Herbs to relieve depression;
◆ Crystal Star WITHDRAWAL SUPPORT™ drops
◆ Medicine Wheel SERENE drops
◆ St. John's wort extract
◆ Wisdom of the Ancients YERBA MATÉ TEA.
◆ Solary EUROCALM caps.
◆ Evening primrose oil 4 daily.

☙ YS ROYAL JELLY 2 teasp. daily. ♀ Bee Pollen 2 teasp. daily. ♂

☙ *Herbal formulas that increase energy and help overcome chronic fatigue:*
◆ Crystal Star RAINFOREST ENERGY™ tea, SUPER GINSENG 6 ENERGY™ capsules and tea.

BODYWORK

In general, avoid the amino acid phenalalanine - as in Nutra-Sweet or amino acid formulas. Many depressed people react allergically to phenol.

▶ Exercise worry and anxiety away. Give yourself plenty of body oxygen. Exercise is a nutrient in itself.

▶ Sunlight therapy - get some on the body every day possible for Vit. D.

▶ Do brain breathing exercises. (See Bragg's book). Yoga stretches or a shiatsu massage can also clear the mind and refresh the body.

▶ Stop smoking. It contracts capillaries and arteries, and slows circulation.

▶ Aromatherapy:
↠ Essential oils of jasmine, geranium, ylang ylang and basil.

Common Symptoms: Feelings of sadness and hopelessness; uncontrollable grief; paranoia; chronic fatigue; insomnia, or conversely, sleeping frequently and for long periods of time; poor appetite alternating with excessive appetite, and resulting in wide swings of weight loss and weight gain; withdrawal from social and family communication; excessive worry, anger and guilt; chronic headaches, backaches and constipation; diminished ability to concentrate; recurrent thoughts of death and suicide.
Common Causes: Hypoglycemia or other sugar imbalance; sugar or alcohol dependency; chemical or food allergies; glandular imbalance with high copper levels; drug abuse; hypothyroidism; prescription drug addiction or intolerance; negative emotions discharging hormonal secretions into the bloodstream; the inability to cope with prolonged and intense stress.

DERMATITIS

Dermatitis is an external skin condition caused by a systemic reaction to an allergen - usually in cosmetics, jewelry metals, drugs or topical medications. It can also be the body's reaction to emotional stress, or to a severe deficiency of essential fatty acids. Its systemic nature means that it can and does spread, and can become quite severe.

FOOD THERAPY

☙ Go on a short 3 day juice cleanse to clear acid waste from the system. Then eat a diet full of leafy greens, and other mineral-rich foods, such as sea vegetables to rebuild healthy tissue and good adrenal function.

☙ Use only poly or mono unsaturated oils. Keep the diet low in both fats and total calories.

☙ Make a mix of 1/4 cup each and take 2 TBS. daily:
♣ Wheat germ
♣ Molasses
♣ Brewer's yeast

☙ Avoid fried foods, red meats, caffeine, chocolate, pasteurized dairy products, and acid-forming refined carbohydrates.

VITAMINS/MINERALS

▶ Biotin 600mcg. daily. ♂

▶ Collagen tabs 6 daily, or Nutrapathic CALCIUM/COLLAGEN tabs as directed.
and/or
Ascorbate vitamin C 3 to 5000mg. daily for collagen/connective tissue growth.

▶ Alta Health SIL-X silica for healthy new growth. ♀

▶ Anti-inflammatories:
♣ Quercetin Plus with bromelain 500mg. 2 daily.
♣ Germanium with suma 30mg.

▶ Zinc 50mg. 2 x daily. ♂

▶ Apply Enzyme Therapy DERMA-CLEAR acne cream.

▶ Apply A D & E oil, and take emulsified A & D or dry A & D, with Vit. E 400IU w. selenium 100mcg.

▶ Beta Carotene 100,000IU daily
with
B Complex 100mg. 2x daily.

▶ Nutribiotic GRAPEFRUIT SEED EXTRACT capsules and spray

HERBAL THERAPY

☙ Ginkgo Biloba extract 3-4x daily
with
Suma caps 3-4 daily. ♀

☙ Apply dandelion tea as a wash.

☙ Crystal Star ADR-ACTIVE™ extract for adrenal cortex formation.
♦ SILICA SOURCE™ for collagen formation.
♦ THERADERM™ capsules or tea as an anti-inflammatory.

☙ Crystal Star BEAUTIFUL SKIN TEA™, applied as a wash to neutralize acids coming out through the skin.

☙ Solaray turmeric caps as an anti-inflammatory.

☙ Apply aloe vera gel or aloe ice gel.

☙ Essential fatty acids:
♦ Evening primrose oil
♦ Omega 3 flax oil
♦ Rainbow Light EFA caps.

BODYWORK

▶ Avoid perfumed cosmetics.

▶ Use Zia PAPAYA PEEL to smooth skin after inflammation is gone.

▶ Apply tea tree oil or Body essentials SILICA GEL.

▶ Use castile non-irritating soap.

▶ Get early morning sunlight on the skin every day possible for healing vitamin D.

▶ Apply and use Aubrey Organics COLLAGEN THERAPY CREAM.

▶ Apply an ascorbate vitamin C with bioflavs. solution in water to the affected areas.

▶ Apply Crystal Star - RAINFOREST RECOVERY™ gel. ☺

Common Symptoms: Inflamed dry, thickened skin patches; scaly, lumpy skin; itching skin.
Common Causes: EFA deficiency; allergic skin reaction to cosmetics, acid-forming foods, pleasure or prescription drugs, or topical medications; emotional stress; poor liver activity resulting in poor metabolism.

DIABETES

Adult-onset diabetes mellitus, Type 2, is a chronic degenerative disease that afflicts more than 12 million Americans. With its complications, it is the third leading cause of death in the U. S. It is a disorder in which the body's ability to use carbohydrates is impaired by disturbances in normal insulin mechanisms. Type 2 diabetics produce insulin, the hormone that helps convert food into energy, but it isn't used properly, and glucose builds up in the bloodstream, and cells can't get the nutrients they need. Type 1 diabetes is usually a juvenile-onset condition, is more severe, and is almost entirely dependent on insulin injections to sustain life. This page deals with Type 2 diabetes.

FOOD THERAPY

Diet improvement is absolutely necessary to overcoming diabetes.

☙ **The ideal diet for Type 2 diabetes is low in fats and total calories, high in complex carbohydrates and fiber to reduce insulin requirements. It should be largely vegetarian - with alkalizing foods, and the main proteins from vegetable sources.** See the DIABETES CONTROL DIET on the following page.

☙ High fiber foods are a key, and in some cases can lead to discontinuation of insulin therapy. Fiber improves control of glycemia and glucose metabolism, lowers cholesterol and triglyceride values, and promotes weight loss.

☙ Chromium-rich foods are a key: whole grains, brewer's yeast, string beans, eggs, cucumbers, soy foods, liver and organ meats, onions and garlic, fresh and dried fruits, shiitake mushrooms, wheat germ, etc. **Have a daily green salad for vegetable fiber.**

☙ **Complete elimination of sugars, alcohol, fried, fatty, refined and high cholesterol foods is imperative.**

☙ Drink only spring water with plenty of minerals.

VITAMINS/MINERALS

Avoid Cysteine, and fish oil capsules.

▶ GTF Chromium or chromium picolinate 200mcg. 3x daily. and/or ProBiologics LIQUID CHROMIUM or ProBiologics GLUCOBALANCE capsules.

▶ To normalize pancreatic activity:
✤ Alta Health CANGEST.
✤ **Twin Labs CSA caps**
✤ Futurebiotics VITAL K.
✤ Glutamine 500mg.
✤ Raw pancreas glandular.

▶ American Biologics VANADIUM 120mcg. daily.

▶ Ener-B Vit. B12 internasal gel or B12 sublingual with carnitine 500mg. ♂

▶ B Complex 100mg. daily with pantothenic acid 500mg. to encourage adrenal activity, niacin 250mg. to stimulate circulation, and zinc 30mg.

▶ Ester C 1000-2000mg. daily to increase insulin tolerance and normalize pancreatic activity.

▶ Magnesium/potassium/bromelain 3 daily to control blood pressure.

▶ Choline/inositol for nerve damage

HERBAL THERAPY

❧ Gymnema sylvestre before meals to help repair the pancreas, and damage to cells in the liver and kidneys.

❧ Crystal Star INSULFORM™ capsules to encourage insulin formation; GINSENG 6 SUPER TEA™ to lower blood sugar levels.

❧ Crystal Star BODY REBUILDER caps for stabilized energy. ADR-ACTIVE™ caps or ADRN™ extract for cortex support. ♀

❧ Sun CHLORELLA 15-20 tabs daily for absorbable germanium; spirulina to stabilize blood sugar.

❧ Effective teas:
◆ Dandelion/licorice ♂
◆ **Fenugreek seed**
◆ Siberian ginseng

❧ Insulin forming herbs:
◆ Pau de arco
◆ Garlic oil capsules
◆ **Bilberry**
◆ Astragalus

❧ Use stevia herb instead of sugar for sweetening. It does not have sugar's insulin requirements.

BODYWORK

▶ Exercise regularly to increase metabolic processes and reduce need for insulin. ♂

▶ A regular deep therapy massage is effective in regulating sugar use.

▶ Don't smoke. Nicotine increases sugar desire.

▶ Avoid phenylalanine. No Nutra-Sweet, etc. (Check labels on colas, diet drinks, etc.)

▶ If overweight, loose the excess. Poor bio-chemistry often results from being overweight. A fiber weight loss drink, such as Crystal Star CHO-LO FIBER TONE™ is effective.

▶ Alternating hot and cold hydrotherapy to stimulate circulation.

▶ Reflexology points:

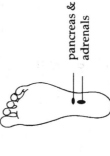

pancreas & adrenals

Common Symptoms: High blood sugar; constant hunger with rapid weight change; dry, itching skin; excessive thirst; lack of energy; kidney malfunction leading to bladder and prostate problems, and excessive urination with high sugar in the urine; obesity; hypertension; accelerated aging.
Common Causes: Poor diet with too many refined foods, fats and carbohydrates; insulin, chromium and HCl deficiencies; glucose and fat metabolism malfunction leading to obesity; pancreas and liver malfunction from excess caffeine, alcohol and stress overloads; inherited proneness usually accompanied by several allergies; hypothyroidism.

BLOOD SUGAR BALANCING DIET FOR DIABETES CONTROL

Although many Type 2 diabetics must take insulin to regulate blood sugar levels, many can successfully do this without drugs by following a controlled diet and getting regular exercise. Diabetic proneness is often hereditary, and can be brought on by eating too much fat, too many sugary foods and refined carbohydrates. Pancreatic activity and other vital organs become damaged, the body loses the ability to produce enough insulin, and high blood sugar results. As less and less insulin is produced, simple carbohydrates and sugars (which require a large secretion of insulin for metabolism) keep accumulating in the body and are stored as fat. Excess body fat and lack of exercise bring on insulin resistance, and energy is prevented from moving into the cells. The following diet, in addition to reducing insulin requirements and balancing sugar function in the bloodstream, has the nice "side effect" of healthy weight loss.

The key to this diet is in supplying slow-burning complex carbohydrate fuels to the body that do not need much insulin for metabolism. Slow-release nutrients, such as legumes prevent quick spikes of blood sugar. Meals are small, frequent, largely vegetarian, and low in fats of all kinds. Proteins come from soy foods and whole grains that are rich in lecithin and chromium. Fifty to sixty percent of the diet is in fresh and simply cooked vegetables for low calories and high digestibility.
All sugars, refined, fried and fatty foods are excluded.

On rising: take two lemons in a glass of water with 1 teasp. spirulina or 2 teasp. chlorella granules.

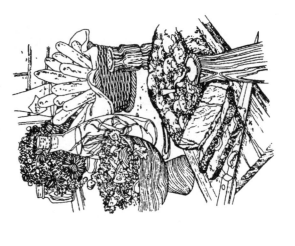

Breakfast: take a heaping teaspoon of Crystal Star CHOL-LO FIBER TONE™ or other natural high fiber drink mix, in apple juice or water, to regulate and balance the sugar curve;
and/or make a mix of 2 TBS. each: brewer's yeast, wheat germ, lecithin granules and rice or oat bran. Sprinkle some daily on your choice of breakfast foods; ◆ poached egg on whole grain toast, ◆ muesli, whole grain or granola cereal with apple juice or vanilla soy milk, ◆ buckwheat or whole grain pancakes with apple juice or molasses; or simply mix into yogurt with fresh fruit.

Mid-morning: have a green drink such as Crystal Star ENERGY GREEN™ or Sun CHLORELLA;
and some whole grain crackers or muffins with a little soy spread or kefir cheese.
and a refreshing, sugar balancing herb tea, such as licorice, dandelion, or pau de arco tea.

Lunch: have a green salad, with celery, sprouts, green pepper, marinated tofu, and mushroom soup;
or baked tofu or turkey with some steamed vegies and rice or cornbread;
or a baked potato with a little yogurt or kefir or soy cheese and some miso soup with sea vegetables;
or a whole grain sandwich, with avocado, low fat or soy cheese and a low fat sandwich spread.

Mid-afternoon: have a glass of carrot juice;
and/or fruit juice sweetened cookies with a bottle of mineral water or herb tea;
or a hard boiled egg with sesame salt, or a vegie dip, and a bottle of mineral water.

Dinner: have a baked or broiled seafood dish with brown rice and peas;
or a Chinese stir fry with rice, vegies and miso soup;
or a Spanish beans and rice dish with onions and peppers;
or a light northern Italian polenta with a hearty vegetable soup, or whole grain or vegie pasta salad;
or a mushroom quiche with whole grain crust and yogurt/wine sauce, and a small green salad.
☙ A little white wine is fine with dinner for relaxation and has surprisingly high chromium content.

Before bed: take another 1 TB. CHOL-LO FIBER TONE™ mix in apple juice;
and/or a VEGEX yeast broth (1 teasp. in water).

☙ *Avoid caffeine and caffeine-containing foods, tobacco, hard liquor, food coloring and sodas. (Even "diet" sodas have phenylalanine in the form of Nutra-Sweet, and will affect blood sugar levels).*
☙ *Avoid tobacco in any form. Nicotine increases sugar and sugary foods desire.*
☙ *Never stop or reduce insulin without monitoring by your physician.*

197

CONTROLLING OTHER PROBLEMS ASSOCIATED WITH DIABETES

Diabetes often leads to other disease conditions - cataracts, glaucoma, high blood pressure, obesity, ulcers and food allergies.

For cataracts, glaucoma, diabetic retinopathy and retinitis and impaired vision resulting from diabetes:

◗ Quercetin Plus with bromelain, Cartilade SHARK CARTILAGE 4 daily and vitamin E 400IU 3 x daily, especially for retinopathy and retinitis.
◗ KAL Pycnogenol, 30mg, 3x daily to reduce vascular fragility.
◗ Raw thyroid glandular (Enzymatic Therapy).
◗ Cartilade shark cartilage capsules for blood vessel and capillary support.
◗ Crystal Star ANTI-HST™ capsules, or ALRG-HST™ extract.

◗ Ascorbate vitamin C or Ester C powder with bioflavonoids, 1/4 teasp. at a time, 4 to 6 x daily, and B Complex.
◗ Bilberry extract, Solaray VIZION capsules, or Solaray MADAGASCAR CENTELLA ASIATICA.

For heart disease/high blood pressure risk, (people with diabetes are 250 times more likely to suffer from stroke):

◗ Vitamin E as an anti-oxidant to increase blood flow and to decrease platelet aggregation.
◗ To help keep arteries and circulatory system free of fats - Omega 3 flax oil 3x daily, with B12 sublingual or internasal gel, and carnitine 500mg.
◗ To help lower cholesterol - niacinamide 500mg, 2x daily, and chromium picolinate 200mcg. daily, or Solaray CHROMIACIN.
◗ KAL Pycnogenol, 30mg, 3x daily to reduce vascular fragility.

For chronic obesity resulting from diabetes:

◗ Lewis Labs FIBER YEAST daily in the morning, and/or Lewis Labs WEIGH DOWN DIET DRINK with chromium picolinate.
◗ Gymnema sylvestre before each meal for pancreatic normalization and increase in insulin output.
◗ Carnitine 500mg. daily.

For kidney disease resulting from diabetic small blood vessel malfunction:

◗ Gymnema sylvestre water soluble extract
◗ Cartilade shark cartilage capsules for blood vessel and capillary support.

For diabetic ulcers:

◗ Emulsified vitamin A & D 25,000/1,000IU (Schiff, Am. biologics). Apply vitamin E oil squeezed from capsules. Note: beta-carotene is not effective for diabetics, who cannot convert it to A in the liver.
◗ Zinc 30mg, 2x daily.
◗ Clean ulcer of necrotic tissue and apply a comfrey poultice or B & T CALIFLORA GEL.
◗ Country Comfort goldenseal/myrrh salve.

For food allergies caused by diabetic sugar imbalance:

◗ When being tested for glucose tolerance, be sure to take food tolerance tests also, to determine food allergies.
◗ HCI with meals, digestive enzymes after meals, such as Solaray DIGEST-AWAY, Alta Health CANGEST.
◗ Keep the diet high in fresh raw fruits and vegetables, with lots of soluble vegetable and grain fiber.
◗ Avoid all acid-forming foods, refined carbohydrates, and preserved foods.

For accelerated aging associated with diabetes:

◗ Chromium picolinate 200mcg. 3x daily.
Caution note: Diabetics progressively lose the ability to heal from cuts and wounds as they age. It is recommended that they cut toenails straight across or have a professional do it.

For diabetic peripheral neuropathy: (damage to the nervous system characterized by numbness, tingling, burning, pain and cramping in the extremities.)

◗ Quercetin plus with bromelain, and gotu kola capsules.
◗ Ginkgo Biloba extract 2 to 3 x daily.. (Also effective for Reynaud's syndrome)
◗ Crystal Star BIOFLAV., FIBER & C SUPPORT™ drink or wafers daily at night.
◗ Biotin 100mcg. daily. (Also shown to lessen insulin requirements.)

DIARRHEA

Uncomfortably frequent, fluid and excessive bowel movements. Diarrhea is one of the body's best methods of rapidly throwing off toxins. Unless diarrhea is chronic, or continues for more than two to three days, it is best to let it run its cleansing course.

FOOD THERAPY

🍃 Go on a short juice fast for 24 hours (pg. 43) to clean out harmful bacteria. Then take daily for 3 days: Miso soup with sea vegetables, papaya juice, a fresh green salad, and brown rice with steamed vegetables.

🍃 Add fiber to your continuing diet. Eat plenty of whole grain brans, brown rice and fresh vegetables. Add yogurt, kefir and cultured foods for friendly flora. Avoid dairy products, fatty and fried foods during healing.

🍃 Drink plenty of liquids to keep from getting dehydrated and losing minerals. Take a potassium broth (pg. 53) or mineral drink such as Crystal Star SYSTEM STRENGTH™ to alkalize, replace lost electrolytes and stimulate enzyme activity.

🍃 To curb symptoms:
♣ Two teasp. roasted carob powder in water with 1 teasp. of cinnamon 2x daily.
♣ Two TBS. cider vinegar in hot water with honey 2 to 3x daily.
♣ Black orange pekoe tea with a lemon and a pinch of cloves.
♣ Alacer MIRACLE WATER.

VITAMINS/MINERALS

▶ Dr. DOPHILUS powder ½ teasp. 3x daily in water or juice.

▶ Niacin therapy 250mg. 3x daily with Future Biotics VITAL K. ♂

▶ Chlorophyll liquid 1 teasp. in water 3x daily before meals.

▶ Source of Life FOOD SENSITIVITY SYSTEM. ♀

▶ Vitamin A 10,000IU. ☺

▶ Lewis Labs FIBER YEAST daily for B vitamins and fiber.

▶ Am. Biologics. DIOXYCHLOR as directed.

▶ Activated charcoal tabs on a temporary basis with Cal/Mag/Zinc caps at night.

▶ Raw pituitary glandular for chronic diarrhea.

▶ Apple pectin capsules 3 daily. ♂ with garlic capsules 6 daily.

▶ Homeopathic *Nux Vomica* and Hylands *Diarrex.*

HERBAL THERAPY

🌿 Crystal Star DIAR-EX™ extract followed in 2 or 3 days by BWL TONE™ capsules for gentle bowel rebalance.
and
SILICA SOURCE™ extract for rebuilding tissue.

🌿 Effective extracts:
◆ Myrrh drops ♀
◆ Horsetail

🌿 Aloe vera juice with herbs 3 x daily.

🌿 Bee pollen, 2 teasp. 2x daily, with kelp tabs 6 daily.

🌿 Kukicha twig tea with ¼ teasp. ginger powder and 1 teasp. tamari daily.

🌿 Effective teas:
◆ Red raspberry - rich in calcium, magnesium and iron.
◆ Peppermint
◆ Crystal Star GREEN TEA CLEANSER™ for body rebalance.
◆ Bayberry/barberry ♀
◆ Slippery elm
◆ Blackberry/elder/cinnamon ☺
◆ Catnip ☺

BODYWORK

▶ Mix 1 TB. each: psyllium husk, flax seed, chia seed, and slippery elm in water. Let soak for 30 minutes. Take 2 TBS. at night for 2 days before bed.

▶ If no inflammation is present, use mild catnip enemas to rid the body of toxic matter.

▶ Apply ice packs to the middle and lower back to stimulate nerve force.

▶ Eat only small meals during healing. Chew food well.

Common Symptoms: Loose, watery, frequent stools , often with abdominal pain and dehydration; sometimes vomiting and fever.
Common Causes: Poor food absorption, and lack of fiber in the diet; enzyme and chronic vitamin A deficiency; intestinal parasites; colitis; food poisoning; reaction to rancid or unripe foods; food allergy - particularly lactose intolerance; chemical allergy reaction; reaction to water and/or foods in foreign countries; too many antibiotics, or a reaction to other drugs; viral/bacterial infection.

DIVERTICULITIS

Diverticular disease mimics many of the symptoms of Irritable Bowel Syndrome. Bowel mucous membranes become inflamed from fermented, uneliminated food residues. The constipated colon forms protruding pouch-like areas in its walls that trap the toxic waste and protect the body from main-canal infection. However, if constipation continues, and the diet is not improved, the pouches (diverticula) themselves become painfully infected, and healing becomes more difficult.

FOOD THERAPY

Diet improvement is the main solution.

- **Start with a short juice diet for 3 days** (pg. 43). Use carrot, apple, grape or carrot/spinach juice.
Add oat or rice bran, and take 2 TBS. molasses with a banana and plain yogurt daily.
Then add mild fruits and vegetables, such as carrots, bananas, potatoes, yams, papayas, broccoli, etc.
Finally, as inflammation subsides and healing begins, add whole grains, rice, tofu, baked fish or sea food for protein.

- See the CONSTIPATION CLEANSING DIET in this book for more information.

- Eliminate dairy products, fatty and sugary foods, red meats and fried foods during healing.

- Eat plenty of cultured foods for healthy G.I. flora; yogurt, kefir, miso, etc.

VITAMINS/MINERALS

Liquid and chewable supplements are preferable for ease and gentleness.

- **Solaray REFRESH caps.**

- Take a food source multiple, such as Living Source, to curb gas and rumbling as fiber combines with minerals.

- Dr. DOPHILUS POWDER - $^1/_2$ teasp. 3x daily with meals.

- **Enzymatic Therapy DGL chewables as needed.** ♂

- Chlorophyll liquid or Green Foods GREEN MAGMA granules before meals.

- Whey complex powder after meals for bowel rebalance. ♂

- Natures Plus chewable BROMELAIN 40mg. or chewable PAPAYA ENZYMES at each meal.

- Twin Lab B Complex liquid with iron.

  and

  Activated charcoal tablets.

HERBAL THERAPY

- ♕ Crystal Star **BWL TONE™** capsules 2-3x daily for 3 months to heal and tone bowel tissue.
  with
  ENERGY GREEN™ drink with sea vegetables for iodine therapy 3x a week.

- ♕ Aloe vera juice *with herbs* to soothe pain and gently aid bowel action.

- ♕ Pau de arco tea 3 cups daily.

- ♕ Sonné liquid bentonite or Crystal Star CHO-LO FIBER TONE™ to gently clean the bowel.

- ♕ Effective teas:
  - ✦ Slippery elm
  - ✦ Comfrey/fenugreek
  - ✦ Alfalfa/mint

BODYWORK

- ➤ Take peppermint or catnip enemas once or twice a week for bowel cleansing and rebalancing.

- ➤ **A massage therapy treatment can often help.**

- ➤ Apply wet hot compresses to abdomen and lower back to stimulate systolic/diastolic action.

- ➤ Avoid drugstore antacids. They eventually make the problems worse by causing the stomach to produce more acids.

- ➤ Diverticulitis area:

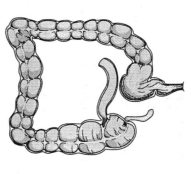

Common Symptoms: Inflammation and soreness in the colon mucous membranes from unpassed food residues and gas; chronic constipation; abdominal pain, cramping and distention; alternating constipation and diarrhea.
Common Causes: Fiber deficiency from too many refined foods, leading to weakening of the colon wall, and formation of pockets like worn tire bulges; chronic constipation; thyroid deficiency; emotional stress causing colon spasms; obesity; causing compressed or prolapsed colon structure.

DOWN'S SYNDROME ▨ MENTAL RETARDATION

Down's syndrome, or mongolism, is a genetic condition caused by an extra 21st chromosome, characterized by both physical and mental retardation. Vanguard nutritional work is being done and clinical knowledge is accumulating about natural therapies. We now know that some retarded dysfunction and behavior is learned, not hereditary. Studies also show that Down's syndrome victims have many immune deficiencies - alterations that are largely reponsible for the accelerated aging progress of the condition. Because of this, most Down's victims do not live very long lives. Those that do almost always fall prey to Alzheimer's disease. Many of the same therapies can help in both cases. See Alzheimer's Disease in this book.

FOOD THERAPY

Better nutrition can improve IQ and physical health in both Down's syndrome, which represents a glycogen storage problem, and in mental retardation.

➢ Eat only fresh foods for 3-4 days to clear the body of toxic waste, and provide a clean working ground for nutritional therapy.

➢ Then, insist on a highly nutritious diet of fresh and whole foods, rich in vegetable proteins and magnesium foods.

➢ **Avoid all refined foods, sugars, pasteurized dairy and alcohol. Reduce high gluten foods.**

➢ See Hypoglycemia Diet suggestions in this book, or "COOKING FOR HEALTHY HEALING" by Linda Rector-Page, for optimal brain nourishment diets.

➢ Make a mix; take 2 TBS. daily:
♣ Brewer's yeast
♣ Lecithin
♣ Wheat germ

➢ Garlic caps 4 daily as brain oxygenators, with kelp tabs 4 daily for brain potassium.

VITAMINS/MINERALS

▶ **Free radical scavengers are a key:**
✦ B15 DMG sublingual 1 daily
✦ Vitamin E 400IU
✦ CoQ 10, 10mg. daily
✦ Ester C 550mg. with bioflavs 4 to 6 daily.

▶ High potency royal jelly 2 teasp. daily. ☺

▶ Country Life MAXI-B with taurine, and extra B6 100mg.
and/or
ENER B intranasal B12 gel every other day.

▶ Mezotrace SEA MINERAL COMPLEX for children. ☺

▶ Choline 600mg. 4 daily, or phosphatidyl choline (PC 55), with niacin 100-500mg. and B6 200mg.

▶ Zinc 50mg. SL daily, with raw thyroid glandular SL.

▶ Country Life RELAXER capsules.
with
Taurine 500mg. for stress symptoms. ☺

HERBAL THERAPY

🌿 **Thyroid balance is a key:**
◆ One to 2 tablespoons of sea veggies daily sprinkled on soup or a salad.
and/or
✦SYSTEM STRENGTH™ drink.

🌿 **Ginkgo biloba extract 2 to 3x daily.**

🌿 Evening primrose oil caps 4-6 daily for 3-4 months for prostaglandin balance.

🌿 Crystal Star MENTAL CLARITY™ caps 1 daily
with
YS ginseng and honey tea 1 cup daily.

🌿 Effective teas: Take 3-4 cups daily for 3-4 months to see noticeable improvement.
✦ Crystal Star CREATIVITEA™
✦ Chamomile ☺
✦ Gotu kola
✦ Sage tea ☺
✦ Siberian ginseng

BODYWORK

▶ Play soothing classical or new age music in the home. It works wonders.

▶ Expose the body to early morning sunshine daily if possible for vitamin D.

▶ Avoid pesticides, heavy metals, (cadmium, lead and mercury), and aluminum.

▶ Do deep breathing exercises every morning to oxygenate the brain.

▶ Reflexology pressure points for the brain:
→ Squeeze all around the hand and fingers.
→ Pinch the end of each toe. Hold for 5 seconds.

Common Symptoms: Slow reactions and motor dysfunction; learning disability; withdrawal from, and poor behavior with, people; thyroid disease; gland and hormone deficiencies giving the person a "retarded" appearance.

Common Causes: Drugs, either given to the child or taken by the mother when pregnant; great susceptibility to free radicals; immune system dysfunction; excess water fluoridation; too much sugar and refined foods; heavy metal poisoning altering brain chemistry; hypoglycemia and glycogen storage deficiency; allergies; great emotional shock or stress; birth trauma.

DRUG ADDICTION & ABUSE
Rehabilitation ✧ Withdrawal

Most people begin taking drugs to alleviate boredom and fatigue, or to relieve physical or psychological pain. In the overwhelming number of cases, habitual drug users suffer from chronic subclinical malnutrition. A healthy, well-balanced number of cases, and from specific, multiple depletions of critical nutrients that set off increasingly addictive chain reactions. Vitamins, minerals, amino acids, fatty acids and enzymes all become debilitated, some by 50 to 60%. Diet and natural supplementation has been very successful in correcting these deficiencies so that the need for getting high by artificial means is diminished. No program will be successful against drug abuse without continued, consistent therapy and awareness.

FOOD THERAPY

Most addictive drugs create malnutrition. A healthy, well-balanced diet is essential for overcoming substance abuse.

🍃 Include plenty of slow-burning complex carbohydrates and vegetable protein in the diet.

🍃 Eliminate refined sugars, alcohol and caffeine from the diet. They aggravate the craving for drugs.

🍃 Make a mix and take 2 TBS. daily in orange juice and honey:
♦ Wheat germ
♦ Brewer's yeast

🍃 The brain is dependent on glucose as an energy source. Drug withdrawals often mean the drop of blood glucose levels and the consequent results of sweating, tremor, palpitations, anxiety and cravings. See and use the Hypoglycemia Diet in this book for more information. See "COOKING FOR HEALTHY HEALING" by Linda Rector-Page for a complete program.

VITAMINS/MINERALS

▶ Take 2 each daily:
✦ Glutamine 500mg.
✦ Tyrosine 500mg.
✦ Cysteine 500mg, with evening primrose capsules 4 to 6 daily.

▶ B Complex 150mg. to control sugar cravings and provide a steadier floor under a glycemic drop.

▶ Vitamin C crystals up to 10,000mg. daily for adrenal health, with niacin 1000mg. 3x daily.
and
Full spectrum pre-digested amino acid compound 1000mg. daily.

▶ Country Life RELAXER (GABA with taurine).

▶ Enzymatic Therapy THYROID/ TYROSINE capsules. ♀

▶ Excel energy formulas as natural non-addictive energizers. Use on a temporary basis to let the body rebuild. ♂

▶ Effective drug withdrawal support:
✦ Methionine for heroine.
✦ Tyrosine for cocaine.
✦ CoQ 10 for prescription drugs.
✦ Logic lithium arginate for uppers and depressants.

HERBAL THERAPY

🍃 Crystal Star ANTI-HST™ capsules or extract to increase circulation.
and
HEAVY METAL™ or DETOX™ capsules 4 daily to help clean the blood.

🍃 For detoxification:
♦ Sun CHLORELLA tabs with chaparral caps 4 daily as an antioxidant.
♦ Crystal Star GREEN TEA CLEANSER™.
♦ Echinacea/myrrh extract.

🍃 Crystal Star RELAX™ capsules or VALERIAN/WILD LETTUCE™ extract to relieve tension. ♀

🍃 Crystal Star WITHDRAWAL SUPPORT™ caps and DETOX™ kit with GINKGO BILOBA extract.

🍃 High potency aged ginseng, especially Lotus Light SAGES GINSENG to uphold energy levels and reduce desire. ♂

🍃 Effective withdrawal support:
♦ Ephedra tea to dilate veins.
♦ Oatstraw for depression.
♦ Chamomile for stess relaxation.
♦ Gotu kola for energy.
♦ Scullcap for nervousness.
♦ Siberian ginseng for cocaine.
♦ Ginkgo biloba for memory loss.

BODYWORK

It takes a year or more to detoxify the blood of drugs.

▶ Biofeedback techniques have been successful in overcoming drug addictions.

▶ Avoid smoking. It increases craving for drugs.

▶ Apply tea tree oil or B&T CALl-FLORA GEL to ulcers in the nose.

▶ Reflexology point:

Drug spot is between the 2nd and 3rd toe *on top of the foot.*

▶ Note: Strong drugs, from LSD to hard alcohol, nicotine to heroin can put one at higher risk for Alzheimer's disease due to microvascular blockage and cerebral dementia.

Common Symptoms: Low blood sugar; irritability; fatigue and unusual drowsiness, shakiness, nervousness, trembling; disorientation; memory loss; wired feeling anxiety and paranoia; headaches; sweating; cramps; palpitations; poor food absorption even when meals are good; deep depression.
Common Causes: Severe metabolic and nutritional deficiencies from too many drugs, either pleasure or prescription - including oral contraceptives; exhausted or underactive adrenals, liver and thyroid; malnourishment from using drugs in place of food for energy.

DYSENTERY

Acute ✧ Amoebic ✧ Giardia

Dysentery is acute, unremitting diarrhea, usually contracted from parasite infested water or food in third world or tropical countries. If you plan to be in a part of the world that has untreated water supplies, a strong immune system is the best defense.

FOOD THERAPY

🍂 Take carrot/beet/cucumber juice once a day for a week to clean the kidneys, so they can rid the body of the infestation more efficiently.

🍂 Take a lemon juice and egg white drink every morning.

🍂 Take 2 TBS. epsom salts in a glass of water to purge the bowels.

🍂 Amaranth grain is used successfully in South America to remove parasites and strengthen the system.

VITAMINS/MINERALS

▶ Natren LIFE START II or Prof. Nutr. Dr. DOPHILUS, 1/2 teasp. 6x daily.

▶ Am. Biologics DIOXYCHLOR liquid as directed.

▶ Nutr. Resource GRAPEFRUIT SEED EXTRACT as directed.

▶ Homeopathic remedy *Ipecac* as directed.

▶ Alta Health CAN GEST. ♀
     or
Solaray DIGEST-AWAY as directed.

▶ Chlorophyll liquid 1 teasp. 3x daily in water with meals.
     or
Sun CHLORELLA granules 2 pkts. in water daily.

▶ Yerba Prima or George's aloe vera juice with herbs, 1 glass daily. ♀

▶ Psyllium husks, and Sonné BEN-TONITE #7 liquid, 2 TBS. morning and evening to clean the colon and bowel.

HERBAL THERAPY

🌿 Cayenne/garlic capsules 6 to 8 daily.

🌿 Crystal Star VERMEX™ capsules as directed.
     with
BITTERS & LEMON™ EXTRACT each morning.

🌿 For giardia: take black walnut or myrrh extract, 10 drops under the tongue every 4 hours.
     or

🌿 Tea tree oil, 4 drops in water 4x daily.
     and/or

🌿 Goldenseal extract in water - particularly for giardia, when used over a 10 day period.

🌿 Effective extracts:
   ✦ Horsetail herb
   ✦ Red raspberry extract. ☺

🌿 Effective teas:
   ✦ Slippery Elm.
   ✦ Nettles
   ✦ Strawberry leaf ☺
   ✦ Calendula flwrs.

🌿 Witch hazel tea, bark and leaf, 4 cups daily.

BODYWORK

▶ Take a garlic enema every other day to combat pathogenic organisms.
     and/or
▶ Take a high colonic irrigation to clean the colon fast.

▶ See Internal Parasites in this book for more information.

Common Symptoms: Frequent and often uncontrollable running of the bowels; irritation, pain, and dehydration; inflammation and infection.
Common Causes: Parasite infestation from bad water, usually contracted in tropical countries; extreme nutritional deficiency from rancid or unsanitary food.

EARACHES

Excessive Earwax ✧ Infections

The most common type of infection in adults is swimmer's ear - inflammation of the outer ear canal. Middle ear infections are most common in children whose eustachian tubes have not fully formed. Frequent use of antibiotics for these types of ear infections are almost never justified, because common use often results in thrush in children and candidiasis in adults. A ruptured eardrum can result from diving, a hard slap on the ear, a loud explosion or a serious middle ear infection. See a doctor if there is extreme weakness or loss of consciousness.

FOOD THERAPY

☙ **If earaches are chronic, keep the diet low in fats and mucous forming dairy products.**

☙ Use castor oil drops in the ear, and hold in with cotton. ☺

☙ Use ice packs instead of heat on the ear to relieve pain. ♂

☙ Press out and strain onion juice. Place in a small cotton plug. Place in the ear for fast, effective relief and infection fighting.

☙ Drink as much water and diluted liquids as necessary to keep mucous secretions thinned. ☺

☙ During healing, eliminate all milk and dairy products, sugars and protein-concentrated foods such as peanut butter. Do not take sweet fruit juices in full strength. The high natural sugars may feed bacteria.

VITAMINS/MINERALS

▶ Use a small dropper and flush ear gently with a food grade *dilute solution of 3% H₂O₂ to cleanse infection.*

▶ Effective homeopathic remedies:

✦ NatraBio EARACHE ☺

✦ *Pulsatilla* and *Kali Mur.* ♂
✦ *Chamomilla* for irritability ☺
✦ *Belladonna* for throbbing pain.

▶ Beta carotene 25,000IU 4x daily.

▶ Zinc lozenges 30mg. under the tongue til dissolved.

or

Cal/mag/zinc caps 4 at night.

▶ Mix warm vegetable glycerine and witch hazel. Soak a piece of cotton and insert in the ear to draw out infection.

▶ Dr. DOPHILUS powder - ¹/₄ to ¹/₂ teasp. in juice 3 to 4x daily.

with

▶ Ascorbate or Ester vitamin C 3-5000mg. daily with bioflavs.

▶ Raw lymph/thymus glandulars.

HERBAL THERAPY

Increasing immune defenses is a primary factor in controlling chronic earaches in both adults and children.

❧ Mullein or garlic oil, or TURTLE ISLAND EAR OIL drops as needed. ☺

❧ Warm garlic oil ear drops. Also take garlic tabs 4x daily to increase immune response.
✦ Drop warm lobelia extract in the ear for pain relief. ☺

❧ Crystal Star ANTI-BIO™ capsules 4 to 6 daily, or extract 4x daily to clear infection. (Extract may also be used as ear drops morning and evening.) ANTI-HST™ capsules as a decongestant to take down swelling and shrink swollen membranes. ASPIRSOURCE™ capsules 4 at a time for pain. ☺

❧ Effective teas:
✦ Chamomile for pain
✦ Yarrow
✦ Angelica rt.

❧ Echinacea extract in water as a gargle.

BODYWORK

While most childhood earaches can successfully be treated at home, there are definite illness signs that indicate medical treatment:
- if acute pain and loss of hearing does not respond within 48 hours.
- if fever does not abate within 3 days.
- if there is dizziness, bloody discharge, or redness around the bony structure of the ear.
- if there is difficulty breathing, or any vomiting.

▶ Massage ear, neck and temples. Pull lobe 10 times on each ear. Fold ear shell over and back repeatedly until blood suffuses area.

▶ Avoid smoking. Keep children away from secondary smoke.

For earwax:
▶ Have the ear flushed for infection by a doctor.

▶ Press firmly but gently behind, then in front of the ear. Pull lobe up and down to work wax out. Fold ear shell in half. Open and fold repeatedly to bring up circulation.

and/or

▶ Put 2-3 drops of warm olive oil in each ear to soften wax, and flush with warm water.

Common Symptoms: Pain in the mastoid, eustacian and ear area; swelling, inflammation, thickness and temporary loss of hearing in the ear; slight fever; discharge from the ear; sharp pain in the ear or extreme tenderness when the earlobe is pulled.
Common Causes: Residue of a cold, flu or bronchial infection settling in the ear; viral infection; too many mucous-forming foods such as dairy products; high altitude, cold and decompression in air travel; in the case of children, often the inner ear structure is not fully developed and canals and eustachian tubes become easy breeding areas for bacterial infection.

EATING DISORDERS
Anorexia Nervosa ✧ Bulimia

To over thirty five percent of American women, and over *seventy-five percent* of American teen-age girls, looking good in today's world means being bone thin. Fashion models are presented as both the aesthetic standard *and* the health standard. Striving to meet this abnormal standard translates to thinness at any cost - specifically to eating disorders that are extremely hard to overcome, and which eventually result in other disabling health problems.

FOOD THERAPY

🍃 Emphasis must be on optimal nutrient foods for body regeneration. Eat a high vegetable protein, high complex carbohydrate diet. See The Forever Diet in "COOKING FOR HEALTHY HEALING" by Linda Rector-Page.

🍃 Crystal Star nutrient-rich LIGHT WEIGHT™ MEAL REPLACEMENT DRINK has been very well-accepted by people struggling with eating disorders - satisfying nutrition requirements without excess calories or any fats.

🍃 NO junk foods, heavy starches or sugars. They disrupt efforts normalize body chemistry.

🍃 Breakfast is important, with whole grain cereals, fruit, yogurt and/or a good protein drink such as Nature's Plus SPIRUTEIN or Nutri-Tech All I, or one from page 63.

🍃 Make a mix of the following and take 2 TBS. daily:
  ❧ Brewer's yeast, or Bio-Strath Liq.
  ❧ Wheat germ
  ❧ Blackstrap molasses

🍃 Have a green drink (pg. 54) or carrot juice often for blood building energy.

🍃 Eat slowly; chew well; have small meals often for best absorption.

VITAMINS/MINERALS

Note: Many minerals are lost from vomiting and laxatives. (Minerals also help to regain normal menstrual periods.)

● Mineral therapy is effective. ✦ Zinc is a key. Severely zinc-deficient individuals can't manufacture a key protein that allows them to taste. Use chewable zinc lozenges or 30mg. capsules 3x daily.
✦ Potassium liquid 3x daily.
✦ Mexotrace SEA MINERAL COMPLEX daily.

● ENER B vit. B12 internasal gel, sublingual B12 or folic acid with B12 for healthy cell growth and energy.

● A good food source multiple daily, such as Living Source MASTER NUTRIENT SYSTEM.

● Gamma Oryzonal (GO) 60mg. for better calorie utilization, with BCAAs for muscle growth.

● A GABA compound for stress relief and nerve building, such as Natrol SAF or Country Life RELAXER.
  with
Ester C with bioflavs. 3000mg. daily for healthy tissue/collagen growth.

● Acidophilus complex powder 1/4 teasp. 3x daily, with an enzyme capsule for digestion/absorption.

HERBAL THERAPY

❦ Crystal Star BODY REBUILDER™ capsules with ADR-ACTIVE™ caps, 2 each daily.
  and
HEARTSEASE/ANEMI-GIZE™ capsules 2 daily for red blood cell rebuilding.

❦ Crystal Star ENERGY GREEN DRINK™, or BIOFLV., FIBER & C SUPPORT DRINK™ - 1 daily for 1 month to help change body chemistry, and establish normal system functions.
  with
RELAX CAPS™, 2 daily to rebuild nerve structure.

❦ Ginseng/Gotu Kola caps to stimulate a healthy appetite.

❦ High potency YS royal jelly 3-4 teasp. daily. ♀
  with
Angelica tea daily.

❦ Alta Health SIL-X silica caps, or Crystal Star SILICA SOURCE™ extract for new collagen/tissue growth. ♀

BODYWORK

Since there is a high correlation between sexual abuse and eating disorders, psychological counseling is often helpful. It can help in understanding the almost universal problem of low self-esteem that triggers this type of harmful behavior, and in beginning to deal with it. Therapy during healing reinforces the idea that destructive thinking and behavior can change , and self-confidence of the patient reestablished.

▶ To improve self-esteem, cultivate relationships with positive people who make you feel important, and whose accomplishments you admire. Don't waste your time on people who are bad for your mental health.

▶ Get some mild exercise every day for lung, heart and muscle rebuilding.

▶ Reflexology point:

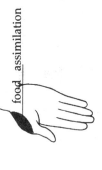

food assimilation

Common Symptoms: Extreme malnutrition from vomiting/laxatives (bulimia) that discharges most nutrients; or refusing to eat (anorexia); belligerent, impolite, aggressive behavior.
Common Causes: Eating disorders are usually caused by complex cultural or emotional problems that end up turning into a form of compulsive psychosis.

ECZEMA ▓ PSORIASIS

Eczema is an itchy, inflammatory skin disease found on the tender areas of elbows, knees, wrists and neck. Afflicted individuals have trouble converting linoleic acid to gamma-linolenic acid. It is most common in infants and children. **Psoriasis** is a common adult skin disorder caused by a too-rapid replication and pile up of skin cells. It usually affects the scalp, and the outsides of the elbows, wrists, knees, etc. Drugs can produce dramatic short-term results, but the problem reappears after they are discontinued. Natural therapies have had notable achievement in both skin conditions because they get to the root of the problem. Natural methods take several months to produce consistent improvement, but they offer lasting results.

FOOD THERAPY

A healthy, low fat diet is a key factor. Most severe psoriasis sufferers are overweight.

▸ A high fiber, high mineral diet with lots of vegetable protein is the key to clearing and preventing troublesome skin conditions.

▸ Go on a short 3 day cleansing diet (pg. 43) to release acid wastes.
♦ Take 1TB. psyllium husk or Sonné bentonite in water morning and evening.
♦ Take a green drink daily, such as Green Foods GREEN MAGMA, Sun CHLORELLA or crystal star ENERGY GREEN.
♦ Take 3 glasses of cranberry or apple juice daily.
♦ Then follow a sugar-free, milk-free, lowfat and alkalizing diet with 60-70% fresh foods, whole grains, seafood and sea vegetables for iodine therapy.

▸ Eliminate refined fatty or fried foods, alcohol and red meats.

▸ Make a mix and take 2 TBS. daily:
♦ Lecithin granules
♦ Brewer's yeast
♦ Unsulphured molasses

▸ Crystal Star BIOFLAV., FIBER & C SUPPORT drink or wafers for tissue integrity.

VITAMINS/MINERALS

Support healthy liver function. It is a key to normalizing skin balance.

▸ Alta Health SIL-X tabs 3 daily with Nature's Plus evening primrose w. E 4x daily for 3 months. ♀

▸ High omega 3 flaxseed oil 3 daily. ♂

▸ Ester C w/ bioflavonoids 3000mg. daily for tissue/collagen regrowth. with Am. Biologics emulsified A & E 4 x daily, and vitamin D 1000IU daily.

▸ Dr. Diamond HERPANACINE capsules as directed. ♀

▸ Cartilade SHARK CARTILAGE capsules 2 daily for 3 months. ♂

▸ Zinc picolinate 50mg. 2x daily as an anti-inflammatory, with germanium 100mg. daily, and Vitamin E 400IU w. selenium 200mg.

▸ B Complex 100mg. with extra pantothenic acid 500mg. & PABA 1000mg.

▸ Apply Enzymatic Therapy SIMICORT CREAM, or Body Essentials SILICA GEL.

HERBAL THERAPY

❧ Crystal Star THERADERM™ caps w. echinacea extract for 3 months. Take THERADERM™ tea internally 2 cups daily, and apply to lesions with soaked cotton balls.

❧ Crystal Star ADRN™ extract drops daily to help form adrenal cortex, RELAX CAPS™ to ease stress, and milk thistle drops 2x daily for better liver function.

❧ Sarsaparilla extract. ♂

❧ Effective topical/internal solutions:
♦ Myrrh/goldenseal rt. extract
♦ Dandelion/licorice/burdock tea
♦ Milk thistle seed extract
♦ Crystal Star SILICA SOURCE™
♦ Nettles tea or extract.
♦ C. Star GINSENG REPAIR gel.

❧ Apply propolis extract to affected areas daily, and take internally.

❧ Apply aloe vera gel and drink aloe vera juice, 2 glasses daily.

❧ Effective GLA sources: *Use for at least 3 to 6 months in decreasing doses.*
♦ Evening primrose oil 4-6 daily
♦ Borage seed oil
♦ Black currant seed
♦ Source Nat. MEGA GLA caps.

BODYWORK

▶ Apply hot ginger, flax seed, golden-seal or fresh comfrey lf. compresses.

▶ Exercise is important to keep circulation healthy - body wastes released.

▶ Apply Advanced Research PAU DE ARCO GEL.

▶ Take a catnip or chlorophyll enema once a week to release acid toxins.

▶ Effective local applications:
→ Enzymatic Therapy SIMICORT CREAM.
→ Aloe ice gel
→ Tea tree oil
→ Calendula gel
→ Jojoba oil (to scalp)
→ Care Plus H2O2 OXYGEL

▶ Expose affected areas to early morning sunlight daily for healing Vit. D. A gradual suntan is ideal.

▶ Stress management is a key. Depression and emotional stress can cause and aggravate psoriasis flare-ups.

▶ Swim or wade in the ocean, or take kelp foot baths for iodine therapy.

▶ Overheating therapy (pg.49ff.) is effective for psoriasis.

Common Symptoms: Chronic silvery red, scaly, skin rash or patches on knees, elbows, buttocks, scalp or chest that flare up irregularly; skin is continually dry and thickened even when not in the weeping, blistered stages; "oil drop" stippling of the nails; sometimes accompanying arthritis.
Common Causes: Overuse of drugs/antibiotics; inherited proneness; eczema is associated with diabetes, asthma and Candida allergies, psoriasis with arthritis; hypothyroidism; EFA deficiency; liver malfunction; thin bowel walls allowing acid waste in the system to be eliminated through the skin; too many fatty, animal foods in the diet, and poor protein digestion.

EMPHYSEMA

Emphysema is a wasting pulmonary disease, characterized by loss of elasticity and dilation ability, and scarring/thickening of delicate lung tissue. The lung exchange of oxygen and carbondioxide is seriously affected to the point of extreme breathlessness and the inability to take a deep breath at all. Neither inhaling nor exhaling are easy, especially during exertion or speaking. The person feels asphyxiated. Chronic, heavy smokers almost always develop emphysema. If they continue to smoke, emphysema is usually fatal.

FOOD THERAPY

ક Go on a short mucous cleansing juice diet for 3-5 days (pg. 42). Then, eat a largely fresh foods diet with *increased vegetable protein*, from whole grains, tofu, nuts, seeds and sprouts. Have a green salad every day and add vitamin B rich foods such as brown rice and eggs frequently.
Add *extra protein* to the diet in the form of sea foods and sea vegetables for additional B12.

ક Have a glass of fresh carrot juice every day for a month, then every other day for a month. Then take Crystal Star SYSTEM STRENGTH drink for 1 mo.

ક Eliminate mucous-forming foods such as pasteurized dairy, red meats, and caffeine.

ક Make a mix - take 1 TB. daily:
♣ Brewer's yeast
♣ Lecithin granules
♣ Unsulphured molasses
♣ Wheat germ

ક See the Mucous Cleansing Diet accompanying the ASTHMA suggestions in this book for more information.

VITAMINS/MINERALS

▶ High B Complex daily with pantothenic acid 500mg.
and
Vitamin C crystals with bioflavonoids, 1/4 teasp. every hour to bowel tolerance daily for a month. (This is an ascorbic acid body flush to neutralize lung poisons and encourage tissue growth and elasticity.)

▶ Enzymatic Therapy LUNG-THYMUS complex and ADRENAL COMPLEX or LIQUID LIVER w. Sib. ginseng caps.

▶ Wakunaga KYO-GREEN or Sun CHLORELLA drink 3x daily with meals.

▶ Propolis extract 3x daily.

▶ Anti-oxidants are key factors:
♦ Co Q10 30mg. daily. ♂
♦ Germanium 100mg., or 150SL
♦ Vit. E 1000IU with selenium ♂
♦ DMG B15 with extra folic acid 800mcg. ♀
♦ Beta or marine carotene 100,000IU
♦ Pycnogenol 50mg. 3x daily.

▶ BioForce ASTHMASAN drops or tablets. ♂

HERBAL THERAPY

ક Crystal Star RSPR™ CAPS *and* TEA 2x daily.

ક Crystal Star SUPER LICORICE™ extract to encourage adrenal activity, and X-PEC-TEA™ to expel mucous congestion.

ક Effective lung healants:
♦ Comfrey/fenugreek tea
♦ Mullein/lobelia extract
♦ Pleurisy root tea
♦ Ma Huang capsules

ક High potency YS Royal Jelly 2 teasp. for pantothenic acid. ♀
with
ક Aloe vera juice, 2 glasses daily.

ક Crystal Star HEAVY METAL™ if chemical pollutants are the cause. Use WITHDRAWAL SUPPORT™ capsules if heavy marijuana smoking is the cause.

ક Rainbow Light GARLIC/ONION caps, 6 daily with 1 teasp. olive oil in juice - to dissolve mucous, and detoxify.

ક Take 5 drops anise oil in 1 teasp. brown sugar 3x daily before meals.

BODYWORK

▶ Avoid smoking and secondary smoke, including smog and other air pollution. (Use Enzymatic Therapy NICOTABS formula to help stop smoking.)

▶ Do deep breathing exercises for 3 minutes every morning when rising to clean out the lungs.
Take a brisk deep breathing daily walk to increase oxygen.

▶ Get some early sunlight on the body every day possible.

▶ Steam head and nasal passages with eucalyptus and wintergreen steams.

▶ Use 1 teasp. food grade 3% solution H_2O_2 in 8 oz. water in the vaporizer at night.

▶ Reflexology point:

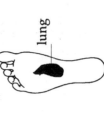

lung

Common Symptoms: Chronic bronchitis with shortness of breath, continuing post-nasal drip and congestion; frequent colds; coated tongue; bad breath; frequent hacking cough, especially during exhalation and speaking; lack of energy and general vitality because of lack of oxygen.
Common Causes: Smoking and secondary smoke; air and environmental pollution; excess refined foods and dairy products; allergies; heavy metal pollution from industry; poor circulation and elimination of poisons by the lungs.

♀ ENDOMETRIOSIS ♣ PELVIC INFLAMMATORY DISEASE ♀

Endometriosis is a condition caused by mislocation and overgrowth of uterine endometrial tissue, and attachment of this tissue to other organs. It is normal tissue growing in abnormal places. Menstrual flow is heavy and painful, and much of the waste blood flows back through the fallopian tubes instead of through the vagina and out of the body normally. Endometriosis significantly increases risk for uterine and breast fibroids. A good natural program will address liver therapy, improve emotional stress and body trauma, and relieve pain.

FOOD THERAPY

Keep weight and body fat down through lower dietary fats, but do not become anorexic, because this affects hormone and lipo-substance balance.

❧ Eliminate all forms of caffeine from the diet permanently. Restrict refined sugars, alcohol, salt, acid-forming foods, red meats and dairy products during healing. Keep all animal fats and high cholesterol foods low, to prevent excess estrogen production - a clear cause of endometriosis. Particularly avoid chocolate, tropical oils, nuts, seeds and saturated fats of all kinds.

❧ Go on a short 24 hour juice diet (pg. 44) to clear out acid wastes. (This helps you to work on the integrity of the liver and digestive system first. Fasting may be returned to as needed.) Then follow a modified macrobiotic diet (pg. 52) - eat plenty of cultured foods, fresh fruits and salads, whole grains and cereals until condition clears.

❧ Have a green drink daily for the first month of healing, or Crystal Star ENERGY GREEN™.

❧ See the Hypoglycemia Diet in this book, or "COOKING FOR HEALTHY HEALING" by Linda Rector-Page for more information.

VITAMINS/MINERALS

Avoid cortico-steroid drugs commonly given for endometriosis - particularly prednisone. Call 1-800-992-ENDO: up-to-date support.

▶ Enzymatic Therapy RAW OVARY and RAW PANCREAS 3x daily. and/or NUCLEO-PRO F for pain relief. Chew tablets for faster results.

▶ Prof. Serv. PRO-GEST CREAM or OIL rubbed on the abdomen.

▶ Future Biotics VITAL K liquid potassium 3 teasp. daily, *with* B Complex 100mg. and extra folic acid 400mcg., B6 100mg. and Floradix liquid iron.

▶ Effective anti-oxidants together:
✦ Marine carotene 100,000IU daily
✦ Nature's Plus Vit. E 800IU
✦ Ester C w. bioflavonoids 3000mg.

▶ Nature's Plus vitamin E 800IU 2 daily. with Solaray LIPOTROPIC complex or SELENOMETHIONINE capsules.

▶ Effective unsaturated fatty acids:
✦ Shark liver oil as an anti-infective.
✦ Omega-rich flax or fish oil
✦ Borage or black currant
✦ Black currant seed oil

▶ Floradix iron 3x daily.

HERBAL THERAPY

Note: Bitters herbs can be excellent cleansers of pelvic congestion, but should be avoided during painful flare-ups.

❧ Evening primrose oil caps 8 daily. with Crystal Star WOMAN'S BEST FRIEND™ caps 6 daily, *and* burdock tea 2 cups daily for 3 months, *or* sarsaparilla or chaste tree berries extract daily for progesterone stimulation/to control pain. Then, Crystal Star WOMEN'S STRENGTH ENDO TEA™ as a body-balancing adaptogen.

❧ Crystal Star ANTI-BIO™ caps or extract to stimulate lymphatic circulation and relieve inflammation.

❧ Crystal Star VITEX™ and ADRN™ extracts for estrogen and adrenal cortex balance, *and* RELAX CAPS for stress reduction - 2 at a time as needed.

❧ Energy-building liver therapy:
✦ Echinacea & milk thistle extracts.
✦ NatureWorks SWEDISH BITTERS or Crystal Star BITTERS & LEMON CLEANSE™ extracts.
✦ Dandelion to help metabolize excess estrogen.

❧ Black cohosh extract to dissolve adhesions of abnormally placed tissue.

BODYWORK

Remember, before you jump into surgery or any drastic treatment decision, endometriosis fibroids often go away when glands and hormones rebalance, such as after pregnancy and birth, or menopause.

▶ Stress reduction is effective, through massage therapy or acupuncture.

▶ Avoid all chlorfluorocarbon products and any other known toxic chemical or environmental pollutants.

▶ Get mild exercise and early morning sunlight on the body every day.

▶ Effective douches:
→ Garlic
→ Mineral water

▶ Avoid all IUDs. They are a major contributor to endometriosis.

▶ Reflexology point: Press both sides of the foot just below the ankle bone, 2x daily for 10 seconds each.

▶ Boluses and vaginal packs are effective in drawing out internal infection. Crystal Star has one available by special order, or use castor oil packs. See CERVICAL DYSPLASIA in this book for more information. Make sure there are long rest times between pack or bolus use - 1 week of use to 3 weeks rest.

Common Symptoms: Severe cramping and extreme abdominal and rectal pain during menses, ovulation and sex; fluid retention; swelling of the abdomen and abdominal bleeding; irritable bowel syndrome and gas; pinched nerve-type pain and insomnia; excessive menstruation and prolonged cycles; infertility.
Common Causes: High levels of imbalanced estrogen, deficient progesterone, and over-all hormone imbalance; sexually transmitted virus; magnesium deficiency; hypoglycemia; EFA deficiency and consequent prostaglandin imbalance; chlamydia; cervical dysplasia or condyloma acuminatum; X-Ray consequences; high fat diet with too much caffeine and alcohol.

ENERGY
Overcoming Fatigue, Nervous Exhaustion and Mental Burn-Out ✧ Increasing Stamina and Endurance

FOOD THERAPY

☙ A basic high energy diet should consist of 65-70% complex carbohydrates, fresh fruits, vegetables, whole grains and legumes; 20-25% protein, from nuts, seeds, whole grains, legumes, soy and dairy products, sea foods and poultry; 10-15% fats from quality sources such as unrefined vegetable, nut and seed oils, eggs and low fat dairy products.

☙ Take a high protein drink every morning (pg. 63). Add spirulina or bee pollen granules if desired.

☙ Foods that fight fatigue include potassium/magnesium-rich foods, complex carbohydrates, high vitamin B and C foods, and iron-rich foods.
◆ Alacer EMERGEN-C granules or HI-K KOLA drink
◆ Braggs LIQUID AMINOS
◆ ALFALCO alfalfa tonic
◆ ALL 1 vitamin/mineral drink
◆ Crystal Star SYSTEM STRENGTH
◆ Sun CHLORELLA tabs
◆ Source Of Life ENERGY SHAKE
◆ Nature's Life SUPER-PRO drink
◆ Bee pollen granules 2 teasp. daily
◆ Nature's Plus SPIRUTEIN
◆ Brewer's yeast or Bio-Strath liquid
◆ Green tea

☙ Eliminate tobacco and prescription drugs. Reduce sugar, caffeine dairy foods and alcohol.

☙ Have a little white wine at dinner for mental relaxation and good digestion.

VITAMINS/MINERALS

Energy areas for supplementation include adrenals, thyroid, liver, minerals.

▶ B Complex 100mg. with extra pantothenic acid 500mg. 2x daily. ♀

▶ Ener-B vit. B12 internasal gel or dibencozide ♂ every three days.

▶ Effective anti-oxidants:
♣ Country Life B15 DMG SL tabs
♣ Germanium 25-30mg.
♣ Co Q10 10mg.
♣ Vitamin C w. bioflavonoids, 3000-5000mg. daily.

▶ Effective raw glandulars:
♣ Adrenal complex
♣ Pituitary
♣ Thyroid
♣ Brain

▶ Phenylalanine 500mg. 1 to 2 x daily.

▶ Full spectrum, pre-digested amino acid compound, 1000mg. daily.

▶ Glutamine 1000mg. daily, with Zinc picolinate 50-75mg. ♂

▶ Rainbow Light ULTRA ENERGY PLUS caplets 3 daily. ♀

▶ Enzymatic Therapy LIQUID LIVER w. SIBERIAN GINSENG or Siberian ginseng extract capsules 2000mg. ♂

HERBAL THERAPY

❧ Effective extracts:
♦ Ginkgo biloba
♦ Ginseng Co. CYCLONE CIDER ♂
♦ Bioforce GINSAVENA ♀
♦ Siberian ginseng
♦ Hawthorne

❧ Congleton LADY PEP tabs. ♀

❧ Effective ginseng combinations:
♦ Lotus Light SAGES GINSENG
♦ Ginseng/gotu kola
♦ Ginseng/damiana
♦ Ginseng/royal jelly vials
♦ Chinese red ginseng ♂

❧ Crystal Star energizers for men:
♦ SUPERMAX™ capsules
♦ HIGH PERFORMANCE™
♦ RAINFOREST ENERGY™ caps
♦ ADRN™ extract
♦ SUPER MAN'S ENERGY™ extr.

❧ Crystal Star energizers for women:
♦ DONG QUAI/DAMIANA extract
♦ BODY REBUILDER with ADR-ACTIVE™ capsules.

❧ Crystal Star energizers - both sexes:
♦ FEEL GREAT capsules and tea
♦ HIGH ENERGY™ tea
♦ GINSENG SUPER 6 ENERGY™ caps and tea
♦ RAINFOREST ENERGY™ tea

❧ Excel energy formulas on a temporary basis.

BODYWORK

If symptoms are chronic for more than 6 months, get a test for EBV, chronic fatigue syndrome, or Candida albicans.

▶ Take a brisk walk or other aerobic exercise every day for tissue oxygen. Aerobic exercise stimulates endorphins and replenishes oxygen in the blood, brain and tissues.

▶ Get some early morning sunlight on the body every day possible.

▶ Have a full spinal massage for increased nerve force.

▶ Alternating hot and cold hydrotherapy to increase circulation.

▶ Acupressure procedure to restore energy:
Squeeze point between the eyes where brows come together.

▶ Stretching program for 5 minutes daily to release energy blocks.

▶ Do not smoke. Avoid secondary smoke. Both restrict circulation.

Common Symptoms: Lack of energy for even everyday tasks; mental depression; lethargy.
Common Causes: Poor eating habits - lack of proper nutrition; protein deficiency caused by extreme "new age" eating beliefs; too much sugar; emotional stress; low thyroid, liver and adrenal activity; anemia; stress; allergies, diabetes, chronic fatigue syndrome, mononucleosis, anemia or Candida albicans conditions; abuse of tobacco, caffeine, drugs or alcohol; pessimistic outlook on life.

ENVIRONMENTAL POLLUTION & TOXICITY
Ways To Guard Against Its Effects In Your Body

Chemical pollutants and toxic byproducts affect every facet of our lives today - from our water and food supply to the workplace and our homes. The major effects of an unhealthy environment are on immune response, particularly in the way that the body's filtering organs, the liver and kidneys are impacted. See ALLERGIES section for more information.

FOOD THERAPY

🍃 Drink only distilled water - 6 glasses daily.

🍃 Eat a high fiber, high vegetable protein diet, low in fats and sugars.

🍃 Eat miso soup and miso foods often to neutralize environmental toxins.

🍃 Take 2 teasp. daily each:
♣ Brewer's yeast
♣ Wheat germ

🍃 Add more green leafy vegetables to the diet, or a green drink, such as Crystal Star ENERGY GREEN™ or Green Foods GREEN ESSENCE several times weekly.

VITAMINS/MINERALS

▶ Beta or marine carotene A 100,000IU daily.
with
▶ Vit. C w. bioflavonoids 5000mg.

▶ Free radical scavengers:
✚ Bio-Genetics BIOGUARD or Biotec CELL GUARD.
✚ Country Life OPC-85, and CELL PROTECTA capsules.

▶ Effective anti-oxidants:
✚ CoQ 10, 30mg, 3 x daily.
✚ Vit. E /selenium 400IU, 2 daily.
✚ Glutathione 50mg. 2 daily.

▶ Zinc 75-100mg, daily. ♂

▶ B Complex 50mg. 2x daily with extra pantothenic acid 250mg. 2x.

▶ Am Biologics OXY-5000 FORTE.

▶ Effective liver/kidney nutrients:
A lipotropic formula w. methionine/choline/inositol, 2x daily.

▶ Immune enhancers:
✚ Enzymatic Therapy RAW THYMUS COMPLEX daily.
✚ Country Life LIFE SPAN 2000.
✚ Germanium SL 150mg.

HERBAL THERAPY

🌿 Crystal Star SYSTEM STRENGTH™ drink mix daily, and/or
HEAVY METAL caps 2 daily. ♂

🌿 Crystal Star FIRST AID™ CAPS - a source of white pine pycnogenol> may be used for preventive measures when taken at 2 daily over several months.

🌿 Garlic 4 tabs daily.

🌿 Propolis extract or lozenges.

🌿 Siberian ginseng extract

🌿 Immune enhancing herbs:
♦ Chlorella 15 tabs daily.
♦ Astragalus extract capsules.
♦ Zand HERBAL INSURE formulas.
♦ Crystal Star HERBAL DEFENSE TEAM™ formulas.

🌿 Effective liver health herbs:
♦ Milk thistle seed extract
♦ Licorice extract
♦ Dandelion extract

🌿 Kelp tabs 6-8 tabs daily. ♀

BODYWORK

▶ Get plenty of tissue oxygen. Take a walk every day, breathing fresh air deeply. Do deep breathing exercises in the morning on rising and in the evening on retiring to clear the lungs and respiratory system.

▶ Use an air ionizer if possible, especially at work where pollutants are heaviest.

▶ Take a hot seaweed bath, or a sweating bath, such as Crystal Star POUNDS OFF BATH™ to remove toxins. Use a dry skin brush after the bath to remove toxins coming out on the skin.

▶ Rub H$_2$O$_2$ food grade OXYGEL on the soles of the feet every 2 or 3 days to keep tissue oxygen high.

▶ A hair analysis is very helpful in determining nutrient deficiencies caused by environmental toxins.

Common Symptoms: Allergy type reactions of coughing, wheezing, congestion, chronic bronchitis, emphysema, respiratory infections; difficulty in breathing headaches; skin itching, eczema and rashes; eyes itching and burning; asthmatic symptoms; depression.
Common Causes: Smoking and being around a smoker; auto engine exhaust; industrial/chemical pollutants; heavy metals carried in the air by winds; agriculture and fossil fuel pollutants; food additives.

EPILEPSY ▨ PETIT MAL

There are several types of seizures. Most people have no memory of an attack. 1) Petit mal - a short seizure characterized by a blank stare. This type is most common in children and may also be accompanied by falling. 2) Grand mal - a long seizure characterized by falling, muscle twitching, incontinence, gasping, and ashen skin. 3) Partial seizures - characterized by muscle jerking, and/or sensing things that do not exist. Many of the currently used anti-convulsant drugs today are so strong and so habit forming that even non-epileptic people have bad reactions and seizures when cut off suddenly. Nutritional medicines can make drugs unnecessary. If you decide to use natural therapies, or try methods other than drugs, taper off gradually. If seizures recur, return to the anti-convulsants briefly to let the body adjust.

FOOD THERAPY

🍃 There must be a diet and lifestyle change for there to be permanent control and improvement.
- Start with a 3 day liquid diet (pg. 42) to release mucous from the system.
- Then follow a diet with at least 70% fresh foods for a month. Have a green salad every day. Add cultured foods such as yogurt and kefir, tofu, brown rice and other whole grains.
- After a month, add eggs, small amounts of low fat and raw dairy, legumes and seafoods.

🍃 See the Hypoglycemia Diet in this book, "COOKING FOR HEALTHY HEALING" by Linda Rector-Page, or P. Airola's rotation diet for more information.

🍃 Eliminate any foods with preservatives or colorings; refined foods, sugars, fried and canned foods, red meats, pork, alcohol, caffeine, and pasteurized dairy products.

VITAMINS/MINERALS

▶ Evening primrose caps 4-6 daily for 2 months, then 3-4 daily for 1 month.
with
Raw thyroid glandular, with taurine 500mg. and B6 100mg. daily.

▶ Country Life MAXI-B w/taurine and B6 as an anti-convulsant.
and
Magnesium 500mg. daily.

▶ Country Life RELAXER caps with GABA and taurine 500mg. 2x daily.
and
Glutamine 500mg. daily or DMG sublingual, 1 daily.

▶ PSI PROGEST CREAM as directed.

▶ Alta Health SL MANGANESE with B12 and cysteine 500mg.

▶ Carnitine 250mg. ☺ with folic acid 400mcg. esp. if taking Dilantin.

▶ Phosphatidyl choline 2-4 daily.

▶ Niacin therapy: 100-250mg. 3x daily, to decrease the need for high doses of anti-convulsants, with tyrosine 500mg. daily.

HERBAL THERAPY

🌿 Crystal Star EPILEX™ extract - an anti-seizure formula for kids,
with
RELAX CAPS™ and ANTI-SPZ™ caps as needed.

🌿 Nature's Way ANTSP tincture, or lobelia tincture under the tongue as emergency measures.

🌿 Effective teas:
◆ Catnip ☺
◆ Scullcap, 3 cups daily - (take with vitamin E 400IU and C 500mg. for best results.)
◆ Siberian ginseng
◆ Hyssop

🌿 Crystal Star HEARTSEASE/ANEMI-GIZE™ capsules to strengthen spleen for tissue oxygen and red blood cell formation.

🌿 Logic lithium arginate capsules.

🌿 Floradix liquid multiple vit./min. complex for body balance. ☺

🌿 Solaray EUROCALM caps.

🌿 Mezotrace SEA MINERAL COMPLEX to resupply deficiencies. ☺

BODYWORK

▶ Take lemon juice or catnip enemas once a month to keep the body pH balanced and toxin-free.

▶ Get some outdoor exercise every day for healthy circulation.

▶ Epileptic seizures are usually short, and there is usually immediate recovery of consciousness.
→ Let the person lie down and get plenty of fresh air.
→ Squeeze the little finger very firmly during a seizure.
→ Do not put anything in the person's mouth or throw water on the face.
→ Turn head to let excess saliva drain out.

▶ Biofeedback has been successful in shortening and limiting seizure attacks.

Common Symptoms: Brief seizures, often with motor disability; loss of memory, and often loss of consciousness; sometimes there is falling down and jerking with foam at the mouth.
Common Causes: Inability of the body to eliminate wastes properly with a resultant overload on the nervous system; heavy metal toxicity; allergies; magnesium and other mineral deficiency; hypoglycemia; deficient metabolic function and prostaglandin formation.

EYESIGHT

Floaters & Spots Before the Eyes ◇ Weak & Failing Eyes ◇ Strain, Blurring & Fatigue ◇ Swollen, Bloodshot & Burning Eyes
See following page for other specific vision problems

The eyes are not only the windows of the soul, but windows to body health as well. Eyes often reflect imbalances elsewhere in the system. As with so many other body systems, the liver is the key to healthy eyes.

FOOD THERAPY

ra Keep plenty of protein in the diet from sea and soy foods, whole grains, low fat dairy foods, eggs, sprouts and seeds.

ra Include lots of vitamin A and high mineral foods, such as leafy greens, endive, carrots, broccoli, sea vegetables and parsley.

ra Other beneficial vision foods:
♣ Sunflower and sesame seeds
♣ Leeks, cabbage and cauliflower
♣ Barley
♣ Blueberries
♣ Watercress

ra Take a good vision drink 2x a week:
Mix 1 cup carrot juice, 1/2 cup eyebright tea, 1 egg, 1 TB. wheat germ, 1 teasp. rosehips powder, 1 teasp. honey, 1 teasp. sesame seeds, 1 teasp. brewer's yeast, 1 teasp. kelp.

ra Reduce sugar intake. Avoid refined foods, pasteurized dairy, and red meats. These foods cause the body to metabolize slowly, use sugars poorly, and form clogging crystallizations.

ra Liver malfunction is the most common cause of eye problems. Keep it clean and well-functioning.

VITAMINS/MINERALS

▶ For general eye health and to lessen risk of disease, take zinc 30-50mg. with taurine 500mg. daily.

▶ Effective bioflavonoids to strengthen eye vessels:
♣ Quercetin Plus w/ Bromelain
♣ Pycnogenol 50mg. with Vit. D.

▶ Beta carotene, up to 150,000IU daily.
with
GTF chromium 200mcg. to regulate sugar use, and Vit. B₂ 100mg. daily.

▶ For spots before the eyes:
♣ Vit. A & D, 25,000mg./400IU.
♣ Panto. acid 500mg. w. B6 250mg.
♣ Ascorbate vit. C or Ester C.

▶ For floaters:
♣ Bioflavonoids 500mg. daily
♣ Vit. K 100mg. 2x daily.
♣ Choline/Inositol

▶ For bloodshot eyes:
♣ Lysine 500mg. 2x daily.
♣ Ascorbate vitamin C 500mg.

▶ For myopia:
♣ Ascorbate C powder 5000mg. daily.
♣ Vitamin D 1000IU.

▶ For itchy, watery eyes:

HERBAL THERAPY

❦ Effective eyewashes:
♦ Crystal Star EYEBRIGHT HERBAL™ tea
♦ Aloe vera juice
♦ Red raspberry tea
♦ Chaparral tea.
♦ Calendula tea for scleroderma.
♦ Ephedra tea.

❦ Crystal Star EYEBRIGHT HERBAL™ capsules 4-6 daily
with
LIV-ALIVE™ capsules 4-6 daily.

❦ Parsley root capsules 4 daily or eyebright tea with kelp tabs 6 daily. ♀

❦ Ginkgo biloba extract to support healthy circulation to the eye area.

❦ For floaters/spots before the eyes:
♦ Rub Care Plus OXYGEL on the feet at night for several months.
♦ Dandelion root tea and eyewash.

❦ Effective liver support:
♦ Enzymatic Therapy SILYMARIN CAPS as a liver cleanser.
♦ Dandelion root tea.

❦ For myopia, strain and eye fatigue:
♦ Ginkgo biloba extract
♦ Passion flower extract
♦ Solaray VIZON or bilberry caps
♦ Enzymatic Therapy VISION-ADE
♦ Pycnogenol caps 50mg. 2x daily

BODYWORK

▶ To relieve eye strain:
↝ Massage temples; pinch skin between the brows
↝ Bathe eyes in a witch hazel solution or chamomile tea.
↝ Bathe eyes in ice water - then squeeze them shut for a few seconds to increase blood flow to the area.
↝ Palm each eye 3 x daily for 10 seconds per time.
(See the Bates Method book for more exercises and information.)

▶ Bad substances for eyes:
↝ Cocaine
↝ Aspirin
↝ Nicotine
↝ Phenylalanine
↝ Excess alcohol
↝ Hydrocortisone

▶ For clarity and brightness, bathe eyes in a rosemary solution. (Better than Visine)

▶ Reflexology point:

eye points - squeeze all around on fingers

Common Symptoms: Poor, often degenerating vision; easily strained eyes, blurring more as the day goes on; frequent headaches over the eyes; spots and floaters before the eyes.
Common Causes: Liver malfunction; environmental pollutants; allergies; poor diet deficient in usable proteins and minerals, excessive in sugars and refined foods; serious illness; prescription and other drug abuse.

THERAPIES FOR SPECIFIC VISION PROBLEMS

❖ **Cataracts - See page 172.**

❖ **Dry Eyes - (Sjögren's syndrome)** - characterized by dryness of eyes, mouth, skin and all mucous membranes, the inability to tear, a vitamin A deficiency, and sometimes lowered immune response. Eliminate common food allergens, such as milk and other pasteurized dairy products, corn, wheat, and nightshade plants (including tobacco and the drug Motrin which is nightshade-based.) Increase green vegetable, whole grain and fiber intake. Reduce all refined sugars, red meats and saturated fats. Increase cold water fish and sea foods. Increase water and healthy fluid intake. Take high omega 3 flax and/or evening primrose oil capsules, 3 to 4 daily, 3000-5000mg. ascorbate vitamin C daily with, emulsified vitamin A and E, to clear and support tear pathways, butcher's broom tea or Crystal Star HEARTSEASE/CIRCU-CLENZ™ tea, vitamin B 6 - 50mg. daily, zinc 30-50mg. daily. Bathe the eyes daily with aloe vera juice.

❖ **Dark Circles Under the Eyes** - usually caused by iron deficiency, but also an indication of liver or kidney malfunction or chronic allergies. Take Floradix liquid iron.

❖ **Dyslexia** - color therapy eyewear has had some success. Pick whatever color glasses make your ability to read easier. Wear for 30 minutes at a time.

❖ **Macular Degeneration** - the macula is the part of the eye responsible for fine vision. In macular degeneration, the blood vessels supplying the macula narrow and harden causing the tissues to break down. Commonly thought of as an age-related disorder, it is the leading cause of blindness in people over 60. It may also be brought on by long-term exposure to ultra-violet and blue light from the sun. Symptoms of developing macular degeneration include blurry or distorted vision, decreased reading ability, even of large lettering. Colors are less bright; there are blind spots when looking straight ahead, even though peripheral vision is good. Driving becomes difficult and vertical lines are wavy. Glasses cannot help. Macular degeneration is often reversible with nutritional therapy. Take vitamin E 400IU with taurine 500mg. daily. for the first 6 weeks of healing. Eliminate red meat from the diet, and take HCl and/or pancreatin tabs for digestion of nutrients, particularly for zinc absorption. Take extra zinc 30mg. 2x daily, and selenium 200mcg. daily. Eat plenty of fish and seafoods, poultry, beans and whole grains for natural zinc sources. Wear ultra-violet protective (not tinted) glasses at all times. Wear amber, or blue-blocking glasses when in bright sunlight and when driving. Carotenoids such as beta or marine carotene up to 100,000IU daily are key factors. Anti-oxidants such as ascorbate vitamins C 3000mg. daily. vitamin E 400IU daily, and ginkgo biloba are important. Quantum SEE is an effective brand name antioxidant product. Omega 3 lipids such as flax oil also help.

❖ **Night Blindness** - Take bilberry extract capsules or liquid, such as Crystal Star BILBERRY extract (do not use for cataracts, near/far-sightedness, or astigmatism) Use amber glasses when driving. Carotenoids such as beta or marine carotene up to 100,000IU daily are key. Take Enzymatic Therapy HERBAL FLAVONOIDS 4 daily.

❖ **Glaucoma - See page 222.**

❖ **Over-sensitivity to Light** - Ascorbate vitamin C, vitamin A or Am. Biologics A & E EMULSION as directed.

❖ **Protruding/Bulging Eyes** - generally denotes a thyroid problem. Iodine therapy has had some success in these cases. See page 85.

❖ **Retinitus Pigmentosa** - Pycnogenol 50mg. 3x daily, Taurine 500mg. daily. Zinc picolinate 50mg. daily. Omega 3 lipids such as flax or fish oils. Vitamin E 400IU 2x daily if retinitis is hemorrhagic.

❖ **Retinal Deterioration** -occurs when the retinal epithelium, the thin layer of cells located behind the receptor cells does not function properly in providing nutrients to or removing wastes from the crucial light receptor cells. The photo-receptors die and vision loss is irreversible. Ginko biloba extract has proven effective.

❖ **Styes/Eye Inflammation and Infection** (See also Conjunctivitis, page 172) - Styes are painful, pimple-like infections of the eyelids. Natural therapies work well when treatment is early. Sometimes origins stem from allergic, viral, herpes-type infections. In these cases, use buffered vitamin C eye drops (must be sterile solution), vitamin A, and zinc. If the cause is a bacterial infection, bathe eyes in aloe vera juice, chamomile tea, raspberry leaf tea, eyebright tea and wash, yellow dock tea wash, or goldenseal capsules and wash. Mix one drop aged garlic extract in 4 drops distilled water and drop into infected eye. Take HCl tabs for extra stomach digestive activity. Take Crystal Star ANTI-FLAM™ or ANTI-BIO™ caps or extract to help reduce inflammation.

FEVERS as CLEANSERS & HEALERS

A slight fever is often the body's own way of clearing up an infection or toxic overload quickly. Body temperature is naturally raised to literally "burn out" the poisons, to throw them off through heat and then through sweating. The heat from a fever can also de-activate virus replication, so unless a fever is exceptionally high (over 103º for kids and 102º for adults) or long lasting (more than two full days), it is sometimes a wise choice to let it run its natural course, even with children. Often they will get better faster. Administer lots of liquids during a fever - juices, water, broths. Bathe frequently. Infection and toxic waste from the illness are largely thrown off through the skin. If not regularly washed off, these substances will just lay on the skin and be partially reabsorbed into the body. As there is usually substantial body odor during a cleansing fever when the toxins are being eliminated, frequent baths and showers help you feel better, too. A cup of hot bayberry or elder flower tea, or cayenne and ginger capsules, will speed up the cleansing process by encouraging body temperature to rise and by stimulating circulation.

Watchwords for fevers and kids: It's probably ok unless - 1) you have an infant with a temperature over 100º; 2) the fever has not abated after three days, and is accompanied by vomiting, a cough and trouble breathing; 3) your child displays extreme lethargy and looks severely ill; 4) your child is making strange, twitching movements.

Remember: Fevers are a result of the problem and a part of the cure.

FOOD THERAPY

- ❧ Stay on a liquid diet during a fever to maximize the cleansing process: bottled water, fruit juices, broths and herb teas.

- ❧ Carrot/beet/cucumber juice is a specific to clean the kidneys and help bring a fever down.

- ❧ Sip on lemon juice with honey all during the morning; grapefruit juice during the evening.

- ❧ After a fever breaks, take hot tonic drinks (pg. 57ff).

VITAMINS/MINERALS

- ▶ Vitamin A 10,000IU. ☺ or Beta-carotene 25,000IU ♂ ♀ every 6 hours as an anti-infective.

- ▶ Vitamin C crystals ¼ teasp. per ½ hour in juice or water to bowel tolerance as an ascorbic acid flush.

- ▶ Effective homeopathic remedies:
  - ✦ Bioforce *Fiebresan* drops
  - ✦ Natra-Bio *Fever* tincture
  - ✦ Hylands *Hylavir* tablets ☺

HERBAL THERAPY

Do not give aspirin to children to reduce a fever. Give herb teas instead - chamomile, peppermint, or catnip.

- ❧ Effective teas:
  - ✦ Catnip/peppermint/ginger
  - ✦ Elder flower/sage
  - ✦ Boneset/white willow
  - ✦ Yarrow
  - ✦ Thyme ☺

- ❧ Lobelia tincture drops in water every few hours. ☺

- ❧ Use a fever to fight a cold or flu. Take Crystal Star FIRST AID CAPS™ until sweating occurs, usually within 24 hours.

- ❧ Crystal Star ANTI-BIO™ caps or drops as an anti-infective. Then, COLD SEASON DEFENSE™ to help rebuild immune strength.

- ❧ Take 2 cups daily, fenugreek or sassafras tea with lemon and honey.

BODYWORK

- ➤ Take catnip enemas to cleanse the elimination channels. ☺

- ➤ Use cool water sponges, or alcohol rubdowns to reduce a fever. Add plenty of extra liquids to the daily diet.

- ➤ Take echinacea tincture to encourage the lymph glands to throw off the toxins. Then sponge off with cool water, and follow with a brisk towel rub.

- ➤ Take a sauna to sweat toxins out.

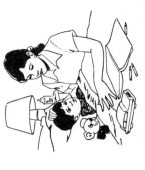

Common Symptoms: Hot, dry, flushed skin; lethargy.
Common Causes: Bacterial or viral infection in the system that the body is trying to throw off; sometimes a sign of more serious problems, such as mononucleosis, Epstein-Barr virus, or diabetes.

♀ FIBROID BREAST GROWTHS ♀

New statistics show that 1 out of 1500 American women between the ages of 35 and 39 are combating fibroid breast growths - the risk of getting them increases dramatically with age. By 75, almost 1 out of 230 women has fibroids. Hormone imbalance, primarily too much estrogen and an under-active thyroid is the normal cause. The usual medical answer is regular mammograms for early detection, surgical biopsies and then removal. Since the tests are often inaccurate (15% false negatives and 30% false positives), and the attendant invasive medical procedures cause great anxiety, pain and expense, many women are turning to alternative methods to reduce breast fibroids. We have found that there is a very real risk in receiving regular doses of radiation through mammograms, even though the dosage is less than that received in the 1970's. Breast tissue is so sensitive and delicate that the time between a mammogram and fibroid growth is sometimes as little as three months. We feel that prevention methods should center on breast self-exams, with mammograms reserved for confirming a doctor's diagnosis. Fibroids are not cancer, and have little chance of becoming cancerous. Natural therapies have been consistently successful in helping a woman avoid surgery.

FOOD THERAPY

ঌ Follow a low fat, vegetarian diet to guard against fibroid formation. High fats mean salt retention and high estrogen production - a common cause of fibroids. Obesity from a high fat diet also increases risk.

ঌ Avoid caffeine and caffeine-containing foods, such as chocolate. Avoid oxalic acid-containing foods, such as cooked spinach, rhubarb, and carbonated or cola sodas.

ঌ Reduce sugar and salt intake. Eliminate smoked or preserved meats and seafoods.

ঌ Eliminate fried foods, especially during the menstrual cycle.

ঌ Take 4 teasp. wheat germ oil daily for a month.

ঌ Add miso, sea vegetables, and alkalizing food to neutralize toxins. Add diuretic foods - cucumber & watermelon to flush them out.

VITAMINS/MINERALS

▶ Nature's Plus Vitamin E 800IU during healing,
with
Schiff emulsified A 25,000IU or marine carotene 3x daily.

▶ High omega 3 oils or shark cartilage - anti-infectives 3x daily.

▶ Ascorbate Vitamin C or Ester C powder with bioflavonoids 5000mg. daily in divided doses,
with
Alta Health SIL-X silica for collagen regrowth.

▶ Care Plus H₂O₂ OXYGEL rubbed directly on the fibroids. Noticeable reduction in 3-6 weeks.

▶ Prof. Serv. PRO-GEST CREAM rub directly on fibrous areas.
with
Germanium 30-100mg. daily or CoQ 10 30mg. as anti-oxidants.

▶ Enzymatic Therapy RAW MAMMARY caps w. vitamin E 400IU.

HERBAL THERAPY

❧ Crystal Star WOMAN'S BEST FRIEND™ 4 daily for 3 months; w. evening primrose oil or borage caps 6 daily, and gotu kola 2 caps for connective tissue.
Then Crystal Star FEMALE HARMONY™ caps or VITEX extract 2x daily as a hormone balancer to prevent return.

❧ Iodine Therapy - often effective in 3-4 months. ATOMODINE, drops, or Crystal Star IODINE THERAPY™ extract, 2-3x daily. Take w. vit. E for best results.

❧ Effective diuretic herbs:
◆ Crystal Star BLDR-K caps
◆ Sarsaparilla extract - 2 dropperfuls in 1 cup water as needed.

❧ Apply a *fresh* comfrey leaf poultice to nodules. Drink 4 cups pau de arco tea daily.

❧ Use an echinacea/goldenseal formula to flush lymph glands; milk thistle seed extract to support better liver function.

BODYWORK

➤ No smoking. Avoid secondary smoke.

➤ Get some outdoor exercise every day for tissue oxygen.

➤ Do not take synthetic estrogen compounds if possible. They keep fibroids growing even after menopause.

➤ Try to avoid mammograms and chest X-rays. Breast tissue is so sensitive that we have seen lumps appear and sometimes grow significantly after even small X-Ray doses. X-rays also contribute to iodine deficiency.

➤ Reflexology point:

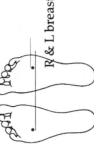

R & L breast points

Common Symptoms: Moveable nodules or cysts near the surface of the breasts; benign growths usually cease after menopause (new growths after menopause can mean breast cancer); sometimes the cause of excessive vaginal bleeding, back and abdominal pain, and bladder infections.
Common Causes: Too much caffeine and too much fat in the diet; EFA deficiency; hormone imbalance with too much estrogen production and an underactive thyroid; obesity; high-dose birth control pills; X-rays; high-stress lifestyle, producing acid wastes in the body.

FROSTBITE ▦ POSSIBILITY of GANGRENE

If untreated, severe frostbite of the extremities can turn into a gangrenous condition, in which blood flow stops, and tissue becomes numb, oxygen-deprived and dies. If treated right away, this type of dry, non-infected gangrene, responds successfully to natural self-therapy.

FOOD THERAPY

🍃 For frostbite: paint on, but do not rub in, warm olive oil. Massage in for gangrene.

🍃 Give the person warm drinks or green drinks, but no alcohol. It constricts blood flow.

🍃 Eat a high protein diet for the next two weeks after exposure, with plenty of whole grains to speed recovery.

VITAMINS/MINERALS

▶ Bach Flowers RESCUE REMEDY every 5 minutes under the tongue as needed for shock.

▶ Vitamin C powder with bioflavs and rutin, $1/4$ teasp. every half hour for 6 days for collagen and tissue rebuilding.

▶ Vitamin E 400IU. Take internally and prick and apply oil to affected areas.
with
Liquid K 3 teasp daily.

▶ Care Plus H2O2 OXYGEL. Rub on affected area several times daily until healing begins.
with
Sun CHLORELLA tabs 20 daily

▶ Effective anti-oxidants:
♣ CoQ 10, 30mg. 3x daily.
♣ Pycnogenol, 50mg. 3x daily
♣ Germanium for wound healing, 150mg. SL for 2 months.

▶ Oral chelation therapy 2 packets daily for 2 months. Then follow with a full-spectrum multi-vitamin complex for 1 month to help redevelop tissue.

HERBAL THERAPY

🌿 Effective herbal compresses mixed with olive oil:
♦ Marshmallow rt.
♦ Slippery elm
♦ Comfrey/plantain
♦ Ginger/cayenne

🌿 Effective tinctures:
♦ Black walnut
♦ Myrrh gum
♦ Witch hazel
♦ Butcher's broom - apply locally mixed in water and take internally.

🌿 Crystal Star RECOVERY TONIC™ or FIRST AID CAPS™, or Ginseng Co. CYCLONE CIDER™ to raise body temperature.

🌿 Apply aloe vera gel often to affected areas - several times daily.

🌿 Crystal Star HEARTS-EASE HAWTHORNE™ caps 4 daily for circulation, with sage tea 2 cups daily.

🌿 Crystal Star GREEN TEA CLEANSER™ or HEARTSEASE/CIRCU-CLENSE™ tea, or ginkgo bilob extract, kukicha tea or butcher's broom caps to stimulate circulation.

BODYWORK

▶ Get the person to a heated room immediately.
↝ Gently rub the kidneys toward the middle of the back.
↝ Cover warmly, so frostbitten areas will warm up gradually.
↝ If case is severe, wrap in gauze so blisters don't break. Elevate legs.

▶ Use alternating warm and cool hydrotherapy to stimulate circulation. No hot water bottles, hair dryers, or heating pads. **Slow warming is the key.**

▶ Apply Body Essentials SILICA GEL.

▶ Effective applied oils:
↝ Cajeput
↝ Mullein
↝ Olive oil
or
↝ Tea tree oil, which sloughs off old and infected tissue, and leaves healthy tissue intact.

▶ If case is very severe, immerse areas in warm water and massage very gently *under water* for 5-10 minutes.

Common Symptoms: Freezing of cold-exposed extremities, and its effects of redness, swelling, blistering, numbness, etc. Gangrene, a painful condition where tissue darkens and dies because of oxygen deprivation, may follow if left unattended.
Common Causes: prolonged exposure of the feet and hands to severe cold; poor circulation; arteriosclerosis.

FUNGAL INFECTIONS

Thrush ✧ Yeast ✧ Ringworm

Fungal infections are characterized by moist, weepy, red patches on the body. Though the causes are many and opportunities for risk seem to be everywhere, fungal infections do not take hold when there is healthy immune response. Stimulating and rebuilding immune response is the key to controlling recurring infections.

FOOD THERAPY

🍃 Eliminate pasteurized dairy products. Keep the diet low in carbohydrates - both simple carbos as in sugar and sweeteners, and complex carbos from whole grains and nuts. (Vegetable carbohydrates are fine).

🍃 Omit red meats, fried and fatty foods during healing.

🍃 Eat plenty of cultured foods such as plain yogurt, kefir and tofu.

🍃 Keep dietary protein high for fastest healing; from sea foods and sea vegetables, sprouts, eggs, soy foods, poultry and vegetables.

🍃 Garlic oil capsules 6 daily. Also apply a garlic poultice to ringworm and cover for 3 days.

🍃 Pat on cider vinegar, or garlic vinegar, or rub papaya skins to affected areas.

VITAMINS/MINERALS

Maintaining healthy bowel flora is crucial to overcoming these conditions.

▶ Effective acidophilus compounds - take before meals.
  ✦ Nature's Plus JUNIOR DO-PHILUS chews. ☺
  ✦ Solaray MULTIDOPHILUS
  ✦ Natren LIFE START ☺
  ✦ Natren LIFE START II
  ✦ Pro. Nutr. Dr. DOPHILUS
  ✦ DDS dairy free capsules

▶ Amer. Biologics DIOXYCHLOR liquid as directed.

▶ Care Plus H2O2 OXYGEL. Rub on affected area, or take a 3% dilution, 1 TB. in 8oz. water for 2 weeks until infection clears.

▶ Solaray CAPRYL caps. ♀

▶ Effective digestive aids:
  ✦ Schiff ENZYMALL
  ✦ Alta Health CANGEST

▶ Stimulating and rebuilding immune response is the second key to preventing recurring infection:
  ✦ Biotin 600mcg.
  ✦ Beta carotene 50,000IU
  ✦ Nutrapathic NUTRAMUNE

HERBAL THERAPY

🌿 Nutrition Resource NUTRIBIOTIC grapefruit seed extract. Mix 1 to 4 drops in 5 oz. water and apply directly.

🌿 Crystal Star WHITES OUT™ #2 caps. May be used internally, 4-6 daily, or opened and applied directly.

or

FUNGEX™ skin gel as needed.

🌿 Crystal Star HERBAL DEFENSE TEAM™ capsules to stimulate better immune strength.

🌿 Black walnut tincture. Apply to affected areas and take a few drops under the tongue daily.

🌿 For bowel health and regulation:
  ✦ Barberry/chaparral tea
  ✦ Sonné #7 Bentonite

🌿 Thuja - take externally and internally for both thrush and ringworm. ☺

🌿 Cartilade SHARK CARTILAGE capsules 3x daily. ♀

BODYWORK

▶ Avoid alcohol, tobacco and sugars as prime culprits for fungal imbalance conditions.

▶ Avoid drug overuse, particularly prolonged courses of antibiotics and cortico-steroids.

▶ Get early morning sunlight on the body every day possible for healing vitamin D.

▶ Apply tea tree oil as an antifungal to affected areas. Rinse mouth with a dilute solution for thrush. ☺

▶ Apply a goldenseal/myrrh solution to area.

▶ Use a mild non-detergent soap to clean skin.

▶ Take Epsom salts baths; use 1 cup salts to bath water, and soak for 20-30 minutes.

▶ Keep all bathroom cups and toothbrushes very clean to prevent re-infection of thrush bacteria. (Or soak toothbrush in H2O2 or grapefruit sed extract solution.)

Common Symptoms: Moist, weepy patches on the body that do not dry out, such as athlete's foot, a non-healing cut, mouth, nail, or vaginal yeast infections; excessive belching and internal gas; loss of sexual desire; anxiety attacks and paranoia; cold hands and feet; mood swings; unexplained allergies; chronic bronchitis; persistent headaches; acne; diaper rash in babies; ringworm.

Common Causes: Broad spectrum antibiotic and prescription drug use that kills friendly digestive flora; synthetic steroid use; birth control pills; low immunity; poor hygiene.

GALLSTONES ❖ GALL BLADDER DISEASE

The gallbladder helps digest fats through production of bile. Gallstones are formed from bile components that become saturated, do not dissolve and precipitate to begin crystallization as stones. The culprit components in the U.S. are inorganic minerals, and a mixture of cholesterol and inorganic bile pigments and salts. As the stones enlarge, the gallbladder becomes inflamed, causing severe pain that feels like a heart attack, and in some cases can be life threatening if left untreated. Stones can also block the bile passage, causing pain and digestive incapacity. High risk factors include poor diet with high cholesterol and low bile acids, obesity, sex, certain drugs, age, and the presence of Crohn's disease. Gallstones are far easier to prevent than to reverse.

FOOD THERAPY

The primary factor in both prevention and control is the elimination of red meats and other unhealthy foods.

🍃 Go on a short juice and gallbladder flush fast for 3 days. (See following page for details.)
♣ In the acute stage, all food should be avoided. Only pure water should be taken until pain subsides.

🍃 After this fast and flush, take a glass of cider vinegar and honey in water each morning for prevention and oxygen uptake.
♣ Take 1 TB. lecithin granules before each meal.
♣ Take 1 TB. brewer's yeast and 1 TB. olive oil daily.
♣ Add yogurt, pears, apples, apple and pear juice to the diet.
♣ Eat small meals more frequently. No large meals. Drink plenty of water for bile maintenance.

🍃 Increase dietary fiber intake. Reduce or avoid animal foods. The main cause of gallstones are fiber-depleted, refined, saturated-fat foods. A vegetarian diet is the best protection.

Note: A predisposing factor for gallstones is excessive sugar consumption. Do not take highly sweetened protein powder drinks.

VITAMINS/MINERALS

◗ Nutritional lipotropics are a key.
✦ Choline/Inositol 2 daily with Vit. E 400IU and Biotin 600mcg.
✦ High Omega 3 flax or fish oils 3 x daily.
✦ Vitamin A 25,000IU & D 1000IU
✦ Methionine before meals.
✦ Solaray LIPOTROPIC 1000.
✦ Phosphatidyl choline 500mg.

◗ Taurine 1000mg. daily to increase bile formation.

◗ Take full-spectrum digestive enzymes with meals to stimulate bile, such as Alta Health CANGEST, Solaray DIGEST-AWAY or Schiff ENZYMALL.
or
Take 2 acidophilus complex caps before meals,
and
1 HCl tablet after meals if needed.

◗ Enzymatic Therapy LIVA-TOX 4-6 daily w. BIO-CALCIUM 4 daily. ♀

◗ Ascorbate vitamin C or Ester C 550mg. with bioflavs. 6 daily. ♂

◗ Glycine caps for sugar regulation, with taurine to keep bile thinned.

◗ Chromium picolinate 200mcg.

HERBAL THERAPY

Increasing bile solubility is the goal.

❦ Effective herbal cholagogues to stimulate bile flow:
◆ NatureWorks SWEDISH BITTERS
◆ Crystal Star BITTERS & LEMON CLEANSE™ extract.
◆ George's ALOE VERA JUICE with HERBS daily, with milk thistle extract drops added to each glass.
◆ Enzymatic Therapy IBS capsules.

❦ Chamomile or gravel root tea 5-7 cups daily for a month to dissolve stones.

❦ Crystal Star STNX™ capsules with lemon juice and water, or LIV-ALIVE™ tea.

❦ Effective gallbladder teas:
◆ Wild yam
◆ Catnip
◆ Peppermint
◆ Dandelion 1f. & rt.

❦ Ginkgo biloba extract 2x daily.

❦ Gynemna sylvestre capsules before meals to reduce dietary sugar.

❦ Crystal Star CHO-LO FIBER TONE™ morning and evening. ♀

BODYWORK

➤ Take coffee, garlic or catnip enemas every 3 days til relief.

➤ Take olive oil flushes for 2-3 weeks until stones pass. (See next page.)

➤ Sedentary lifestyle is a major high risk factor. Get mild regular exercise and reduce body fat to keep the system free and flowing.

➤ Apply cold milk compresses to the abdomen area.

➤ Reflexology point: right foot only

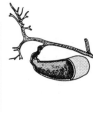

liver & gallbladder

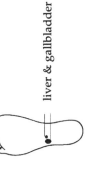

➤ Gallbladder area:

Common Symptoms: Intense pain in the upper right abdomen during an attack, sometimes accompanied by fever and nausea; chronic gas, belching, pain, and bloating, especially after a heavy meal; headache and bad temper; sluggishness, nerves.
Common Causes: Too many fatty and fried foods, and lack of ability to digest them; chronic indigestion and gas from too much dairy and refined sugars; food allergies; parasite infections can lead to calcium composition stones; high cholesterol sediment (coagulated serum fats that do not pass); birth control pills; lack of regular exercise.

THERAPEUTIC GALLSTONE FLUSHES ◼ GALLBLADDER HEALING DIET

Gallbladder cleansing flushes have been very effective in passing and dissolving gallstones. Depending on the size of the stones and the length of time they have been forming, the flushing programs may last from 3 days to a month. Have a sonogram before embarking on a flush to determine the size of the stones. If they are too large to pass through the bile and urethral ducts, *they must be dissolved first, using the STONEX™ program for 1 month,* or other surgical methods must be used. **Note: If olive oil is hard for you to take straight, sip it through a straw.** ✴ See previous page or "COOKING FOR HEALTHY HEALING" by Linda Rector-Page for a complete diet program to prevent gallstones.

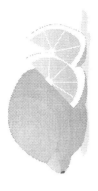

✴ **NINE DAY GALLSTONE FAST & FLUSH** - This 9 day program has often been successful in passing gallstones without surgery. **After stones have been passed, the next diet phase should concentrate on healing the liver/gallbladder area, and preventing further stone formation.**

Start With A Mild 3 Day Olive Oil & Lemon Juice Flush: Repeat for 3 days.
On rising: take 2 TBS. olive oil and the juice of 1 lemon in water;
Breakfast: take a glass of carrot/beet/cucumber juice; **or** a potassium juice or broth. (pg. 53)
Mid-morning: have 1 to 2 cups of chamomile tea.
Lunch: take another glass of lemon juice in water with 2 TBS. olive oil; **and** a glass of black cherry juice, carrot juice or organic apple juice.
Mid-afternoon: have 1 to 2 cups of chamomile tea.
Dinner: have another glass of organic apple, carrot or black cherry juice.
Before bed: take another cup of chamomile tea.

Follow with a 5 day Alkalizing Diet: ❧ Drink 6-8 glasses of bottled water each day.
On rising: take 2 TBS. cider vinegar in water with 1 teasp. honey; **or** 2 TBS. lemon juice in water, or a glass of fresh grapefruit juice.
Breakfast: take glass of carrot/beet/cucumber juice, **and** a glass of organic apple juice.
Mid-morning: have 1 to 2 cups of chamomile tea, **and** a glass of organic apple juice.
Lunch: take a green drink - Sun CHLORELLA, Green Foods GREEN MAGMA, or Crystal Star ENERGY GREEN ™ **and** a small fresh green salad with lemon/oil dressing. Have a cup of dandelion root tea after lunch.
Mid-afternoon: have 1 - 2 cups of chamomile tea, and another glass of grapefruit juice or apple juice.
Dinner; have a small green salad with lemon/oil dressing **or** some steamed vegies with brown rice or millet; **and** another glass of organic apple juice.
Before bed: have another cup of chamomile or dandelion tea.

Finish with a One Day Intensive Olive Oil Flush:

Starting around 7 P.M. on the evening of the 5th day of the alkalizing diet, make a mix of 1 pint of pure olive oil and 9-10 juiced lemons; take $^1/_4$ cup of this mix every 15 minutes til it is gone, (about 3-4 hours). Lie on the right side for better assimilation if desired.

❧ ❧ ❧ ❧ ❧

✴ **4 DAY INTENSIVE OLIVE OIL FLUSH:**
On rising, and every 2 hours throughout the day for three days: take a glass of apple or pear juice. Take a coffee, catnip or garlic enema each day.

Before bed on the 3rd day: take $^1/_2$ cup olive oil mixed with $^1/_2$ cup lemon or grapefruit juice. Sip slowly. Sleep on the right side with a pillow under the hip to concentrate the remedy in the gallbladder area.
On the morning of the 4th day, take a garlic enema. The stones will often pass during the day.
❧ Take 6-8 glasses of bottled water throughout each day.

Follow With A Two Day Alkalizing Diet: To rebalance the system and build a preventive environment against gallstones. Repeat for 2 days. ❧ Drink 6-8 glasses of bottled water each day.
On rising: take 2 TBS. cider vinegar or lemon juice in water, or a glass of fresh grapefruit juice.
Breakfast: take a potassium juice or essence (pg. 53).
Mid-morning: take a cup of chamomile tea and a glass of pear or apple juice.
Lunch: have a green drink (pg. 54ff) or Sun CHLORELLA or Green Foods GREEN MAGMA granules in water; and a small fresh green salad with lemon/oil dressing.
Midafternoon: take a cup of dandelion root tea, and a glass of apple, pear or black cherry juice.
Dinner: have a small green salad, and some steamed vegetables with brown rice or millet and a glass of apple juice.
Before bed: have a cup of chamomile or dandelion root tea.

GASTRITIS ▓ GASTROENTERITIS ▓ GASTRIC ULCERS

These conditions refer to a group of ulcerative disorders of the upper gastro-intestinal tract. Stomach acids and some enzymes can damage the lining of the G.I. tract if natural protective factors are not functioning normally. Current medical treatment for these problems focuses on reducing stomach acidity - a symptom - rather than addressing the long term cause of the problem. Many of these treatments are extensive, with definite side effects, and a tendency to alter the normal structure of the digestive tract walls. The alternative approach focuses on rebuilding the integrity of the stomach lining and normalizing G.I. pH and function.

FOOD THERAPY

🍃 Include plenty of soluble fiber foods in the diet: whole grains, brown rice, fresh fruits and vegetables, etc. Eat cultured foods for friendly G.I. flora. Have a leafy green salad daily.

🍃 Effective juices for stomach acid balance:
  ♣ Carrot
  ♣ Carrot/cabbage
  ♣ Pineapple/papaya
  ♣ Have a glass of non-carbonated mineral water every evening.

🍃 Take 2 teasp. brewer's yeast flakes daily.

🍃 Avoid alcohol, except a little wine at dinner. Eliminate caffeine, tobacco, aspirin and all fried foods.

🍃 Eat small meals more frequently. No large meals. Chew everything well.

🍃 See Colitis and Diverticulitis pages for more diet information.

VITAMINS/MINERALS

▶ Prof. Nut. Dr. DOPHILUS complex before meals.
  or
Liquid chlorophyll 1 tsp. before each meal.

▶ Effective aids to rebalance digestive activity:
  ♣ Activated charcoal for gas
  ♣ HCl for stomach acid
  ♣ Pancreatin for fat digestion
  ♣ Magnes. to soothe membranes
  ♣ Raw pancreas for enzymes
  ♣ Schiff ENZYMALL w. ox bile

▶ Enzymatic Therapy BROMELAIN before meals. ♂

▶ Living source FOOD SENSITIVITY SYSTEM.

▶ Body Essentials SILICA GEL 1TB. in 3 oz. water 3x daily.

▶ Co. Garden DIGESTIVE FORMULA.

▶ Ester C 550mg. with zinc 75mg. daily. ♂

▶ Calcium citrate 4 daily for low stomach acid. ♀

HERBAL THERAPY

🍃 Enzymatic Therapy chewable DGL tabs.

🍃 Hyland's BILIOUSNESS tabs after meals. ♀

🍃 Crystal Star RELAX CAPS™ for nerve stress as needed.
  with
MINERAL SPECTRUM caps 4 daily.

🍃 Hops/Valerian/Scullcap tea to relax esophagus.

🍃 Effective teas w / mineral water:
  ✦ Pau de arco
  ✦ Chamomile
  ✦ Slippery elm
  ✦ Ginger to tone intestinal walls

🍃 Twin Lab propolis tincture
  or
Goldenseal/myrrh tincture 3x daily for a month. ♂

🍃 Aloe vera juice with magnesium/potassium/bromelain capsules 2 before meals. ♂

🍃 Ginkgo biloba extract 2-3x daily for a month.

BODYWORK

▶ Remember that Tagamet and Zantac, both drugs prescribed regularly (one billion dollars in sales yearly) for ulcers and other gastric problems, can be addictive. They also inhibit bone formation and proper liver function. **DGL normalizes these functions after drugs.**

▶ Avoid cortico-steroid drugs. They often result in ulcers.

▶ Acupressure points:
Pull middle toe on each foot for 1 minute.

▶ Reflexology point:

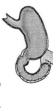
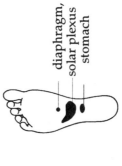

diaphragm,
solar plexus
stomach

▶ Upper gastro-intestinal tract:

Common Symptoms: Chronic poor digestion, with sharp abdominal and chest pains; heartburn and tenderness; nausea and acid bile reflux in the throat; asthma-like symptoms, hoarseness and chronic cough.
Common Causes: Poor diet with too many fried, fatty foods, sugars, and refined foods; poor food combining, and drinking with meals; overeating - esp. of highly spiced foods; eating too fast, too much and too often; acidosis; intestinal parasites; food allergies; too much caffeine and alcohol; steroid use; stress.

GLANDS
Health ◇ Regulation ◇ Balance

The health of the endocrine system interacts directly with our foundation genetics, determining genetic potential. Proper gland function gives us a basis for living life to the fullest. See individual pages for information on specific glands.

FOOD THERAPY

Glands need greens!

🌿 For best results in a gland balance program, start with a 24 hr. detox diet - watermelon only - to rapidly flush and cleanse. Then eat a high vegetable protein diet for at least a month, with whole grains, brown rice, nuts, seeds and sprouts.

🌿 Include "good gland foods": Sea foods and sea vegies, fresh figs and raisins, pumpkin and sesame seeds, green leafy vegetables, broccoli, avocados, yams, and dark fruits.

🌿 Drink 6 glasses of bottled water daily. The glands are affected first by dehydration. ♂

🌿 Make a mix and take 2 TBS. daily in juice or on a salad:
♦ Brewer's yeast
♦ Wheat germ
♦ Sesame seeds

🌿 Avoid red meats, preserved and all refined foods.

🌿 See COOKING FOR HEALTHY HEALING by Linda Rector-Page, for gland and organ target diets.

VITAMINS/MINERALS

Raw glandular extracts offer biochemical nutritional support for stress and fatigue affecting glands. They can improve gland health dramatically by delivering cell-specific and gland specific factors.

▶ Effective pre-dig. raw glandulars:
♦ Strength Systems ♂
♦ Enzymatic Therapy ♀

▶ Effective mineral complexes:
♦ Mezotrace SEA MINERAL COMPLEX tabs 2-4 daily.
♦ Prof. Nutr. Dr. SUPER MINERALS.

▶ Future Biotics VITAL K LIQUID.

▶ Atomodine drops 2-3x daily, with Vit. E 400IU 2 daily for iodine therapy.

▶ Co. Life WELL-MAX or LIFE-SPAN 2000.

▶ Vit. B6 250mg. 2x daily, with vit. A & D caps daily.

▶ High potency YS royal jelly 2 teasp. daily. ♂
and/or

▶ Superior bee secretion ½ dropperful 2x daily. ♀

HERBAL THERAPY

Herbs work through the glands, at the deepest levels of the body processes. The complex, holistic nature of herbal activity make them ideal support for endocrine health.

🌿 Crystal Star ENDO-BAL™ caps.
and
MINERAL SOURCE™ extract or MINERAL SPECTRUM™ caps twice daily.

🌿 Crystal Star ENERGY GREEN™ and/or HEAVY METAL™ capsules if pollutants are prevalent. The glands are very sensitive to chemical pollutants and toxins.

🌿 Effective capsules:
♦ Kelp 6 daily
♦ Wild Yam 4 daily
♦ Saw Palmetto 2 daily

🌿 Effective extracts:
♦ Siberian ginseng
♦ Lobelia
♦ Mullein

🌿 Effective balancing teas:
♦ Horsetail/blue malva
♦ Lemon balm
♦ Sarsaparilla
♦ Burdock rt.

BODYWORK

▶ Avoid air and environmental pollutants. The glands go first.

▶ Get a regular 20 minute "gland" walk every day.

▶ Acupressure points: stroke the top of the foot on both feet for 5 minutes each to stimulate endocrine and hormone secretions.

▶ Reflexology points:

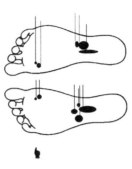

pituitary, pancreas, spleen, thyroid, parathyroid, adrenals, thymus. (*Thump the thymus point briskly each morning 6 times to stimulate immune response.*)

Common Symptoms: Poor assimilation of nutrients; adrenal and pancreas exhaustion; constant tiredness; hypoglycemia.
Common Causes: Mineral deficiency; stress; hypothyroidism; environmental pollutants; too much sugar, alcohol, caffeine, tobacco and drugs.

GLAUCOMA

While glaucoma affects over 2 million people in America, it is often undetected. Chronic glaucoma, often asymptomatic in the early stages, is characterized by increasing inner eye pressure because of fluid imbalance in the eye. If the pressure is not relieved, the eyeball may harden, harm the retina and damage the optic nerve. Collagen, as the most abundant and necessary protein in the eye, is responsible for eye tissue strength and integrity. Improved collagen metabolism and use by the body can be a key to the relief of pressure on the eye. Glaucoma is also often the result of, and accompanied by, liver malfunction. The liver must be cleansed for there to be real advancement against the problem.

FOOD THERAPY

🍃 Go on a fresh foods diet for 2 weeks to clear the system of inorganic crystalline deposits. Take one of the following every day during these 2 weeks:
 ❀ Carrot/beet/cucumber/parsley juice
 ❀ Fresh carrot juice
 ❀ Potassium broth (pg. 53)

🍃 Effective vit. A rich foods for eyes:
 ❀ Endive and leafy greens
 ❀ Carrots
 ❀ Sea foods and sea vegetables
 ❀ Broccoli

🍃 Effective Vit. C sources for eyes:
 ❀ Citrus juice
 ❀ Green peppers
 ❀ Cucumbers
 ❀ Carrot juice
 ❀ Beets

🍃 Crystal Star BIOFLAV., FIBER & C SUPPORT™ drink.

🍃 Avoid all refined sugars, caffeine and foods containing caffeine.

VITAMINS/MINERALS

▶ Quercetin Plus w. bromelain 6 daily. and/or
Ascorbate Vit. C *with bioflavonoids and rutin*, 10,000mg. or more daily.

Take ¼ teasp. at a time in water every hour as an ascorbic acid flush.
and
Bathe eyes daily with a weak ascorbate C and bioflavonoid solution in water.

▶ Pycnogenol 50mg. 6 daily with vitamin D 1000IU. ♂

▶ Evening primrose oil caps 4 daily.

▶ Vital Health GOLDEN PRIDE oral chelation with EDTA 2 -3 daily. ♂

▶ Beta carotene 150,000IU daily, with glutathione 50mg. 2x daily.

▶ B Complex 100mg. with extra B2 100mg, B6 250mg,, and niacin 250mg.

▶ Effective glandulars:
 ✚ Raw liver
 ✚ Raw adrenal complex
 ♣ Raw orchic ♂

HERBAL THERAPY

🐑 Crystal Star EYEBRIGHT HERBAL™ capsules 4 daily to strengthen eyes, with RELAX CAPS™ to ease tension.

🐑 Effective eye washes:
 ◆ Crystal Star EYEBRIGHT™ tea
 ◆ Weak goldenseal solution
 ◆ Aloe vera juice.
 ◆ Calendula tea

🐑 Effective herbal "greens":
 ◆ Sun CHLORELLA
 ◆ Spirulina tabs 6 daily
 ◆ Crystal Star ENERGY GREEN™ capsules
 ◆ Soloray ALFAJUICE capsules

🐑 Kelp tabs 6 daily, or black walnut tincture for iodine imbalance. ♀

🐑 For formation of collagen and tissue integrity:
 ◆ Bilberry extract
 ◆ Solaray VIZION caps w. bilberry.
 ◆ Gotu kola/ginseng
 ◆ Enzymatic Therapy HERBAL FLAVONOIDS.

🐑 Cayenne capsules to increase circulation to optical system.

🐑 Beet root capsules 6 daily, or Crystal Star BITTERS & LEMON CLEANSE™ as a liver cleanser.

BODYWORK

▶ Relax more. Cultivate a calmer lifestyle. Stop smoking. It constricts eye blood vessels and increases fluid pressure.

▶ Get a good spinal chiropractic adjustment or massage therapy treatment.

▶ Avoid **cortico-steroid drugs, tranquilizers, epinephrine-like or atropine drugs, aspirin and over-the-counter antihistamines. These drugs tend to inhibit or destroy collagen structures in the eye.**

▶ Reflexology point: Important in breaking up crystalline deposits:

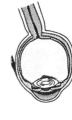

eyes

▶ Eye interior:

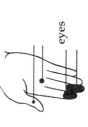

Common Symptoms: Colored haloes around lights; eye inflammation - great eye area pain and headaches; tunnel vision - loss of peripheral vision; inability to tear; increased eye fluid pressure with fixed and dilated pupil.
Common Causes: Overuse of cortico-steroid and other drugs - see list above; diabetes; food allergies that raise eyeball pressure; poor collagen metabolism and use; too much caffeine and sugar in the diet; prolonged emotional stress; allergies; adrenal exhaustion and liver malfunction; long TV watching in the dark; thyroid imbalance; arteriosclerosis.

GOUT

Gout is primarily suffered by adult males with arthritic symptoms. The natural healing approach is simple and successful. It involves diet change to eliminate high purine foods and heavy alcohol that causes precipitates to form. It reduces dietary fat for weight loss and cholesterol reduction. It advocates cleansing of the kidneys to normalize uric acid release and levels in the blood and tissues. It uses herbal support to take down inflammation and enrich body flavonoids.

FOOD THERAPY

Low fats, low meat proteins, low grains are the diet key.

☙ Go on a short 3 day liquid cleansing diet (pg. 42) to rid the body of acid wastes quickly. Then follow with a diet of 75% fresh foods for a month to rebalance uric acid formation.

☙ **Drink 4 glasses of black cherry juice *and* 6 glasses of water daily. Add plenty of dark fruits to the diet.**

☙ Eat high potassium foods: fresh cherries, bananas, strawberries, celery, broccoli, potatoes, and greens to put acid crystals in solution so they can be eliminated.

☙ Avoid high purine foods. These include red meats, red meat extracts, rich gravies, broths and bouillon, sweetbreads, organ meats, mushrooms, asparagus, dry peas, cooked spinach and rhubarb, sardines and anchovies. Eliminate alcohol during healing because it inhibits uric acid secretion from the kidneys.

☙ **Avoid high levels of fructose in any food or drink. Reduce caffeine, fried foods, and all saturated fats.**

VITAMINS/MINERALS

◗ Ascorbate vitamin C powder with bioflavs. and rutin, ¼ teasp. every 4 hours daily for a month.

◗ Quercetin with bromelain 3 to 4 daily until relief. (For both acute and preventive benefits.)

◗ Enzymatic Therapy ACID-a-CAL capsules as needed. ♂

◗ B Complex 100mg. with *extra* B₆ 250mg., and folic acid 800mcg, 3x daily.

◗ Biogenetics BIOGUARD PLUS w with SOD, 6 daily.

◗ Apply DMSO for pain. ♂

◗ Twin Lab Liquid K 3 teasp. daily with vitamin E 400IU and niacin 500mg. to increase circulation. ♂

◗ Vital Health FORMULA 1 oral chelation with EDTA to help dissolve heavy metal, inorganic calcium and cholesterol build-up.

◗ Glycine 500mg. daily. w. chromium picolinate to regulate sugar levels.

HERBAL THERAPY

Many herbs are rich in anthocyanosides and flavonoids - a key to overcoming gout.

♣ Herbs with effective anthocyanosides and flavonoids:
  ◆ Hawthorne extract 4x daily
  ◆ Bilberry extract 4x daily
  ◆ Crystal Star BIOFLAV., FIBER & C SUPPORT drink daily.
  ◆ Enzymatic Therapy HERBAL FLAVONOIDS caps.

♣ Solaray ALFAJUICE tabs.
  and
  Enzymatic Therapy CHERRY JUICE extract tabs 6 daily. ♂

♣ Crystal Star AR EASE™ or ANTI-FLAM™ capsules with
  ADRN™ extract 2x daily. ♂

♣ Crystal Star ENERGY GREEN™ drink 2-3x weekly for absorbable potassium and greens.

♣ Effective anti-inflammatory teas:
  ◆ Dandelion/yarrow
  ◆ Horsetail
  ◆ White willow/scullcap

♣ BioForce DEVILS CLAW extract to reduce uric acid and cholesterol levels.

BODYWORK

▶ Weight reduction is a key factor to ease pressure on feet and legs.

▶ Apply plantain, ginger, or fresh comfrey compresses to inflamed area.

▶ Check your high blood pressure medicine. Several of them cause formation of inorganic crystal sediments.

▶ Crystal Star ALKALIZING ENZYME HERBAL BODY WRAP™ to neutralize acids and balance body pH right away.

▶ See ARTHRITIS DIET suggestions in this book for more information.

Common Symptoms: Extremely painful joints in the foot and big toe; tenderness, redness, swelling - sometimes chills and fever; gradual joint destruction with longer and longer attacks.
Common Causes: Increased uric acid in blood and body fluids caused by overeating, too much red meat, refined food, alcohol, sugar, caffeine, etc.; overuse of drugs, such as thiazide diuretics causing potassium deficiency; lead toxicity; obesity; hypoglycemia.

GRAVES' DISEASE ■ HYPERTHYROIDISM

An auto-immune disease involving thyroid imbalance and characterized by an overactive metabolism. Since the thyroid affects all glands, every body process seems to speed up - digestion, nervous energy and irritability, shakiness and perspiration, the onset of tiredness but the inability to rest adequately, hair loss, unhealthy weight loss, rapid heartbeat, climate sensitivity, and more. Overactive thyroid conditions respond very well to diet improvement and natural supplementation. Drugs for these conditions have dangerous side effects.

FOOD THERAPY

🍃 For the first month of healing, follow a diet of at least 75% fresh foods. Include plenty of vegetable proteins from sprouts, sea vegetables soy foods and whole grains. Add B vitamins and complex carbohydrates from brown rice and vegetables for stabilizing energy.

🍃 Have a potassium broth or green drink frequently (pg. 53ff.).

🍃 Make a mix and take 2 TBS. daily:
   ♣ Brewer's yeast
   ♣ Wheat germ
   ♣ Lecithin

🍃 Eat plenty of cultured foods for friendly G.I. flora.

🍃 Avoid stimulant foods such as caffeine and carbonated drinks.

🍃 Nature's Plus SPIRUTEIN protein drink or NutriTech ALL 1 daily for increased energy levels.

VITAMINS/MINERALS

▶ Living Source MASTER NUTRIENT SYSTEM food source multiple daily.

▶ Ester C with bioflavs. 550mg. 6 daily.
      with
   Zinc picolinate 50-75mg. daily.

▶ **Stress B Complex with extra B₂ 100mg. and B₆ 100mg. with Marine carotene daily.**

▶ CoQ 10, 10 mg. 2x daily.

▶ Twin Lab liquid K, 2 teasp. daily.

▶ Enzymatic Therapy THYROID / TYROSINE COMPLEX 4 daily.

▶ To calm thyroid storms:
   ✤ Calcium citrate 4 daily
   ✤ Lecithin 1900gr. daily
   ✤ Vitamin E 800IU daily

HERBAL THERAPY

🌿 Crystal Star META-TABS™ capsules 2-4 daily as balancers, with LIV-ALIVE™ tea or MILK THISTLE extract for 2 months.

🌿 Effective extracts:
   ◆ Ginkgo biloba
   ◆ Echinacea
   ◆ Mullein/lobelia
   ◆ Hawthorne

🌿 Astragalus capsules 4 daily.

🌿 Evening primrose or borage oil caps 4 to 6 daily.

🌿 Effective potassium sources:
   ✦ Crystal Star POTASSIUM SOURCE™ capsules.
   ✦ Crystal Star SYSTEM STRENGTH™ drink.

BODYWORK

▶ Exercise daily to the point of breathlessness and mild sweating.

▶ Get some early morning sun on the body every day possible. Wade and swim in the ocean frequently to balance thyroid minerals.

▶ Acupressure points: press points on both sides of the spinal column at the base of the neck, 3 times for 10 seconds each.

▶ Reflexology point:

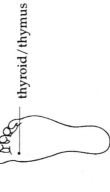

thyroid/thymus

▶ Eliminate over-the-counter diet pills. Their ingredients can both bring on and aggravate a thyroid imbalance.

Common Symptoms: Bulging eyes and blurred vision; fatigue; restlessness and irritability; insomnia; nervous tension; sweating and tremors; unhealthy weight loss; systolic hypertension, mood swings, and sometimes mental psychosis during a "thyroid storm".

Common Causes: Auto-immune disease; stress; overuse of diet pills; mental burnout and fatigue; zinc deficiency; anorexia syndrome.

GUM DISEASE

Periodontal Disease ✧ Gingivitis ✧ Pyorrhea

Almost 50% of the U.S. population over 35 has some form of periodontal disease. But gum problems can occur at any age. Today, many children show signs of gingivitis. Gum disease is an outward sign of an internal imbalance of body chemistry. The warning signs include ▶red, swollen, tender gums that bleed when you brush; ▶chronic bad breath that no amount of mouthwash will help; ▶loose or shifting teeth; ▶pus between the teeth and gums; ▶receding gums that leave the root surface of teeth exposed; ▶the loss of even cavity-free teeth. In most cases, holistic therapies are highly successful alternatives to surgery, involving body chemistry change through diet improvement, supplements and natural irrigation solutions.

FOOD THERAPY

Alert: New findings are showing that risk of gum and mouth cancers are related to highly fluoridated water.

🐾 Avoid acid-forming foods, such as tomatoes, sugars, refined foods, colas and carbonated drinks.

🐾 Eat raw crunchy foods to stimulate the gums; apples, celery, Grape Nuts cereal, seeds, high fiber grains. Have a green salad every day.

🐾 Eat high vitamin C foods, such as broccoli, green peppers, papaya, cantaloupe, and citrus fruits.

🐾 Eat vitamin A and carotene-rich foods, such as dark green leafy vegetables, yellow and orange vegetables and fruits, fish and sea vegetables

🐾 Rub gums with halved fresh straw - berries, or honey, or lemon juice.

🐾 Eat cultured foods for friendly digestive bacteria.

🐾 Crystal Star BIOFLAV., FIBER & C SUPPORT™ drink (no sugars).

VITAMINS/MINERALS

▶ **Ascorbate vitamin C powder with rutin and bioflavonoids. Make into a solution with water. Rub directly onto gums, and take 1 teasp. daily.**

▶ **CoQ 10 30mg. 2x daily for almost immediate relief. Continue for prevention.**

▶ **Am. Biologics DIOXYCHLOR gel. Rub directly on gums.**
   or
   Body Essentials SILICA GEL 1 TB. in 3 oz. water 3x daily. Also rub directly on gums as an anti-inflammatory.
   or

▶ Vitamin E oil caps 400IU. Take internally; prick to rub directly on gums.

▶ Quercetin Plus with bromelain to control inflammation, *with* Lysine 500mg. 2x daily.

▶ Biogenetics BIO-GUARD w. SOD for anti-oxident enzymes.

▶ Effective homeopathic remedies:
   ✦ *Arsenicum Album*
   ✦ *Ferrum Phos.*
   ✦ *Hypericum*

▶ Nature's Life LIQUID CALCIUM PHOS. FREE w/ D. ♀

HERBAL THERAPY

🐾 Effective herbal solutions to apply to the gums to stop bleeding and counter infection:
   ◆ Goldenseal/myrrh powder
   ◆ Tea tree oil
   ◆ Witch hazel
   ◆ Comfrey tincture
   ◆ Cayenne extract
   ◆ Aloe vera juice/myrrh

🐾 **Crystal Star ANTI-FLAM™ caps for gingivitis and abscesses.**

🐾 St. John's wort tea or mouthwash solution to promote healing.

🐾 Crystal Star MINERAL SPECTRUM™ capsules to strengthen gums.
   and
   Open up an ANTI-BIO™ capsule or use ANTI-BIO™ extract, and rub directly on gums to counter infection.

🐾 Siberian ginseng or echinacea extract drops 2-3x daily. ♂

🐾 Evening primrose oil caps as an effective EFA source, 4 daily.

▶ Chlorophyll liquid 3 teasp. daily before meals. Also make into a solution with water and apply directly to gums daily.

BODYWORK

▶ Chew propolis lozenges. ♂ Use propolis toothpaste. Rub on propolis tincture.

▶ Effective gum massages to control pain and soothe inflammation:
   ↠ Clove oil - dilute
   ↠ Eucalyptus oil - dilute
   ↠ Sage oil - dilute
   ↠ Baking soda
   ↠ Lobelia extract

▶ Put 4-5 drops of Nutrition Resource GRAPEFRUIT SEED EXTRACT or Rainbow Light HERBADENT extract in a Water Pik and use daily for recurring gum infections.

▶ Daily watchwords for gum health:
   ↠ Brush teeth well twice a day.
   ↠ Floss well once a day.
   ↠ Eat sugarless, low fat snacks.
   ↠ Rinse your mouth immediately after eating.

▶ Reflexology point:

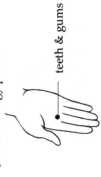

teeth & gums

Common Symptoms: Red, swollen, bleeding gums; bad breath and bad taste in the mouth; loose teeth, change in the bite; hot and cold sensitivity in the mouth.
Common Causes: A sign of nutritional deficiencies, (especially vitamins A, C, and D). Low intake of dietary calcium and other minerals are evidenced first in the gums and jawbone. Allergies or lack of fresh foods; too much red meat, refined foods, sugar, alcohol and soft drinks; poor tooth brushing; diabetes.

HAIR GROWTH ☒ HEALTHY SCALP ☒ GRAYING HAIR

Healthy hair is a mirror of both good nutrition and common sense. Hair consists of protein layers called keratin. In healthy hair, the cell walls of the hair cuticle lie flat like shingles, leaving hair soft and shiny. In damaged or dry hair, the cuticle shingles are broken and create gaps that make hair porous and dull. Hair problems are never isolated conditions. They are the result of more basic body imbalances. In fact, changes in hair are often the first indication of nutritional deficiencies. They let you know right away that diet improvement is needed.

FOOD THERAPY

Nutrition is the real secret to healthy hair.

❧ Feed your hair a high vegetable protein diet. Make a mix of the following hair foods and take 3 TBS. daily:
  ✦ Wheat germ (oil or flakes)
  ✦ Blackstrap molasses
  ✦ Brewer's yeast
  ✦ Sesame seeds

❧ Have a low fat protein drink every morning. It can have a dramatic effect on dry hair texture.

❧ Good hair foods:
Carrots, green peppers, lettuces, bananas, strawberries, apples, peas, onions, eggs, green peppers, cucumbers and sprouts. **Avoid saturated fats, sugars, refined foods.**

❧ Kitchen cosmetics for hair:
  ◆ Wet hair, blot, and apply 4 TBS. mayonnaise. Wrap head in a towel for 30 minutes. Rinse and shampoo.
  ◆ Mix yogurt and an egg. Apply to hair. Wrap in a towel for 30 minutes. Rinse and shampoo.

❧ Poor liver function is often the cause of unhealthy hair. Too much alcohol, caffeine and drugs put a heavy load on the liver and rob the body of B vitamins. See Liver Health pages in this book.

VITAMINS/MINERALS

▶ For color and growth, take together daily:
  ✦ PABA 1000mg.
  ✦ Molasses 2 TBS.
  ✦ Pantothenic acid 1000mg.
  ✦ Folic acid 800mcg. ♂

▶ Alta Health SIL-X silica tabs 2 daily for growth.
  with
  Cysteine 500mg. 2 daily, vitamin C w. bioflavs. 6 daily,
  and/or
  Tyrosine 500mg. 2x daily.

▶ Mezotrace SEA MINERAL COMPLEX 3 daily with boron 3 mg. or mineral uptake.

▶ Homeopathic *Silicea.*

▶ Biotin 600mcg. daily
  with
  Choline/inositol capsules

▶ B Complex 100mg. daily with extra B6 100mg. and folic acid 800mcg. ♀

▶ Ener B B12 internasal gel every 3 days.

▶ Rainbow Light HAIR SENSATION tablets.

HERBAL THERAPY

❧ Take rosemary tea steeped in wine for maximum uptake of minerals.

❧ Effective extracts to blend through hair and scalp:
  ◆ Camocare concentrate for dazzle.
  ◆ New moon HAIR RUSH for shine and elasticity.
  ◆ Jojoba oil to dissolve sebum deposits.

❧ Crystal Star SILICA SOURCE™ capsules 2x daily for a month for strength and growth.
  ◆ HEALTHY HAIR & NAILS™ tea as a rinse and shine.
  ◆ ADR-ACTIVE™ caps and ADRN™ extract to prevent graying.

❧ Effective teas and rinses:
  ◆ Horsetail & oatstraw for strength.
  ◆ Nettles for shine and to darken graying hair.
  ◆ Japanese green tea
  ◆ Alfalfa/sage
  ◆ Dab on witch hazel for oily hair.

❧ Crystal Star IODINE THERA-PY™, 2 capsules, or 6 kelp tablets daily. Sea vegetables are excellent for hair health. Try Crystal Star SYSTEM STRENGTH™ drink mix.

BODYWORK

▶ Massage the scalp every morning for 3 minutes to waken the brain and stimulate hair growth.

▶ Use alcohol-free gels as style holders, not hair sprays that coat hair and pollute the atmosphere.

▶ Wash hair in warm, not hot water. Rinse in cool water for scalp circulation. Condition regularly.

▶ Effective shampoos, containing:
  → Aloe vera
  → Jojoba for damaged, brittle and over-processed hair ♂
  → Wheat germ oil

▶ Effective hair rinses:
  → Nettles to darken.
  → Rosemary/sage to shine dark hair.
  → Kelp or sea water for strength and body.
  → Cider vinegar for acid/alkaline pH balance.
  → Calendula/lemon to tint blonde hair.
  → For hair shine, rub drops of coconut oil between palms and apply.
  → Chamomile to brighten hair.
  → 1 egg yolk with the second shampooing for bounce/protein.
  → Mix olive oil with drops of lavender and rosemary oil and use as a hot oil treatment

Common Symptoms: Too dry or too oily hair; lots of falling hair; flaky deposits on the scalp; brittle hair with split ends; lack of bounce and elasticity.
Common Causes: Poor diet with several mineral deficiencies; lack of usable protein; poor circulation; recent illness and drug residues; liver malfunction resulting in loss of hair.

HAIR LOSS ▦ MALE PATTERN BALDNESS ▦ ALOPECIA

Over 30 million men and 20 million women have thinning or falling hair. Although androgenic alopecia is hereditary and not easily reversible, there are other factors, both internal and external, involved in most hair loss that can indeed result in hair improvement, thickness and regrowth. Hair health depends on blood supply, circulation and nutrition. Your therapy choice must be vigorously followed. Occasional therapy will have little or no effect. Two months is usually the minimum for really noticeable growth.

FOOD THERAPY

🍃 Take daily: 2 TBS. or more blackstrap molasses

with

PABA 1000mg. and pantothenic acid 1000mg. for 2 months.

🍃 Diet is very important. Reduce salt, sugar and caffeine - avoid fat, refined and preserved foods.

🍃 Eat foods rich in silica and sulphur, such as onions, garlic, sprouts, horseradish, green leafy vegies, carrots, bell peppers, cucumbers, rice, and seeds.

🍃 Eat foods rich in iodine and potassium, such as sea vegetables and sea foods for growth and thickness.

🍃 Make a mix and take 2 TBS. daily in food:
   ◆ Wheat germ flakes
   ◆ Brewer's yeast flakes
   ◆ Pumpkin seeds
   ◆ Chopped dulse

🍃 Drink 6 glasses of water daily.

🍃 Use vinegar rinses for thickness and body.

VITAMINS/MINERALS

Discontinue commercial hair coloring and hair dryers.

▶ Biotin 1000mcg. daily with Choline/inositol 1000mg. daily.

▶ High B Complex daily with extra niacin 500mg. daily, Ester C with bioflavonoids and rutin 550mg, 4 daily. Vit. E 400IU daily as an antioxidant, and Pancreatin 1300mg. at meals. ♀

▶ Mezotrace SEA MINERAL COMPLEX 2x daily.

▶ High Omega 3 fish or flax oils 3 daily.

▶ Nature's Plus ULTRA HAIR tabs.

▶ Alta Health SIL-X tabs.

▶ Cysteine 500mg. daily with zinc 75mg. daily, and CoQ 10 30mg. daily, esp. if hair loss is related to low thyroid with zinc deficiency. ♂

HERBAL THERAPY

🌿 Crystal Star SILICA SOURCE™ extract daily.

and/or

HEALTHY HAIR & NAILS™ tea both as a drink and hair rinse.

🌿 Effective teas to drink and rinse hair:
   ◆ Comfrey/alfalfa
   ◆ **Nettles**
   ◆ **Horsetail**
   ◆ Rosemary/dulse
   ◆ **Sage for thinning hair**

🌿 Reishi mushroom tea daily.

🌿 Crystal Star MINERAL SPECTRUM™ caps or MINERAL SOURCE COMPLEX extr. for 4 - 6 weeks.

🌿 Phyto-estrogen and hormone balancing herbs can help hair loss in women: ♀
   ◆ Borage oil capsules
   ◆ Licorice rt.
   ◆ Black cohosh rt.
   ◆ Dong quai/burdock rt.

🌿 Cayenne extract: Apply 2x daily. Rub directly onto scalp before shampooing. Leave on for 30 minutes.

BODYWORK

External factors that cause hair loss are tight hairstyles and curlers, hot rollers, and chemicals for perming or straightening.

▶ Effective scalp conditioners:
   → Biotin treatments
   → Jojoba oil and shampoo to relieve sebum build-up.
   → Aloe vera oil and shampoo

▶ Head circulation is the key.
   → Massage scalp vigorously for 3 minutes every morning.
   → Brush dry hair well.
   → Rinse for several minutes with alternating hot and cold water.
   → Use a slant board once a week for 15 minutes.

▶ Get some outdoor exercise every day possible for body oxygen.

▶ Rinse hair with sea water when possible for thickness.

▶ Reflexology point:

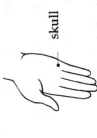 skull

Common Symptoms: Thinning or complete loss of hair.

Common Causes: Poor circulation; poor diet with excess salt and sugar; dandruff or seborrhea; plugs of sebum, cholesterol; heredity; gland imbalances in women from postpartum changes or discontinuance of birth control pills and overproduction of male sex hormones - (hair loss above the temples in women can mean a possible ovarian or adrenal tumor); chemotherapy and high blood pressure drugs; B vitamin deficiency; prolonged emotional stress and anxiety; severe illness or anemia; mineral deficiencies; hypothyroidism.

HEADACHES ■ TENSION & SINUS HEADACHES

Tension headaches: muscle contractions of the scalp and back of the head. Sinus headaches: congestion and inflammation of the nasal sinuses.

FOOD THERAPY

ه Go on a short 24 hour juice fast (pg. 44) to remove body clogs. Drink lots of water, lemon and green drinks (pg. 54ff) and potassium broth. (pg. 53).

ه Follow the next day with a very alkaline diet: apples and apple juice, cranberry juice, sprouts, salads and some brown rice.

ه Make a mix and take 2 TBS. daily to restore body balance:
♦ Brewer's yeast
♦ Lecithin granules
♦ Cider vinegar and honey

ه Avoid refined foods, salty, sugary foods, and chemical foods.

ه See LIVER CLEANSING and hypoglycemia diet suggestions in this book.

ه Apply cold black tea bags to the eyes for 15 minutes.

VITAMINS/MINERALS

▶ Country Life MAXI-B w. taurine
and
Ester C 550mg. with bioflavs and rutin 3 - 4 daily.

▶ Niacin therapy 100mg. or more as needed daily to keep blood vessels and circulation open.

▶ DLPA 500-750mg. or a GABA compound such as Country Life RELAXER caps for brain relief.

▶ Bromelain 500mg. as needed. Acts like aspirin without the stomach upset.

▶ Magnesium 800mg. daily.

▶ Nature's Plus germanium 25mg. with suma. ♂
and
Evening primrose caps 3–4 daily.

▶ Homeopathic remedies:
✚ Hylands *Calms Forte*
✚ *Kali Phos. or Mag. Phos. for frontal headaches.*
✚ *Kali Sulph., Kali Mur or Ferr. Phos for back of the head aches.*
✚ Hylands *Hylavir.* ☺

HERBAL THERAPY

❦ Crystal Star RELAX™ caps 2 as needed to rebuild nerve sheath, HEADACHE DEFENSE™ extract, ASPIRSOURCE™ capsules (for frontal pain), or STRESS RELIEF™ extract for pain relief, DEPRESS-EX™ extract for brain relief.

❦ Effective extracts:
♦ Valerian/wild lettuce
♦ Feverfew
♦ Ginkgo biloba
♦ Quantum MIG-RELIEF

❦ Effective teas:
♦ Wisdom Of The Ancients Yerba Maté
♦ St. John's wort
♦ White willow bk.
♦ Chamomile
♦ Catnip/sage

❦ Use rosemary as a tea, or mix the essential oil in hot water and inhale as an effective steam; or take the extract under the tongue as an anti-oxidant.

❦ Dong quai/damiana caps or extract for prevention. ♀

BODYWORK

▶ Take a brisk walk. Breathe deeply for oxygen. The more brain oxygen, the fewer headaches.

▶ Lie down with the head higher than the body.

▶ Apply an ice massage on the back of the neck and upper back. It will dramatically reduce pain.

▶ Have a chiropractic adjustment shiatsu massage, or massage therapy treatment if headaches are chronic. Take CSA 250mg. daily, if spinal misalignment is the cause.

▶ Aromatherapy:
➥ Lavender essential oil.
➥ Apply peppermint oil to the temples. ♀

▶ Reflexology point:

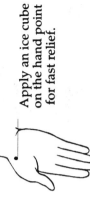

Apply an ice cube on the hand point for fast relief.

Common Symptoms: Pain over the eyes, forehead and temples; inability to sleep; irritability.
Common Causes: Emotional stress; food sensitivities; eyestrain; muscle tension; constipation; too much caffeine, salt, sugar or MSG intake; hypoglycemia; allergies; water retention; TMJ dysfunction syndrome; poor circulation; sluggish liver; jawbone misalignment; arthritis; Candida albicans; drug toxicity.

CLUSTER HEADACHES

Cluster headaches are two or more sudden and extremely painful headaches a day, localized over the eyes or a spot on the forehead, usually coming in cycles for several days, with long periods of remission - recurring every few months. There are no advance warning symptoms. Vasodilation is a key factor, but cluster headaches are not migraines. Sometimes called atypical facial neuralgia, or histamine cephalgia, these headaches appear to stem from imbalance in the frontal part of the brain, and affect the nerves in the face.

FOOD THERAPY

❧ Food allergens appear to be a main factor in onset. Eliminate the following foods: pickled fish and shellfish, smoked meats and other nitrate-containing foods, aged cheeses, red wines, avocados, caffeine and chocolate.

❧ Eat high magnesium foods to reduce throbbing and contractions: dark leafy greens, fresh sea foods and sea vegetables, nuts, whole grains, molasses.

❧ Eat vitamin C rich foods: broccoli, green peppers, hot peppers, sprouts, cherries, citrus, etc.

❧ The food sensitivities accompanying this type of headache are often a favorite food that one craves. Watch out for these "trigger foods" and avoid them.

❧ Bancha Green tea or Crystal Star GREEN TEA CLEANSER™ every morning as a preventive. A good cleansing, colon health program is very effective in stopping headaches.

VITAMINS/MINERALS

Note: Although niacin therapy is helpful for other types of headache, it is not recommended for cluster headaches.

▶ DLPA 750mg. for natural endorphin formation.
and/or
Twin Lab GABA PLUS, or Country Life RELAXER capsules for brain stress control.

▶ Anti-oxidants can be a key: Nature's Plus GERMANIUM 25mg. with SUMA, and Extra strength ginkgo biloba extract capsules.

▶ Glutamine 500mg. 2 or more times daily. ♂

▶ Quercitin Plus 500mg. 2x daily with magnesium 500mg. 2x daily.

▶ Natrol Ester C with bioflavonoids 2000mg. activity daily.

▶ Omega 3 fish or flax oils 3x daily.

▶ Nature's Life CAL/MAG preacidified liq. 3 teasp. daily. ♂

HERBAL THERAPY

❧ Feverfew extract capsules or liquid as needed for pain, and as a preventive when used on a regular basis. ♀

❧ Crystal Star CLUSTER CAPS™ and/or STRESS RELEASE™ or Quantum MIGR™ extract.
with
ASPIRSOURCE CAPS™ for frontal lobe pain.

❧ Capsicum/ginger capsules, 2 daily, or Crystal Star RECOVERY TONIC™ drops in water as needed. ♂

❧ Evening primrose oil, 4 daily for prostaglandin balance.

❧ Crystal Star VALERIAN/WILD LETTUCE extract.

❧ Medicine Wheel SERENE or Crystal Star DEPRESS-EX™ extract as needed. ♀

❧ Alcohol-free goldenseal extract or capsules 2 to 3x daily with garlic tabs 4 daily.

BODYWORK

▶ Biofeedback and other relaxation techniques such as meditation, help; especially in conjunction with deep breathing exercises.

▶ Chiropractic manipulation, acupuncture, and massage therapy are also effective.

▶ Apply an ice pack on the back of the neck and upper back to reduce swelling and pain.

▶ Reflexology point:

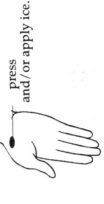

press and/or apply ice.

Common Symptoms: Severe pain, usually localized around one eye; dilated blood vessels with irritated adjacent nerve endings; localized histamine reaction; nasal stuffiness, sensitivity to light; restlessness.
Common Causes: Vascular changes in the brain; eating allergen foods; caffeine withdrawal; prostaglandin deficiency and hormone imbalance, sometimes related to birth control pills; magnesium deficiency; glare, esp. from computer screens.

MIGRAINE & VASCULAR HEADACHES

Migraines appear to be a primary disorder of the brain, involving a drop in estrogen levels, and characterized by neurologic inflammation. They are a common problem, affecting 15% of American men and 30% of American women. A migraine usually indicates vascular instability, cranial artery constriction and inadequate blood supply to the brain. Chronic stress is a potentiator of migraines. Platelet aggregation, build-up of histamine levels, and serotonin (a vaso-constrictor) release are also abnormal in migraine sufferers. The resulting inflammation, vasodilation, serotonin release and histamine reactions can be successfully addressed by natural healing methods. Indeed, sometimes these work when nothing else does.

FOOD THERAPY

Nutritional awareness is a must for preventing migraines.

🍃 Food allergies or intolerances are always involved in migraines. Trigger foods include: **citrus juices, red wine, nitrates in foods, chocolate, aged meats, canned fish, refined sugars, and cultured foods, such as yogurt and cheeses.**

🍃 At the first signs of a migraine: take 1-2 cups of strong coffee to prevent blood vessel dilation; (avoid excess caffeine on a regular basis) or a glass of carrot/celery juice if possible.

🍃 Avoid animal fats, (especially in red meats and dairy products), excess caffeine, (withdrawal can be a precipitator) soft drinks, (the phosphorus binds up available magnesium) MSG containing foods and hard liquor.

🍃 The diet should include plenty of whole grains, fresh leafy greens, fiber foods and fish for prevention.

🍃 See HYPOGLYCEMIA DIET in this book to help blood sugar regulation.

🍃 Take Schiff GARLIC/ONION caps regularly as a brain anti-oxidant.

VITAMINS/MINERALS

Take only hypo-allergenic supplements.

▶ Niacin therapy: up to 500mg. as needed to normalize circulation. Take with Stress B Complex and extra B6 for best preventive results.

▶ **Quercetin Plus and bioflavonoid and rutin caps 500mg. 4 daily.**

▶ DLPA 1000mg. for pain control. ♀

▶ Effective body balancers:
   ♣ Germanium 30mg. daily
   ♣ Omega 3 flax oil 3x daily
   ♣ **PSI PROGEST oil** - apply to temples every 1/2 hour, take 1/4 teasp. SL.
   ♣ Alta Health magnesium chloride
   ♣ Logic LITHIUM complex
   ♣ 1 aspirin daily as a preventive.

▶ Evening primrose oil caps *or* royal jelly caps, 4 daily for prevention. ♀

▶ Magnesium 400mg. 2x daily to prevent nerve twitching. ♀

▶ ENER B internasal B12 gel and 1 aspirin every other day.

▶ Twin Lab CSA caps w. Rainbow Light GARLIC & GREENS caps.

HERBAL THERAPY

🌿 Crystal Star **MIGR-EASE™** and **RELAX CAPS™** as needed for pain and preventive activity,

or

MIGR™ extract with feverfew, or RECOVERY TONIC with capsicum to normalize circulation.

🌿 Feverfew extract capsules or tea as needed before and during an attack to inhibit inflammatory secretions and excess serotonin, and decrease blood vessel reaction to vasoconstrictors.

🌿 Crystal Star **RAINFOREST ENERGY™** tea with kola nut.

🌿 Take 1 ginger capsule dissolved in water at first sign of visual disturbance - 4x daily thereafter. ♀ ☺

🌿 Effective extracts:
   ♦ **Valerian/wild lettuce**
   ♦ Lobelia
   ♦ **Ginkgo biloba**
   ♦ Angelica rt.
   ♦ Alcohol-free goldenseal

🌿 Effective teas:
   ♦ **Ginger rt.**
   ♦ Scullcap
   ♦ **Rosemary/sage**

BODYWORK

▶ Physical therapies to decrease intensity of attacks:
   → Biofeedback/relaxation training
   → Chiropractic adjustment
   → Acupuncture and acupressure
   → Massage therapy treatment
   → Fresh air and exercise
   → Soft melodious music
   → Red color therapy eyewear

▶ Apply Pro. Serv. PROGEST OIL. to pain areas every 1/2 hour - *and* take 1/4 teasp. under the tongue.

▶ Use ice packs on the neck to draw blood out of the head.

▶ Apply pressure to the inside base of the big toe 3 times for 10 seconds each time. Massage temples for 5 minutes. Breathe deeply. Do 10 neck rolls. Pull ear lobes for 5 seconds. Rub back and all around ear shell.

▶ Aromatherapy: Lavender essence - also apply lavender to the temples.

▶ Avoid smoking and secondary smoke. It constricts blood vessels.

▶ **Take a coffee enema to stimulate liver and normalize bile activity for almost immediate results.**

Common Symptoms: Constriction/dilation of blood vessels in the brain, scalp and face - lasts 4 hours to two days - recurrent several times a month; a preceding aura, light sensitivity, visual problems and halos appearing around lights; nausea, made worse by light and movement; intense, long-lasting pain, usually on one side of the head; water retention.
Common Causes: Vascular instability; arterial neuron disorder brought on by severe emotional distress; poor diet, with too much caffeine, junk and fast foods, fats and refined sugars; pituitary/hormone imbalance; platelet aggregation/serotonin imbalance; viral infection; over-acid system stripping away protective nerve sheathing; food allergies/sensitivities and deficiency of friendly intestinal organisms; liver toxicity; poor circulation; menstrual dysfunction; over-use of drugs; hereditary weakness.

HEARING PROBLEMS & HEARING LOSS

Tinnitus ◊ Ringing In The Ears

Hearing problems are the consequence of a wide spectrum of causes (see below). The ones addressed here are the result of externally or nutritionally-based causes - as opposed to internal bone fusions that need surgical attention. See Hypoglycemia Diet pages in this book for additional diet suggestions.

FOOD THERAPY

Lose excess weight. Fat clogs the head, too.

🐾 Reduce dietary fats, cholesterol and mucous-forming foods. Avoid refined sugars, heavy starches and concentrated foods. See HEALTHY HEART DIET in this book.

🐾 Eat light to hear better - plenty of vegetable proteins, sprouts, whole grains, fruits, and cultured foods .

🐾 Take fresh grated horseradish in a spoon with lemon juice. Hang over a sink to release excess mucous and clear head passages.

🐾 Take a green drink (pg. 54ff) or a Sun CHLORELLA drink daily.

🐾 For ringing in the ears:
◆ Go on a short 3 day mucous cleansing diet (pg. 42). Then eat fresh foods for the rest of the week. Have plenty of salads and citrus fruits.
◆ Then, for a month, eat a mildly cleansing diet. Avoid all clogging, saturated fat foods. Reduce dairy products. Add plenty of fiber foods from vegetables and whole grains.
◆ Have a glass of lemon juice and water each morning.
◆ Drink only bottled water.
◆ Keep the diet very low in sugars, salt, and dairy foods.

VITAMINS/MINERALS

One of the common high-dose aspirin side effects for arthritic sufferers is ringing in the ears.

▶ Take a good hearing vitamin mix - one of each:
✚ Emulsified A 25,000IU
✚ Ester C with bioflavonoids
✚ Mezotrace MULTIMINERAL
✚ Methionine
✚ Glutamine 500mg.

▶ Mega C therapy: Use ascorbate or Ester C crystals $1/4$ teasp. every half hour to bowel tolerance for 1 week.

▶ Nature's Plus GERMANIUM w/ Suma 30mg. daily. ♂

▶ Vital Health ORAL CHELATION FORMULA 1 w. EDTA, two packs daily to open clogged arteries and stimulate blood flow to the brain. ♂ with
Body Essentials SILICA GEL 1 TB. in 3 oz. liquid 3x daily.

▶ For ringing in the ears:
✚ Beta carotene 150,000IU daily
✚ Niacin therapy: 500mg. daily. ♂
✚ **Vitamin C *with bioflavonoids*, 3000-5000mg. daily for 3 months.**
✚ Alta Health manganese and B₁₂ lozenges. ♂

HERBAL THERAPY

🌿 Ginkgo biloba extract 2 - 3x daily.

🌿 Mullein oil drops in the ears for 2 weeks to relieve pain. ☺

🌿 Crystal Star ANTI-HIST™ caps to relieve pressure in ears and sinus canals.

🌿 Echinacea extract liquid*with* Siberian ginseng extract caps 4 daily. ♂

🌿 Other effective ear extracts: (Dilute in water to use as drops).
◆ Lobelia
◆ Angelica ♀
◆ Peppermint

🌿 Put 6 drops garlic oil and 3 drops goldenseal extract in the ear. Hold in with cotton. Repeat daily for a week. Flush out with vinegar and water.

🌿 For ringing in the ears:
◆ **Ginkgo biloba extract 3-4x daily.**
◆ Licorice rt. extract
◆ Summer savory and rose water tea. May be used internally and also as drops in the ear.

🌿 Other effective teas:
◆ Yellow dock
◆ Yarrow flower
◆ Bayberry bark

BODYWORK

▶ Massage neck, ear and temples. Pull ear lobes - top front and back to clear passages of excess wax or mucous.

▶ Use dilute 3% H₂O₂ to gently clean out excess ear wax or obstructions.

▶ Avoid continuous loud noise. (Listening to loud rock music through headphones on a regular basis results in major ear problems.)

▶ Acupressure point:
Squeeze the joints of the ring finger and the 4th toe, covering all sides for several minutes each day.

▶ For ringing in the ears:
→ Avoid high doses of aspirin.
→ Massage the ear as above.
→ Acupressure: stroke gently downward from the top of the temple to the bottom of the cheek with the nails for 30 seconds on each side.

▶ Reflexology point:

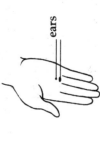

ears

Common Symptoms: Degenerative hearing loss; feeling of fullness and clogging in the ear; obstructed ear passages; no pain, but extremely annoying ringing sound in the head.
Common Causes: Arteriosclerosis; thickening of the passages or fluid congestion in the middle ear so that there is no vibration; excess ear wax or other obstruction; mucous clog infection or inflammation; swelling and congestion; chronic bronchial mastoid and sinus inflammation; hypoglycemia (raised blood insulin causing poor carbohydrate metabolism); poor diet with too many mucous-forming foods; poor circulation; high blood pressure; imbalance in the inner ear; allergies; lowered immune defenses; raised copper levels; metabolic imbalance.

HEART ARRYTHMIA ▦ TACHYCARDIA

Atrial Fibrillation ✧ Palpitations

Arrythmia: Electrical disruptions that affect the natural rhythm of the heart. Palpitations: the heart beating out of sequence. Atrial fibrillation: heart flutter and the uncomfortable awareness of the beating of the heart, sometimes accompanied by dizziness or fainting. Tachycardia: rapid beating of the heart coming on in sudden attacks.

FOOD THERAPY

🍃 Keep your diet low in fats, salt and calories. Have a fresh green salad and some whole grain protein every day.

🍃 Add sunflower and sesame seeds, miso soup, rice and oat bran, green leafy vegetables, or a green drink frequently.

🍃 Take a low fat protein drink every morning such as Natures Plus SPIRUTEIN for prevention.

🍃 Take a glass of mineral water and/or a Crystal Star MINZYME-MINOS™ drink daily for potassium.

🍃 Avoid hard liquor, caffeine and tobacco.

🍃 Make a mix and take 2 TBS. daily in a salad, soup or protein drink.
   ♦ Lecithin granules
   ♦ Toasted wheat germ
   ♦ Brewer's yeast
   ♦ Chopped sea vegetables

🍃 See the Healthy Heart Diet in this book for more information.

VITAMINS/MINERALS

▶ Future Biotics VITAL K or Enzymatic Therapy HERBAL K 3 teasp. daily.

Liquid chlorophyll 1 teasp. daily in water before each meal.

▶ Taurine 500mg. 2x daily w. Ester C 550mg. 2x daily for stability.
   and
Solaray CHROMIACIN 3x daily to normalize circulation. (Do not take high doses of isolated niacin.)
   and

▶ Country Life RELAXER capsules and/or CALCIUM/MAGNESIUM/POTASSIUM capsules.

▶ Effective preventives:
   ♦ Vit. E 400IU w/Selenium ♂
   ♦ Stress B Complex 150mg. w. extra B6 100mg.
   ♦ Carnitine 500mg. 2x daily ♀
   ♦ Cal/Mag/Bromelain ♂
   ♦ CoQ 10 30mg. 3x daily.

▶ Magnesium 800mg. daily
   or
Rainbow Light CALCIUM PLUS w. high magnesium, 4 daily. ♀

▶ Omega 3 fish or flax oils 3 daily.

HERBAL THERAPY

🌿 Crystal Star HEARTSEASE/HAWTHORNE™ caps as a preventive measure.
   and
Hawthorne leaf and flower extract as needed to regulate.

🌿 Cayenne/ginger caps or Solaray COOL CAYENNE 2 daily.

🌿 Ginkgo biloba extract as needed 2-3x daily.

🌿 Emergency measures:
   ♦ Cayenne extract drops
   ♦ Ginseng Co. CYCLONE CIDER
   ♦ Hawthorne extract drops
   ♦ Crystal Star RECOVERY TONIC™ as directed.

🌿 Effective capsules:
   ♦ Siberian ginseng 2 daily
   ♦ Garlic oil capsules 6 daily.
   ♦ Bee pollen 2 daily ♀
   ♦ Crystal Star POTASSIUM SOURCE™ 2 daily.

🌿 Evening primrose or borage oil caps - 4 daily.

🌿 Effective teas:
   ♦ Butcher's broom
   ♦ Rosemary
   ♦ Wild cherry
   ♦ Peppermint/sage

BODYWORK

▶ Plunge the face into cold water when arrhythmia occurs to stop palpitations.

▶ Avoid soft drinks. The phosphorus binds up magnesium and makes it unavailable for heart regularity.

▶ See How To Take Your Own Pulse in the Appendix of this book, pg. 347. If your pulse is over 80 and remains that way, you should make some diet improvements and get a further heart diagnosis.

▶ Reflexology point:

heart points

▶ Heart artery area:

Common Symptoms: Irregular and/or rapid heartbeat; uncomfortable awareness of your heartbeat; shortness of breath, and a feeling that you cannot breathe.
Common Causes: Poor diet with refined sugar and too many saturated fats; lack of exercise and aerobic strength; obesity; smoking; stress; high blood pressure; diabetes.
Note: DIGOXIN, often given for irregular heartbeat problems, has side effects that include G.I. irritation, hearing and visual distrubances, headaches, and dizziness. A lifestyle and diet change is a better way to avoid these conditions.

HEART DISEASE ■ CARDIOVASCULAR DISEASE
Angina ◇ Coronary ◇ Stroke ◇ Heart Attack

Almost unknown at the turn of the twentieth century, today, two-thirds of America suffers from heart disease. The term **heart disease** covers all ailments of the heart from heart attacks to congenital defects. **Cardiovascular disease** refers to disorders of both the heart and circulatory system, including hypertension, athersclerosis, stroke, rheumatic heart disease,etc. (See the following page for a more definitive discussion.) Nutritional measures and natural therapies are proving to reduce mortality far better than even aggressive medical intervention with the most advanced drug treatment. Indeed some of the favored drugs for heart disease have serious side effects and can even shorten life. ❀ In other recent tests on women - surprise, surprise - women have different problems of the heart than men. Heart attacks in women are hormone-dependent. Estrogen and hormone balance can be a major protective factor.

FOOD THERAPY

See the HEALTHY HEART DIET on the following pages.

▲*No more than 10% of total daily caloric intake from fat.*
▲*70% calories from complex carbohydrates.*
▲*20% calories from low fat protein. sources.*
▲*Less than 100mg. per day of dietary cholesterol. Keep cholesterol below 160.*

🍃 A healthy heart diet has plenty of magnesium and potassium rich foods:
fresh greens, sea vegetables,pitted fruits, sea food and fish, tofu, brown rice and whole grains, garlic and onions.

🍃 Make a mix and take 2 TBS. daily:
◆ Lecithin granules
◆ Toasted wheat germ
◆ Brewer's yeast
◆ Chopped sea vegetables
◆ Molasses

🍃 Pay conscious attention to omitting red meats, caffeine and caffeine - containing foods, refined sugars, fatty, salty and fried foods, prepared meats and soft drinks. The rewards are worth the effort.

🍃 Drink at least 1 cup of mineral water daily. (Remember that chlorinated/ fluoridated water destroys vitamin E in the body).

🍃 A glass or two of wine with dinner can relieve stress, improve digestion and raise HDLs.

VITAMINS/MINERALS

▶ Vital Health FORMULA 1 advanced chelation w/ EDTA 2 packs daily.

▶ Effective cardio-tonic anti-oxidants:
◆ CoQ 10, 60mg. daily
◆ Inosine 150mg.
◆ Bioflavonoids to preserve arterial integrity and prevent little strokes. ♀
◆ DMG B15 125mg. SL
◆ Vitamin E with selenium
◆ B1 50mg. esp. if taking diuretics
◆ BioChem CARDIO-FACTORS

▶ Carnitine 500mg. daily. Use liquid carnitine for myocardial infarction during an attack.

▶ Effective preventives:
◆ Ascorbate or Ester C with bioflavonoids, up to 5000mg. daily for interstitial tissue elasticity.
◆ Chromium picolinate or Solaray CHROMIACIN and HEARTHORN to control arterial plaque and counteract insulin resistance.
◆ Omega 3 fish and flax oils 3x daily.

▶ Biogenetics BIO-GUARD enzymes to decrease free radical activity.

▶ CSA for congestive heart failure.

▶ Germanium, 150SL daily or 1 gm. powder in 1 qt. water, take 2-3 TBS. daily. ♂

▶ Evening primrose oil caps 4 daily. ♀

HERBAL THERAPY

🌿 In an emergency; 1 teasp. cayenne powder, or drops of cayenne tincture in water will often bring a person out of a heart attack or coronary.

🌿 Effective emergency aid: Take a few drops of Crystal Star RECOVERY TONIC™ on the back of the tongue every 15 minutes or as needed.
or
Take 1/2 dropperful Hawthorne extract every 1/2 hour.

✦ Take 1/2 dropperful daily as preventive support.

🌿 Crystal Star HEARTSEASE HAW-THORNE™ caps, or HEART-SEASE/CIRCU-CLENSE™ tea.

🌿 Effective heart tonics:
◆ Cayenne/ginger capsules
◆ Liquid chlorophyll
◆ Ginseng Co. CYCLONE CIDER
◆ Garlic oil capsules
◆ Wheat germ oil caps
◆ Gotu kola

🌿 Effective phyto-estrogen herbs for postmenopausal women:
✦ Crystal Star FEMALE HARMO-NY™ capsules and tea.
✦ Dong quai/damiana extract
✦ Vitex extract
✦ Licorice rt. extract, caps or tea

🌿 Siberian ginseng extract caps 2000mg. or tea 2 cups daily. ♂

BODYWORK

▶ **Apply hot compresses and massage chest of the victim to ease a heart attack.**

▶ When administered immediately following symptoms of a heart attack, aspirin has been shown to reduce mortality through its ability to reduce arterial blockage.

▶ Take alternate hot and cold showers frequently to increase circulation.

▶ Stop smoking. Tobacco constricts circulation.

▶ Take some mild regular daily exercise. Do deep breathing exercises every morning for body oxygen, and to stimulate brain activity.

▶ Consciously add relaxation and a good daily laugh to your life. A positive mental outlook does wonders for stress.

▶ Reflexology points:

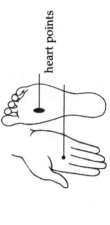

heart points

DIAGNOSING HEART PROBLEMS

Call an emergency room or urgent care center immediately if you are experiencing a serious heart attack of any kind.

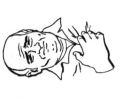

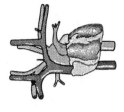

❖**Angina:** Chest pains or pressure usually brought on by emotional stress, exposure to cold, or overexertion. A warning of a heart attack - the result of degeneration of the artery walls.
✛ Major Symptoms: Recurring, sudden, intense chest pains, lasting 30 seconds to 1 minute, with a vise-like grip of pressure across the chest.

❖**Arteriosclerosis/Atherosclerosis:** Hardening and loss of elasticity of the arteries resulting from degeneration of the artery walls narrowed by multiple fat and cholesterol plaque lesions. Possible embolism when these break loose into the bloodstream.

❖**Ischemic Heart Disease:** Obstruction of the blood flow to the heart and cell starvation, caused by fatty deposits along the coronary artery walls. Leads to angina, coronary or congestive heart failure.
✛ Major Symptoms: High blood pressure; poor circulation brought on by ischemia (cell nutrient starvation); aching feet, legs and muscles, or numbness and weakness in the legs; gradual mental deterioration, weakness and unsteadiness; diagonal earlobe crease.

❖**Congestive Heart Failure:** A damaged heart weakened by arteriosclerosis or other disease such as hypothyroidism, ceases to pump effectively. Circulation is inefficient and organs and tissues become clogged with blood.
✛ Major Symptoms: Early symptoms include abnormal fatigue, and shortness of breath after exertion. Breathing is impaired, ankles and feet usually swell, and there is nausea and gas. Later symptoms are greater heart exhaustion and fluid in the lungs.

❖**Myocardial Infarction/Coronary Occlusion/Coronary Thrombosis:** Permanent damage or death to the heart muscle, resulting from fatty plaque obstructions, and/or narrowing of the coronary artery walls by atherosclerosis, reducing or cutting off oxygen to the heart. The heart stops beating; the blood supply to the brain is cut off.
✛ Major Symptoms: Excruciating pain, starting in the lower chest and spreading throughout the upper half of the body; weak and rapid pulse with perspiring, pale skin; blood pressure drops dangerously, there is dizziness, and then unconsciousness. Fever usually follows this kind of attack.

❖**Stroke:** A cerebro-vascular condition affecting the blood supply to the brain. It is a result of blocked blood vessels - similar to that of a coronary, the difference being cell death in the brain. A stroke occurs when an artery to the brain becomes clogged cutting off oxygen supply to a part of the brain. A stroke can disorder the senses, speech, behavior, thought patterns and memory. Since oxygen-deprived brain tissue dies within minutes, the part of the body controlled by those cells cannot function. It may result in paralysis, coma and death.
✛ Major Symptoms: Sudden weakness or numbness of the face arm and leg, usually on one side of the body; loss of speech - trouble talking or understanding speech; impaired or fluctuating state of consciousness, tingling sensations; dimness or loss of vision, particularly in one eye; sudden severe headache; dizziness, unsteadiness or sudden fall.

❦

Quick Heart Rehabilitation Check Program - *This program is especially for those of you who have survived a heart attack or major heart surgery. Coming back is tough. Beginning and sticking to a new lifestyle that changes about everything about the way you eat, exercise, handle stress, and even the smallest details of your life is a challenge. The following mini-rehabilitation program is a blueprint that you can use with confidence. It has proven successful against heart disease recurrence.*

❥ Reduce fats to at least 15% of your diet; less if possible. Limit polyunsaturates (margarine, oils) to 10%. Add mono-unsaturates (olive oil, avocados, nuts, seeds)
❥ Eat potassium-rich foods for cardiotonic activity: fresh spinach and chard, broccoli, bananas, sea vegetables, molasses, cantaloupe, apricots, papayas, mushrooms, tomatoes, yams.
 or take a high potassium drink regularly, such as potassium broth (pg. 53), Crystal Star SYSTEM STRENGTH™ drink, or Future Biotics VITAL K. (a serving of high potassium fruits or vegetables offers about 400mg. of potassium; a serving of the above drinks offers approx. 1000-1250mg. of potassium)
❥ Eat plenty of complex carbohydrates, such as broccoli, peas, whole grain breads, vegetable pastas, potatoes, sprouts, tofu and brown rice.
❥ Have several servings of cold water fish or seafood every week for high omega 3 oils.
❥ Have a fresh green salad every day.
❥ Add miso and oat or rice bran to your diet regularly.
❥ Have a glass of white wine before dinner for relaxation and better digestion.
❥ Eat magnesium-rich foods for heart regulation: tofu, wheat germ, bran, broccoli, potatoes, lima beans, spinach, chard.
❥ Eat copper-rich foods for clear arteries: oysters,clams, crab, fish, brewer's yeast, fresh fruit and vegetables, nuts, seeds.
❥ Eat high fiber foods for a clean system and alkalinity: whole grains, fruits and vegetables, legumes and herbs.
❥ Choose several of the following supplements as your individual daily micro-nutrients:
 ✛ Heart regulation and stability: Sun CHLORELLA tabs 15 daily; magnesium 400mg.; carnitine 500mg.; evening primrose oil 4 daily.
 ✛ Clear arteries: Solaray CHROMIACIN; selenium; omega 3 flax or fish oils 3x daily; advanced oral chelation w. EDTA.
 ✛ Anti-oxidants: Wheat germ oil raises oxygen level 30%; chlorophyll; vitamin E 400IU with selenium; pycnogenol; CoQ 10, 30mg.; ginkgo biloba extract, rosemary, chaparral.
 ✛ Cardiac tonics: Hawthorne extract; cayenne; or cayenne/ginger capsules; garlic; Siberian ginseng extract; gotu kola.
 ✛ Anti-cholesterol/blood thinning: Ginger; butcher's broom; taurine 500mg.; oral chelation with EDTA.
 ✛ Healthy blood chemistry: Chromium picolinate; Ester C 500mg. with bioflavonoids.
❥ Get regular daily exercise. To be effective for heart, circulation and artery health, the heart rate and respiration must rise to the point of mild breathlessness for 5 minutes each day.

Diet For A Healthy Heart

Diet is the single most influential key to heart health. In general, refined, high fat and high calorie foods create cardiovascular problems, and natural foods relieve them. Fried foods, salty foods, sugar, low fiber foods, pasteurized dairy products, red meats and processed meats, tobacco, hard liquor and caffeine all contribute to clogged and reduced arteries, LDL cholesterol, high blood pressure and heart attacks. Almost all circulatory disease can be treated and prevented with improvement in diet and nutrition. You can carve out health with your own knife and fork. The following diet is for long-term heart and circulatory health. It's easy to live with, but has all the necessary elements to keep arteries clear, and heart action regular and strong. It emphasizes fresh and whole fiber foods, high mineral foods with lots of potassium and magnesium, oxygen-rich foods from green vegetables, sprouts and wheat germ (wheat germ oil can raise the oxygen level of the heart as much as 30%), and vegetable-source proteins. Conscious attention must be paid at first to avoid red meats, caffeine, fried and fatty foods, soft drinks, refined pastry, salty foods and prepared meats, but the rewards are high - a longer, healthier life - and control of your life.

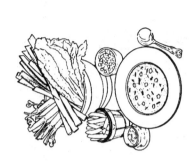

On rising: take a high protein or high vitamin/mineral drink such as NutriTech ALL 1 or Nature's Plus SPIRUTEIN in orange or grapefruit juice, or a cup of Japanese green tea.

Breakfast: Make a mix of 2 TBS. each: lecithin granules, wheat germ, brewer's yeast, honey, and sesame seed. Sprinkle 2 teasp. every morning on fresh fruits, such as apricots, peaches, apples or nectarines, or mix with yogurt;
and/or have a poached or baked egg with bran muffins or whole grain toast and kefir cheese; or some whole grain cereal or pancakes with a little maple syrup.

Mid-morning: have a green drink (pg. 54ff.), or Sun CHLORELLA, a potassium drink (pg. 53), Crystal Star SYSTEM STRENGTH™, or all natural V-8 juice (pg. 54ff) or Green Foods GREEN ESSENCE drink;
and/or some crunchy raw vegies with a kefir cheese or yogurt dip; and/or a cup of miso soup with sea vegies snipped on top.

Lunch: have a cup of fenugreek tea with additions: 1 teasp. honey, 1 teasp. wheat germ oil, 1 teasp. lecithin granules or liquid;
then have a tofu and spinach salad with some sprouts and bran muffins;
or a high protein salad or sandwich with nuts & seeds and a black bean or lentil soup;
or an avocado, low fat cheese or soy cheese sandwich on whole grain bread;
or a seafood and whole grain pasta salad with a light tomato sauce;
or a light vegie omelet and small green salad;
or some grilled or braised vegetables with an olive oil dressing and brown rice.

Mid-afternoon: have a cup of mint tea, or Crystal Star Chinese ROYAL MU™ tonic tea;
and/or a cup of miso soup with a hard boiled egg. or whole grain crackers; or a glass of carrot juice, or Personal V-8 (pg. 55).

Dinner: have a broccoli quiche with a whole grain or chapati crust; and a cup of onion soup;
or a baked seafood dish with brown rice and peas;
or a whole grain and steamed vegetable and tofu casserole;
or an oriental stir fry with light soup and rice;
or grilled fish or seafood and a small green salad and baked potato;
or a salmon or vegie souffle with a light sauce and salad.
•A little white wine before dinner is fine for relaxation, digestion and tension relief. Avoid commercial antacids, that neutralize natural stomach acid, and invite the body to produce even more acid, thus aggravating stress and tension.

Before bed: have another cup of miso soup, or a cup of VEGEX yeast paste broth, apple or pear juice, or chamomile tea.

▲**Daily prevention supplementation should include:** Vitamin E 400IU, Solaray CHROMIACIN, or niacin, 250mg. daily; CoQ 10, 60mg., and flax oil 3x daily; Siberian ginseng extract caps, 2000mg. or extract, 1/2 dropperful daily; Vitamin C 3000mg. daily with bioflavonoids, or Crystal Star BIOFLAV., FIBER & C SUPPORT™ drink; evening primrose oil caps, 2 to 4 daily; hawthorn extract 1 dropperful daily as a heart tonic.

➤**Preventive bodywork should include:** a regular daily walk, or other aerobic exercise, such as dancing swimming or jogging to strengthen the heart muscle.

It all adds up to today's definition of living well. Pleasure is derived from improved health and vitality instead of rich food and drink. See "COOKING FOR HEALTHY HEALING" by Linda Rector-Page for a complete heart diet and healing program.

HEMORRHAGING ■ INTERNAL BLEEDING
Excessive Bleeding ✧ Blood Clotting Difficulty

FOOD THERAPY

☙ Make a variety of sprouts a regular part of your diet for natural Vitamin K.

☙ Have a glass of carrot/spinach juice frequently.

☙ Eat plenty of papayas.

☙ Take a green drink (pg. 54ff), or use Crystal Star ENERGY GREEN™ drink at least once a week to build healthier blood.

☙ Crystal Star BIOFLAV, FIBER & C SUPPORT™ drink for tissue integrity and strength.

VITAMINS/MINERALS

► Solaray CALCIUM CITRATE caps 4 daily. ♀

► Vitamin C therapy for collagen and interstitial issue formation: use Ester C or ascorbic acid crystals with bioflavs, and rutin. Take up to 5000mg. daily. and/or

Quercetin Plus with bromelain 4 daily.

► Vitamin K 100mg. 3x daily.

► Propolis tincture; apply directly, and take internally 4x daily. ♂

► Liquid chlorophyll 3 teasp. daily with vitamin E 400IU and selenium 200mcg. for blood building.

► Effective homeopathic remedies - especially for clotting difficulties from dental or cosmetic surgery:
♣ *Ferrum Phos.* for bright red bleeding.
♣ *Arnica* for bleeding accompanied by bruising.
♣ *Phosphorus* for persistent bleeding.

HERBAL THERAPY

❦ Capsicum, take 1 teasp. in a cup of hot water to stop bleeding. (Take with an eyedropper on the back of the tongue if it is too hot to swallow.)

❦ External clotting agents:
♦ Plantain and water paste
♦ Witch hazel
♦ Cayenne powder
♦ Buckthorne tincture

❦ Internal bleeding control:
♦ Pau de arco tea
♦ Turmeric capsules
♦ Comfrey root
♦ Shepherd's purse ♀

❦ Herbal astringents/flavonoids to tighten and strengthen veins and capillaries. All may be used both externally and internally:
♦ White oak bark ♂
♦ Citrus peel
♦ Peony rt.
♦ Bilberry
♦ Cranesbill ♀
♦ Rosehips
♦ Goldenseal extract

❦ Clotting agent tea combo:
Licorice rt., comfrey rt., shepherd's purse, goldenseal rt., cranesbill.

BODYWORK

► Acupressure point: Press the insides of the thighs with the fingers just above the knees, for 10 seconds at a time.

► Body pressure points:
→ Hold arm in the air on the side of the bleeding to decrease pressure.
→ Pull knuckle of the middle finger on either hand until it pops, to lower blood pressure and tension.

► Apply direct pressure to a vein or artery. Get a doctor and treat for shock. See SHOCK TREATMENT page in this book for more information.

► Don't use aspirin or other blood-thinning drugs if you are at risk for internal hemorrhaging.

Common Symptoms: Inability to clot even small wounds; internal pain as with a rupture or ulcer; easy bruising and ulcerations; broken blood vessels; black stools when there are stomach ulcers.
Common Causes: Broken blood vessels; weak vein and vessel walls; internal wounds from a blow or accident; lack of vitamin K in the body, from heredity, or accident; over-use of aspirin or other blood thinning drugs.

HEMORRHOIDS ▦ PILES ▦ ANAL FISSURE

Swollen, inflamed veins and capillaries around the anus that often protrude out of the rectum. There is usually constipation and thus, because of straining, rectal bleeding. The pain and discomfort of hemorrhoidal itch and swelling are well known. A change in diet composition and natural therapies can help you avoid drugs and surgery.

FOOD THERAPY

Diet improvement is the key to permanently reducing hemorrhoids.

☙ Take 1 TB. olive oil before each meal. Include plenty of soluble fiber foods in the diet, particularly lots of vegetable cellulose, such as stewed and dried fruits, brans, vegetables.
Avoid refined, low fiber foods, and acid forming foods, such as caffeine and sugar.

☙ **Include a variety of sprouts and dark greens for vitamin K.**

☙ Take 2 TBS. cider vinegar mixed with honey each morning.

☙ Wisdom of the Ancients YERBA MATÉ tea.

☙ **Drink plenty of healthy liquids throughout the day.**

☙ Keep meals small, so the bowel and sphincter area won't have to work so hard.

☙ **Apply papaya skins or lemon juice directly to inflamed area to relieve itching.**

☙ See DIET FOR CONSTIPATION & COLON HEALTH in this book.

VITAMINS/MINERALS

► Vitamin C therapy for collagen and interstitial issue formation: use Ester C or ascorbic acid crystals with bioflavs. and rutin. Take up to 5000mg. daily, and make a solution in water to apply directly.
and/or
Quercetin Plus with bromelain **4 daily, or Pygnogenol 2 daily.**

► Vit. K 100mg. 2x daily with Vit. B6 250mg. daily.

► NatureAde SOFT-EX tablets, or flax seed oil to soften stool. ♀

► Enzymatic Therapy HEMTONE capsules to stop rectal bleeding. ♀

► Vitamin E 400IU daily. Also apply to inflamed area for healing.

► BioForce *Hemorrhoid* homeopathic.

► Bromelain 500mg. with lecithin caps 1900gr. daily. ♂

► **Apply aloe vera gel.**

► Evening primrose or borage oil caps 4 daily for a month.

HERBAL THERAPY

☙ **Apply calendula ointment. Take stone root tea, 3 cups daily for a month.** ♂

☙ Crystal Star HEMR-EASE™ capsules for 2 weeks to relieve inflammation and encourage healing. (May also be used as a suppository)
Add LIV-ALIVE™ tea to clear sluggishness, and BWL TONE™ capsules or butcher's broom tea for gentle healing.

☙ Effective suppositories in cocoa butter:
◆ Goldenseal/myrrh
◆ Slippery elm in cocoa butter
◆ Garlic/comfrey
◆ Cranesbill/yarrow
◆ White oak bark/yarrow ♂

☙ Hemorrhoid tea: mix equal parts comfrey root, wild yam, and cranesbill. Take internally and apply directly.

☙ For anal fissure: take internally and apply externally. Crystal Star ANTI-BIO™ caps and YSK WAKASA CHLORELLA extract.
or
Dilute horsetail extract - apply externally and take internally.

BODYWORK

► Effective applications:
→ Ice packs
→ **Witch hazel**
→ **Hylands PILE OINTMENT**
→ Crystal Star HEMR-EASE GEL™ w. VITAMIN C.

► Effective enemas:
→ Nettles
→ Chlorella or spirulina
→ Cayenne/garlic
→ Nut. Res. GRAPEFRUIT SEED extract - 20 drops per gal. water.

► Use a bee pollen 1000mg. tablet as a suppository. Insert 1 daily.

► Effective compresses:
→ Alternating hot and cool water to stimulate circulation.
→ Horsetail tea - frequently
→ Elder berry
→ Butcher's broom ♂

► **Take a good half hour walk every day for circulation.**

► Reflexology points:

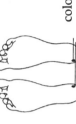

colon & rectum

Common Symptoms: Pain, itching and rectal bleeding with bowel movements; inflamed anal fissure; protruding swellings.
Common Causes: Junk food diet with too many refined, fried, fatty, low residue foods and not enough healthy hydrating liquids; constipation; pregnancy; overeating; lack of exercise, too much sitting; Vit. B 6 deficiency; acid/alkaline imbalance; liver exhaustion; allergies.

HEPATITIS
Jaundice ◇ Viral Liver Infection

There are several types of viral hepatitis. **Type A:** a viral infection passed through blood and feces; **Type B:** a sexually transmitted viral infection carried through blood, semen, saliva and dirty needles. Occasionally develops into chronic hepatitis. See page 308 for more information. **Type D:** caused by Epstein-Barr virus and cytomegalovirus; **Non-A, non-B:** a higher mortality virus passed through transfusion blood products. Frequently develops from chronic fatigue to serious liver damage and even to death from liver failure. Natural therapies have had outsanding success in hepatitis cases, both in arresting viral replication, and in regeneration of the liver and its functions.

FOOD THERAPY

See *LIVER CLEANSING DIET in this book for more information.*

☙ **Hepatitis Healing Diet:**
For 2 weeks: Eat only fresh foods: salads, fruits, juices, bottled water.
Take a glass of carrot/beet/cucumber juice every other day.
Take a glass of lemon juice and water every morning.
Take Sun CHLORELLA granules daily, or liquid chlorophyll 3 teasp. daily at meals.

☙ **Then for 1 to 2 months:** Take carrot/ beet/cucumber juice every 3 days, and papaya juice w/ 2 teasp. spirulina each morning.
Eat a high vegetable protein diet, with steamed vegetables, brown rice, tofu, eggs, whole grains and yogurt. Avoid meat protein.

☙ **Then for 1 more month:** Take 2 glasses of tomato juice/wheat germ oil/brewer's yeast/lemon juice every day.
Take a daily glass of apple/alfalfa sprout juice.
Continue with vegetable proteins, cultured foods, fresh salads and complex carbohydrates for strength.

☙ Avoid refined, fried and fatty foods, sugars, heavy spices, alcohol and caffeine during healing. No amphetamines, cocaine, barbiturates, or tobacco *at all.*

VITAMINS/MINERALS

▶ Beta carotene 150,000IU daily, with B Complex 150mg. and Ener B internasal B12 gel daily for 1 month. Then reduce beta carotene to 50,000IU, and B Complex to 100mg. daily, and add a strong multiple vitamin/mineral

▶ Alta Health CANGEST if detection is early. Take 1 teasp. powder in water 2-3x daily for 7 days; then 1 teasp. 4x daily at meals and bedtime for 7 days.

▶ Natren LIFE START II daily for 1 month, *with* raw thymus extract 2x daily as a liver detoxifier.

▶ Solaray LIPOTROPIC 1000 caps.

▶ Ascorbate Vit. C crystals, up to 10,000mg. daily in water, to bowel tolerance for 1 month.

▶ Enzymatic Therapy LIVA-TOX, *with* IMMUNO-PLEX 402A capsules *and* RAW THYMUS COMPLEX caps.

▶ Nutricology GERMANIUM SL or powder (1gm. to 1 qt. water) Shake before each use. Take 2 teasp. liquid daily.
or
Germanium, 200mg. capsules daily.

HERBAL THERAPY

❧ Crystal Star LIV-ALIVE™ capsules 4-6 daily, with LIV ALIVE™ tea 2 cups daily for 1 month.
Reduce dose to half the 2nd month.
Add HEARTSEASE/ANEMIGIZE™ caps for blood building, and ANTI-HST™ caps as needed to control histamine reactions.

❧ Enzymatic Therapy SILYMARIN PHYTOSOME. ♂

❧ Liver detoxifying teas:
♦ Oregon grape
♦ Gotu kola
♦ Pau de arco/calendula; also apply Crystal Star GINSENG SKIN REPAIR GEL™ to lesions.
♦ Licorice rt./red clover

❧ Effective extracts:
♦ Dandelion root and leaf
♦ Astragalus
♦ Milk thistle seed 3x daily
♦ Lobelia
♦ Reishi mushroom
♦ Sarsaparilla

❧ Nutribiotic GRAPEFRUIT SEED ext. 10 drops 3x daily for 1 month

❧ Take 2 glasses of aloe vera juice w. herbs, *with* spirulina 6 tabs daily. ♀

BODYWORK

▶ Count on 2 weeks for emergency detox measures; 1-3 months for healing the liver and rebuilding blood and body strength.

▶ Get plenty of bed rest, especially during the acute infectious stages.

▶ Overheating therapy has been effective for Hepatitis. See P. Airola, "How To Get Well" or page 49 in this book.

▶ Use chlorophyll implants twice weekly for the first two critical weeks of healing to detoxify.

▶ Reflexology point:

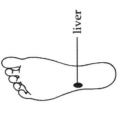

liver

Common Symptoms: Great fatigue and exhaustion; enlarged, tender, congested, sluggish liver; loss of appetite, nausea and flu-like symptoms; dark urine, gray stools; skin pallor and histamine itching; depression; skin jaundice; cirrhosis of the liver.
Common Causes: Infectious hepatitis is primarily a lifestyle disease - with almost 90% of intravenous drug users, and 85% of homosexuals infected. Others at risk include dental and medical workers, and over 25% of people receiving blood transfusions. Hepatitis can lead to liver cancer, cirrhosis and is sometimes itself fatal.

HIATAL HERNIA ■ ESOPHAGEAL REFLUX

A hiatal hernia occurs when a part of the stomach protrudes through the diaphragm wall, causing difficulty swallowing, acid burning and reflux in the throat, and great nervous anxiety. Today's American diet habits mean that a hiatal condition is common. Esophageal reflux is due to leaking of stomach acid back into the lower esophagus and acid coming up into the throat. This can also occur in severe cases of osteoporosis, when the rib cage and upper body have collapsed to the point where normal food transit is impeded.

FOOD THERAPY

❧ Eat only raw or lightly steamed vegetable-source fiber foods during healing. Drink 2 glasses of fresh carrot or apple juice every day.

❧ Avoid nuts, seeds, acidic juices and gas-producing foods during healing.

❧ Eat smaller meals more frequently. No large meals. No liquids with meals.

❧ When digestion has normalized, follow a low fat, low salt, high fiber diet. Avoid stimulant foods, such as caffeine, red meats, fried and spicy foods, and carbonated drinks.

❧ Take 1-2 glasses of mineral water or aloe vera juice daily.

❧ Remember that commercial antacids often do more harm than good as they upset stomach pH causing it to produce even more harmful acids.

VITAMINS/MINERALS

➤ Quercetin Plus 3 daily for inflammation, with
    Enzymatic Therapy BROME-LAIN or CHEWABLE DGL as needed.

➤ Schiff EMULSIFIED A 25,000IU 2x daily.

➤ Liquid chlorophyll 3 teasp. daily at meals. ♂

➤ Pancreatin 1400mg. with meals.

➤ Chewable enzymes as needed.

➤ Alta Health CANGEST caps or powder 3x daily. ♀

➤ Zinc gluconate lozenges under the tongue as needed.

HERBAL THERAPY

❧ Crystal Star ANTI-FLAM™ caps 4 daily, and ANTI-SPZ™ caps 2 with each meal.

❧ Aloe vera juice or slippery elm tea daily as needed to soothe inflamed tissue.

❧ Psyllium husk 1-2 TBS. morning and evening to provide gentle cleansing fiber.
    or
    Crystal Star CHO-LO FIBER TONE™ drink. ♂

❧ Crystal Star CRAMP BARK COMBO™ extract 1/2 dropperful at a time as needed for pain and spasms.

❧ Propolis extract 1/2 dropperful every 4 hours during an attack.

❧ Pau de arco tea daily. ♀

BODYWORK

➤ No smoking. Avoid all tobacco.

➤ Lose weight. Tone the abdomen with exercise. Watch posture to avoid slouching.

➤ Wear loose comfortable, non-binding clothing.

➤ Apply a green clay pack to the area.

➤ Reflexology point:

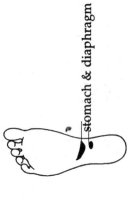

stomach & diaphragm

➤ Yellow color therapy eyewear - wear until hernia is gone, esp. during meals.

➤ Have a chiropractic adjustment to the area.

➤ To prevent night time reflux, elevate head of bed on 6 to 8" blocks.

Common Symptoms: Chest pains and heartburn; belching, excess gas and bloating; difficulty swallowing and a full feeling at the base of the throat; hiccups and regurgitation; pressure behind the breast-bone; raised blood pressure; diarrhea; inflammation and gastro-intestinal bleeding, usually with a stomach ulcer; mental confusion and nerves.

Common Causes: Food allergies; short esophagus; overeating; obesity; enzyme deficiency; constipation from a low residue diet and too many refined and acid-forming foods; osteoporosis and bone collapse of upper body structure; tobacco; too tight jeans or underclothing.

HIGH-BLOOD PRESSURE ■ HYPERTENSION

High blood pressure is a major problem in today's fast-paced, high-stress world. It is a silent disease that steals health and is a precursor to serious cardiovascular disease that can steal life. Most cases of high blood pressure can be brought under control by improvement in diet and lifestyle. In fact, recent clinical studies are showing that people with hypertension who make the necessary life changes actually fare much better than those on anti-hypertensive prescription drugs.

FOOD THERAPY

❧ Go on a liquid juice diet for 1 day every week for 2 months to improve body chemistry and reduce excess blood fats:
  ♦ Have some citrus juices or a potassium essence (pg. 53) in the morning;
  ♦ A green drink (pg. 54ff.) V-8, or carrot juice at mid-day;
  ♦ Apple, pear or papaya juice at dinner;
  ♦ Chamomile tea or vegex broth at bedtime.

❧ Then follow the HIGH BLOOD PRESSURE DIET on the next page, including plenty of vitamin C, magnesium and potassium-rich foods.

❧ Avoid refined foods, caffeine, salty, sugary, fried and fatty foods, prepared meats, heavy pastries and soft drinks. All cause potassium depletion and allow arterial plaque build-up.

❧ Make a mix and take 2 TBS. daily:
  ♦ Wheat germ
  ♦ High omega 3 flax oil
  ♦ Brewer's yeast
  ♦ Aloe vera juice

❧ Consciously add these fiber, mineral and vitamin C-rich foods to your diet: broccoli, bananas, dried fruits, potatoes, seafood, buckwheat, green peppers, cherries, avocados, cauliflower, brown rice and leafy greens.

VITAMINS/MINERALS

Most high blood pressure medicines cause potassium and magnesium deficiency. If you are taking diuretics, supplement with vitamin C, potassium and B C complex.

▶ Vitamin E therapy: Take 1 100IU. capsule daily for 1 week, then 4 capsules daily for 1 week, then 2 400IU capsules daily for 2 weeks. ♂
  Add 1 selenium 100mcg. and 1 Ester C with bioflavonoids each time. ♂
  Sufficient organic selenium intake is the best preventive measure - esp. for hypertension caused by toxic, heavy metals.

▶ B Complex 100mg. daily with extra B6 100mg. and niacin 100mg. 3x daily. ♀

▶ Omega 3 fish or flax oils 3 daily, or Choline 600mg. daily, with bromelain 500mg. to digest fats, and chromium picolinate 200mcg. daily to combat insulin resistance.

▶ Vitamin C 3000mg. daily with bioflavonoids and rutin for venous integrity.

▶ Co Q 10 30mg. 2x daily, and Country Life RELAXER capsules with GABA.

▶ Rainbow Light CALCIUM PLUS capsules w. high magnesium 6 daily.

▶ Vital Health ORAL CHELATION w. EDTA; extra magnesium 400mg.

HERBAL THERAPY

❧ Crystal Star HEARTSEASE H.B.P.™ capsules or tea daily, with POTASSIUM SOURCE™ caps and HAWTHORNE extract daily.

❧ Crystal Star TINKLE™ caps to clear edema; ADR-ACTIVE™ capsules or extract to combat fatigue.
  Crystal Star RELAX CAPS™ as needed for tension.

❧ Effective herbal capsules:
  ♦ Garlic oil, 8 daily
  ♦ Bee pollen, 6 daily
  ♦ Evening primrose oil 4-6
  ♦ Cayenne/ginger 4 daily
  ♦ Suma 6 daily
  ♦ Bilberry for herbal flavonoids
  ♦ Siberian ginseng extract caps. ♂

❧ Effective tension reducing products:
  ♦ Hyland's calms forte
  ♦ Solaray EUROCALM caps.
  ♦ Medicine Wheel SERENE extract

❧ Effective diuretic herbs:
  ♦ Crystal Star BLDR-K™ extract
  ♦ Uva ursi extract
  ♦ Dandelion extract

❧ Sun CHLORELLA drink daily to lower blood fats, *with* 1 TB. Body Essentials SILICA GEL mixed in the drink.

BODYWORK

You have high blood pressure with a repeated reading over 150/90mmHg.
If you have a high blood pressure problem, monitor your progress often with a home or free drugstore electronic machine reading.

▶ Keep body weight down. One of the biggest risk factors is increased fat storage.

▶ Avoid tobacco in all forms. It aggravates hyperinsulemia. Eliminate caffeine and hard liquor. (A little wine at night with dinner is fine, and can lower stress.)

▶ Take a brisk 1/2 hour walk every day, with plenty of deep lung breathing.

▶ Use a dry skin brush all over the body frequently to stimulate circulation.

▶ Reflexology point:
  → Pull middle finger on each hand 3x for 20 seconds each, daily.

▶ Avoid phenylalanine (esp. as found in Nutra-Sweet) and over-the-counter antihistamines.

Common Symptoms: Headaches; irritability; dizziness and ringing in the ears; flushed complexion; red streaks in the eyes; fatigue and sleeplessness; edema; frequent urination; depression; heart arrhythmia; chronic respiratory problems.
Common Causes: Clogging arterial fats and increased fat storage; calcium/fiber deficiency; thickened blood from excess mucous and waste; insulin resistance and poor sugar metabolism; obesity and lack of aerobic exercise; too much salt and red meat, causing raised copper levels; kidney malfunction; auto-toxemia from constipation; prostaglandin deficiency.

High Blood Pressure Prevention Diet

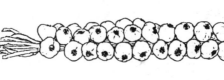

Eighty-five percent of high blood pressure is both treatable and preventable without drugs. The most beneficial change you can make to reduce high blood pressure is a diet change. Reduce and control salt use. (See About Low Salt Diets, pg. 73) Eat smaller meals more frequently, and consciously undereat. Avoid large meals, caffeine, and red meats. It is worth noting that vegetarians have less hypertension and fewer blood pressure problems. Lifestyle change must be made for there to be permanent control of high blood pressure. Conscious attention must be paid at first to avoid red meats, caffeine, fried and fatty foods, soft drinks, refined pastry, salty foods and prepared meats, but the rewards are high - a longer, healthier life - and control of your life.

On rising: Have a glass of lemon water and honey, and/or a high vitamin/mineral drink such as Nutri-Tech ALL 1 or Crystal Star SYSTEM STRENGTH™ drink.

Breakfast: Make a mix of 2 TBS. **each:** lecithin granules, wheat germ, brewer's yeast, honey, and sesame seeds. Sprinkle some on fresh fruit or mix with yogurt;
and/or have a poached or baked egg with bran muffins or whole grain toast, and kefir cheese or unsalted butter;
or some whole grain cereal or pancakes with a little maple syrup.

Mid-morning: Have a green drink (pg. 54ff.) or Sun CHLORELLA, a potassium drink (pg. 53), Crystal Star SYSTEM STRENGTH™ broth, or Green Foods GREEN ESSENCE drink, or natural V-8 juice (pg. 55) or mint tea:
and/or a cup of miso soup with sea vegies snipped on top, or ramen noodle soup;
and/or some crunchy raw vegies with a kefir cheese or yogurt dip.

Lunch: Have one cup daily of fenugreek tea with 1 teasp. honey, and 1 teasp. wheat germ oil;
then have a tofu and spinach salad with some sprouts and bran muffins;
or a large fresh green salad with a lemon oil dressing. Add plenty of sprouts, tofu, raisins, cottage cheese, nuts, and seeds as desired;
or have a baked potato with yogurt or kefir cheese topping, and a light vegie omelet;
or a seafood and vegetable pasta salad;
or some grilled or braised vegetables with an olive oil dressing and brown rice;
or a high protein whole grain sandwich, with avocados and low fat or soy cheese.

Mid-afternoon: Have a mineral water, a cup of mint tea, or an herb tea such as Crystal Star LICORICE MINTS™, or ROYAL MU™ tonic tea.
and/or a cup of miso soup with a hard boiled egg, or whole grain crackers;
or some dried fruits, and an apple or cranberry juice.

Dinner: Have a baked vegetable casserole with tofu and brown rice, and a small dinner salad;
or a baked fish or seafood dish with rice and peas, or a baked potato;
or a vegetable quiche (such as broccoli, artichoke, or asparagus), and a light oriental soup;
or some roast turkey and cornbread dressing, with a small salad or mashed potatoes with a little butter;
or an oriental vegetable and seafood or chicken stirfry, with a light, clear soup and brown rice;
☛ A little white wine is fine with dinner for relaxation, digestion and tension relief.

Before bed: Have a cup of miso soup, or vegex yeast paste broth, apple juice, or some chamomile tea.

Note: Particular foods to avoid if you have high blood pressure: canned and frozen foods, cured, smoked and canned meats, and fish, commercial peanut butter, soy sauce, bouillon cubes and condiments, fried chips and snacks, canned and dry soups.
Note: Avoid commercial antacids, that neutralize natural stomach acid, and invite the body to produce even more acid, thus aggravating stress and tension.

◗ **Suggested supplements for the High Blood Pressure Prevention Diet**

✤ Siberian ginseng extract caps, 2000mg, or extract, $1/2$ dropperful daily.
✤ Vitamin C 3000mg. daily with bioflavonoids, or Crystal Star BIOFLAVONOID, FIBER & C SUPPORT™.
✤ Evening primrose oil caps, 2 to 4 daily with Vitamin E with selenium 400IU daily.
✤ High Omega 3 oils, from flax or cold water fish, 1000mg. daily.
✤ Sun CHLORELLA, 1 packet granules, or 15 tabs daily.
➤ Regular exercise is a key factor in circulatory health.

HORMONE IMBALANCE

Effective for Men After Prostate and Related Problems, or Surgery ✧ Effective for Women After Hysterectomy, Childbirth, D & C, or Suction Curretage

Hormones help regulate everything from energy flow to inflammation to a woman's monthly cycle to a man's hair growth. Natural therapy focus for hormone balance is to gently stimulate body regulatory functions after trauma, stress or serious illness - rather than to regulate hormone levels by injection. This allows the body to make its own hormones, and bring itself to its own balance at the deepest level of the body processes.

FOOD THERAPY

➥ Start with a modified macrobiotic diet for 2 weeks (pg. 52) with seasonal fresh foods, whole grains, brown rice and vegetable protein.

➥ Take a protein drink such as Nature's Plus SPIRUTEIN each morning, or a green drink (pg. 54ff) or Crystal Star ENERGY GREEN™ drink daily.

➥ Avoid sugar, refined and canned foods.

➥ Drink 6-8 glasses of unchlorinated bottled water daily.

➥ Add complex carbohydrate-rich, building foods to your diet: broccoli, peas, cauliflower, tofu, wheat germ, brewer's yeast, nuts and seeds, and whole grains.

VITAMINS/MINERALS

For male balance: ♂
▶ Cal/mag/zinc 4 daily, or zinc 75mg. daily.

▶ Green Foods GREEN MAGMA daily.

▶ Effective raw glandular therapy:
✦ Raw Pancreas glandular
✦ Raw Orchic glandular
✦ Raw Pituitary glandular

▶ Bee pollen 2-4 daily.

For female balance: ♀
▶ Prof. Serv. PROGEST CREAM applied as directed.

▶ B Complex 100mg. daily.

▶ Pantothenic acid 1000mg.

♂ *For both sexes:* ♀
▶ High potency YS royal jelly 1 teasp. daily with 6 kelp tabs daily.

▶ Vitamin E 800IU daily.

▶ Effective GLA sources
✦ Evening primrose oil 2-4 daily.
✦ BioSource black currant oil
✦ Source Natural GLA 240

HERBAL THERAPY

For male balance: ♂
☙ Siberian ginseng extract daily.

☙ Crystal Star PROX CAPS™ and PROX™ extract.

☙ Effective combinations:
✦ Ginseng/Damiana
✦ Ginseng/Sarsaparilla
✦ Licorice/Dandelion

☙ Smilax extract 10-15 drops daily for testosterone production.

☙ Crystal Star MALE PERFORMANCE™ capsules for 1 month.

For female balance: ♀
☙ Crystal Star DONG QUAI/DAMIANA extract, or dong quai capsules as a nutritive tonic.

☙ Evening primrose oil 2-4 daily.

☙ Crystal Star FEMALE HARMONY caps or EST-AID™ extract.

☙ Burdock, wild yam, or peony root tea 2 cups daily.

♂ *For both sexes:* ♀
☙ Crystal Star ADR-ACTIVE™ capsules or extract.

BODYWORK

If you are taking synthetic estrogen or progesterone for glandular problems, it can destroys vitamin E in the body, allowing greater risk for heart, cancer and other diseases. Supplementation is advisable to counteract this.

▶ Applied kinesiology (muscle testing) is successful in hormone balance healing to determine which specific products are suitable for individual problems.

▶ Get morning sunlight on the body every day possible, especially on the male genitalia. ♂

▶ Take a good brisk exercise walk every day.

▶ Chiropractic adjustment or massage therapy treatment are excellent to reestablish unblocked meridians of energy and increase circulation for healing and hormone balance.

Common Symptoms: ❙ Women: Painful, difficult menstruation, or absence of menstruation; spotting between periods; depression; mood swings and irritability; water retention ❙ Men: Prostate pain and inflammation; lack of abdominal tone; poor urinary and sexual function.

Common Causes: Birth control pills or vasectomy; adrenal exhaustion due to stress; severe dieting or body building; surgery or illness; protein or iodine deficiency; calcium deficiency; B Complex or EFA deficiencies; synthetic steroid use.

Controlling Other Problems Associated With Hormone & Gland Imbalance

Erratic or deficient hormone secretions can be caused by, or can lead, to, other conditions, such as hot flashes, night sweats, contraceptive side effects, synthetic hormone side effects, frigidity, low libido and prostaglandin deficiency.

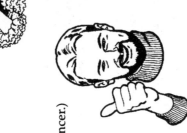

For Hot Flashes and Night Sweats:
❖ Crystal Star EST-AID™ capsules, and IODINE THERAPY™ capsules, and/or DONG QUAI/DAMIANA extract, or SUPER LICORICE™ extract.
❖ Black cohosh and kelp capsules, and vitex extract.
❖ Nature's Plus vitamin E 800IU.
❖ Evening primrose oil capsules 4 daily.
❖ B Complex 100mg. daily with ascorbate or Ester C 1 to 3000mg. daily.

To Overcome Side Effects from Contraceptives and Birth Control Pills:
❖ Nature's Plus vitamin E 800IU.
❖ Country Life MAXINE capsules 2-3 daily.
❖ B Complex 100mg. daily, with extra B6 250mg., B12 and folic acid capsules, and Ester C 550mg. with bioflavonoids 3-4x daily.
❖ Emulsified A & D 25,000IU/1,000IU.
❖ Women's Health RELEAF capsules.

To Overcome Side Effects from Synthetic Hormones: (Substances that can increase the risk of uterine, ovarian and breast cancer.)
❖ Nature's Plus vitamin E 800IU with B Complex 100mg. daily.
❖ Ester C 550mg. with bioflavonoids, 6x daily.
❖ Solaray CALCIUM CITRATE SUPREME capsules, 4-6 daily.
❖ Sarsaparilla extract 2-3x daily.

For Frigidity, Painful Intercourse, or Dry Vagina: (See MENOPAUSE page in this book for more information.)
❖ High potency YS or Premier 1 royal jelly 2 teasp. daily, and/or YS ginseng tea w. honey, 1 cup daily.
❖ Natures Plus vitamin E 800IU, or vitamin H with selenium 400IU 2x daily.
❖ Evening primrose oil, 4 daily for essential fatty acids, with extra B6 250mg.
❖ PSI PRO-GEST cream, rubbed on the abdomen regularly.
❖ Country Life MAXINE capsules for women, 2-3 daily.
❖ Crystal Star WOMEN'S DRYNESS™ extract, LOVE CAPS FEMALE™, DONG QUAI/DAMIANA extract, LOVE BATH FOR WOMEN, and CUPID'S FLAME™ tea.
❖ Country Life ADRENAL w. TYROSINE, or Enzymatic Therapy THYROID w. TYROSINE capsules, 4 daily.

To Rebalance Prostaglandin Formation: (Prostaglandin deficiency can lead to breast and uterine fibroids, arthritis, eczema, menstrual difficulties, high blood pressure and cholesterol, and a tendency to gain weight.)
❖ Avoid saturated fats, especially from red meats and pasteurized full fat dairy products.
❖ High Omega 3 oils from cold water fish and flax seed oil 3x daily.
❖ Effective GLA sources: Evening primrose or borage oil, black currant, or Source Naturals MEGA GLA 240 capsules 4-6 daily for 3 months.

To Rebalance Male Hormonal Energy and Libido:
❖ Evening primrose oil, 4 daily.
❖ Country Life MAX capsules daily.
❖ Sarsaparilla extract 2-3x daily.
❖ Crystal Star LOVING MOOD EXTRACT FOR MEN™, SUPER MAN'S ENERGY TONIC™ and LOVE CAPS MALE™.

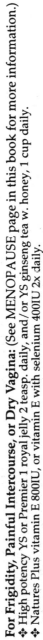

Note: Muscle Testing (Applied Kinesiology), is effective and useful in showing which hormonal herbs or supplements are specific to an individual problem. Once the simple technique is learned, (see a nutritional consultant, a holistic chiropractor, or a massage therapist), it can easily be done at home to determine which herbs are right for your condition.

HYPERACTIVITY ■ HYPERKINETIC BEHAVIOR IN CHILDREN

Attention Deficit Disorder ◇ Minimal Brain Dysfunction ◇ Learning Disabilities ◇ Autism

Hyperactivity is probably the best-known disorder affecting children since the fifties. It is the behavioral expression of either hypoglycemia or allergy or both. **Attention Deficit Disorder** is slow learning caused by any or all of these three disorders, and can be successfully treated in the same way. **Autistic** children are born with a brain malfunction that creates a barrier between them and the rest of the world. Autism is characterized by withdrawn behavior, lack of emotion and speech, extreme sensitivity to sound and touch and sometimes hyperactivity. We know, however, that hyperkinetic behavior is not so much the food or allergen, but the child's poor immune response. Children at greatest risk are male, with a history of

FOOD THERAPY

Diet change has been found to be the key factor in relieving hyperactive behavior. Diet improvement results are almost immediately evident, most within one to three weeks.When behavior has normalized maintain the improved diet to prevent reversion.

🍃 Since food sensitivities play a large part in these disorders, test common allergen foods - milk, wheat, corn, chocolate, and citrus with an elimination challenge diet; avoid all foods with sugar, dyes, colors, or additives. Eliminate all red meats (nitrates) and canned or frozen foods (too much salt). Reduce carbonated drinks.

🍃 The ongoing diet should be high in vegetable proteins and whole grains, with plenty of fresh fruits and vegetables, with no junk or fast foods. Have a green salad every day. Include tryptophan-rich foods; turkey, fish, wheat germ, yogurt, eggs.

🍃 Read labels carefully. Avoid all foods with preservatives, (BHT, MSG, BHA, etc.) additives or colors.

VITAMINS/MINERALS

Avoid aspirin and amphetamine of all kinds if your child has these disorders.

▶ Stress B Complex with extra pantothenic acid 100mg. and B6 100mg. to activate serotonin in the brain.

with

Vitamin C with bioflavonoids, 1-3000mg. daily. Best in powder form, 1/4 teasp. every 2 hours in juice.

▶ Twin Lab GABA plus or Country Life RELAXER CAPS as needed.

▶ Effective homeopathic remedies:
✦ Hylands CALMS tablets
✦ *Argenticum nit.*
✦ *Arsenicum*

▶ Taurine 500mg. daily. ☺

▶ Choline/inositol for brain balance. ♂
with
Magnesium 400mg. and Co. Life DMG sub-lingual 125mg.

▶ Glycine powder in liquid with passion flower extract drops to restore homeostasis.

▶ Logic LITHIUM ARGINATE as directed.

HERBAL THERAPY

🌿 Effective GLA sources to improve body "electrical connections".
✦ Evening primrose oil daily.
✦ BioSource black currant oil
✦ Source Naturals GLA 240
✦ High omega 3 flax oil.

🌿 Ginkgo biloba extract for inner ear balance problems often present.

🌿 Crystal Star RELAX CAPS™ as needed.

🌿 Planetary CALM CHILD drops or capsules as needed. ☺

🌿 Effective teas:
✦ Catnip
✦ Hops/lobelia
✦ Scullcap
✦ Passion flower

🌿 Effective extracts:
✦ Valerian/wild lettuce
✦ Black walnut as an anti-fungal
✦ Crystal Star CALCIUM SOURCE™ as a calmative.

BODYWORK

▶ Ritalin, Cylertor, and Atarax are short-term sedative drugs that often prove to make the condition worse over long use. They have side effects of nervousness, insomnia, unhealthy weight loss, stunted growth, stomach aches, skin rashes, headaches and hallucinations. Avoid them if you can. Try diet improvement first.

▶ Applied kinesiology is effective in determining allergic substances.

▶ Avoid fluorescent lighting and pesticides.

▶ See Hypoglycemia and Epilepsy Diets in this book, or the Optimal Eating For Children Diet in "COOKING FOR HEALTHY HEALING" by Linda Rector-Page, for more information.

Common Symptoms: *Behavioral Deficit:* Extreme emotional instability; compulsive, aggressive, destructive behavior; short attention span; can't sit still; self-mutilation; chronic liar; doesn't follow directions or listen; impatient and defiant. *Muscular Incoordination:* Poor motor coordination; speech problems; dyslexia; accident prone. *Cognitive/Perceptual Disorders:* slow learning and reasoning; unusual chronic thirst; chronic "cold", with sneezing and coughing.
Common Causes: Mineral and EFA deficiencies, prostaglandin imbalance; general malnutrition from too many refined and junk foods; food intolerances to preservatives and additives; hypoglycemia; heavy metal (esp. lead) poisoning causing excess ammonia waste in the brain; prescription drugs that make the condition worse by blocking EFA conversion in the brain.

HYPOGLYCEMIA ■ LOW BLOOD SUGAR

Hypoglycemia is a condition in which the pancreas over-reacts to sugar intake by producing too much insulin. Excess insulin results in lowering blood sugar too much as the body strives to achieve proper glucose/insulin balance in the blood. This is particularly harmful to the brain, the most sensitive organ to blood sugar levels, which requires glucose as an energy source to think clearly. Hypoglycemia causes a change in the way the brain functions. Small fluctuations disturb one's feeling of well-being. Large fluctuations cause feelings of depression, anxiety, mood swing fatigue and even aggressive behavior. Sugar balance is also needed for muscle contractions, the digestive system and nerve health.

FOOD THERAPY

🍃 Sugar and refined carbohydrates must be avoided. Omit natural sugars such as honey, molasses, maple syrup, and alcohol until sugar balance is achieved.
Reduce full fat dairy foods, fried and fatty foods, fast foods, pastries, prepared meats and saturated fats. Eliminate refined foods, caffeine, preserved foods and red meats permanently.

🍃 Include some vegetable protein at every meal. Add whole grains, fresh fruits and vegetables, low fat dairy products, sea vegetables, soy foods and brown rice frequently. Eat plenty of cultured foods such as yogurt and kefir for G.I. flora.

🍃 Include plenty of high fiber foods to help stabilize blood sugar swings.

🍃 Take 2 TBS. brewer's yeast flakes or Crystal Star SYTEM STRENGTH™ drink daily for glucose stability.

🍃 Go on a 24 hour liquid diet (pg.44) whenever low blood sugar symptoms seem to be appearing regularly. Add a good, high nutrient, no sugar protein powder. A feeling of well-being will return rapidly.

VITAMINS/MINERALS

Glucose homeostasis depends on a wide range of micro-nutrients - many of which are in short supply in the American diet.

▶ Effective chromium therapy choices:
✦ GTF Chromium 200mcg.
✦ Solaray CHROMIACIN
✦ Chromium picolinate
✦ ProBiologics GlucoBalance caps or LIQUID CHROMIUM
and add
✦ DMG B₁₅ 125mg.
✦ Am. Biologics VANADIUM.

▶ B Complex 100mg. 2x daily with extra B6 100mg. and panto. acid 500mg.
and
Vit. C 3000mg. w. bioflavs. daily. (Take vitamin C immediately during an attack).

▶ CoQ 10 30mg. daily for 3-6 weeks, with
Mezotrace minerals 1 daily. ♀

▶ Country Life GLYCEMIC FACTORS *and* MOOD FACTORS capsules as needed. ♂

▶ Glutamine 500mg. daily.

▶ Enzymatic Therapy HYPO-ADE caps, and LIQUID LIVER w. Sib. ginseng.

HERBAL THERAPY

🌿 Crystal Star SUGAR STRATEGY LOW™ capsules and tea.
with
ADR-ACTIVE™ caps or ADRN™ extract.
and
GINSENG 6 DEFENSE RESTORATIVE™ TEA to help remove sugar from the blood.

🌿 High potency YS royal jelly for adrenal stimulation.

🌿 Effective teas:
♦ Dandelion/licorice ♂
♦ Juniper
♦ Yarrow flowers

🌿 Crystal Star CHO-LO FIBER TONE™ or other good fiber cleanse morning and evening to absorb unnecessary carbohydrates and balance sugar curve.   with
1 teasp. each:
♦ Spirulina granules
♦ Bee pollen granules

🌿 Sun Chlorella daily as a liver nutrient.

🌿 Alta Health CANGEST or HI-LO BALANCE caps.

BODYWORK

▶ Eat small meals frequently throughout the day to keep blood sugar levels up. Large meals throw sugar balance way off.

▶ Eat relaxed, never under stress.

▶ Get some exercise every day to work off unmetabolized acid wastes.

▶ Some oral contraceptives can cause glucose intolerance and poor sugar metabolism. Ask your doctor.

▶ Reflexology point:

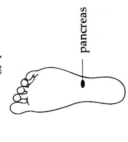
— pancreas

▶ Pancreas area:

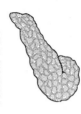

Common Symptoms: Manic/depressive psychological states; irritability, often violence; restlessness, insomnia; anxiety, depression and a feeling of going crazy; dizziness, shakes, and trembling; ravenous hunger and craving for sweets; headaches; lethargy or hyperactivity; nausea; blurry vision; great fatigue.
Common Causes: Poor diet or excess dietary sugar causing abnormally low levels of glucose in the blood, affecting brain, nerves, digestive system and muscles; food allergies; too much alcohol, caffeine or nicotine; stress; exhausted adrenals and liver damage; hypothyroidism; too large meals.

DIET FOR HYPOGLYCEMIA CONTROL

The two key factors in hypoglycemia are stress and poor diet. Both are a result of too much dietary sugar and refined carbohydrates. These foods quickly raise glucose levels, causing the pancreas to over-compensate and produce too much insulin, which then lowers body glucose levels too far and too fast. The following diet supplies the body with high fiber, complex carbohydrates and proteins - slow even-burning fuel, that prevents these sudden sugar elevations and drops. Small frequent meals should be eaten, with plenty of unrefined, fresh foods to keep sugar levels stable. Other watchwords: 1) Eat potassium-rich foods, such as oranges, broccoli, bananas, and tomatoes. 2) Eat chromium-rich foods, such as brewer's yeast, mushrooms, whole wheat, sea foods, beans and peas. 3) Eat some high quality vegetable protein at every meal.

On rising: take a "hypoglycemia cocktail": 1 teasp. <u>each</u> in apple or orange juice to control morning sugar drop: glycine powder, powdered milk, protein powder, and brewer's yeast;
or a protein/amino drink, such as Nature's Plus SPIRUTEIN or Crystal Star SYSTEM STRENGTH™.

Breakfast: a very important meal for hypoglycemia, should include ⅓ of daily nutrients; have some oatmeal with yogurt and fresh fruit;
or poached or baked eggs on whole grain toast with a little butter or kefir cheese;
or a whole grain cereal or granola with apple juice, soy milk or fruit yogurt and nuts;
or some whole grain pancakes with an apple or fruit sauce;
or some tofu scrambled "eggs" with bran muffins, whole grain toast and a little butter.

Mid-morning: have a green drink (page 54), Sun CHLORELLA or Green Foods GREEN MAGMA with 1 teasp. Bragg's LIQUID AMINOS, or Crystal Star ENERGY GREEN DRINK™; **and/or** a balancing herb tea, such as licorice, dandelion, or Crystal Star SUGAR STRATEGY LOW™; **and** some crisp, crunchy vegetables with kefir or yogurt cheese;
or cornbread or whole grain crackers, or bran muffins with butter or kefir cheese.

Lunch: have a fresh salad, with a little cottage cheese or soy cheese, nut, noodle or seed toppings, and lemon oil dressing; **and/or** a high protein sandwich on whole grain bread, with avocados, low fat cheese, and mayonnaise;
or a bean or lentil soup with a tofu or shrimp salad or sandwich;
or a seafood and whole grain pasta salad;
or a vegetarian pizza on a chapati crust with low fat or soy mozzarrella cheese.

Mid-afternoon: have a hard boiled egg with sesame salt, and whole grain crackers with yogurt dip; **and/or** an herb tea, such as Crystal Star LICORICE MINTS, a green drink, or small bottle of mineral water,
or yogurt with nuts and seeds.

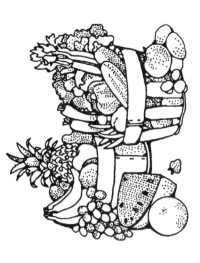

Dinner: have some steamed vegies with tofu, or baked or broiled fish and brown rice;
or an oriental stir fry with seafood and vegetables, and miso soup with sea vegetables;
or a whole grain or vegetable Italian pasta dish with a verde sauce and hearty soup;
or a Spanish beans and rice dish, or paella with seafood and rice;
or a vegie quiche on whole grain crust and a small mushroom and spinach salad;
or roast turkey with cornbread stuffing and a light soup.

Before bed: have a cup of VEGEX yeast paste broth; **or** papaya juice with a little yogurt.

◗ **Suggested supplements for the Hypoglycemia Control Diet**
❖ To support adrenal glands depleted by stress and hypoglycemic reactions, take B complex 100mg. and vitamin C 3000-5000mg. daily, (or immediately during a sugar drop attack). **or** Crystal Star ADR-ACTIVE™ caps or ADRN™ extract, or Enzymatic Therapy RAW ADRENAL extract; **and/or** add 2 teasp. daily of YS royal jelly to a protein or green drink.
❖ To balance sugar use in the bloodstream, take GTF chromium or chromium picolinate 200mcg. or Solaray CHROMIACIN daily.
❖ To improve carbohydrate digestion, take Alta Health CANGEST, with Spirulina or Bee Pollen granules, morning and evening.
❖ To increase oxygen uptake and add minerals, take CoQ10 10-30mg. and Mezotrace SEA MINERAL COMPLEX daily.
➤ Get regular aerobic exercise every day to work off unmetabolized acid wastes.
➤ Eat relaxedly, never under stress.

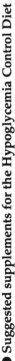

LOW BLOOD SUGAR SELF-TEST

The importance of correct diagnosis and treatment of sugar instabilities is essential. The human body possesses a complex set of checks and balances to maintain blood glucose concentrations within a narrow range. Blood sugar control is influenced by the pituitary, thyroid and adrenal glands, as well as the pancreas, liver, kidneys and even the skeletal muscles. Hypoglycemia symptoms are often mistaken for other problems. Low blood sugar is the biological equivalent of a race car running on empty. It is not so much a disease as a symptom of other disorders. The symptoms can be improved right away by eating something, but this does not address the cause.

Children are also subject to hypoglycemia which has been indicated as a cause of both hyperactivity and learning disorders. (See page 243.) Chronic negativism, hyperkinesis, and obstinate resentment to all discipline are reasons for at least the self-test below and probably a Glucose Tolerance Test. (With children, the condition can only be managed by a diet from which all forms of concentrated sugars have been removed, including fruit juices, until the body achieves glucose homeostasis.)

The following questionnaire is for self-determination, reprinted from the Enzymatic Therapy Notebook. It can help you decide, in cooperation with a health care professional, whether you need low blood sugar support, and whether professional help is necessary.

Mark the following symptoms as they pertain to you: (1) for mild symptoms, occurring once or twice a year; (2) for moderate symptoms, occurring several times a year; (3) severe symptoms, occurring almost constantly.

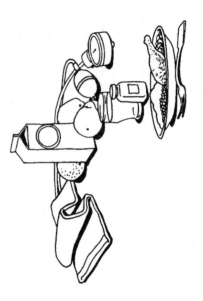

( ) Irritability
( ) Anti-social behavior
( ) Craving for sweets
( ) Blurred vision
( ) Heart palpitations
( ) Rapid pulse
( ) Mental confusion, spaciness
( ) Forgetfulness
( ) Constant phobias, fears
( ) Constant worry and anxiety
( ) Nightmares
( ) Cold sweats and shaking
( ) Frequent headaches
( ) Faintness and dizziness
( ) Nervousness
( ) Convulsions, trembling
( ) Poor concentration
( ) Crying spells
( ) Weak spells
( ) Extreme fatigue, exhaustion
( ) Lots of sighing and yawning
( ) Insomnia; inability to return to sleep after awakening
( ) Twitching, involuntary muscle jerks
( ) Digestive problems
( ) Indecisiveness
( ) Unexplained depression
( ) Nervous breakdown
( ) Suicidal intent

A score of 6 or more signifies a need for sugar balancing and nutritional support. A score of 12 -18 indicates a need for therapeutic measures several times daily.

HYPOTHYROIDISM

Goiter ✧ Sluggish Metabolism ✧ Parathyroid Disease

Thyroid gland hormones affect every cell of the body. Hypothyroidism, low thyroid function, results in a large number of symptoms. The brain is quite sensitive to low thyroid levels and the primary signs of the disease are slowed brain functions. To determine your thyroid condition: Take your basal temperature for 10 minutes on rising in the morning. Do not move while taking temperature. It should be between 97.8 and 98.2 for health. Below this, and a sluggish thyroid exists. Repeat temperature taking for three days. Temperature will return to normal as treatment begins to work. If menstruating, take temperature on the 2nd, 3rd and 4th day of menses. (See THYROID HEALTH page for more information.)

FOOD THERAPY

🍃 Follow a 75% fresh foods diet for a month to rebalance metabolism. Have a green salad twice a day.

🍃 Eat plenty of iodine-rich foods, such as sea vegetables, sea foods, fish, mushrooms, garlic, onions and watercress.

🍃 Eat vitamin A-rich foods such as yellow vegetables, eggs, carrots, dark green vegetables, raw dairy.

🍃 Take a green drink (pg. 54ff) or a potassium broth (pg. 53) or Crystal Star ENERGY GREEN™ drink several times weekly.

🍃 Take 2 TBS. brewer's yeast, 1 teasp. wheat germ oil and 1 teasp. cod liver oil every day.

🍃 Use an herb salt instead of table salt.

🍃 Avoid refined foods, saturated fats, sugars, white flour and red meats.

🍃 Avoid "goitrogens", foods that prevent the use of iodine: cabbage, turnips, peanuts, mustard, pine nuts, millet and soy products. (Cooking these foods inactivates goitrogens.)

VITAMINS/MINERALS

▶ Emulsified A 25,000IU 3x daily, or Beta carotene 100,000IU daily.
Vitamin E 400IU daily.

▶ Cal/mag/potassium caps 2 daily, with zinc 50mg. daily. ♂

▶ Tyrosine 500mg. with lysine 500mg. 2x daily.

▶ **Enzymatic Therapy thyroid/tyrosine complex. ♀ or Nutrapathic Thyroid.**

▶ Ascorbate vitamin C with bioflavonoids 3000mg. daily.

▶ B Complex 100mg. with extra B₂ 100mg., B₁ 500mg., and B₆ 200mg.

▶ CoQ 10 30mg. daily with B₁₂ SL.

▶ Raw glandular therapy:
  ✚ **Raw Thyroid complex**
  ✚ **Raw Pituitary**
  ✚ Raw Adrenal substance or Country Life ADRENAL COMPLEX with tyrosine 2-3 daily. ♀

▶ Spirulina or Chlorella 8 tablets daily.

HERBAL THERAPY

🍃 Crystal Star IODINE THERAPY™ capsules or extract 2x daily.
or
META-TABS 2 daily.
or

🍃 **Heritage ATOMODINE drops. ♀**

🍃 Evening Primrose oil 3x daily.

🍃 Effective teas:
  ◆ Pau de arco, 3 cups daily
  ◆ Sarsaparilla extract tea ♂
  ◆ Bayberry bark
  ◆ Gotu kola
  ◆ Irish moss
  ◆ Calendula
  ◆ Dulse
  ◆ Alfalfa/dandelion
  ◆ Parsley/watercress

🍃 **Kelp tabs 10 daily, with Cayenne caps 2 daily. ♂**

🍃 Crystal Star SYTEM STRENGTH™ drink mix daily.

🍃 For goiter, apply black walnut tincture as a throat paint, and take 1/2 dropperful 2x daily.

BODYWORK

▶ Take a brisk half hour walk daily to oxygenate the tissues and stimulate circulation.

▶ Sun bathe in the morning. Sea bathe and wade whenever possible.

▶ Acupressure point:
Press hollow at base of the throat to stimulate thyroid, 3x for 10 secs. each.

▶ Avoid fluorescent lights and fluoride toothpaste. They deplete vitamin A in the body.

▶ Reflexology point:

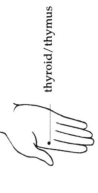 thyroid/thymus

▶ For goiter, apply calendula compresses twice a day for a month.

▶ The drug levothyroxine, frequently given for hypothyroidism, can cause significant bone loss. Ask your doctor. Avoid antihistamines and sulfa drugs.

Common Symptoms: Mental depression, and emotional instability; muscle weakness and great fatigue; poor memory; lethargy; headaches; deep, slow speech; hoarseness; goiter; coarse hair and loss of hair; swollen hands and feet; constipation; pale and sallow skin; cold hands and feet; coarse, dry skin; swelling of the face, tongue and eyelids; excessive and painful menstruation; nervousness and heart palpitations; unexplained weight gain. In children, hypothyroidism also results in retarded growth and mental development. Goiter common symptoms: Enlargement of the thyroid gland. This is usually a woman's problem.
Common Causes: Iodine deficiency; Vitamin E, A and zinc deficiency; overuse of iodine-depleting prescription diet pills; pituitary and thyroid malfunction; environmental pollution.

IMMUNITY
Building It ◇ Strengthening It

The immune system is the collection of organs, cells and molecules which are responsible for both protective and adverse response to substances encountered in the environment. White blood cells are the vital components - containing anti-bodies (immunoglobulins), B-cells, T-cells, and their helper lymphocytes that act as the body's primary defense against viral infection. Prostaglandins regulate the immune system with particular influence on the white cells and their involvement in activating and controlling antibodies.

FOOD THERAPY

🍃 The American diet of processed foods, 20% sugars, and 37% fat, suppresses immunity. Saturated fats, such as those in pastries, fried foods, and red meats are particular culprits. Refined foods offer little nutrition. Avoid junk and processed foods. Reduce dairy and sugary foods.

🍃 Take a balanced protein drink every morning for strength. See Pg. 63, or Natures Plus SPIRUTEIN.

🍃 Eat a generally cleansing/building, low fat diet, with plenty of fresh foods, fiber foods, whole grains, sea foods, eggs and cultured dairy foods, such as yogurt and kefir for friendly G.I. flora.

🍃 Effective immune-stimulating drinks:
   ◆ BioStrath YEAST ELIXIR w. HERBS
   ◆ Nutri-Tech ALL 1.
   ◆ Crystal Star BIOFLAV., FIBER & C SUPPORT™ drink
   ◆ Crystal Star SYSTEM STRENGTH™
   ◆ George's aged ALOE VERA JUICE
   ◆ Sun CHLORELLA 1 packet daily
   ◆ Crystal Star GINSENG 6 DEFENSE RESTORATIVE™ TEA or Celestial Seasonings GINSENG PLUS tea.

🍃 Effective food immune enhancers: kelp, papaya, garlic, sea vegetables.

VITAMINS/MINERALS

▶ Biogenetics BIO-GUARD ♂ daily for 3-6 weeks, with B Complex 100mg., Ener B internasal gel for B12, and Mezotrace SEA MINERAL complex.

▶ Effective immune-stimulants:
   ✦ Source Naturals WELLNESS
   ✦ Enzym. Therapy IMMUNO-PLEX
   ✦ Am. Biologics OXY-FORTE 5000
   ✦ Co.Life WELL-MAX w. pycnogenol, and LIFE SPAN 2000
   ✦ Rainbow Light DEEP DEFENSE SYSTEM or ADVANCED DEFENSE SYSTEM
   ✦ Future Biotics VITAL K

▶ Effective anti-oxidants prevent thymus shrinkage:
   ✦ Pycnogenol 2-4 daily.
   ✦ Germanium 50mg. 2x daily.
   ✦ Beta or marine carotene 25,000IU
   ✦ Glutathione 50mg.
   ✦ CoQ 10 30mg. daily. ♂
   ✦ Vitamin E 400IU w. selenium. ♂

▶ Raw Thymus extract or SL tabs, and/or Homeopathic *Aconite* tabs.

▶ Vitamin C or Ester C with bioflavonoids 3000mg. with zinc 50mg. daily.

▶ Dr. DOPHILUS capsules, or ¹/₂ teasp. in water 2x daily.

HERBAL THERAPY

🍂 Crystal Star HERBAL DEFENSE TEAM™ capsules, extract or tea, for at least 1 month.
then
🍂 Crystal Star FEEL GREAT™ tea and caps to rebuild strength and a feeling of well-being. ♀

🍂 Zand HERBAL INSURE extract .

🍂 Effective immuno-modulating adaptogen herbs:
   ◆ Siberian ginseng
   ◆ Propolis
   ◆ Echinacea rt.
   ◆ Pau de arco
   ◆ Ginkgo biloba
   ◆ Health Concerns ASTRA 8

🍂 Effective anti-oxidants:
   ◆ Reishi mushroom tea or Health Concerns POWER MUSHROOMS or Planetary REISHI MUSHROOM SUPREME for production of interferon.
   ◆ Milk thistle seed
   ◆ Green tea or Crystal Star GREEN TEA CLEANSER™

🍂 Effective immune enhancers:
   ◆ Echinacea/myrrh
   ◆ Royal jelly ♂
   ◆ Licorice rt.
   ◆ Suma/schizandra
   ◆ Chaparral/burdock capsules

BODYWORK

▲ Tobacco/nicotine in any form is an immune depressant. The cadmium content causes zinc deficiency. Note: It takes 3 months to get good immune response even after you quit.

▲ Get regular exercise every day to keep system oxygen high. Disease does not readily attack in a high oxygen, high potassium environment.

▲ The mind affects the immune system. A positive mental attitude can make a big difference in how the body fights disease. Creative visualization to establish belief and optimism is effective, and allows you to take an active part in your own wellness.

▲ Environmental pollutants, particularly pesticides, lower immunity. Eat organically grown foods whenever possible.

▲ Eliminate recreational drugs. Reduce prescription drugs, especially antibiotics and cortico-steroids that depress immunity.

Common Symptoms: Chronic and continuing infections, colds, respiratory problems; Candida yeast overgrowth; chronic fatigue; chronic allergies.
Common Causes: Glandular malfunction, usually because of poor diet and nutrition; staph infection; prolonged use of antibiotics and/or cortico-steroids. (Long use of these drugs can depress the immune system to the point where even minor illness can become life-threatening.); some immunization shots; Candida albicans yeast overgrowth; great emotional stress; food and other allergies; environmental and heavy metal pollutants; radiation.

About The Immune System & Maintenance Checkpoints

The immune defense system is the most complex in the human body. Only recently, because of the great rise of opportunistic diseases in the world today are we beginning to understand its nature and comprehensive dynamics. A strong immune system is absolutely necessary for prevention of modern opportunistic diseases such as Cancer, AIDS, Herpes, Lupus, Candida albicans, and Chronic Fatigue Syndrome (EBV). Primarily involving the thymus gland, lymph glands, and bone marrow, it is a wonderful autonomic, subconscious defense system that can hold off and neutralize infection so the body can heal itself. It is this quality of being a part of us, yet not under our conscious control, that manifests its greatest power. And its greatest problem. When immune response is continually involved in fighting a "rear guard" action against a constant immune-depressing overload of antibiotics, cortisones, and antacids, etc. that destroy vital enzymes, and foods full of pesticides, chemical foods and preservatives with poor nutrition, it gets to a point where it cannot distinuish harmful cells from healthy cells, and attacks everything (as in cases of AIDS or some cancers today). In many instances, when we can limit overkill from drugs and anti-biotics, the immune system functions at its best when we just "get out of the way" by keeping the body well nourished and clear of toxic wastes. Immune energy is then directed toward rebuilding and maintaining strength against outside invasions of harmful bacteria, viruses or pollutants.

The immune system is the body system most sensitive to nutritional deficiencies. Most disease is caused by lack of sufficient minerals and oxygen in the vital fluids, which allows a pathogenic environment to take hold. Things that reduce normal immune response include air and water pollution, toxic household substances, drugs, stress, and poor nutrition. Providing optimum nutrition at the first sign of infection or loss of health vastly improves the defense shield. Immune rebuilding is not easy. It takes time and commitment, but it is worth it. The inherited immunity and health of you, your children and your grandchildren is laid down by you.

The following checkpoints can help maintain strong immunity in today's world.

1) Take some high potency, concentrated, green, "superfoods" several times a week, such as Sun CHLORELLA, Green Foods GREEN MAGMA, wheat grass, spirulina, alfalfa or Solaray ALFAJUICE, liquid chlorophyll, or Crystal Star ENERGY GREEN™ drink. Remember that the composition of chlorophyll is very similar to that of human hemoglobin, so these foods provide a "mini-transfusion" for your bloodstream.

2) Include sea vegetables, such as kelp, hijiki, dulse, kombu, wakame, and sea palm, in your daily diet for their therapeutic iodine, high potassium, and sodium alginate content (see page 85); or take Crystal Star POTASSIUM SOURCE™, SYSTEM STRENGTH™ drink, or IODINE THERAPY™ complexes.

3) Take a high potency lactobacillus or acidophilus complex, such as Natren LIFE START II, Dr. DOPHILUS, or Solaray MULTI-DOLPHILUS for friendly G.I. flora, and good food assimilation.

4) Include one or more anti-oxidant supplements, such as vitamin E with selenium, beta carotene, zinc, CoQ 10, germanium, pycnogenol and vitamin C. The highest potency anti-oxidants are in enzyme form, such as Biotec CELL GUARD, or Biogenetics BIOGUARD PLUS.

5) Several herbs also have strong anti-oxidant qualities: echinacea, chaparral, goldenseal, Siberian ginseng, rosemary, astragalus, suma, burdock, and pau de arco.

6) New extract forms of silica may now be taken internally to strengthen immunity. Take 1 TB. in 3 oz. water in a full course for three months.

7) Protect the thymus gland from shrinking with age, and to nourish the immune organs with a raw thymus glandular supplement.

8) Regular aerobic exercise keeps system oxygen high, and circulation flowing. Remember that disease does not readily overrun a body where oxygen and organic minerals are high in the vital fluids.

9) The immune system is stimulated by a few minutes of early morning sunlight every day. Avoid excessive sun. Sun *burn* depresses immunity.

See "COOKING FOR HEALTHY HEALING" by Linda Rector-Page for a complete diet to build and maintain strong immunity.

* *Laughter lifts more than your spirits. It also seems to boost the immune system. Laughter decreases cortisol, an immune suppressor, allowing immune boosters to function better.*

♂ MALE IMPOTENCE ▦ SEXUAL PROBLEMS ▦ STERILITY ♂

Many are concerned about their ability to achieve or maintain an erection, premature ejaculation, the frequency with which they are able to have intercourse and the recovery period in between. Male infertility is also reaching alarming proportions from modern lifestyles and environments. Stress reduction techniques and natural therapies for reversing infertility have been notably successful, as well as being far less invasive and expensive than medical treatment.

FOOD THERAPY

Most impotency originates in poor diet and nutrition - a problem of the dinner table, not the bedroom. The first step is to lose weight if you are overweight.

❧ The problem can often be corrected simply by improving the diet. Junk, chemical, and processed foods are a key factor today in male impotency.

❧ Eat a high vegetable protein diet. Take a high protein drink every morning. Include a green leafy salad every day. Add plenty of potassium and selenium-rich foods.

❧ Have a "potent-C" drink every morning for several months: For 4 drinks, mix in the blender:
1 cup sliced strawberries
1 sliced banana
1 cup papaya chunks
1 cup pineapple/coconut juice
1 cup amazake rice drink
2 TB. honey or barley malt
2 TB. toasted wheat germ
2 TB. pumpkin seeds
2 TB. lecithin
2 TB. brewer's yeast
1 egg
1 TB. sesame seeds
2 teasp. vanilla

❧ Avoid red meats (they sometimes contain female hormones); prepared meats that contain nitrates; reduce dietary salt and sugar.

VITAMINS/MINERALS

▶ Zinc 50mg. 2x daily.
with
Germanium 100mg. daily.

▶ Effective raw glandulars:
✦ Strength Systems orchic extract
✦ Pituitary
✦ Male
with
✦ vitamin E 400IU 2x daily, and Carnitine 500mg.

❦ Strength Systems yohimbe capsules *with* tyrosine 500mg. daily.

▶ Highest potency royal jelly 2 teasp. daily.

▶ Niacin (not niacinimide), up to 3000mg. daily for circulation.

▶ B15 DMG sublingual daily.

▶ Alta Health magnesium chloride 6 daily on a full stomach, for 1 week, then 3 daily for 3 weeks.

▶ Vitamin C 3000mg. daily if there is sperm agglutination.

▶ Country Life MAX tabs as a good male multi-vitamin.

HERBAL THERAPY

❦ Damiana/kola nut/saw palmetto capsules.

❦ Crystal Star LOVE MALE™ capsules, or LOVING MOOD™ extract.

❦ Crystal Star MALE PERFORMANCE™ for long term hormone building.

❦ Effective Ginseng formulas:
◆ Ginseng/Royal Jelly ampules
◆ Siberian Ginseng extract
◆ Chinese Red Ginseng caps
◆ Ginseng/Sarsaparilla caps
◆ Ginseng/Damiana caps
◆ Ginseng/Cayenne capsules
◆ Ginseng/Gotu Kola caps
◆ Ho-Shou-Wu
Remember that ginseng is a regenerative herb. It does not make the normal body "supernormal".

❦ Licorice/damiana caps to increase sperm count. Take with pineapple juice for 6 days in a row, then rest for 6 days, then resume, and etc.

❦ Effective male stimulants:
◆ BioForce GINSAVENA extract
◆ Scandanavian EXSATIVA
◆ Smilax extract 10x strength, for increased testosterone production.
◆ PEP COBRA tabs as desired.

BODYWORK

The other key factor in impotency is life style - stop smoking, using hard liquor, and recreational drugs.

▶ Take alternating hot and cool showers to increase circulation.

▶ Crystal Star LOVE BATH FOR MEN for a sexy, masculine feeling.

▶ Squeeze the testicles every day to stimulate, once for every year of your life.

▶ Breathe deeply. Get regular exercise. Get some early morning sunlight on the body and genitals every day possible.

▶ Try hypnotherapy as an effective relaxation technique.

▶ Avoid clothing that holds the testes too close to the body. (Body heat hampers sperm production.) Also avoid electric blankets, hot tubs and saunas because of too much heat.

▶ Reflexology point:

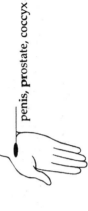

penis, **prostate**, coccyx

Common Symptoms: Inability to have or maintain an erection during intercourse; premature ejaculation; inability to impregnate a woman.
Common Causes: Poor diet and nutrition; psychological or emotional stress; depression; hypoglycemia; diabetes; gland imbalance; protein deficiency.

arteriosclerosis; environmental or heavy metal poisoning; too much alcohol and tobacco; low sperm count;

INDIGESTION

Heartburn ◇ Gas ◇ Flatulence

Good food digestion and assimilation is at the "heart" of health. When digestion is not optimum, problems go beyond the usual symptoms of gas and bloating. Energy is reduced, constipation results from metabolic byproducts that are not eliminated, allergic reactions, diarrhea and fatigue can all ensue. In cases of chronic indigestion, the immune system suffers drastically, allowing viral and other infections, such as candidiasis and chronic fatigue to take hold. Good digestion is important! **See page 29 for a complete discussion of enzyme therapy.**

FOOD THERAPY

Get a food combining chart so you can be aware of good food combining.

☙ Make sure you are eating an alkalizing diet, with plenty of cultured foods such as yogurt, kefir and miso soup, high fiber foods such as whole grains, fresh vegetables and fruits, and enzyme-rich foods such as papaya and pineapple.
Avoid fatty, spicy, and acid-forming foods. Omit fried foods, red meats, refined sugars, sodas and caffeine.

☙ To cleanse the digestive system and establish good assimilation and enzyme production:
Start with a cleansing high pectin mono diet of apples and apple juice for 2 days.
Then for 4 days use a diet of 70% fresh foods and steamed brown rice for B vitamins and to rebalance digestion.

☙ Take one of these daily:
♦ 1 tsp. cider vinegar in water
♦ 2 lemons in water
♦ a green drink (pg. 54ff)

☙ Avoid the following foods until digestion is better balanced: beans, full fat dairy products, cabbages, bagels, dried fruits, and onions.

VITAMINS/MINERALS

▶ Enzymatic Therapy MEGA-ZYME, or Living Source FOOD SENSITIVITY SYSTEM after eating.

▶ Solaray SUPER DIGEST AWAY ♀ Dr. DOPHILUS caps, or 1 teasp. chlorophyll liqid before eating. ♂

▶ **If there is belching and burping:**
♦ Betaine HCl after meals
♦ Schiff super enzymall
♦ AkPharma BEANO drops
♦ Hyland's *Biliousness* after meals
♦ Co. Life DIGESTIVE FORMULA

If there is gas and bloating:
♦ Pancreatin capsules 1400mg.
♦ Biotec BIOGESTIN for protein
♦ HCl capsules after meals
♦ Activated charcoal - short term
♦ BioForce *Flatulence* tabs

If there are ulcers:
♦ Glutamine 500mg.
♦ Enzymatic Therapy DGL

If there is diarrhea:
♦ Activated charcoal tabs
♦ Apple pectin tabs ♂

If there is acute indigestion:
♦ Papaya chewables
♦ Alta Health manganese lozenges
♦ Enzymatic Therapy DGL

▶ Sun chlorella or barley green on a regular basis for prevention.

▶ Solaray ALFAJUICE caps.

HERBAL THERAPY

❦ To relieve gas quickly; put pinches of cinnamon, nutmeg, ginger and cloves in water and drink down.

❦ Crystal Star HERBAL ENZ™, tea or MEDITATION™ tea as needed.

❦ Crystal Star SYSTEM STRENGTH™ drink mix for good enzyme activity and system alkalizing.

❦ Aloe vera juice with herbs after meals, and bee pollen or royal jelly 2 teasp. daily. ♂

❦ Good digestion teas:
♦ Catnip/fennel ☺
♦ Slippery elm
♦ Peppermint/spearmint
♦ Wild yam
♦ Sage
♦ Alfalfa/mint

❦ Effective digestive caps:
♦ Turmeric ♀
♦ Garlic/parsley
♦ Nature's Plus chewable bromelain 40mg. or papaya enzyme chewables after meals. ♂
♦ Turmeric or ginger capsules.

❦ NatureWorks SWEDISH BITTERS, or Crystal Star BITTERS & LEMON CLEANSE™ extract.

BODYWORK

▶ Apply ginger compresses to abdominal area. Take 2 ginger capsules as needed to break up gas.

▶ Take peppermint oil drops in a cup of water as needed. (also helpful if there is irritable bowel syndrome).

▶ Lie on the back and draw knees up to chest to relieve abdomen pressure.

▶ Try to eat when relaxed. Meals eaten in a hurry and under stress all contribute to poor digestion. Life isn't going to slow down, so a conscious effort must be made to break this "vicious digestive circle". Try a short walk before eating.

▶ For flatulence: take a catnip or slippery elm enema for immediate relief.

▶ Eat smaller meals. Chew food very well. No smoking with meals. No fluids with meals. A little white wine is OK for better absorption.

Note: Commercial antacids neutralize stomach acid, inviting the stomach to produce even more acid, and therefore usually making the condition worse in the long run. In fact, some tests are now showing that chronic use of aluminum-containing antacids causes bone loss. Also avoid over using antibiotics. They destroy friendly flora in the digestive tract.

Common Symptoms: Gnawing, burning pain and tenderness occurring directly after food consumption; excess gas and abdominal distention; passing foul gas; poor food assimilation.
Common Causes: Poor food combining; eating too much, and too many refined, fatty and spicy foods; allergies to sugar, wheat or dairy; enzyme deficiency; overeating; candida yeast overgrowth; food allergies; too much caffeine, sodas and acid-forming foods; constipation; diverticulitis; vegetable protein deficiency; HCl deficiency.

INFECTION & INFLAMMATION

Staph ◇ Viral ◇ Bacterial

A staph infection involves a staphylococcus micro-organism, is usually quite virulent, and is often food-borne. Antibiotic measures are usually effective. A bacterial infection involves pathogenic microbial bacteria. Antibiotic agents are effective for this type of infection. A viral infection involves one of myriad virus organisms that can infiltrate the deepest regions of the body, and that live off the body's cell enzymes. They are virulent, deep-reaching and tenacious. Antibiotic agents do not kill viruses. Antiviral agent treatment must be specific and vigorous, since viruses can both mutate and move to escape being overcome. All infections regularly cause painful inflammation as the body reacts to isolates and overcome the infection. Chronic recurring infections can indicate low thyroid function. See also **Fungal Infections** in this book for more information

FOOD THERAPY

♨ Eat only fresh foods and brown rice for three days during acute stages of any infection to keep the body alkaline and free flowing.

♨ Take a glass of lemon juice and water each morning to stimulate kidney filtering.

♨ Take vegetable juices frequently during healing, with a potassium broth (pg. 53), Future Biotics VITAL K liquid, or Crystal Star SYSTEM STRENGTH™ drink daily.

♨ Include plenty of vegetable source proteins for faster healing; sea vegetables and sea foods, whole grains, sprouts, and soy foods.

♨ Avoid all sugars, refined foods, caffeine, colas, tobacco and alcohol (except for a little wine) during healing.

♨ Sun CHLORELLA or a good green drink (pg. 54) to restore body balance.

♨ Honey has antiseptic, antibiotic and antimicrobial properties. It may be taken internally and applied locally for infections.

VITAMINS/MINERALS

Viral infection:
▶ Dr. DOPHILUS 2 caps 3x daily with meals.
▶ Cartilade SHARK CARTILAGE to take down inflammation.
▶ Vitamin C crystals with bioflavs, 1/2 teasp. in water every hour during acute stages, reducing to 5000mg. daily.
▶ Body Essentials SILICA GEL 1 teasp. internally as an anti-inflammatory.
▶ Hylands *Hylavir* tablets as needed.
▶ Cntry. Life PYCNOGENOL caps.

Staph infection: See above.
▶ Nut. Res. GRAPEFRUIT SEED extract
▶ Vitamin C crystals with bioflavs. See above.
▶ Strength Systems FIRST AID.
▶ Raw Thymus drops and/or propolis capsules or extract 3-4x daily to restore immune defenses.

Bacterial infection: See above.
▶ Grapefruit Seed extract
▶ Dr. DOPHILUS 2 caps 3x daily with meals.
▶ Cartilade SHARK CARTILAGE to take down inflammation
▶ Beta Carotene 100,000IU daily, w. vit. E 800IU daily, for 2 weeks.
▶ Kal pycnogenol caps as a source of super bioflavonoids.
▶ Vitamin C crystals with bioflavs.

HERBAL THERAPY

Herbs are well suited to management of infective conditions that are resistant to medical treatment.

Viral infection:
❦ Destroy the active virus. Use Crystal Star ANTI-VI™ or ANTI-BIO™, or lomatium, goldenseal, myrrh, astragalus propolis or St. John's wort extracts; or Cartilade shark cartilage capsules.
❦ Limit bacterial harm with echinacea/myrrh, garlic, Siberian ginseng chaparral caps, or Crystal Star ANTI-FLAM™.
❦ Raise immunity with reishi mushroom, or Health Concerns MUSHROOM POWER capsules, calendula tea, and echinacea extract.
❦ Restore homeostasis with Crystal Star GINSENG 6 SUPER caps or tea.

Staph infection: See above.
❦ Echinacea extract, and see sbove.
❦ Raise immunity with propolis extract to stimulate thymus activity.

Bacterial infection: See above.
❦ Destroy the active microbe. Crystal Star ANTI-BIO™ extract or capsules, and orFIRST AID CAPS in acute stages.
❦ Raise immunity with propolis and echinacea extract, and reishi mushroom extract capsules.
❦ Flush out released lymphatic toxins

BODYWORK

▶ Overheating therapy is extremely effective in controlling virus replication. Even slight temperature increases can lead to considerable reduction of infection.
See page 50 or P. Airola "How To Get Well" for the proper technique.

▶ Blood temperature may also be raised by taking a hot sauna, and by hot ginger/cayenne compresses applied to the affected area.

▶ Use alternating hot and cold hydrotherapy, pg. 49, to stimulate circulation.

▶ Get some early morning sunlight on the body every day possible.

▶ Activate kidney cleansing with a chamomile or chlorophyll enema.

▶ Flush any open wound with food grade H$_2$O$_2$ 3% solution, tea tree oil, or grapefruit seed extract spray.

▶ Get plenty of rest.

Note: For children: use osha root or horsetail/oatstraw teas. ☺

Common Symptoms: Inflammation, boils, sores, and abscesses; breakdown of tissue into waste matter and pus; sore throat, cough, and headache; high temperature and fever; reduced vitality; chronic fatigue and lethargy.
Common Causes: Lowered immunity; over use of antibiotics; chronically low nutrition diet with too many refined foods and too few green vegetables; food or environmental allergies.

♂ INFERTILITY ♀

In America today, one in six married couples of child-bearing age has trouble conceiving and completing a successful pregnancy. Poor nutrition seems to be at the foundation of most infertility problems. In men, the main hindrances are zinc deficiency, excessive alcohol and tobacco; in women, the primary inhibitors are anxiety, emotional stress, severe anemia, and being underweight from athletic or workout activity. There seems to be a link with infertility and vitamin C deficiency in both sexes. **See Having A Healthy Baby in this book for more information.**

FOOD THERAPY

Diet is an all-important key. The body does not readily allow conception without adequate nutrition. Consciously follow a healthy diet and lifestyle for at least six months before trying to conceive.

For both sexes:
🍃 Eat plenty of whole grains, cultured foods such as yogurt, sea foods and sea vegetables, fresh fruits and vegetables.

🍃 Avoid tobacco, alcohol, except moderate wine, caffeine, red meats (synthetic hormones), and refined foods.

🍃 Reduce dairy products, fried and fatty foods, sugary and junk foods.

🍃 Take a daily morning protein drink, such as one from page 63 or Nature's Plus SPIRUTEIN. Make a mix and blend 2 teasp. into each drink:
　◆ Brewer's yeast
　◆ Bee pollen granules
　◆ Wheat germ
　◆ Pumpkin seeds

🍃 See "COOKING FOR HEALTHY HEALING" by Linda Rector-Page for a complete diet for infertility.

VITAMINS/MINERALS

Female: ♀
▶ Enzymatic Therapy
　◆ NUCLEO-PRO F
　◆ STEREOPLEX MF
　◆ RAW OVARIAN extract
　◆ RAW FEMALE glandular

▶ Vitamin E 400IU 2x daily, with C 1000mg. daily and A & D 25,000IU daily.

▶ B Complex 100mg. with extra B6 100mg., PABA 1000mg. and folic acid 800mcg.

Male: ♂
▶ Enzymatic Therapy
　◆ NUCLEOPRO M caps
　◆ STEREOPLEX MF

▶ Carnitine 500mg. daily *with* chromium picolinate for increased sperm count and motility.

▶ Vitamin E 800mg. with selenium 200mcg. daily.

▶ **Vitamin C 3000mg. daily and niacin 500mg., esp. for sperm clumping.**

▶ Zinc 75mg. daily with vitamin C 3000mg. daily.

HERBAL THERAPY

Female: ♀
❧ Crystal Star
　◆ FEMALE HARMONY™ caps or WOMANS BEST FRIEND™
　　with
Evening primrose oil 4-6 daily
　　and
High potency YS royal jelly 2 teasp. daily.

❧ Effective teas:
　◆ Scullcap tea
　◆ Red raspberry tea

❧ Effective extracts:
　◆ Echinacea extract
　◆ Vitex
　◆ Dong Quai - discontinue after pregnancy is achieved.

Male: ♂
❧ Crystal Star
　◆ ADRN™ extract daily with highest potency YS royal jelly 2 teasp. daily.

❧ **Smilax extract 2-3x daily.**

❧ Effective capsules:
　◆ Damiana/licorice
　◆ Ginseng/damiana
　◆ Kelp tabs
　◆ Propolis tabs 2 daily.

BODYWORK

▶ Alternate hot and cold sitz baths to stimulate circulation in the reproductive area.

▶ Sun bathe in the early morning, nude if possible for 15 minutes. ♂

▶ Consciously relax your life more during this time. Get some regular mild exercise every day.

▶ Do not smoke; avoid secondary smoke. Avoid areas with smog and pollutants as much as possible.

▶ Men: avoid bikini underwear, hot electric blankets, and hot water beds.

▶ For vaginal pH balance douche right before intercourse: use baking soda/honey for over-acid, vinegar/water for over-alkaline.

▶ Reflexology points:

penis, coccyx, prostate
uterus

Common Symptoms: Inability to have a child, a condition of both man and woman.
Common Causes: ▮ Female: Nutrient deficiency and hypoglycemia from too many refined foods; emotional stress; chlamydia or pelvic inflammatory disease; obstruction in the fallopian tubes; toxicity from drugs or environmental pollutants; birth control pill causing hormone imbalance; vaginal pH imbalance and allergic reaction to partner's sperm.
　▮ Male: Low sperm production; prolonged marijuana or other drug use; radiation or heavy metal poisoning; steroid use; poor nutrition and lack of protein; hypoglycemia; physical obstruction in the genital/urethral area; glandular malfunction; chlamydia.

INSECT BITES & STINGS

Bees ✧ Wasps ✧ Mosquito ✧ Non-poisonous Spiders

Insect bites can be annoying, painful, and even dangerous, because of the diseases transmitted through them. Natural therapies provide time-proven defense against insect bites and stings. Chemical repellents have racked up many reports of toxic side effects in the last few years. The following are recommendations for persons mildly affected by insect poisons. If you are violently allergic, get emergency medical treatment immediately.

FOOD THERAPY

❧ Food-source applications to take down swelling:
- ✦ raw onion slice
- ✦ raw potato slice
- ✦ lemon juice and vinegar
- ✦ wet mud pack
- ✦ tobacco and water paste
- ✦ toothpaste
- ✦ cologne or toilet water
- ✦ rubbing alcohol
- ✦ honey
- ✦ baking soda
- ✦ sea salt
- ✦ ice packs
- ✦ charcoal tabs or burnt toast
- ✦ wheat germ oil
- ✦ chlorophyll liquid.

❧ Avoid meats and sweets for faster healing.

❧ Avoid consuming sugar and alcohol for 24 hours before you are going to be in mosquito territory.

❧ Apply cold or ice pack compresses, and see shock suggestions in this book if reaction is severe.

❧ Take sun CHLORELLA to reestablish body balance.

VITAMINS/MINERALS

▶ Vitamin C therapy: Use calcium ascorbate powder. Take 1/4 teasp. every 15 minutes right after the bite, then 1/4 teasp. every few hours until pain and swelling are gone.
  ✦ Also mix some powder to a paste with water and apply directly.

▶ Pantothenic acid 1000mg, as an antihistamine for swelling.

▶ Quercetin Plus with bromelain. Take every 4 hours to take down inflammation.

▶ Put Am. Biologics DIOXYCHLOR on a piece of cotton and apply as needed.

▶ Dissolve PABA tablets in water and apply.

▶ For prevention, take vitamin B1 for a month during high risk seasons - 100mg, for children, ☺ 500mg, for adults.

▶ Homeopathic remedy Ledum palustre tincture to relieve swelling and stinging.

HERBAL THERAPY

❧ Effective local applications:
- ✦ B&T SSSTING STOP gel. ☺
- ✦ Comfrey poultice.
- ✦ Aloe vera gel.
- ✦ Witch hazel.
- ✦ Pau de arco gel

❧ Effective compresses:
- ✦ Hot parsley leaf
- ✦ Black cohosh
- ✦ Chamomile

❧ Crystal Star ANTI-HST™ and ANTI-FLAM™ caps as needed to take down rash or swelling.

❧ Take a few drops of cayenne extract in warm water every 1/2 hour to stimulate the circulatory defense mechanism.

❧ Mix the following oils and apply to exposed areas for prevention:
- ◆ citronella, pennyroyal, eucalyptus, in a base of safflower oil.

❧ For prevention: rub fresh elder leaves or elder/chamomile tea on the skin every 20 minutes.

❧ Apply Wright Pathways NO SCRATCH-UM, or Body Essentials SILICA GEL as needed.

BODYWORK

▶ Environmental preventives:
- → Sprinkle garlic powder around the house.
- → Sprinkle sassafras tea or dried tomato leaves around the house.
- → Sprinkle eucalyptus leaves around the house.
- → Wear light colors and try to remain cool and dry.
- → Cover up in the early morning and evening.

▶ To lessen the effect of the bite, keep quiet, and keep the affected area below the level of the heart.

▶ Avoid flowery scents and perfume to escape bees. They think you are a source of pollen!

▶ Natural repellents: Re-apply often - repellency is based on aroma. Don't use on fine fabrics.
- → Citronella for mosquitoes and flies.
- → Cedarwood for fleas and ticks.
- → Eucalyptus for most flying insects.
- → Lemon grass for a broad range of insects.
- → Pennyroyal for fleas (don't use if pregnant)
- → Peppermint, rosemary, thyme, geranium and lavender for flies.

Common Symptoms: Pain, swelling, itching, and redness around the bite area; more severe reactions include nausea, dizziness, headache, chills, fever, allergic and histamine side-effects.

255

INSOMNIA ■ SLEEP DISORDERS

Millions of Americans suffer from insomnia, twisting, turning and agonizing through the night, battling anxiety and rumpled bedding. Insomnia itself seems to be due largely to psychological, rather than physical factors. Maintaining sleep involves nighttime blood glucose levels. A blood sugar drop promotes awakening by sugar-regulatory hormones. Avoid commercial sleeping pills. They interfere with the ability to dream, and interrupt natural sleeping patterns. They interact adversely with alcohol and tranquilizers because the nervous system never really relaxes. Eventually they lose their sleep promoting effectiveness in as little as 3-5 days of use. Natural therapies are conservative, non-addictive and effective.

FOOD THERAPY

🍃 Eat only a light meal at night. Good late night "sleepytime" snacks about an hour before bedtime: bananas, celery and celery juice, wheat germ and wheat germ oil, brown rice, a little warm milk, lemon water and honey, brewer's yeast, VEGEX yeast paste broth, 1 TB. Bragg's LIQUID AMINOS in water.

🍃 Have a glass of wine at dinner for minerals, digestion and relaxation.

🍃 Have a glass of bottled mineral water at bedtime. ♂

🍃 Don't take caffeine drinks except in the morning.

🍃 Avoid a heavy meal in the evening. Avoid salty and sugary foods before bed. Don't drink a lot of liquids before bed.

🍃 Alfalco homeopathic *Alfalfa tonic* drink before bed.

VITAMINS/MINERALS

A lack of balanced calcium and magnesium in the blood can cause one to wake up at night and not be able to return to sleep.

▶ Rainbow Light CALCIUM PLUS, w. high magnesium 2 before bed, with Country Life MAXI-B capsules or other B Complex, or Lexon B BLEND.

▶ Hyland's CALMS FORTE

▶ Source Naturals NUTRA-SLEEP

▶ Country Life RELAXER capsules, with Alta Health mag. chloride. ♂

▶ One each for sleep when there is pain:
  ✚ Tryptophan 500mg.
  ✚ DLPA 500mg.
  ✚ Calcium/magnesium ♀

▶ Pantothenic acid 500mg. and Inositol 500mg. 1/2 hour before bed.

▶ GABA 500mg. and glycine capsules before bed, esp. if hypoglycemic.

▶ For nightmares:
  ✚ B1 500mg.
  ✚ Niacinimide 500mg.

▶ Restless legs/nocturnal myoclonus:
  ✚ Vitamin E 400IU before bed.
  ✚ Folic acid 800mcg daily.

HERBAL THERAPY

It takes several days of common-sense therapy to establish good sleep patterns.

🌿 Crystal Star RELAX CAPS™, NIGHT CAPS™, NIGHT ZZZ™ extract or GOOD NIGHT™ tea.

🌿 Passion flower capsules or extract, especially for weaning away from sleeping pills.

🌿 Solaray EUROCALM caps.

🌿 Effective teas:
  ◆ Licorice rt. ♀
  ◆ Chamomile
  ◆ Catnip/lemon balm
  ◆ Reishi mushroom/ginseng
  ◆ St. John's wort
  ◆ Siberian ginseng

🌿 Effective extracts:
  ◆ Floradix HERBAL REST liquid
  ◆ Crystal Star CALCIUM SOURCE™
  ◆ Crystal Star NIGHT ZZZZ™
  ◆ Scullcap
  ◆ Wild lettuce/valerian

🌿 For quality sleep and dream recall: Crystal Star INCREDIBLE DREAMS™ tea before bed.

🌿 Make a hops and rosemary sleep pillow. Sprinkle with a little alcohol to enhance aromatherapy. ♀

BODYWORK

Don't worry about "making up" lost sleep. One good night's sleep repairs fatigue.

▶ Snoring - which causes insomnia for your mate, has two causes: 1) an obstruction or narrowing of the airway; 2) sleep apnea, where the snorer actually ceases to breathe because the tongue blocks the throat.
→ Get off your back. Elevate your head. Lose some weight. Cut back on alcohol at night. Clear your nose before bed. Avoid tranquilizers and CNS depressants at night.

▶ Effective stress reduction techniques:
  ↟ Biofeedback and Yoga exercises
  ↟ Hypnotherapy
  ↟ Massage therapy care
  ↟ Gazing at a lighted candle for 3 minutes before retiring.
  ↟ Before bed stretch: take 10 deep breaths; wait 5 minutes; take 10 more.

▶ Sleep stealers:
  ↟ Too much alcohol - interrupts normal sleep patterns.
  ↟ Nicotine - a long-lasting stimulant.
  ↟ Too much coffee and caffeine (also in foods and some drugs)
  ↟ Too much stress

▶ Exercise in the morning, outdoors if possible, to release prostaglandins, to promote sleep 12 hours later, and to keep circadian rhythm regular. Take a "constitutional walk" before bed.

Common Symptoms: Chronic inability to sleep; prematurely ended or interrupted sleep; difficulty falling asleep.
Common Causes: Stress, tension, depression and anxiety; the inability to "turn your mind off"; too much caffeine; pain; hypoglycemia; overeating; too much salt and sugar; B Complex deficiency; nicotine or other drugs; asthma; indigestion and toxic liver overload; too high copper levels.

ITCHING SKIN ■ MINOR RASH

Skin itch and rash symptoms can come from a wide variety of causes, ranging from systemic to emotional stress, from food allergies to topical infective reactions to cosmetics. Investigate the cause of your symptoms thoroughly before you attempt treatment to get best results. See Liver Malfunction, Insect Bites and Eczema pages in this book for more information.

FOOD THERAPY

🍃 Drink lemon water in the morning to neutralize acids if the condition is chronic body imbalance.

🍃 Keep the liver clean and functioning well with a carrot juice or green drink frequently (pg. 54ff).

🍃 Eat cultured foods frequently for healthy G.I. flora.

🍃 Effective food applications:
♦ Wheat germ oil
♦ Baking soda solution
♦ Apple cider vinegar

🍃 Since a rash is regularly a symptom of food allergy, avoid common allergens, such as milk and wheat products, eggs, meats (that usually have nitrates), refined foods, sugar and fried foods.

VITAMINS/MINERALS

▶ Amer. Biologics DIOXYCHLOR liquid as directed.
with
Lysine 500mg. 3-4x daily.

▶ Nutrition Resource NUTRIBI-OTIC grapefruit seed extract. Mix 1 to 4 drops in 5 oz. water and apply directly.

▶ Vitamin C therapy: use Ester C or Ascorbate C powder and mix with water to a solution. Apply to area, and take 1 teasp. every hour, and/or
Crystal Star GINSENG SKIN RE-PAIR GEL™ WITH C.

▶ Vitamin E 400IU and emulsified A&D. Prick capsules and apply locally. ♂

▶ Prof. Nutr. Dr. DOPHILUS or DDS dairy free acidophilus.

▶ Apply Wright Pathways NO SCRATCH-UM, or Body Essentials SILICA GEL as needed.

▶ Quercetin Plus with bromelain as an anti-inflammatory agent.

▶ Homeopathic Nat. Phos.

HERBAL THERAPY

🌿 Crystal Star ANTI-HST™ capsules, 4-6 daily as needed for liver stimulation to relieve a typical histamine weal rash. Very effective.
and/OR
ANTI-FLAM™ caps 4-6 daily,
and
THERADERM™ tea. Drink and pat onto affected areas with cotton.

🌿 Thirty min. before going outdoors, take 3 caps of liquid aged garlic extract (contains B1).

🌿 Black walnut tincture. Apply to affected areas and take a few drops under the tongue daily.

🌿 Effective teas, for internal and topical use:
♦ Crystal Star CLEANSING & PURIFYING™ tea to neutralize.
♦ Comfrey
♦ Chamomile
♦ Chickweed
♦ Red Clover/hops

🌿 Crystal Star P.O. #2™ capsules 2-6 daily as needed to calm the itch.

BODYWORK

▶ Avoid using detergents on the skin. Use mild castile soap.

▶ Apply fresh comfrey leaf compresses.

▶ Effective applications:
→ B & T CALIFLORA gel
→ Crystal Star CALENDULA gel
→ Crystal Star LYSINE/LIC-ORICE gel
→ Care Plus H₂O₂ OXYGEL
→ Cocoa butter
→ Tea tree oil if fungus is the cause.
→ Aloe vera gel
→ Pau de arco gel

Common Symptoms: Tingling, unpleasant skin prickling; redness, rash; scaling and bumps on the skin.
Common Causes: Liver malfunction or exhaustion; allergic reaction; stress and anxiety; detergents; over-acid system; drug after-and side-effects; poor diet with too many refined and chemical foods.

KIDNEY MALFUNCTION
Nephritis ✧ Bright's Disease ✧ Urinary Tract Infection

Kidney infections are usually severe and serious, and should be attended to immediately. Nephritis involves the chronic inflammation of the kidney filtering tissue. Bright's disease is also inflammatory with blood in the urine, high blood pressure, and water retention. The bloodstream becomes toxic from the overload of unfiltered wastes, and uremia develops.

FOOD THERAPY

See Kidney Stone Diet on the next page for more information.

- Go on a short 3 day liquid kidney cleanse to clear out toxic infection: Each morning take 2 TBS. cider vinegar or lemon juice in water. Take 1 each of the following juices every day: carrot/beet/cucumber, cranberry, potassium broth (pg. 53), and a green drink (pg. 54ff).

- Then eat a very simple low salt, low protein, vegetarian diet with 75% fresh foods for the next 2 weeks.

- Then add sea foods and sea vegetables, whole grains and *vegetable proteins*. Have a Sun CHLORELLA or spirulina drink daily for the rest of the month. Drink 8 glasses of bottled water a day.

- Avoid heavy starches, red and prepared meats, dairy products (except yogurt or kefir), refined, salty, fatty and fast foods during healing. They all inhibit kidney filtering.

- Kidney healing foods include garlic and onions, papayas, bananas and watermelon, sprouts, leafy greens and cucumbers.

VITAMINS/MINERALS

Eliminate iron supplements during healing.

- B Complex 100mg. daily with extra B6 100mg. 3x daily and magnesium 400mg. 2x daily.
  and
  Natren LIFE START II or Dr. DOPHILUS $1/2$ teasp. 3-4x daily.

- Am. Biologics A & E EMULSION.
  and
  Ascorbate vitamin C powder 3-5000mg. with bioflavs and rutin 1000mg. daily.

- Choline/Inositol caps 4x daily.

- Future Biotics VITAL K or Co. Life CAL/MAG/POTAS. caps. ♂

- Enzymatic Therapy LIQUID LIVER w. GINSENG, 2x daily. ♂

- Activated charcoal or liquid chlorophyll tabs with meals. ♂

- Zinc 50mg. 2x daily. ♂

- Body Essentials SILICA GEL 1 TB. gel in 3oz. liquid 3x daily for 1 month for urinary tract infection.

HERBAL THERAPY

- ☙ Crystal Star ANTI-BIO™ capsules 4 daily til infection clears; then BLDR-K™ capsules and tea for a month. Then take GREEN TEA CLEANSER™ every morning for one more month.

- ☙ Crystal Star HERBAL ENZ™ capsules before each meal and hawthorne or bilberry extract 2x daily.

- ☙ Evening primrose oil caps 4 daily w/ echinacea extract 4x daily.

- ☙ Solaray ALFAJUICE daily.

- ☙ Effective teas:
  - ◆ Parsley/cornsilk ♀
  - ◆ Watercress
  - ◆ St. John's wort if incontinent.
  - ◆ Watermelon seed ♀
  - ◆ Marshmallow rt./licorice rt.

- ☙ Effective kidney detoxifiers:
  - ◆ Burdock rt.
  - ◆ Dandelion extract esp. for nephritis.
  - ◆ Ginger rt.

- ☙ Garlic/cayenne caps 6-8 daily.

BODYWORK

- ➤ Apply white flower oil or tiger balm to kidney area 2-3x daily.

- ➤ Avoid smoking and secondary smoke. Take a daily brisk walk to keep kidney function flowing.

- ➤ Apply moist heat packs, comfrey compresses, and/or alternating hot and cold compresses on the kidney area.

- ➤ Capsicum, spirulina or catnip enemas 2-3x weekly as needed to stimulate better kidney function.

- ➤ Reflexology points:

kidney points

- ➤ Kidney cross section:

Common Symptoms: Painful urination, irritation and frequency; chronic lower back pain and fatigue; chills and fever as with a cold or flu; sometimes nausea and vomiting; accumulation of excess fluid.

Common Causes: Excess sugar, red meat and oxalic acid-forming foods in the diet; diabetes; EFA deficiency; adrenal exhaustion; kidney stones; overuse of prescription or pleasure drugs.

KIDNEY STONES

Kidney stones form when too many mineral molecules, calcium and oxalate, combine into crystals in the kidneys. These minerals usually float freely in the the kidney fluids, but when there is an overload of inorganic mineral waste and too little fluid, the molecules can't dissolve and eventually form sharp-edged stones. It takes from 5 to 15 hours of vigorous and urgent treatment to dissolve and pass small stones. Kidney stones are extremely painful, but very preventable. Prevention through improved diet and exercise is the best medicine.

FOOD THERAPY

Kidney stones plague people who eat a rich, high fat diet. A vegetarian diet is best.

❧ Go on a 3 day intensive kidney cleansing diet until pain clears:

♦ **On rising:** take 2 TBS. lemon juice or cider vinegar in water.
♦ **Breakfast:** take a glass of cranberry, apple or watermelon juice.
♦ **Mid-morning:** take a carrot/beet/cucumber juice.
♦ **Lunch:** take potass. broth (pg. 53).
♦ **Midafternoon:** take a green drink (pg. 54ff).
♦ **Dinner:** take 2 cups watermelon seed tea.
♦ **Before bed:** take a glass of aloe vera juice.

Take plenty of water through the day.

❧ Take 2 TBS. olive oil through a straw every 4 hours during this intensive stage as a kidney stone flush.

❧ Then follow the Kidney Cleansing Diet on the next page for 2 more weeks to normalize kidney activity.

❧ **Avoid all refined, fried and fatty foods, and baked breads during healing. Avoid salts, sugars and oxalic acid-forming foods, such as red meats and caffeine-containing foods. Eliminate dairy products and commercial antacids. Reduce intake of all animal protein. (It produces too much mineral waste that results in kidney stones.)**

VITAMINS/MINERALS

If you have kidney stones or have a history of them, avoid L-cystine. It aggravates crystallization in the kidneys. Do not use TUMS for indigestion. They have a history of increasing risk for stone formation.

▲ Ascorbate or Ester C powder in water; 1/4 teasp. every hour to bowel tolerance daily until stones pass - about 5000mg. Take for a month to acidify urine and prevent further stones.

▲ Beta carotene 100,000IU with high Omega 3 flax oil daily, and
Solaray LIPOTROPIC 1000 daily.

▲ Enzymatic Therapy ACID-A-CAL caps 2-4 daily to help dissolve sediment. ♂
and/or
Solaray CALCIUM CITRATE caps 4 daily. ♀

▲ Vit. B Complex with extra B6 100mg. *and* magnesium 400mg. 2x daily, *and* Vitamin K 100mg.

▲ Golden Pride ORAL CHELATION w. EDTA 1 daily. ♂

▲ Future Biotics VITAL K liquid, with raw kidney glandular.

HERBAL THERAPY

❦ Crystal Star BLDR-K™ caps and tea with ginkgo biloba extract as needed for both healing and prevention.

❦ Drink a quart daily of any of the following teas til stones dissolve:
♦ Chamomile
♦ Rosemary ♀
♦ Rosehips

❦ Other effective teas:
♦ Watercress
♦ Cleavers
♦ Couch grass ♀
♦ Uva Ursi/juniper ♂

❦ Apply a hot ginger/oatstraw compress to kidney area.

❦ Crystal Star POTASSIUM SOURCE capsules daily if taking diuretics.

❦ George's ALOE VERA JUICE w. herbs, or Sun CHLORELLA drink 2 glasses daily.
or
Solaray ALFAJUICE caps.

❦ **Body Essentials SILICA GEL, internally, 1 TB. gel in 3oz. liquid 3x daily for 1 month.**

BODYWORK

▶ Effective compresses:
→ Cayenne/ginger
→ Mullein/lobelia
→ Hot ginger/oatstraw

▶ Take hot and cold, or Epsom salts sitz baths to stimulate circulation.

▶ Take a warm catnip enema daily til pain subsides.

▶ Reflexology points:

kidney points

In addition, press on the back, on the tops of both hip bones, 3x for 10 seconds each.

Common Symptoms: Usually no symptoms are apparent except a dull ache in the lower back, until the stone blocks the urinary tract, which results in excruciating pain that starts in the hip and radiates. Then there is frequent and painful urination; nausea, fever and vomiting.
Common Causes: B vitamin and magnesium deficiency; excess uric and oxalic acids in the elimination system from foods such as red meat, carbonated drinks, sugars and caffeine; excess aspirin, salt and chemical diuretics; potassium and kidney fluid deficiency from too many diuretics.

Kidney Cleansing & Rebuilding Diet

Follow this diet after the 3 day liquid cleanse on the preceding page. Intense pain should have ceased. The diet is recommended for at least two to three weeks after acute stage has passed. Keep salt and protein low for at least 3 weeks. This diet may be used for 2 to 3 months, or longer for chronic problems. It is a vegetarian diet emphasizing fresh and cultured foods to alkalize the system. It is very low in proteins, starches and carbohydrates, allowing the body to spend more energy on healing than on dealing with heavier foods. It is high in soluble fiber, which results in lowering urinary calcium waste. It eliminates acid-forming foods, such as caffeine and caffeine-containing foods, salty, sugary and fried foods, soft drinks, alcohol, and tomatoes. It also avoids mucous-forming foods, such as pasteurized dairy products, heavy grains, starches and fats – to relieve irritation and sediment formation, to continue cleansing activity, and to normalize kidney function. The ongoing diet should be low in cholesterol and saturated fats forever to prevent further kidney stone formation.

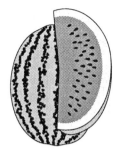

On rising: take a glass of lemon juice in water with 1 teasp. honey; **or** 2 TBS. apple cider vinegar in water with 1 teasp. honey;
or 2 TBS. cranberry juice concentrate in water with ¹/₄ teasp. ascorbate vitamin C crystals added;
or Crystal Star GREEN TEA CLEANSER™.

Breakfast: have a glass of papaya or apple juice;
or a glass of fresh watermelon juice, or a bowl of watermelon chunks;
then some fresh tropical fruits, such as papaya, mango, or banana.

Mid-morning: have a green drink such as Sun CHLORELLA or Green Foods GREEN MAGMA, or Crystal Star ENERGY GREEN™;
or a glass of apple juice; **or** dandelion, watermelon seed, or parsley tea, or Crystal Star BLDR-K™ tea.

Lunch: have a green salad with lots of cucumbers, spinach, watercress and celery, with lemon/oil or cottage cheese dressing
and/or baked or marinated tofu with sesame seeds and wheat germ;
or a Chinese vegetable salad with bok choy, daikon, pea pods, bean sprouts and other Chinese greens, with a cup of miso or ramen noodle soup with sea vegies.

Mid-afternoon: have a cup of alkalizing, sediment-dissolving herb tea, such as cornsilk, plantain, dandelion leaf or oatstraw, or another cup of Crystal Star BLDR-K™ tea;
or some celery and carrot sticks with kefir or yogurt cheese; **or** fresh apples and pears with kefir or yogurt dip.

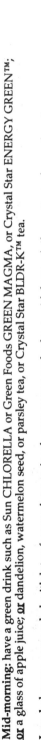
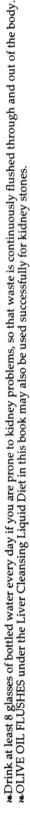
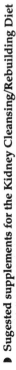

Dinner: have some brown rice with tofu and steamed vegies;
or steamed asparagus with miso soup and sea vegies;
or a baked potato with kefir cheese or 1 teasp. butter, and a spinach salad;
or baked or broiled salmon with millet and baked onions.
▸A glass of white wine is fine at dinner for alkalizing and relaxation.

Before bed: have another apple or papaya/mango juice;
or miso soup with sea vegetables snipped on top; **or** VEGEX yeast broth in hot water.

▸Drink at least 8 glasses of bottled water every day if you are prone to kidney problems, so that waste is continuously flushed through and out of the body.
▸OLIVE OIL FLUSHES under the Liver Cleansing Liquid Diet in this book may also be used successfully for kidney stones.

See "COOKING FOR HEALTHY HEALING" by Linda Rector-Page for a complete diet for kidney health.

◗ **Suggested supplements for the Kidney Cleansing/Rebuilding Diet**

✦ Continue with 3-5000mg. ascorbate vitamin C daily in juice or water (about ¹/₂ teasp. every 4 hours) **and** beta carotene, or emulsified A 25,000IU 4x daily).
✦ Take chlorophyll liquid, or other concentrated green food supplement, such as Green Foods GREEN MAGMA, or Crystal Star ENERGY GREEN™ in water before meals.
✦ Take Enzymatic Therapy ACID-A-CAL caps to dissolve sedimentary waste, with bromelain 500mg. daily.
✦ Take Crystal Star ANTI-BIO™ caps **with** BLDR-K™ caps or tea as needed for inflammation or irritation.
✦ Take DDS milk-free acidophilus powder in juice or water, as needed 2-3 times daily, **with** garlic oil caps 6 daily.

➤ **Bodywork for the Kidney Cleansing/Rebuilding Diet**
→ Continue with wet, hot compresses and lower back massage when there is inflammation flare up.
→ Take hot saunas when possible to release toxins and excess fluids, and to flush acids out through the skin. A swim after a sauna is wonderful for body tone.

LEUKEMIA ▦ BLOOD & BONE MARROW CANCER

Leukemia is a disease characterized by excessive production of white blood cells and their precursors in the tissues. It seem to result from a failure of the bone marrow to function adequately. The spleen and liver are infiltrated and damaged by the excess leukocytes. The lymph nodes and nervous system are also affected. Natural treatments, and natural treatment in conjunction with cytotoxic drugs have improved the remission rate of this type of cancer to over 50%.

FOOD THERAPY

Food healing value is lost very quickly in this disease. Make sure the diet is very nutritious to make up for this.

🥬 Start with a cleansing/detoxification program (pg. 48) for 2 months. Follow with a macrobiotic diet program (pg. 52) for 3 to 4 months with no animal protein and lots of alkalizing foods.
◆ High vegetable proteins are the key after initial detoxification.

🥬 To clean vital organs, take a glass of carrot/beet/cucumber juice every day for the first month of healing; every other day for the second month; once a week the third month.

🥬 Eat lots of green leafy vegetables on a continuing basis for red blood cell formation. Include plenty of potassium-rich foods.

🥬 Take 2-3 glasses of cranberry juice (no high sugar content) and George's ALOE VERA JUICE with herbs daily.

🥬 Avoid all alcohol, junk and chemically processed foods. Omit all refined sugars and red meats.

🥬 See the CANCER DIET suggestions in this book, and/or "COOKING FOR HEALING" by Linda Rector-Page for a complete healing diet.

VITAMINS/MINERALS

▶ Germanium 150mg. SL daily.

▶ ENER B internasal B12 every other day.

▶ Enzymatic Therapy LIQUID LIVER W. GINSENG 4 daily.

▶ Niacin therapy: 250mg 4x daily all during healing.

▶ B Complex 100mg. with extra folic acid, and B6 250mg. ♀

▶ Glutathione 50mg. 2x daily. ♂
with
Vitamin E 800IU with selenium 200mcg. and zinc 50mg.

▶ Beta or marine carotene 150,000IU daily for at least 6 weeks.
and/or
Sun CHLORELLA 20 tabs daily for 6 weeks. ♂

▶ Ascorbate vit. C or Ester C powder, up to 10,000mg. daily with bioflavonoids and rutin for several months.

▶ Mezotrace SEA MINERAL COMPLEX 4 daily. ☺
and
Am. Biologics DIOXYCHLOR as directed.

HERBAL THERAPY

🌿 Crystal Star DETOX™ caps with GREEN TEA CLEANSER™ 2x daily for 2 months.
Then HEARTSEASE/ANEMIGIZE™ caps to rebuild marrow.

🌿 Effective red blood cell builders:
◆ Wakasa liquid CHLORELLA
◆ Liquid chlorophyll
◆ Floradix LIQUID IRON ☺
◆ Crystal Star GINSENG 6 DEFENSE RESTORATIVE™ tea.
◆ Crystal Star IRON SOURCE™.

🌿 Effective extracts:
◆ Crystal Star PAU DE ARCO/ ECHINACEA™
◆ Siberian ginseng
◆ Hawthorne
◆ Carnivora herb

🌿 Effective teas:
◆ Yellow dock
◆ Chaparral
◆ Pau de arco
◆ Astragalus

🌿 Propolis 4 daily, and/or high potency royal jelly ½ teasp. 4x daily.

🌿 Garlic/cayenne caps 8-10 daily.

🌿 Health Concern POWER MUSHROOMS caps. 4 daily.

BODYWORK

Cortico-steroid drugs given to relieve symptoms of leukemia, over a long period of time greatly weaken immunity and bone strength.

▶ Overheating therapy is effective for leukemia. See P. Airola "How To Get Well", or page 49 in this book.

▶ Avoid pesticides, X-rays, and radiation of all kinds if possible.

▶ See Lymphatic Health/Spleen in this book for additional information.

Common Symptoms: Increase in white blood cells, with no red blood cell production; extreme tiredness and anemia; pallor, easy bruising, bone pain, thinness and weight loss; chronic infections - esp. in children; spleen malfunction or loss; symptoms similar to pernicious anemia.
Common Causes: Indiscriminate use of X-rays and some drugs, especially in children and pregnant women; severe malnutrition with too many refined carbohydrates (especially in children); overfluoridation of the water; thyroid malfunction; deficiencies of vitamin D, iron, B12 and folic acid; chronic viral infections; hereditary proneness. See Cancer causes in this book.

LIVER DISEASE ■ JAUNDICE

The health and vitality of the body depend to a large extent on the health and vitality of the liver. It is the body's most complex and useful organ - a powerful chemical plant that converts everything we eat, breathe and absorb through the skin into life-sustaining substances. The liver is a major blood reservoir, filtering out toxins at a rate of over a quart of blood per minute. It manufactures bile to digest fats and prevent constipation. It metabolizes proteins and carbohydrates, and secretes hormones and enzymes. Be good to your liver!

FOOD THERAPY

Avoiding a high fat diet is crucial for liver health and regeneration. Optimum nutrition is the best liver protection.

☙ If condition is acute, go on a 3 day liquid detoxification diet (see next page) to clean out toxic waste. Then follow with an alkalizing rebuilding diet for a month with high quality vegetable protein. (A brief version is in "COOKING FOR HEALTHY HEALING" by Linda Rector-Page.)

☙ Take daily during healing: 1 TB. each lecithin granules and brewer's yeast, 2-3 glasses cranberry or apple juice and 6-8 glasses of bottled water.

☙ Avoid red meats and other acid-forming foods such as caffeine, alcohol, refined starches and dairy products during all healing phases. Reduce sugars, saturated fats and fried foods permanently.

☙ Liver health foods include:
  ♣ Fiber and plant foods that absorb excess bile and increase regularity.
  ♣ Potassium-rich foods, such as sea foods, dried fruits and brewer's yeast.
  ♣ Chlorophyll-rich foods, such as leafy greens and sea vegetables.
  ♣ Cultured, high enzyme foods, such as yogurt and kefir.
  ♣ Sulphur-rich foods like garlic and onions.

VITAMINS/MINERALS

The liver is a vast storehouse for vitamins, minerals, and enzymes. It secretes them as needed to build and maintain healthy cells.

▶ A "spring cleaning" inositol cocktail: Supreme B BLEND 1/2 teasp. 3x daily, and/or a good lipotropic daily, such as Solaray LIPOTROPIC 1000 - esp. if taking contraceptives.

▶ Natren LIFE START II, or Dr. DO-PHILUS, 1/4 teasp. 3-4x daily.

▶ Natrapathic PURE & REGULAR. ♂

▶ Beta Carotene 100,000IU with Carnitine 500mg. and CoQ 10 30mg. daily, and
Ascorbate vitamin C or Ester C 1500mg. every hour during acute stages, then 3000mg. daily.

▶ Enzymatic Therapy PHOS./CHOL. and IMMUNO-PLEX complexes.

▶ Alta Health CANGEST w/chromium picolinate 200mcg. ♀

▶ **Germanium 100mg. or pycnogenol 50mg. daily as anti-oxidants.**

▶ High omega 3 flax seed oil 3x daily with liquid chlorophyll 3 teasp. daily, or Sun CHLORELLA 15 daily. ♂

HERBAL THERAPY

A complete liver renewal program can take from three months to a year.

☙ Crystal Star LIV-ALIVE™ caps and LIV-ALIVE™ tea, and/or BITTERS & LEMON CLEANSE™ extract for intense cleansing.
  or
LIV ALIVE™ or milk thistle seed extract in aloe vera juice for gentler, longer range cleansing.

☙ Royal jelly 2 teasp. daily, with Floradix LIQUID IRON.

☙ Solaray TURMERIC extract caps to stimulate bile flow.

☙ Take a liver rebuilding tea: Mix 4 oz. hawthorne berries, 2 oz. red sage, 1 oz. cardamom. Steep 24 hours in 2 qts. of water. Add honey. Take 2 cups daily.

☙ Crystal Star HEARTSEASE/ ANEMIGIZE™ caps to rebuild liver and spleen activity ♂ and/or IRON SOURCE™ extract. ♀

☙ Effective liver herbs:
  ◆ Pau de Arco
  ◆ Roast dandelion and burdock root
  ◆ Barberry for jaundice
  ◆ Siberian and Panax ginsengs
  ◆ Reishi mushroom

BODYWORK

The liver is very dependent on the amount and quality of oxygen coming into the lungs. Exercise, air filters, time spent in the forest and at the ocean, and drinking pure water are important.

▶ Overheating by raising blood temperature is effective. See Airola "How To Get Well", or pg. 49 in this book.

▶ Good liver lifestyle practices: eat smaller meals, minimize eating late at night; get adequate regular sleep; exercise every day, with a good brisk aerobic walk.

▶ Take one coffee enema during your detoxification cleanse; (1 cup coffee to 1 qt. water.)

▶ Take several saunas if possible during a liver cleanse for faster, easier detoxification.

▶ Reflexology point:

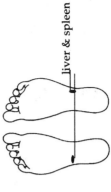

liver & spleen

Common Symptoms: Sluggish system; general depression and melancholy; unexplained weight gain and great tiredness; poor digestion; food and chemical sensitivities; PMS; constipation and congestion; nausea and shakes; dizziness; dry tongue and mouth; jaundiced skin and/or liver spots; skin itching.
Common Causes: Too much alcohol and/or drugs; too much sugar, refined, low nutrition foods, and preservatives; overeating - esp. too much animal protein; low vegetable diet; exposure to toxic chemicals and pollutants; stress; hepatitis virus; long-term use of prescription drugs (especially antibiotics and tranquilizers).

Liver Detoxification Diet

Since any toxic substance can harm the liver, and since most of us are continually assailed by toxins in our food, water and air, it is generally realized that none of us has a truly healthy liver. The good news is that the liver has amazing rejuvenative powers, and can continue to function when as many as 80% of its cells are damaged. A clean, functioning liver produces natural antihistamines to keep immunity high, neutralizes and destroys poisons in the body, cleanses the blood and discharges waste into the bile, metabolizes and helps excrete fat and cholesterol, helps form and store red blood cells and iron, aids digestion, maintains hormone balance, and remarkably enough, regenerates its own damaged tissue. A liver cleanse and detoxification twice a year in the spring and fall is highly recommended to maximize its abilities, using the extra vitamin D from the sun to help. See "COOKING FOR HEALTHY HEALING" by Linda Rector-Page for a complete liver cleansing and healing diet.

On rising: take a glass of 2TBS. lemon juice or cider vinegar in water with 1 teasp. honey, and 1 teasp. royal jelly; or Crystal Star BITTERS & LEMON CLEANSE™ extract in water .
If an olive oil flush or coffee enema are to be included in the cleanse, now is the time to take them.

Breakfast: take a glass of carrot/beet/cucumber juice, or a potassium broth (pg. 53); or a glass of organic apple juice. Add ¹/₂ teasp. dairy free acidophilus powder.
Mid-morning: have an apple or cranberry juice; or a cup of Crystal Star LIV-ALIVE™ tea; **or** a green drink (page 54ff). **or** Sun CHLORELL, or Crystal Star ENERGY GREEN™ drink.
Lunch: have a glass of fresh carrot juice, or another glass of organic apple juice.
Mid-afternoon: have a cup of peppermint, pau de arco, or roasted dandelion root tea; or another green drink, or Crystal Star GREEN TEA CLEANSER™, or LIV-ALIVE™ tea.
Dinner: have another glass of organic apple juice; **and/or** a Crystal Star SYSTEM STRENGTH™ drink or another potassium broth if cleansing action is not too stressful.
Before bed: take another glass of lemon juice or cider vinegar in water. Add 15 drops of milk thistle seed extract.

✤ Suggested supplements for the Liver Detoxification Diet:

✿ Add one teasp. royal jelly, ascorbate vitamin C crystals, ¹/₄ teasp. at a time, or 15 drops milk thistle seed extract to any of the above liquids for increased cleansing benefit.
✿ Drink six to eight glasses of bottled water every day to encourage maximum flushing of liver tissues.

➤ Bodywork for the Liver Detoxification Cleanse:

➙ Only mild exercise should be undertaken during the fast. ➙ Get plenty of early morning sunlight every day possible. ➙ Make a point to get adequate rest and sleep during the cleanse. ➙ Take a hot sauna each day of this cleanse for optimum results.

✤

Alkalizing Rebuilding Diet

This diet is high in alkalizing fresh foods (60%), and vegetable proteins, dairy free, and low in fats. All alcohol, caffeine and caffeine-containing foods, saturated fats, and red meats should be avoided while on this diet. It may be used for 1 month, after the Liver Detox Diet above to rebuild healthy liver function, or by itself for a week or more, as a mild "spring cleaning" for the organs at any time. A continuing diet for liver health should be lacto-vegetarian, low fat, and rich in vegetable proteins and vitamin C foods for good iron absorption.

On rising: take a glass of lemon juice and water with 1 teasp. honey.
Breakfast: Make a mix of 2 TBS. **each:** brewer's yeast, lecithin, and high omega 3 flax oil. Take 2 teasp. each morning in prune, organic apple or cranberry juice;
and have some fresh fruits, such as grapefruit or pineapple; **and/or** a whole grain cereal or muesli with apple juice or fruit yogurt on top.
Mid-morning: have a green drink (pg. 54ff). Sun CHLORELLA or Green Foods GREEN MAGMA;
and/or a cup of miso soup with 2 TBS. sea vegies snipped on top; **or** a cup of Crystal Star GREEN TEA CLEANSER™, or SYSTEM STRENGTH DRINK™.
Lunch: have a large fresh green salad with lemon/olive oil dressing; **and** a glass of fresh carrot juice and some whole grain crackers with a yogurt, kefir or soy spread;
or have some marinated, baked tofu with brown rice or millet, and a small spinach/sprout salad with a light olive oil dressing.
Mid-afternoon: have a cup of miso soup, or an alkalizing herb tea, such as chamomile, dandelion root, or pau de arco; **and/or** a hard boiled egg and cup of yogurt.
Dinner: have a baked potato with kefir cheese or soy cheese dressing, and a large dinner salad with mayonnaise dressing;
or a light vegetable steam/stir fry with vegetables, seafood or tofu; **or** some steamed vegies with a light Italian or tofu dressing, and brown rice, millet or bulgur;
or a vegetable souffle or casserole with a light noodle broth.
Before bed: have an herb tea, such as dandelion root, chamomile or Crystal Star ROYAL MU TEA™; **or** a glass of apple juice or prune juice, **or** a cup of VEGEX yeast paste broth. ➤Drink six to eight glasses of bottled mineral water every day. ➤Take small meals more frequently all during the day, rather than any large meals.

✤ Suggested supplements for the Liver Rebuilding Diet:

✿ Add one teasp. royal jelly, ascorbate vitamin C crystals, ¹/₄ teasp. at a time, or 15 drops milk thistle seed extract to any of the above liquids for increased cleansing benefit.
✿ Take a green drink (pg. 54ff), Sun CHLORELL, Cystal Star ENERGY GREEN™ drink, or Green Foods GREEN MAGMA frequently for chlorophyll and red blood cell formation.
✿ Take beta-carotene 100,000IU with ascorbate vitamin C or Ester C - 3000mg., and vitamin E 400IU daily for anti-infective and anti-oxidant activity.

➤ Bodywork for the Liver Rebuilding Diet:

➙ Take a brisk walk every day to cleanse the lungs, increase circulation, and oxygenate the blood. Stretching exercises are particularly helpful to liver tissue tone.

LOW BLOOD PRESSURE ▣ HYPOTENSION

Even though we hear much less about it, marked and chronically low blood pressure is also a threat to good health. It is usually a sign that arterial system walls and tissue are weak, allowing blood and fluid to leak or abnormally distend them - and preventing strong circulation.

FOOD THERAPY

☙ Follow a fresh foods diet for a week, with plenty of green drinks (pg. 54ff), potassium broth (pg. 53), brewer's yeast, and green salads. Take a lemon and water drink every morning with 1 teasp. honey.
Then, follow a modified macrobiotic diet for 1-2 months, stressing vegetable proteins, green salads, miso, onions, garlic and other alkalizing foods, and dried or fresh fruits.

Bioflavonoids are the key

☙ Effective drinks:
♦ Citrus juices
♦ Grape juice
♦ Celery juice
♦ Pineapple juice
♦ Kukicha/Bancha twig tea
♦ Knudsen's RECHARGE drink

☙ Avoid canned and refined foods, animal fats, red meats, and caffeine. Reduce high cholesterol, and starchy foods.

☙ Include complex carbohydrates, such as peas, broccoli, potatoes and whole grains are effective.

VITAMINS/MINERALS

Avoid the amino acids phenylanine and tyrosine.

◗ B Complex 100mg. daily with extra B1 500mg., and pantothenic acid 1000mg.

◗ **Germanium 50mg. 2x daily.**

◗ **Pycnogenol for high flavonoids and anti-oxidant properties.**

◗ Enzymatic Therapy LIQUID LIVER with SIBERIAN GINSENG.

◗ Future Biotics VITAL K, up to 6 teasp. daily during healing.

◗ Magnesium 400mg. 4x daily.

◗ Vitamin E therapy for 8 weeks: work up from 100IU daily the first week, to 800IU daily, adding 100mg. daily each week. ♂

◗ Vitamin K 100mg. 2 daily.

◗ **Vitamin C with bioflavs and rutin 3000mg. daily.**

◗ Floradix LIQUID IRON, with raw thymus extract.

◗ Cal/mag/zinc 4 daily. ♂

HERBAL THERAPY

❧ Crystal Star HEARTSEASE/ ANEMIGIZE™ capsules 2-4 daily for a month, with 6-8 garlic/ parsley caps daily.
Then, ADR-ACTIVE™ capsules 2x daily for a month.
Then ENDO-BAL™ caps for a month.

❧ Take Crystal Star GREEN TEA CLEANSER™ during entire healing period.

❧ **High flavonoid herbs for tissue integrity:**
♦ **Hawthorne extract 2-3x daily during healing.**
♦ Bancha or kukicha twig
♦ Bilberry extract
♦ Gotu Kola extract
♦ Lemon Peel
♦ Hibiscus
♦ Rosehips

❧ Effective capsules:
♦ Siberian ginseng 4-6 daily
♦ Cayenne/ginger 4 daily
♦ Garlic 6-8 daily
♦ Kelp 8-10 daily
♦ Dandelion rt. 4 daily

❧ Crystal Star HEARTSEASE/ CIRCU-CLENSE™ tea for prevention.

BODYWORK

▶ Acupressure, chiropractic spinal manipulation and shiatsu therapy are all effective in normalizing circulatory function.

▶ Alternating hot and cold hydro therapy (pg. 49).

▶ Avoid tobacco and secondary smoke.

▶ Consciously try to relax the whole body once a day with short meditation and rest.

▶ Do deep breathing exercises (See Bragg's book) to stimulate circulation and oxygenate the system.

Common Symptoms: Malfunction of the circulatory system's systol/diastol action; thinning of the blood; great fatigue and easy loss of energy; low immunity and susceptibility to allergies and infections - particularly opportunistic disease like candida yeast overgrowth.
Common Causes: Poor diet with vitamin C and bioflavonoid deficiency causing a "run-down" condition; kidney malfunction causing system toxemia; emotional problems; anemia; over-use of drugs that lower immunity.

LUNG DISEASES
Sarcoidosis ✧ T.B. ✧ Cystic Fibrosis

Chronic pulmonary diseases have increased dramatically in the last decade. Three that have been part of this unusual rise are discussed here. Sarcoidosis is a systemic viral infection involving widespread lesions on tissue or organs. The lungs and liver are both usually affected. Tuberculosis is a highly contagious disease on the rise in America. It is characterized by bloody sputum, a chronic cough, shortness of breath and fatigue, night sweats, serious weight loss and chest pain. Cystic fibrosis is an inherited childhood disease characterized by recurring lung infections and severe malnutrition from lack of absorption.

FOOD THERAPY

☙ Go on a short mucous cleansing liquid diet (pg. 42). Then, use the following cleansing diet for at least two weeks:
♠ Lemon or grapefruit juice and water each morning with 1 tsp. honey.
♠ Fresh carrot juice or potassium broth (pg. 53) daily.
♠ Two fresh green salads daily.
♠ Steamed vegetables with brown rice and tofu or seafood for dinner.
♠ Cranberry or celery juice before bed.

☙ A continuing diet for lung health should be high in vegetable proteins and whole grains, low in refined carbohydrates and starches.
♠ Include cultured foods such as yogurt and kefir for friendly G.I. flora.
♠ Include pitted fruits - apricots, peaches, plums are lung specifics.
♠ Include brewer's yeast 2 teasp. daily.

☙ High quality protein is needed to heal lung diseases. Take a protein drink each morning. (pg. 63) and Crystal Star SYSTEM STRENGTH™ drink daily.

☙ See ASTHMA DIET suggestions in this book or "COOKING FOR HEALTHY HEALING" by Linda Rector-Page for a complete healing diet.

VITAMINS/MINERALS

▶ Beta-carotene 100,000-150,000IU daily, with B Complex 100mg., extra B6 100mg., and B12 internasal gel.

▶ Effective anti-oxidants are a key: *(They may also be given to children in reduced dose to protect them from lung diseases as adults.)*
♣ Vit. C 3-5000mg. with bioflavs
♣ Vit. E 400IU with selenium
♣ Germanium 100-150mg. daily.
♣ Pycnogenol 50mg. 3x daily.
♣ Am. Biologics OXY-5000.

▶ Care Plus 3% *dilute* H2O2 1 Tbl. to 1 glass liquid, 2x daily for 1 month. Rest for a month; resume if needed. *There will be intense and prolonged coughing, as accumulated waste is released. H2O2 works to destroy chronic infection in the lung systems and provide nascent oxygen to the tissues.*

▶ For T.B. - on the rise in America:
♣ Beta-carotene 150,000IU
♣ CoQ 10 30-100mg. daily
♣ Solaray LIPOTROPIC 1000
♣ Garlic caps 6-8 daily
♣ Vit. C to bowel tolerance daily.

▶ Enzymatic Therapy AIR POWER and LUNG/THYMUS complex.
♣ RAW PANCREAS extract for cystic fibrosis to help absorption. ☺

HERBAL THERAPY

☙ Crystal Star ANTI-BIO™ caps or extract 4x daily for 1 week; then 2x daily with RSPR™ caps 4 daily for 1-2 months. Add RSPR™ TEA, DEEP BREATHING™ tea or GREEN TEA CLEANSER™, 2 cups daily for increased results.

☙ High potency royal jelly 2 teasp. daily. ♂

☙ Crystal Star PAU DE ARCO/ ECHINACEA extract or pau de arco tea 3 cups daily.
with
Evening primrose oil capsules 4-6 daily. ♀

☙ George's ALOE VERA JUICE with herbs 1 glass daily, ♂
and
Crystal Star HEAVY METAL™ caps if lungs are subject to lots of environmental pollution.

☙ Effective lung healing herbs:
♦ Red clover
♦ Sarsaparilla/licorice rt. ♀
♦ Comfrey/fenugreek
♦ Mullein/lobelia
♦ Pleurisy rt.
♦ Echinacea/goldenseal for cystic fibrosis.

BODYWORK

▶ Avoid all chlorofluorocarbons. They are as harmful to your lungs as they are to the atmosphere.

▶ Avoid tobacco and secondary smoke. Get plenty of fresh air and sunshine, away from air pollution.

▶ Scratch the arm lightly, for 5 minutes daily, along the meridian line from the shoulder to the outside of the thumb to clear and heal lungs.

▶ Take a catnip or chlorophyll enema once a week to clear body toxins out faster.

▶ Reflexology points:

lung points

▶ Apply Body Essentials SILICA GEL to the chest - may also be taken internally, 1 TB. in 3 oz. water daily.

Common Symptoms: Constant coughing, inflammation and pain; bloody expectoration; difficult breathing; difficulty performing even simple activities without shortness of breath.
Common Causes: Environmental and heavy metal pollutants, such as chlorofluorocarbons and smoking; malnutrition, and vitamin A deficiency; suppressive over-the-counter cold and congestion remedies that don't allow the lungs to eliminate harmful wastes properly.

LUPUS ■ S.L.E.

Lupus erythematosus is another in the growing list of modern auto-immune diseases. It is a systemic type of viral infection characterized by chronic inflammation of the organs. In lupus, the immune system becomes disoriented and develops antibodies that attack the body's own connective tissue. Joints and blood vessels become affected producing arthritis-like symptoms. The kidneys and lymph nodes become inflamed, and in severe cases lupus causes degeneration in the heart, brain centers and central nervous system. More than 80% of those afflicted are women. Orthodox treatment has not been very successful in controlling lupus. Natural therapies are effective in rebuilding a stable immune system. Our experience indicates that you feel worse for a month or so until all toxins are neutralized. Then, suddenly, as a rule, you will feel much better. Stick with your program. It is working, but requires

FOOD THERAPY

Dietary therapy has had notable success in reducing the symptoms of lupus.

- Follow the ARTHRITIS CLEANSING DIET in this book for three months: The diet should be 60-75% fresh foods during this time.
  - ◆ Take a potassium broth (pg. 53) every day for a month, then every other day for a month, then once a week for the 3rd month.
  - ◆ Then, follow a modified macrobiotic diet (pg. 42) until blood tests clear, (sometimes 2-3 years, but healing success rate is good). Take aloe vera juice 1-2 glasses daily.
  - ◆ Make sure the continuing diet is very low in fat. A vegetarian diet is strongly recommended to increase fatty acid levels and decrease harmful fat levels.

- Crystal Star BIOFLAV., FIBER & C SUPPORT™ drink to re-establish damaged tissue integrity; GREEN TEA CLEANSER™ to re-establish homeostasis.

- Avoid all red meats, refined sugars and high starch foods.

- See "COOKING FOR HEALTHY HEALING" by Linda Rector-Page for a complete, effective healing diet.

VITAMINS/MINERALS

- ▶ Twin Lab EGG YOLK LECITHIN with Enzymatic Therapy LIQUID LIVER w. SIBERIAN GINSENG. and Source Naturals MEGA GLA caps.

- ▶ Ascorbate vit. C 5000mg. daily with bioflavonoids and rutin, and/or Quercetin Plus with bromelain 3x daily as an anti-inflammatory.

- ▶ High omega fish or flax oil capsules to reduce inflammation.

- ▶ Future Biotics VITAL K 4 teasp. daily.

- ▶ Ener B internasal B12 *and* CoQ 10, 60mg. daily to rebuild cell structure.

- ▶ Immune building supplements:
  - ✦ Germanium 100-150mg. daily, with Sun CHLORELLA 1 pkt. daily.
  - ✦ Beta carotene 100,000IU and Vit. D 1000IU daily.
  - ✦ Raw thymus glandular, or Enzymatic Therapy THYMUS SL, or LYMPH/SPLEEN complex.
  - ✦ Cartilade SHARK CARTILAGE

- ▶ Alta Health MANGANESE with B12 2x daily, *with* CANGEST caps or powder for pancreatic enzymes.

HERBAL THERAPY

- ❦ Crystal Star LIV-ALIVE™ caps and LIV-ALIVE™ tea daily for 1 month. with BODY REBUILDER, GINSENG 6 DEFENSE RESTORATIVE™ tea, and ADR-ACTIVE™ capsules to re-build energy.

- ❦ Pau de Arco tea 3-4 cups daily.

- ❦ Carnivora extract daily.

- ❦ Gotu Kola capsules 4 daily as a central nervous stimulant.

- ❦ Effective immune stimulants:
  - ✦ High potency royal jelly, 40,000mg or more, 2 teasp. daily.
  - ✦ Crystal Star GINSENG 6 DEFENSE RESTORATIVE tea or caps.
  - ✦ Zand IMMUNE HERBAL extract

- ❦ Crystal Star ANTI-BIO™ caps or extract, with AR EASE™ ro ANTI-FLAM™ caps as needed. with Sun chlorella 15 tabs daily. and Garlic caps 8 daily.

- ❦ Effective anti-inflammatory herbs:
  - ✦ Solaray TURMERIC extract
  - ✦ Black walnut extract

BODYWORK

- ▶ Over-medication for lupus, especially by cortico-steroid drugs is dangerous; they weaken the bones and eventually suppress immune response.

- ▶ Avoid birth control pills, penicillin, allergenic cosmetics, and phototoxins from UV rays. Any of these can result in a flare-up of lupus.

- ▶ Get plenty of rest and quality sleep.

Common Symptoms: Great fatigue and depression; rough, "butterfly" skin patches; chronic nail fungus - red at cuticle base; skin pallor; photosensitivity to light; low grade chronic fever; rheumatoid arthritis symptoms; kidney problems; anemia and low leukocyte count; pleurisy; inflammation, esp. around the mouth; seizures, amnesia and psychosis; low immunity. **Common Causes:** Viral infection; degeneration of the body, often caused by too many antibiotics or prescription drugs from Hydrazine derivatives; alcoholism; emotional stress; reaction to certain chemicals; latent diabetes; overgrowth of Candida albicans yeasts; chronic fatigue syndrome; affects mostly black and Hispanic women.

LYME DISEASE

Lyme disease is caused by a micro-organism that is transmitted to humans by the deer tick, which rides on rodents, birds and mammals. It is a serious, steadily debilitating, degenerative disease, difficult to guard against, especially with children. While antibiotics are the current medical treatment of choice, and seem to work in the initial phases, symptoms recur after the drugs are withdrawn, and they do not work in the later stages at all. Natural therapies that address the disease as if it were a virus have had the best success. Strong immune enhancement is the best defense.

FOOD THERAPY

🐾 A modified macrobiotic diet (pg. 52) is recommended for 2-3 months to strengthen the body while cleaning out and overcoming the disease.

🐾 Have a green drink (pg. 54ff) or a fresh green salad every day.

🐾 Avoid alcohol, tobacco, all refined and caffeine-containing foods, and sugars. Omit red meat, high gluten and starchy foods.

🐾 Take a potassium broth or essence (pg. 53) twice a week.

🐾 Take 1 teasp. each daily:
♣ Liquid whey for orotic acid
♣ Wheat germ oil for body oxygen
♣ Jarrow EGG YOLK LECITHIN
♣ Royal jelly 40,000mg. or more.

VITAMINS/MINERALS

▶ Beta or marine carotene 100-150,000IU daily as an anti-infective, *with* Quercetin Plus with bromelain as an anti-inflammatory.

▶ Solaray pancreatin 1300mg. 4x daily on an empty stomach.

▶ **Vitamin C or Ester C powder, 1/4 teasp. every hour to daily bowel tolerance as an anti-oxidant and toxin neutralizer, especially during acute attacks and recurrences.**

▶ Germanium 30mg. daily, (or dissolve 1 gram powder in 1 qt. water and take 3 TBS. daily).

or

▶ Apply Care Plus OXYGEL H2O2 gel to the bite area, *and* take internally Nutri-biotic GRAPEFRUIT SEED extract, 10 drops 3x daily in water.

▶ Cartilade SHARK CARTILAGE to enhance leukocytes and help overcome the virus, with raw thymus glandular to help restore immunity.

▶ Natren LIFE START ☺, or LIFE START II, ♂ ♀ to overcome digestive damage from long courses of antibiotics and to restore nutrient assimilation.

HERBAL THERAPY

🌱 Crystal Star LIV-ALIVE™ caps or LIV-ALIVE™ extract to enhance liver cleansing activity for a month. Then HEARTSEASE/ANEMI-GIZE™ caps to rebuild blood strength.

🌱 Crystal Star ANTI-BIO™ capsules 4-6 daily (with ANTI-FLAM™ caps to reduce inflammation), for the first week, to clean out infection. Then ANTI-VI™ extract in water 2x daily, one week on and one week off to overcome the virus. Then GINSENG 6 DEFENSE RESTORATIVE™ tea or capsules *with suma* to reestablish homeostasis.

🌱 Effective extracts:
♦ Echinacea/goldenseal extract 3x daily.
♦ St. John's wort extract 2-3x daily.

🌱 Crystal Star RELAX CAPS™ to rebuild nerve structure,

with

Evening primrose oil caps 4-6 daily for prostaglandin support,

and

Solaray TURMERIC caps as an anti-inflammatory.

🌱 Use myrrh oil to both repel and kill lyme ticks. Pennyroyal and mountain mint are also effective.

BODYWORK

▶ Regular exercise for plenty of body oxygen and stress relaxation is a key.

▶ Take a hot bath or spa to discourage organism replication, and to relieve pain.

▶ Environmental preventive measures:
→ Keep lawns cut short and shrubbery to a minimum where children play.
→ When walking through tall grass or brush, wear long-sleeved shirts and pants, and tape pant legs into socks. Use *natural* tick repellent oils on exposed areas of the body. *Note: DEET chemical repellent, while effective, can be fatal if ingested, and can cause adverse reactions in children.* Put suspicious clothing in the dryer to kill ticks by dehydration. Simply washing clothes is not effective.
→ Do a meticulous, daily body inspection if you have been out in the woods or live in an infested area. Look for louse-sized arachnids or dark freckle-sized nymphs behind knees, in scalp and pubic hair, in armpits and under watchbands. Remove the tick with tweezers as close to the skin as possible. Do not squeeze or twist it. Apply alcohol to bite area. Enlist the help of a partner for best results. Time is critical. The longer the tick is attached the greater are the risks of serious disease.
→ Check outdoor pets for ticks regularly.

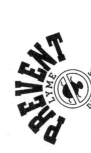

Common Symptoms: A large red "bullseye" rash near the site of the bite that becomes as large as 10 to 20 inches; initial flu-like symptoms of chills and aches; unusual fatigue and malaise, head aches and joint pain, especially in children; later symptoms of heart arrythmia, muscle spasms with racking pain, meningitis (brain inflammation), chronic bladder problems, arthritis, facial paralysis and other numbing nerve dysfunctions, and extreme fatigue. Note: Lyme disease symptoms mimic several other disease conditions. Have a simple test done by a prompt care clinic if you feel that you are at risk.

LYMPHATIC SYSTEM & SPLEEN HEALTH

To stimulate the greatest immune strength, first enhance the spleen and lymphatic systems. The lymphatic system flushes waste from the body, filtering and engulfing foreign, harmful particles and rendering them harmless. The spleen is the largest mass of lymphatic tissue in the body. It destroys worn out and ineffective red blood cells, renews and stores healthy cells, and provides oxygen for the bloodstream and brain. Spleen function is a necessity in times of hemorrhage or shock trauma to prevent shock.

FOOD THERAPY

🥬 To revitalize through diet:
♣ Take a carrot/beet/cucumber juice every day for 1 week, then every other day for another week to "spring clean" these glands of stored toxins.
♣ Then, build up red blood cells with a potassium broth (pg. 54ff), a green drink (pg. 53), Sun CHLORELLA drink, or Crystal Star ENERGY GREEN™ drink, and a leafy green salad every day. Include brown rice and alfalfa sprouts frequently.

🥬 Take a glass of lemon juice and water regularly in the morning, and a glass of papaya juice in the evening.

🥬 Include plenty of potassium-rich foods regularly, such as sea vegetables, broccoli, bananas and seafood.

🥬 Avoid caffeine, sugar and alcohol during healing.

🥬 See the LIVER CLEANSING & DIET suggestions in this book for more details.

VITAMINS/MINERALS

▶ Marine carotene 50-100,000IU daily.
with
Liquid chlorophyll 3 teasp. daily with meals.

▶ Cartilade SHARK CARTILAGE for leukocyte production.

▶ Body Essentials SILICA GEL 1 TB. in 3 oz. water daily for 1 month.

▶ Alta Health CANGEST daily
with
Evening primrose oil caps 4 daily. ♀

▶ Enzymatic Therapy formulas:
✤ Raw spleen glandular
✤ Raw thymus glandular SL
✤ HERPILYN PLUS ♀
✤ LYMPH/SPLEEN complex
✤ LYMPH SYSTEM 25
✤ LIQUID LIVER W. GINSENG ♂

▶ Vitamin E 400IU daily for red blood enhancement.

▶ Zinc picolinate 30mg. or Solaray BIO-ZINC 2x daily, ♂
and
Natren LIFE START #2, 1/2 teasp. in water 2x daily.

HERBAL THERAPY

🌿 Crystal Star ANTI-BIO™ caps or extract for white blood cell formation; HEARTSEASE/ANEMI-GIZE™ caps with hawthorne extract for blood building and tone, SUPER GINSENG 6 DEFENSE RESTORATIVE™ tea for continued health.

🌿 Effective extracts:
♦ Crystal Star SUPER LICORICE™
♦ Hawthorne lf. flr. and bry.
♦ Siberian and panax ginsengs
♦ Floradix HERBAL IRON
♦ Astragalus

🌿 Effective capsules:
♦ Golden seal
♦ Oregon grape rt.
♦ Chaparral/dandelion
♦ Garlic/cayenne
♦ Solaray ALFAJUICE
♦ Echinacea rt.

🌿 Effective oxygenating teas:
♦ **Barberry**
♦ Chaparral
♦ Yellow dock//sage
♦ **Burdock rt.**

🌿 Spleen enhancing tea:
4oz. hawthorne, 1oz. cardamom, 1oz. safflowers, 1oz. lemon balm, 1oz. red sage; take 2 cups daily.

BODYWORK

▶ To stimulate lymph flow:
↠ Activate muscles through regular exercise and stretching. Start every exercise period with deep, diaphragmatic breathing.
↠ Elevate feet and legs for 5 minutes every day.
↠ Massage lymph node areas.
↠ Take a hot and cold hydrotherapy treatment at the end of your daily shower. (pg. 49)

▶ Eliminate aluminum cookware, food additives, and alum-containing foods or deodorants.

▶ Reflexology point;

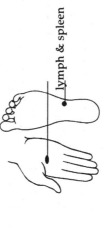

lymph & spleen

▶ Spleen area:

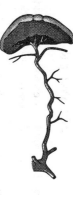

Common Symptoms: Depletion symptoms include anemia, pallor, extreme slimness; lack of energy and memory; sluggishness.
Common Causes: Too many saturated fats and refined carbohydrates reduce activity of these glands; liver exhaustion and stress; protein and B12 deficiency all affect efficiency.

MEASLES ■ RUBELLA

Measles is a viral infection that attacks a lowered immune system. The first symptoms appear as an upper respiratory cold or flu, followed by a red rash. While usually thought of as a childhood disease, measles also affects adults whose immunity to the virus has not been established. Measles is extremely infecting in the acute stages. Rubella is a more severe, and even more contagious form of viral measles, infecting a wider area of the body. Disease effects can be permanent. Keep immunity high for the best defense. Take great care if you are pregnant. Measles can cause birth defects. See remedies for young children on page 112 for more information.

FOOD THERAPY

🍃 Start with a liquid foods diet for at least 24 hours to increase fluid intake as much as possible. Use fresh fruit and vegetable juices, miso soup, bottled water and herb teas such as catnip, chamomile or rosemary, that will mildly induce sweating and clean out toxins faster.

🍃 Then follow with a simple, basic diet featuring vitamin A and C-rich fresh foods.

♣ Give 1 teasp. acidophilus liquid in citrus juice each morning.

♣ Offer fresh fruits all through the morning, with yogurt if desired.

♣ Have one or two fresh green salads each day.

♣ Have a cup of miso or clear soup with 1 teasp. brewer's yeast and snipped sea vegies daily.

♣ Have 2-3 cups of therapeutic herb tea during the day, and a cup of vegex yeast broth before bed.

VITAMINS/MINERALS

▶ Effervescent EMERGEN-C 2-4x daily in juice, or ascorbate vitamin C 1/4 teasp. 3-4x daily in juice or water.

▶ Natren LIFE START or Solaray acidophilus for children 3-4x daily, to replace friendly G.I. flora and rebuild immunity. ☺

▶ Emulsified vitamin A & D 10,000IU/400IU for children as soon as the rash appears. Stronger dosage should be used for rubella - up to 100,000IU in divided doses. ☺

▶ Enzymatic Therapy VIRAPLEX with raw thymus complex SL.

▶ Zinc gluconate lozenges 3x daily.

HERBAL THERAPY

🌿 Crystal Star ANTI-VI™ caps to curb infection, up to 4 daily, and ANTI-FLAM™ caps to reduce inflammation, 2 at a time, up to 6 a day.

and/or

FIRST AID CAPS™ 2 daily for 2 days to break out the fever and rash, and start the healing process.

🌿 Catnip, rosemary, and chamomile tea, 3-4 cups, to break out the rash; raspberry, gotu kola or lobelia tea to heal the skin sores.

🌿 St. John's wort extract or capsules, or mullein/lobelia tincture during acute stage. ☺

🌿 Effective herbal body washes to soothe and heal:

♦ Elder flower ☺
♦ Peppermint
♦ Chickweed
♦ Pleurisy rt./ginger rt.
♦ Safflower herb or turmeric

🌿 Marjoram tea internally to sweat out rash; externally to soothe skin.

BODYWORK

▶ Use hydrotherapy baths with comfrey or calendula flowers to induce sweating and neutralize body acids.

▶ Take tepid oatmeal baths to relieve skin itch and rash. ☺

▶ Apply ginger/cayenne compresses to the rash areas.

▶ Frequent hot baths will often release poisons through the rash.

▶ Take garlic or catnip enemas 1-2 times during acute stages to lower fever and clean out infection fast (person should be 10 years or older).

Common Symptoms: Cold and flu-like symptoms of sneezing, runny nose, red eyes, headache, cough and fever; lymph nodes are usually swollen; fever is followed by a red rash on the face and upper body which sloughs off when the fever drops. With rubella, there is heavy coughing, the rash covers the body; light hurts the eyes; white spots appear in the mouth and throat; there is usually a middle ear infection, and sometimes hearing is affected permanently.
Common Causes: Low immunity from a poor diet, or too many immune-depressing antibiotics or cortico-steroid drugs.

MENINGITIS ▧ ENCEPHALITIS

Meningitis is an infectious, viral disease that attacks and causes inflammation of the nerves and spine, and thus damages brain tissue. It is characterized by deficient blood supply to these areas and therefore deficient oxygen to the brain. Children are especially at risk, and permanent brain damage and/or paralysis and coma or death may ensue if prompt treatment is not undertaken. Medical treatment has been successful with meningitis, but only if received early enough. Nutritional therapies increase the healing and success rate substantially.

FOOD THERAPY

There must be diet and lifestyle change for there to be permanent improvement.

🍃 A 24 hour liquid diet (pg. 44) should be used one day each week to keep the body flushed and alkaline.

🍃 The diet should be 50-75% fresh foods and vegetable juices, with fresh carrot juice and a potassium broth (pg. 53) or green drink (pg. 54ff) 2 to 3x a week.

🍃 **Reduce mucous-forming foods, such as dairy products, red meats, caffeine-containing and refined foods. No sugar, fried, or junk foods at all.** ☺

🍃 Add cultured foods, such as yogurt and kefir, for friendly G.I. flora establishment. ☺

🍃 Drink only bottled water, 8 glasses daily.

VITAMINS/MINERALS

▶ Anti-oxidants are a key both in supporting treatment and for prevention:
✦ Germanium 100mg. daily, or 150mg. SL.
✦ Pycnogenol 50mg. 3x daily.
✦ Beta carotene 50,000IU
✦ Quercetin Plus with bromelain to control inflammation.
✦ **Twin Lab CSA for degeneration.**
✦ **Country Life DMG SL daily.**

▶ Niacin therapy: 100-500mg. daily. (If a child, give a baby aspirin first to avoid niacin flush). ☺

▶ **Enzymatic Therapy raw thymus SL.**

▶ Phosphatidyl choline (PC 55), to nourish brain tissue. ♂

▶ Ascorbate vitamin C or Ester C powder with bioflavonoids, 1/4 teasp. every hour during acute phase. Reduce by 1/2 for maintenance until remission.

▶ Vital Health FORMULA ONE oral chelation with EDTA to increase blood flow to the brain. ♂

▶ B Complex 50mg., with extra B6 100mg. and B12 SL lozenges 2000-3000mcg. daily.

HERBAL THERAPY

🌿 Effective anti-inflammatory herbs:
◆ Crystal Star ANTI-FLAM™ caps.
◆ Fresh comfrey tea 5 cups daily.
◆ Sun CHLORELLA for inflammation and healthy tissue growth.

🌿 Evening primrose oil or Source Naturals MEGA-GLA 240 caps 4-6 daily.

🌿 Kelp tabs 6-8 daily.

🌿 Scullcap tea for nerve support. ♀

🌿 Enzymatic Therapy VIRAPLEX caps, 4 daily.

🌿 Crystal Star ANTI-VI™ extract one week on, one week off to control infection. with

🌿 SYSTEM STRENGTH™ drink to strengthen a weakened system.

🌿 High omega 3 flax oil 3 teasp. daily.

🌿 Lobelia

BODYWORK

▶ Immerse back of the head in warm epsom salts solution several times daily to draw out inflammation. ☺

▶ Alternate hot and cold packs on the neck and back of the head to stimulate circulation to the area.

▶ Use catnip enemas during acute phase to clear body quickly of infection. ☺

▶ Avoid aluminum cookware, deodorants, and other alum containing products.

▶ Get some fresh air and early morning sunshine every day.

▶ Cortico-steroid drugs taken for a long period of time weaken both bone structure and immunity.

Common Symptoms: Lethargy, and slowness of thought and movement; sore throat, with a dark red skin rash; constant, chronic colds and respiratory conditions, with symptoms of high fever, stiff neck, chills, sensitivity to light and nausea; risk of brain retardation - a change in temperature and sleep patterns usually precedes a coma.
Common Causes: Infection by a wide array of viruses; nutritional depletion, especially in children; too many mucous-forming foods; heavy metal or chemical poisoning; constipation; cerebro-vascular disease; psychological trauma.

Menopause is intended by nature to be a gradual reduction of estrogen secretion by the ovaries with few side effects. In a well-nourished, vibrant woman, the adrenals and other glands pick up the job of estrogen secretion to keep her active and attractive after menopause. Unless you are absolutely sure you need synthetic estrogen replacement, choose a natural menopause. Most menopausal problems today stem from exhausted adrenals. Most post-menopausal cancer conditions stem from poor liver function where it does not process estrogens safely. See following page for a discussion of Estrogen Replacement Therapy.

FOOD THERAPY

See Hypoglycemia Diet suggestions in this book, and a complete diet for health during menopause in "COOKING FOR HEALTHY HEALING" by Linda Rector-Page.

◆ Maintain a high level of nutrition to reduce unpleasant menopausal symptoms. Compose the diet of 50% fresh foods, *with vegetable, instead of meat proteins and complex carbohydrates.* ◆ Keep the diet low in fats, and mucous-forming foods such as red meats and dairy products. Steam and bake foods - never fry.
◆ Reduce refined sugars and alcohol intake.
◆ Eliminate carbohydrated drinks that are loaded with phosphates and deplete the body of calcium and other minerals.

◆ Avoid refined foods, excess caffeine, and hard liquor (a little wine is fine).

◆ Avoid chlorinated water. It leaches Vit. E. Drink bottled mineral water.

◆ Make a mix and add 2 TBS. to the daily diet:
 ❧ Brewer's yeast
 ❧ Wheat germ
 ❧ Crushed dried sea vegetables

◆ Eat a calcium-rich diet - from non-fat dairy products, corn, seeds, tofu, broccoli and leafy greens.

VITAMINS/MINERALS

▶ Stress B Complex 100mg. with extra B6 100mg., pantothenic acid 250mg. and PABA 500mg., with flax oil 2 caps 3x daily.

▶ Rainbow Light CALCIUM PLUS, or Enzymatic Therapy OSTEOPRIME.

▶ Co. Life MAXINE multiple vitamins.

▶ Effective raw glandulars:
 ✦ Enzymatic THYROID/TYROSINE
 ✦ Enzymatic MAMMARY
 ✦ Enzymatic OVARY/UTERUS
 ✦ Co. Life ADRENAL w/TYROSINE

▶ Anti-oxidants are important:
 ✦ Pycnogenol 50mg, 2x daily.
 ✦ Nature's Plus vitamin E 800IU for several months.
 ✦ Solaray TRI-O2 capsules.

▶ Ester C with bioflavs. 550mg, 4x, and Am. Biologics emulsified A & D 2x daily esp. in low solar months.

▶ Body Essentials SILICA GEL for tissue integrity and collagen formation.

▶ Enzymatic Therapy NUCLEO-PRO F caps, 2 daily. Chew for immediate results.
  and
PSI PROGEST CREAM daily.

HERBAL THERAPY

Herbal combinations are far better for menopausal symptoms than single herbs.

❦ Crystal Star EST-AID™ caps 4 daily the first month, 2 daily the 2nd and 3rd month, to control hormone imbalances and bone weakness accompanying estrogen changes.
 ◆ Then take EASY CHANGE™ caps as needed for the year or so of the change; RELAX™, ADRN™, or FEMALE HARMONY™ caps for a continued feeling of well-being.

❦ Evening primrose oil caps 4 daily - for prostaglandin balance, with Dong Quai/Damiana caps or extract 2x daily or vitex extract for long term balance.

❦ Effective menopause herbs:
 ✦ Dong quai
 ✦ Red Raspberry
 ✦ Licorice rt.
 ✦ Black cohosh
 ✦ Siberian ginseng for energy
 ✦ Chaste tree berries for 6 months

❦ Kelp tabs 8 daily, or ATOMODINE, or Crystal Star IODINE THERAPY™ caps or extract for thyroid balance.

❦ YS Ginseng tea with honey, 1 cup daily, or royal jelly 2 teasp. daily, or Crystal Star GINSENG 6 SUPER ENERGY™ caps or tea.

BODYWORK

Note: Beware of hormone replacement therapy. Breast, bone and uterine cancer have all been involved with post-menopausal estrogen replacement. New studies are beginning to indicate that menopause is one of nature's ways of decreasing estrogen production and protecting women from cancer.

▶ Take a daily brisk walk to keep the system free and flowing. Do deep stretches on rising and each evening before bed.

▶ Weight training 3x weekly during menopause along with aerobic exercise is a perfect way to keep tissue and skin from sagging and to keep the muscle while you lose the fat - one of the nice advantages of natural menopause. When estrogen levels drop, so does some of the body fat and water retention.

▶ Get a massage therapy treatment once a month during menopause for energy restoration, a body tune-up and a feeling of well-being.

▶ Smoking contributes to cancer, emphysema, osteoporosis, wrinkling and early menopause. Now is the time to quit!

Common Symptoms: Erratic estrogen and other hormone secretions by the glands causing hot flashes, insomnia and fatigue; low libido, irritability, calcium imbalance, unstable behavior, mood swings, palpitations; calcium metabolism disturbances causing osteoporosis; skin and vaginal dryness and sometimes atrophy; occasional appearance of male characteristics.
Common Causes: Deficient nutrition and lack of exercise; thyroid imbalance; exhausted adrenals; poor food absorption; B vitamin deficiency; emotional stress.

Natural Therapies For Other Problems Associated With Menopause

There is a big difference between just surviving menopause and being prepared for it - understanding what to expect and what can help you adjust. Many of the common problems can easily be avoided with natural therapies. These demand that you take responsibility for your well-being, but also give you the control of your health during an individual life change.

❖ **Hot Flashes and Night Sweats** - the body's temperature-regulating mechanism becomes unstable during the shifting hormone balance of menopause. As estrogen levels drop, the pituitary responds by increasing other types of hormones to re-establish hormone homeostasis. The thermostat function of the hypothalamus gland that regulates the pituitary is affected during menopause hormonal transition. Hot flashes will subside as the body becomes adjusted to lower levels of hormones. Stress, excess caffeine and excess alcohol trigger hot flashes. Bioflavonoids are an effective estrogen substitute, exerting chemical activity in the body very similar to that of estrogen.
+ **Natural therapies:** Vitamin E 800IU daily, Dong Quai, Motherwort and Vitex extracts, bioflavonoids 500mg. 2x daily, or Crystal Star BIOFLAV, FIBER & C SUPPORT ™ drink, Siberian ginseng extract, or Crystal Star GINSENG 6 DEFENSE RESTORATIVE™ super tea, PSI ES-GEN CREAM and or PROGEST OIL, Homeopathic *Lachesis or Sepia*, Crystal Star IODINE THERAPY™.

❖ **Sagging Internal Tissue and Organs** - Herbal combinations are particularly well-suited to elasticizing tissue and toning prolapsed organs.
+ **Natural therapies:** Crystal Star WOMAN'S BEST FRIEND ™ or combinations including the following herbs - black cohosh, dong quai, licorice rt., false unicorn, fennel, bupleurum, red raspberry, vitex, Siberian ginseng, peony rt.; a good multi-vitamin for women.

❖ **Dry Vagina** - Reduced estrogen levels sometimes cause the mucous membranes of the vagina to become dry, resulting in discomfort or pain during intercourse - just at a time of life when you can be more spontaneous, without fear of pregnancy. See suggestions above for hot flashes and also those below.
+ **Natural therapies:** PSI ES-GEN CREAM, Crystal Star WOMEN'S DRYNESS™ extract with EST-AID™ extract ro FEMALE HARMONY™ capsules, Women's Health LUBRICATING GEL, Vit. E suppositories, Vit. B6 500mg. daily; vitamin E 800IU daily, and apply Vit. E, or A, D & E oil, or take Solaray A, D & E caps; apply pure aloe gel.

❖ **Depression, Irritability, Insomnia and Fatigue** - These are psychological symptoms that are distressing to many normally practical, well-balanced women. Indeed, many women feel that their lack of energy during menopause is the number one disruption in their lives.
+ **Natural therapies:** Crystal Star GINSENG 6 SUPER ENERGY™ capsules for long, stable energy, vitamin E 800IU, up to 2x daily, chaste tree berry, Siberian ginseng, passion flower extract, ginseng/damiana capsules or dong quai/damiana extract; a good multi-vitamin for women; reduce caffeine intake (it affects the body and mood more during menopause).

❖ **Osteoporosis, Post-menopausal Bone Loss - see page 289.** A mineral-rich diet, with natural supplementation, *and* weight-bearing and aerobic exercise is the best prevention.

❖ **Body Shape Changes** - If you have never exercised, now is the time - at least 3x weekly to retain muscle and gain body tone. Weight training along with moderate aerobic exercise and pre-workout stretches three times a week realizes excellent results during menopause.

About Estrogen Replacement Therapy:

Synthetic estrogen therapy is often prescribed by the medical community. Be very careful and ask before you agree to this. It can be a lifetime drug. It can destroy Vit. E in the body, and can increase the risk of endometrial or breast cancer, heart disease and other diseases. It is not recommended for those with high blood pressure, fibrocystic breast disease, high cholesterol, migraines, or endometriosis. Also avoid synthetic estrogen if there is a history of breast or uterine cancer or fibroids, thrombosis, gallbladder or liver disease. Synthetic estrogen increases appetite, causes fluid retention, aggravates mood swings and depression, and localizes fat deposits on the hips and thighs. Many women are never told that they don't have to be on estrogen replacement therapy forever. In fact most women only need it for a year. Reduce dosage very gradually so that symptoms don't return, and body elasticity is not lost before your body can adjust.

In a nutshell: Things to consider about hormone replacement therapy: **Estrogen Replacement Therapy pros:** 1) reduces risk of osteoporosis. 2) helps vaginal dryness. 3) eliminates hot flashes. 4) decreases risk of heart disease by raising HDL cholesterol levels. 5) decreases risk of uterine cancer when combined with progesterone replacement. **ERT cons:** 1) artificial manipulation of the natural menstrual cycle - continuation of menses. 2) increases growth of uterine and breast fibroids. 4) contra-indicated if there is a history of breast or uterine cancer, endometrosis, high blood pressure, migraines or thrombosis. 5) expense of ERT treatments and doctor visits. **Progesterone Replacement Therapy pros:** 1) decreases risk of uterine cancer when used *with* ERT. **PRT cons:** 1) increases risk of breast cancer. 2) increases risk of heart disease by decreasing HDL levels.

Phyto-estrogens, or plant estrogens are only 1/400th as potent as synthetic estrogen, with no side effects, but have all the balancing advantages of controlling hot flashes and osteoporosis if the body is not producing enough estrogen on its own. Phyto-estrogens simply work with the body to help it stabilize its own estrogen levels better - raising them if estrogens are too low for balance; lowering them if they are too high. Naturally-occurring flavonoids in many of these herbs also exert a similar balancing effect on other hormones. As the inherent estrogen hormone itself does, phyto-estrogen plants also help elevate the body's good cholesterol HDL's, and keep arterial pathways clear. The mineral riches in phyto-estrogens help stave off osteoporosis, and stimulate the companion hormone progestin to promote proper cell growth and replacement.

In addition to phyto-estrogen effects, many of these plants increase uterine and organ tone by improving blood flow. In this way they are also body tonics for women. Examples of phyto-estrogen herbs are licorice rt., dong quai, chaste tree berry, and black cohosh. A good herbal estrogen tonic will include them.

Excessive ✧ Inter-period Spotting

Progesterone is the factor that assures uniform shedding of the uterine lining - low levels of this hormone result in tissue buildup. At the same time, the relatively high level of estrogen stimulates the uterine lining, causing even more endometrial tissue formation. The combination of these two factors leads to abnormally heavy flow during menstruation, and/or spotting between periods as excess tissue is shed. A low progesterone-to-estrogen ratio also causes PMS symptoms of bloating, irritability and depression during the cycle. See MENOPAUSE pages for more information.

FOOD THERAPY

☙ Consciously work on nutrition improvement, with emphasis on vegetable proteins, mineral-rich foods and high fiber foods.
Add plenty of leafy greens, seafood, fish and sea vegetables to regulate metabolism.

☙ Avoid caffeine and caffeine-containing foods, hard liquor (a little wine is fine), and red meats (most are loaded with the hormone DES that has a definite effect on human blood).

☙ Reduce fried, saturated fatty foods, sugars, and high cholesterol foods.

☙ Make a mix and add 2TBS. to the diet daily:
♦ Brewer's yeast flakes
♦ Wheat germ flakes
♦ Amaranth grain
♦ Lecithin granules

☙ Crystal Star BIOFLAV., FIBER & C SUPPORT™ drink daily for tissue strength and integrity,
and/or
A green drink (pg. 54ff) or Crystal Star ENERGY GREEN™ once a week.

VITAMINS/MINERALS

▶ PSI PROGEST CREAM applied to the abdomen as directed.

▶ Enzymatic Therapy RAW MAMMARY caps 2-3 daily for almost immediate results; BIO-CAL or FEM PLUS capsules if periods are too frequent.

▶ Nature's Plus Vit. E 800IU with Floradix LIQUID IRON daily.

▶ Rainbow Light CALCIUM PLUS capsules 4 at a time daily,
with
Octacosanol 1000mg. Clorella 15 tabs daily for breakthrough bleeding.

▶ Vitamin K 2 daily, with Twin Labs citrus bioflavonoids and rutin 500mg./500mg.

▶ Body Essential SILICA GEL for connective tissue strength.

▶ Bee pollen capsules 1000mg. 2 daily.

▶ Mezotrace SEA MINERAL COMPLEX 4 daily, with
Raw adrenal glandular and Source Naturals MEGA GLA caps.

HERBAL THERAPY

☙ Crystal Star FEMALE HARMONY™ caps 2 daily with 2 bayberry capsules, for 2 months to normalize hormone production.
and
FLOW-XS™ tea.

☙ Then WOMAN'S BEST FRIEND™ caps 3x daily with VITEX extract as a tissue toner.

☙ Atomodine, or Crystal Star IODINE THERAPY™ for thyroid balance.

☙ Dong Quai/damiana caps or extract 4x daily, with
♦ Shavegrass or burdock tea.
♦ Crystal Star SILICA SOURCE™ extract for connective tissue.
♦ Milk thistle seed extract as a mild liver cleanse for spotting.
♦ Sarsaparilla extract daily as a source of balancing progesterone.

☙ Effective teas:
♦ Shepherd's purse 3 cups, 3x daily during and before period. Add cranesbill, red raspberry, periwinkle and agrimony for more balanced hormone activity.
♦ Angelica/raspberry
♦ Bayberry bk.
♦ Nettles

BODYWORK

▶ Acupressure: Press on the insides of the legs about 5" above the knees; 5 minutes each leg to decrease bleeding.

▶ Apply icepacks to the pelvic area.

▶ Get extra sleep during this time.

▶ Get daily regular exercise to keep system and metabolism flowing.

▶ Reflexology point:

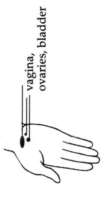

vagina, ovaries, bladder

▶ Avoid drugs of all kinds, even aspirin and prescription drugs if possible. Many inhibit Vitamin K formation.

Common Symptoms: Excessive bleeding for 2 or more days, with large dark clots, spotting between periods.
Common Causes: Nutrition deficient diet with too much caffeine, salt and red meat, causing hormone and glandular imbalance; uterine fibroids, endometrial polyps or hyperplasia; endometriosis; overproduction of estrogen; too much aspirin or other blood-thinning medications; calcium or chronic iron deficiency; underactive, lazy or low thyroid; Vit. K deficiency.

♀ MENSTRUAL PROBLEMS ♀

Suppressed ♦ Delayed ♦ Irregular

Heavy body building and training for marathon or competition sports definitely affects menstruation because the amount of body fat is extremely reduced. Women who exercise competitively sometimes experience total cessation of menses. The body will not slough off tissue when it feels at risk in forming more. In young girls, menses may be delayed because of abnormally low estrogen levels due to low blood calcium levels. Irregular menses due to prolonged emotional stress should be addressed with relaxation and exercise techniques.

FOOD THERAPY

❧ Make sure the diet is very nutritious, with plenty of vegetable proteins and complex carbohydrates. (The body will often not menstruate or conceive if it is malnourished).

❧ Have some brown rice and other B Complex-rich foods every day.

❧ Have a green drink (pg. 54ff), Green Foods GREEEN MAGMA, or Crystal Star ENERGY GREEN™ drink several times a week for healthy blood building.

❧ Drink plenty of pure water daily.

❧ Take 2 TBS. each daily:
♣ Wheat germ
♣ Lecithin granules
♣ Brewer's yeast

❧ Avoid caffeine and caffeine-containing foods, such as chocolate and sodas.

VITAMINS/MINERALS

▶ PSI PROGEST CREAM applied to the abdomen as directed.

▶ B Complex 100mg. daily, with extra folic acid 400mcg. and
ENER B internasal gel vit. B12 every other day.

▶ Nature's Plus Vit. E 800IU.

▶ Enzymatic Therapy NUCLEO-PRO F caps with
ADRENAL COMPLEX, RAW OVARY and RAW MAMMARY glandulars.

▶ For delayed menses:
♣ A good calcium/magnesium supplement *with* zinc 50-75mg. daily *and* kelp tabs 8 daily for 2 months.

HERBAL THERAPY

❧ Crystal Star FLOW EASE™ tea - one cup daily,
and
EST-AID™ caps or EST-AID™ extract,
or
WOMAN'S BEST FRIEND™ caps 4 daily.

❧ Crystal Star FEMALE HARMO-NY™ caps and tea.
or
Burdock tea 2 cups or vitex extract 2x daily.

❧ Evening primrose or borage oil caps 4-6 daily.

❧ Dong quai/damiana caps or extract 2x daily - esp. for young girls with delayed menses.

❧ Effective teas:
♦ Black cohosh
♦ Butcher's broom
♦ Ephedra for delayed menses
♦ Mugwort
♦ Licorice/echinacea

❧ Spirulina and bee pollen caps 2 each daily for metabolic balance.

BODYWORK

▶ Apply horehound compresses to the pelvic area.

▶ Alternating hot and cold sitz baths to stimulate pelvic circulation.

▶ Regular mild exercise to keep system free and flowing.

▶ Do knee-chest position exercises for retroverted uterus.

Common Symptoms: Absence of menses; delayed menses in young girls; irregular menses.
Common Causes: Poor health or nutrition; gland and hormone imbalance; too much caffeine and too many carbonated drinks; poor organ and abdominal tone; lack of exercise or too much exercise (marathoner's syndrome); extreme, or very low protein weight loss diet foods; anorexia or excess dieting for weight loss; hypoglycemia; low blood calcium levels; IUD-caused cervical lesions or cysts; venereal disease; stress, emotional shock or depression; adrenal exhaustion; previous birth control pill use causing irregularity; pregnancy aftermath.

♀   MISCARRIAGE ▦ FALSE LABOR   ✿

To Prevent and Strengthen

Poor diet is the single biggest factor in miscarriage and the inability to carry a pregnancy to full term. Forty-five percent of chronic aborters have low levels of vitamin C complex.

FOOD THERAPY

☙ A good prevention/building diet should include plenty of magnesium and potassium-rich foods; leafy greens, brown rice, green and yellow veggies, tofu, sprouts, molasses, etc.
  ✦ Add sea vegetables for naturally occurring vit. B₁₂ and protein.
  ✦ NO soft drinks; they bind magnesium and make it unavailable.

☙ Be sure to get enough good vegetable protein for the baby's growth: whole grains, sprouts, low fat dairy foods, sea foods, seeds, etc.

☙ Make a mix; take 2 TBS. daily:
  ✦ Lecithin
  ✦ 4 teasp. wheat germ oil
  ✦ Brewer's yeast
  ✦ Molasses

☙ Avoid alcohol, caffeine, and drugs. Reduce sugars and refined foods of all kinds.

☙ Crystal Star BIOFLAV., FIBER & C SUPPORT™ drink daily for tissue strength and integrity.

☙ Nature's Plus SPIRUTEIN drink for extra quality protein.

VITAMINS/MINERALS

▶ Take a strengthening prenatal formula such as Rainbow Light PRENATAL all through pregnancy for a healthier baby and to help prevent miscarriage and birth defects.

▶ Bioflavonoids and C are a key:
  ✦ Vitamin C with rosehips or Ester C with bioflavs. and rutin to strengthen veins and blood vessels 2-3000mg. daily.
  ✦ Alacer SUPER GRAM 2 or 3.
  ✦ Quercetin Plus with bromelain
  ✦ Twin Lab CITRUS BIOFLAVS. w. rutin 500mg.

▶ Vitamin E 400IU and germanium 30mg. daily during pregnancy as protection against miscarriage.

▶ Rainbow Light CALCIUM PLUS w. high magnesium.

▶ B Complex 50mg. with Kal B12 with folic acid 2x daily.

▶ Apply PSI PROGEST CREAM, and take emulsified A & D daily.

▶ Solaray ALFAJUICE caps for chlorophyll and oxygen.

HERBAL THERAPY

❧ For false labor:
Take 2 caps each cayenne and bayberry, or take lobelia and cayenne extracts together, and get to a hospital or call your midwife immediately.

❧ Crystal Star HERBAL PRENATAL™ capsules for strength and tone during pregnancy. Then, 5 WEEK FORMULA™ caps in the last stages of pregnancy as directed for an easier birth. (above products are by special order only)

❧ Effective teas:
  ◆ Cramp bark
  ◆ Wild yam
  ◆ False unicorn
  ◆ Mugwort

❧ Red raspberry and catnip tea, or Crystal Star MOTHERING TEA™ all through pregnancy 2-3 cups daily with kelp tabs 6 daily.

❧ Crystal Star ANTI-SPZ™ caps or CRAMP BARK COMBO™ extract to help stop bleeding, and nettles tea for uterine hemorrhage.

BODYWORK

▶ Have the woman lie very still and give a cup of false unicorn tea every ½ hour. As hemorrhaging decreases, give the tea every hour, then every 2 hours. Add 5 or 6 lobelia extract drops as a relaxing agent to the last cup.

▶ Give comfrey/wild yam/cranesbill tea every hour until bleeding is controlled.

▶ Give hawthorne extract ½ dropperful, and bee pollen 2 teasp. every hour until bleeding is controlled.

▶ To determine if the fetus is still alive: take body temperature first thing upon waking. Have a thermometer by the bed, already shaken down, move as little as possible, and take temperature before getting up. The fetus is alive if body temperature is 98.6 or above, unless normal body temperature is low due to abnormally low thyroid metabolism)

▶ Don't smoke. Smokers are twice as likely to miscarry and have low birth weight babies as non-smokers.

Common Symptoms: Spotting to profuse bleeding during pregnancy, usually with cramps and severe pain.
Common Causes: Deficient uterine muscle tone; weak blood vessels and capillaries; lack of protein and sufficient nutrition for both mother and child; improper fixing of the fetus to the womb walls; allergic reaction to drugs; overload of prescription and/or recreational drugs.

MONONUCLEOSIS

Mono is an opportunistic viral disease that attacks the respiratory and lymphatic systems with severe flu-like infection. Glands, lymph nodes, bronchial tubes, liver, spleen are all affected. The virus is virulent and highly infectious. Immune response is very weak. The whole body feels the symptoms of fever, sore throat, headache, swollen glands, jaundice, muscle aches and general long-term fatigue. Medical antibiotics are not effective for this virus. Liver, lymph and spleen systems are the main organs involved in healing. At least three months of rebuilding are needed to effect restoration of strength.

FOOD THERAPY

High quality vegetable proteins are a key to healing and prevention of further infection.

🍠 Begin healing with plenty of cleansing/flushing fruit juices and bottled water for 1 week. Do not fast. Strength and nutrition are too low.
 ◆ Particularly use apple/alfalfa sprout, papaya/pineapple, and pineapple/coconut juices for strength and enzyme enhancement.
 ◆ Then, follow with a week of green drinks, potassium broth (pg. 53), and vegetable juices to cleanse, strengthen and rebuild liver function.
 ◆ Then eat a diet high in vegetable proteins; (brown rice, tofu, nuts, seeds, sprouts, etc.), and cultured foods; (yogurt, kefir, etc.) for rebuilding friendly flora.

🍠 Add vitamin A and vitamin C rich foods.

🍠 Drink plenty of pure water daily.

🍠 See Liver Cleansing Diet suggestions in this book for more information.

VITAMINS/MINERALS

▶ Sun CHLORELLA or Green Foods GREEN MAGMA, or Solaray ALFA-JUICE during entire healing time.
 Add Natren LIFE START II, 1/4 teasp. 3-4x daily to any juice for 3 months.
 and
 Germanium 100-150mg. or CoQ10 30mg. 2x daily.

▶ Beta or marine carotene 150,000IU daily for 1 month,
 with
 Vitamin C powder w. bioflavonoids, 1/4 teasp. every hour in water to bowel tolerance daily for 1 month. (Reduce dosage on both the 2nd and 3rd months.)

▶ Biotec CELL GUARD 6 daily.
 and
 ENER B internasal B₁₂ gel daily for 1 month, then every other day for a month.

▶ YS royal jelly 2 teasp. daily. ♀

▶ Future Biotics VITAL K 3X daily ♂

▶ Enzymatic Therapy raw thymus SL.
 with
 THYROID/TYROSINE capsules for energy and metabolic increase.

HERBAL THERAPY

🌿 Crystal Star ANTI-BIO™ caps or extract, 4-6x daily for 2 weeks to flush toxins from the lymph glands, with CLEANSING & PURIFYING™ or LIVALIVE™ tea.
 Then, ADR-ACTIVE™ caps with BODY REBUILDER™ caps 2 *each* daily.
 Then, SYSTEM STRENGTH™ *or* ENERGY GREEN™ drinks daily for solid immune building blocks; and/or GINSENG 6 DEFENSE RESTORATIVE SUPER TEA™ for body homeostasis.
 Then, take hawthorne extract 3-4x daily with FEEL GREAT™ tea and SUPER GINSENG 6™ capsules to reestablish strength.

🌿 Effective immune enhancement:
 ◆ Siberian ginseng extract ♂
 ◆ Astragalus extract
 ◆ Reishi mushroom capsules ♀
 ◆ Pau de arco tea
 ◆ Milk thistle extract
 ◆ St. John's wort extract

🌿 Echinacea/goldenseal rt. and garlic to clear lymph glands of infection.

🌿 Planetary REISHI MUSHROOM SUPREME. ♀

BODYWORK

▶ Bed rest during the acute stages, and regular mild exercise during the rebuilding stages are critical to successfully overcoming mono.

▶ Get early morning sunlight; on the body every day possible.

▶ Avoid all pleasure drugs, caffeine and chemical stimulants. These are often the substances that reduce immunity to its infective point.

▶ Reflexology point:

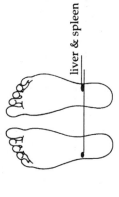

liver & spleen

Common Symptoms: Severe flu/pneumonia/lung symptoms; extreme fatigue; totally run-down condition; pallor; jaundice as the liver throws off body poisons.
Common Causes: An opportunistic disease allowed by a weak immune system; overuse and abuse of pleasure drugs and/or alcohol; liver malfunction.

MORNING SICKNESS ■ NAUSEA ■ VOMITING

Over 50% of pregnant women experience high frequency nausea during the first trimester. While it is quite understandable that the wide variety of sudden hormone and metabolic changes is contributing to the condition, there are also many natural, traditional treatments that can lessen the severity. Other nausea causes that involve allergic, infection or nervous reactions can also be helped with natural, soothing therapies.

FOOD THERAPY

๛ Keep soda crackers or dry toast by the bed, and take some before rising to soak up excess acids; eat ice chips to calm spasms; drink a little fresh fruit juice for alkalinity. Cucumbers soaked in water and eaten will relieve congestion fast.

๛ For breakfast, have orange juice sweetened with honey; then a little bran or barley cereal. Sip slowly.
Take only yogurt in the morning, if friendly flora are needed to settle digestive imbalance.

๛ Take 2 TBS. brewer's yeast flakes in juice or on a salad every day for absorbable and non-toxic B vitamins.

๛ Eat plenty of fiber from vegetables and whole grains to keep bowels clean and flowing.

VITAMINS/MINERALS

▶ Acidophilus powder - 1/4 teasp. 3x daily, or chewable papaya enzymes to settle stomach imbalance.

▶ Premier 1 or YS royal jelly 1 teasp. each morning on rising.

▶ Homeopathic *Nat. Sulph., Nux Vomica*, or *Ipecac* as needed.

▶ Stress B complex 50mg. daily, with extra B6 50mg., B2 200mg., and magnesium 400mg. with
Rosehips vitamin C 500mg. daily.

▶ Country Life RELAXER capsules as needed.

▶ Cal/mag/zinc 2 at a time as needed to settle.

HERBAL THERAPY

๛ **Ginger capsules, tea or extract on rising.**

๛ Crystal Star FEMALE HARMONY™ capsules 2 daily, or vitex extract 1/2 dropperful daily.
and
MOTHERING™ TEA daily a needed. (Helpful all during pregnancy for balance.) ♀

๛ Catnip tea with 1 goldenseal capsule on rising. ♀

๛ Solaray EUROCALM caps and ALFAJUICE caps to calm and balance the stomach.

๛ Effective liver decongestants:
   ◆ Dandelion/yellow dock
   ◆ Milk thistle seed

๛ Peppermint oil, a small drop on the tongue.

๛ Effective teas:
   ◆ **Ginger/peppermint**
   ◆ **Red raspberry**
   ◆ **Alfalfa/mint**
   ◆ **Spearmint/chamomile**
   ◆ **Wild yam**

BODYWORK

▶ Deep breathing exercises every morning, and a brisk deep breathing walk every day, for body oxygen.

▶ Acupressure points: Press the hollow of each elbow 3x for 10 seconds each.

▶ Both biofeedback and hypnotherapy have been effective. See a qualified chiropractor or massage therapist, esp. if nerve reactions are part of the cause.

▶ Soft classical or new age music in the morning will help calm you and the baby. ♀

Common Symptoms: Nausea and heaving in the morning or night during the first trimester of pregnancy; gland and hormone upset causing digestive inbalance; sensitivity to food substances.
Common Causes: Gland and hormone imbalance as the body adjusts to a new biorhythm; congested liver if yellow bile is vomited; low blood sugar.

MOTION SICKNESS ■ JET LAG

Inner ear imbalance is usually at the root of the problem. Deaf people do not get motion sickness. Jet lag is the inability of the internal body rhythm to rapidly resynchronize after sudden shifts in the timing. The internal clock is set by one's hormonal rhythm and by being in light. The system tries to maintain stability and resist time change, causing a psycho-physiological impairment of well-being and performance.

FOOD THERAPY

🔸 Before departure:
  ♣ Take a cup of Vegex yeast broth with a pinch of cayenne.
    or
  ♣ A bowl of brown rice mixed with 3 TBS. brewer's yeast.
    or
  ♣ One egg white mixed with lemon juice
    or
  ♣ Suck on a lemon or lime during the trip whenever queasiness strikes.

🔸 During the trip, munch soda crackers to soak up excess acids. Take sugar-free, carbonated sodas. Avoid eating salty, sugary or dairy foods. They can easily cause digestive imbalance.

For jet lag:
  ♣ Drink plenty of water, juices and herb teas – but avoid alcohol when flying. It can upset the delicate bio-chemistry of the nervous system-Drink before you are thirsty to combat dehydration on a flight.
  ♣ During re-adjustment, eat high vegetable protein meals when you are trying to stay awake; high carbohydrate meals when you are trying to sleep. Eat complex carbohydrates if you are traveling to high altitude places.

VITAMINS/MINERALS

◆ B Complex 100mg. for several weeks prior to travelling, for better "B" balance, and extra folic acid 400mcg. and vit. B12 2000mcg. SL.

◆ Glutamine 500mg. 2-3x before departure.

◆ Activated charcoal tablets 2-3x before departure to soak up acids.

◆ Take vitamin B1, thiamine, 500mg. like Dramamine before a trip.

◆ Nutrition Res. GRAPEFRUIT SEED EXTRACT to overcome the effects of bad food and water or a trip.

◆ Ctry. Life TRAVELLERS SUPPORT caps before a trip, with vitamin E 400IU w. selenium. ♂

For jet lag:
  ♣ Am. Biologics OXY-5000 FORTE
  ♣ Tyrosine 500mg. 2 to 3 daily a few days before a trip and during the trip as needed.
  ♣ Vitamin C 500mg. chewable 6 daily, *with* B Complex 2 daily while traveling.
  ♣ Raw pituitary extract for 2x daily for 8 days before traveling.
  ♣ Homeopathic Hyland's *Calms Forte* as needed.

HERBAL THERAPY

🌿 Take 2-3 ginger caps, or ginger/cayenne caps, or Crystal Star TRAVEL EASE™ extract an hour before traveling. May also take as needed during the trip.

🌿 Ginkgo biloba extract drops on a regular basis before and during traveling for inner ear balance.

🌿 Strong Japanese green tea or Crystal Star GREEN TEA CLEANSER™ each morning for a week before a trip, and during a trip to set up good stomach enzyme balance. ♀
    and/or
    Crystal Star MINERAL SPECTRUM™ caps for about a month before a trip, and herbal enzymes as needed for better stomach balance.

🌿 Peppermint tea before and during a trip.

For jet lag:
  ✦ Ginkgo biloba extract for inner ear balance.
  ✦ Use calming herb teas, such as chamomile or passion flower.
  ✦ Siberian ginseng extract before and as needed during a trip.

BODYWORK

▶ During an attack:
  → Massage knee caps for 3 minutes.
  → Massage little finger for 10 mins.
  → Massage back of head at base of skull, and behind ears on mastoids.

▶ Do conscious deep breathing for 1 minute. Get fresh air and oxygen as soon as possible.

▶ Reflexology point:

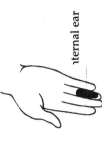

internal ear

For jet lag:
  → Start shifting your sleep/wake cycle in advance to the new time. When traveling long distances, schedule a stop-over if you can.
  → Don't smoke. Stay away from secondary smoke in the airport. Inhaling smoke can keep you toxic for hours.
  → Walk about in the plane to promote circulation and prevent blood stagnation.
  → As soon as you arrive at your destination, get out in the sunlight to help reset your biological clock.
  → Use meditative relaxation tapes to minimize stress.

Common Symptoms: Nausea, upset stomach and/or vomiting during a vehicle trip; unsettled stomach; queasiness; cold sweats; sleepiness; dizziness; poor appetite. For jet lag: fatigue; lethargy; poor performance; dehydration; inability to sleep well.
Common Causes: Inner ear imbalance; mineral deficiency; fear or stress about the trip. For jet lag: circadian rhythm upset.

M.S. ■ MULTIPLE SCLEROSIS ■ A.L.S.

Multiple sclerosis is a chronic, central nervous system disease thought to be triggered by allergens. The disease itself results from damage to the sheaths of nerve cells in the brain and spinal cord and has been incurable because the immune system fights against itself. More women than men seem to be affected, usually experiencing onset between 25 and 40. M.S. must be treated vigorously. A little therapy does not work, but long lasting remission and cure are possible if you catch it in time. Natural therapies take 6 months to a year.

FOOD THERAPY

🍃 Follow a cleansing diet for 2 months, similar to a diet for Candida albicans (see pg. 168). Then follow a modified macrobiotic diet (pg. 52) for 3 to 6 months.

🍃 The diet should be 70-80% fresh foods, with plenty of salads and green drinks; 15-20% fresh fruits; and 5-10% vegetable proteins from sprouts, legumes and seeds. Eat a bowl of brown rice every day for B vitamins. Eat fish at least three times a week.

🍃 Take a potassium broth (pg. 53) at least twice a week.
Then take Crystal Star SYSTEM STRENGTH™ and BIOFLAV, FIBER & C SUPPORT™ drinks to rebuild nerve and tissue .

🍃 Jarrow EGG YOLK LECITHIN 2-3x daily, with high potency royal jelly, 40-50,000mg. 2 teasp. daily.

🍃 Take 2 teasp. each daily:
  ◆ Wheat germ oil
  ◆ Liquid Whey ♂

🍃 Avoid all refined and fried foods, sugars, full-fat dairy foods, and caffeine-containing foods. Eliminate meats except fish. Reduce starchy and high gluten foods.

VITAMINS/MINERALS

▶ Phosphatidyl choline (PC55) 2-3x daily with pancreatin 1300mg. daily.

▶ Antioxidants are a key:
  ◆ Pycnogenol 50mg. 3x daily
  ◆ CoQ 10 30mg. 2x daily to help regeneration of myelin sheath. ♀
  ◆ Germanium 150mg. SL
  ◆ Octacosanol 1000mg.
  ◆ Co. Life DMG B15 SL.
  ◆ Vit. E 800IU w/ selenium 200mcg.

▶ Twin Lab CSA for degenerative spine improvement and threonine as needed for energy, with Ctry. Life MAXI-B capsules. ♂

▶ Niacin therapy, 500mg. 3-4x daily, with B6 500mg. for nerves and circulation, and B1 500mg. ♂

▶ Beta or marine carotene 100,000IU with

Ascorbate vitamin C powder, 1/4 teasp. every hour to bowel tolerance - daily for a month; then reduce to 5000mg. daily.

▶ Ener B internasal B12 every day for 1 month, then every other day for 2 months; with Dr. DOPHILUS, 1/2 teasp. 3x daily or Alta Health CANG-EST caps with meals for assimilation.

HERBAL THERAPY

Treat both M.S. and A.L.S. for nerve damage first, then work on restoring muscle function.

🌿 Crystal Star RELAX CAPS™ to feed and rebuild nerve structure. with
ANTI-SPZ™ caps or ginkgo biloba extract for tremor control. ♀

🌿 Essential fatty acids are a key:
  ◆ Evening primrose oil caps 4-6
  ◆ Omega 3 flax oils 3 daily
  ◆ Borage seed oil caps 4-6 ♀
  ◆ Source Naturals MEGA GLA

🌿 Sun chlorella 2 packets daily.

🌿 Crystal Star LIV-ALIVE™ caps and LIV-ALIVE™ tea to clean out toxins, and
HEARTSEASE/ANEMIGIZE™ caps and/or Ener B internasal B12 every day to build blood strength. ♂

🌿 Solaray ALFAJUICE caps with TURMERIC caps as an anti-inflammatory.

🌿 Mezotrace SEA MINERAL COMPLEX daily, and/or scullcap capsules for nerves.

BODYWORK

▶ Overheating therapy is effective for M.S. See page 49 in this book, or P. Airola "How To Get Well" for effective technique.

▶ Take a catnip enema or spirulina implant once a week for several months.

▶ Avoid emotional stress, poor diet and excessive fatigue. These trigger the onset of M.S. attacks.

▶ Avoid smoking and secondary smoke. You need all the oxygen you can retain.

▶ Mild daily exercise, chiropractic adjustment, massage therapy and mineral baths have been useful in controlling M.S. and A.L.S.

▶ Reflexology points:

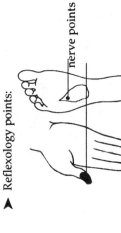

nerve points

Common Symptoms: Numbness; great fatigue and weakness; visual disturbance and loss; breathing difficulty; slurred speech and mental disturbance; poor motor coordination and staggering; tremors; dizziness; nerve degeneration.
Common Causes: Too many refined carbohydrates and saturated fats, causing poor food assimilation and toxemia from constipation and poor bowel health; lead or heavy metal poisoning; hypoglycemia; Vitamin B6, B12, and B1 deficiency; food allergies triggering auto-immune reaction; Candida albicans overgrowth; gland imbalance.

MUSCLE CRAMPS & SPASMS

Leg Cramps ✧ Involuntary Tics

Muscle spasms, cramps, twitches and tics are usually a result of body vitamin and mineral deficiencies. A good diet and natural supplements have been very successful in fortifying and strengthening the body against nutrient shortages. Improvement is noticeable within one to two weeks.

FOOD THERAPY

🍃 Eat vitamin C-rich foods; leafy greens, citrus fruits, brown rice, sprouts, broccoli, tomatoes, green peppers, etc.

🍃 Eat potassium-rich foods; bananas, broccoli, sun seeds, beans and legumes, whole grains and dried fruits.
Add sea vegetables to the diet for extra iodine and potassium (or take Crystal Star SYSTEM STRENGTH™ drink).

🍃 Eat magnesium-rich foods; lettuce, bell pepper, green leafy vegetables, molasses, nuts and seafoods.

🍃 Take a green drink (pg. 54ff) or Sun CHLORELLA drink w. 1 teasp. kelp powder twice a week.

🍃 Avoid refined sugars, processed and preserved foods. Food sensitivities to these are often the cause of tics and spasms.

🍃 Take an electrolyte drink often, such as Knudsen's RECHARGE for good mineral salts transport.

VITAMINS/MINERALS

▶ Vitamin C or Ester C, up to 5000mg. daily with bioflavs and rutin for collagen formation.

▶ Am Biologics INFLAZYME FORTE, or Hyland's homeopathic *Mag. Phos.* to reduce pain.♀

▶ Country Life LIGATEND as needed, MAXI-B COMPLEX w/ taurine and vit. E 400IU daily.

▶ B Complex 100mg. daily, with extra B6 250mg. and pantothenic acid 250mg. for nerve repair.

▶ For eye tics; CoQ 10, 30mg. daily.

▶ Magnesium/potass./bromelain 3 daily, with zinc 75mg.♂

▶ Future Biotics VITAL K 3 teasp. daily, with Vit. E 800mg.

▶ Solaray CAL/MAG CITRATE 4-6 daily, with vitamin D 1000IU.

▶ Mezotrace SEA MINERAL COMPLEX, with bromelain 500mg. and pycnogenol 50mg. for leg cramps, *and*

▶ Phos. Chol for nerve tranquility.

HERBAL THERAPY

🍃 Crystal Star ANTI-SPZ™ caps 4 at a time, or CRAMP BARK COMBO™ extract, with
ANTI-FLAM™ caps daily, 2 at a time as needed.

🍃 Crystal Star RELAX CAPS™ daily as needed to rebuild nerve health. with
POTASSIUM SOURCE™ caps for deficient minerals.♀

🍃 Alta Health SIL-X silica caps 3-4 daily.

🍃 Evening primrose oil 4 daily for essential fatty acids.

🍃 Effective muscle support herbs:
♦ Horsetail/oatstraw ♀
♦ Rosehips ♀
♦ Passion flower
♦ Scullcap
♦ Alfalfa or Solaray ALFA-JUICE caps.
♦ Butcher's broom tea
♦ Spirulina 4 daily
♦ Ginger rt. 2 - 2x daily
♦ Crystal Star VALERIAN/WILD LETTUCE extract.

BODYWORK

Note: If you taking high blood pressure medicine and have continuing muscle spasms, ask your doctor to change your prescription. Some have sodium imbalance that upsets mineral salts in the body.

▶ Take vinegar or epsom salts baths.

▶ Effective applications:
↝ Arnica tincture
↝ Lobelia extract

▶ Massage the legs; elevate the feet, and slap soles and legs hard with open palm to stimulate circulation.

▶ Use alternating hot and cold hydrotherapy, or hot and cold compresses applied to the area to ease pain, promote circulation and healing.

▶ Shiatsu and massage therapy are effective in re-aligning the body's "electrical" impulses, and releasing and relieving muscle cramps.

Common Symptoms: Uncontrollable spasms and twitches of the legs, facial muscles, etc.; unexplained leg cramps at night.
Common Causes: Metabolic insufficiency of calcium, magnesium, potassium, iodine, trace minerals, and vitamins E, D and B6; lack of sufficient HCl in the stomach; Vitamin C and silicon deficiency causing poor collagen formation; food allergies to preservatives and colorants.

MUSCULAR DYSTROPHY ▦ SPINA BIFIDA

Spina bifida is a condition where there is a defect in the nerve growth and development of the spinal column. Children born with spina bifida have poor motor ability and coordination, and are essentially paralysed from the waist down. **Muscular dystrophy** is a severe weakening of the muscles due to abnormal development - it also affects nerve growth and atrophy. Also usually affecting children, muscle and nerve degeneration prohibits the ability to support body weight. Natural therapies have been successful in increasing nutrient assimilation, in overcoming EFA deficiency, in rebuilding nerve and muscle tissue, and in balancing prostaglandin formation.

FOOD THERAPY

🍃 Go on a short 6-10 day cleansing diet to release accumulated toxins (pg. 43).
◆ Then follow an *intensive* macrobiotic diet for degenerative disease for 2 months, and a *modified* macrobiotic building diet (pg. 52) for 6 months or more.
See "COOKING FOR HEALTHY HEALING" by Linda Rector-Page for complete details of this diet.

🍃 Take a potassium broth (pg. 53) daily for the first 6-8 weeks of healing. Reduce to once a week for the next 6 months. Add at least 1 green drink (pg. 54ff) every week.

🍃 Jarrow EGG YOLK LECITHIN 2x daily, with highest potency royal jelly 50-100,000mg. 2 teasp. daily.

🍃 Make a mix and take 2 TBS. daily:
◆ Lecithin granules
◆ Brewer's yeast flakes
◆ Wheat germ

🍃 Avoid all refined foods, caffeine-containing foods, and salty foods.

VITAMINS/MINERALS

▶ Phosphatidyl choline (PC55) 4 daily, with Future Biotics VITAL K 4 to 6 teasp. daily.

▶ Antioxidants are a key:
◆ Pycnogenol 50mg. 3x daily
◆ CoQ 10 60mg. daily to help regeneration of myelin sheath. ♀
◆ Germanium 150mg. SL
◆ Octacosonal 1000mg.
◆ Vit E 800IU with selenium

▶ Twin Lab CSA for degenerative spine improvement and threonine as needed for energy.

▶ Predigested liquid amino acids 1-2 teasp. daily for immediately usable protein building blocks.

▶ Vital Health FORMULA 1 chelation with EDTA with extra niacin 500mg. for increased circulation.

▶ Country Life THREONINE and GLYCINE caps with CARNITINE 500mg. 4-6 daily, and ENER B internasal B12.

▶ Beta carotene 100,000IU with Ester C, 550mg. with bioflavs. and rutin 6 daily.

HERBAL THERAPY

🌿 Crystal Star RELAX CAPS™ as needed to rebuild nerve sheath damage,
    with
High omega 3 flax oil 3x daily, and
BONZ™ caps and tea to support muscle atrophy.

🌿 Essential fatty acids are a key:
◆ Evening primrose oil caps 4-6
◆ Omega 3 flax oils 3 daily ♀
◆ Borage seed oil caps 4-6 ♀
◆ Source Naturals MEGA GLA

🌿 Hawthorne extract 2-4x daily for circulatory tone.

🌿 Crystal Star SYSTEM STRENGTH™ drink and dried, chopped sea vegetables in a soup or salad for rebuilding mineral and enzyme strength.

🌿 Effective teas: three cups daily:
◆ Dandelion
◆ Fennel
◆ Siberian ginseng from extract
◆ Scullcap

BODYWORK

▶ Overheating therapy has been successful in controlling muscular dystrophy. See page 49 in this book or P. Airola "How To Get Well" for technique.

▶ Avoid tobacco and alcohol. Question high blood pressure drugs containing sodium.

▶ Use hot and cold hydrotherapy to stimulate circulation (pg. 49). Use mineral and therapeutic baths for cleansing and muscle support.

▶ Get early morning sunlight on the body every day possible to rebuild muscle strength.

▶ Reflexology point:

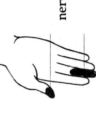

nerves & muscles

Common Symptoms: Muscle weakness and atrophy; nerve damage and atrophy; tremor and palsy; degeneration in ability to walk; occasional loss of bladder control.
Common Causes: Inherited genetic fault - often because of folic acid deficiency in the mother; poor food assimilation causing deficient minerals; too many refined foods and junk foods; EFA and prostaglandin deficiency.

MYASTHENIA GRAVIS

Myasthenia gravis is a debilitating muscle disease, characterized by progressive weakness and fatigue. All muscle action is affected, including breathing and swallowing. Complete exhaustion and paralysis are usually the final results. Many of the symptoms as well as successful treatments are the same as for muscular dystrophy. Remission from this wasting disease has shown marked success with improved diet. See page 281 for more information.

FOOD THERAPY

๛ SEE ARTHRITIS AND HYPO-GLYCEMIA DIET suggestions in this book for effective diet information.

๛ Avoid nightshade plants: tomatoes, eggplant, white potatoes, green peppers, etc.

๛ Eat potassium and magnesium-rich foods: from whole grains, leafy greens, and green or potassium drinks (pg. 53ff), such as Crystal Star SYSTEM STRENGTH™ or ENERGY GREEN™ drinks.

๛ Take Twin Lab EGG YOLK LECITHIN 2-3x daily, with
High potency royal jelly 40-50,000mg. 2 teasp. daily.

๛ Take 2 teasp. wheat germ oil daily in juice or water.

VITAMINS/MINERALS

◗ PSI PROGEST CREAM as directed with thyroid complex glandular. Rapid improvement.

◗ Alta Health MANGANESE W. B12 SL, and Future Biotics VITAL K 3-4 teasp. daily. ♂

◗ Glycine 500mg. and/or chromium picolinate 200mcg. ♂

◗ Effective neuro-transmitters:
✦ Choline 600mg. ♂
✦ Choline/inositol ♀
✦ Lecithin 3x daily
✦ Phosphatidyl choline (PC 55)

◗ Effective antioxidants:
✦ Octacosanol ♂
✦ Vitamin E 800mg. ♀
✦ Ctry. Life DMG sublingual
✦ Pre-digested amino acid complex capsules

◗ Twin Lab CSA capsules as directed. Excellent results.

◗ B Complex 100mg. daily, with extra pantothenic acid 500mg. and B6 250mg. daily.

HERBAL THERAPY

❧ Evening primrose oil caps 4-6 daily for prostaglandin balance.

❧ Take cayenne/ginger capsules 2 at a time as needed to increase circulation. Apply cayenne and ginger compresses to affected areas to help prevent atrophy.

❧ Crystal Star RELAX CAPS to feed and rebuild nerve strength, with POTASSIUM SOURCE™ caps for strengthening minerals.

❧ Ginkgo bilboa extract 2-3x daily if there is muscle tremor. ♂

❧ Siberian ginseng extract 3-4x daily for circulation increase,
with
Sun CHLORELLA for blood building and oxygen. ♂

BODYWORK

➤ Avoid smoking, secondary smoke, and oxygen-depleting pollutants as much as possible.

➤ Get some mild outdoor exercise every day for fresh air and aerobic lung and muscle tone.

➤ Massage therapy and shiatsu are both effective in increasing oxygen use and strengthening nerves and muscles.

➤ Reflexology points:

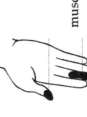 muscles & nerves

Common Symptoms: Severe muscle weakness and fatigue, especially in the upper body; inability to perform even small tasks because of lack of strength; progressive inability, paralysis and exhaustion; double vision; choking; difficult breathing and swallowing; poor articulation and speech.
Common Causes: Chemistry failure between the nervous system and the muscles; choline and prostaglandin deficiency causing poor neurotransmission; chronic constipation causing poor elimination of toxins; chronic sugar regulation imbalances.

NAILS
Nail Fungus

Nails can be very useful as an "early warning system" in diagnosing illness and evaluating health. If the eyes are the "windows of the soul", the nails are considered the "windows of the body". They are one of the last body areas to receive the nutrients carried by the blood, and show signs of trouble before other better-nourished tissues do. Healthy nails are pink, smooth and shiny. Changes in their shape, color and texture signal the presence of disease in the body. Disorders of the blood, glands, circulation and organs as well as nutritional deficiencies all show up in nail conditions.

FOOD THERAPY

Good nutrition and a well-balanced diet are the keys for nail health. Give your program at least a month to show improvement. We have found that nothing seems to happen for 3 weeks, and then noticeable changes appear in the 4th week.

🐾 Eat plenty of vegetable protein and calcium foods, such as whole grains, sprouts, leafy greens, molasses, and seafood. Eat sulphur-rich and silicon-rich foods, such as onions, sea vegetables, broccoli and fish.

🐾 To restore color and texture; mix a little honey, avocado oil, egg yolk, and a pinch of salt. Rub onto nails.

Leave on 1/2 hour. Rinse off.

🐾 To clear discolored nails; rub fresh lemon juice around the nail base. Take extra chewable papaya enzymes.

🐾 To strengthen weak nails; soak daily for 5 minutes in warm olive oil or cider vinegar.

🐾 For hangnails/splitting nails; take 2 TBS. brewer's yeast, or 2 teasp. wheat germ oil daily for a month.

HERBAL THERAPY

If your nail problem is a mineral deficiency; herb and plant minerals are the best choice for supplementation.

🌿 Horsetail tea or extract 3x daily for a month, or Alta Health SIL-X silica caps 2-4 daily.

🌿 Kelp tabs 6-8 daily.

🌿 Crystal Star MINERAL SPECTRUM™ capsules, or MINERAL SOURCE COMPLEX™ extract for a month.

🌿 Effective teas:
 ◆ Rosemary/sage
 ◆ Dulse/oatstraw
 ◆ Pau de arco

🌿 Evening primrose oil caps 4 daily for a month to strengthen nails.

🌿 *For nail fungus:*
 ◆ Apply tea tree oil 3-4x daily.
 ◆ Soak nails in a Nutri-biotic GRAPEFRUIT SEED EXTRACT solution - 3 to 4 drops in 8 oz water til fungus clears.
 ◆ Soak nails in Am. Biologic DIOXYCHLOR or Care Plus *dilute* OXYGEL.
 ◆ Apply a garlic/honey paste to nails

VITAMINS/MINERALS

◗ Mezotrace SEA MINERAL COMPLEX 2 daily, or cal/mag/zinc capsules 4 daily with boron for better uptake. ♀

◗ Body Essentials SILICA GEL - take internally as directed for 1 month; apply directly daily.

◗ Nature's Plus ULTRA NAILS with extra biotin 600mcg. 2x daily,
or
Enzymatic Therapy ACID-A-CAL.

◗ Zinc 50-100mg. daily for spots or poor growth.

◗ Vit. E 400IU daily for breaking nails, ingrown or hangnail infections.

◗ Vit. A&D for poor growth, ridges and crusty skin around nails.

◗ Betaine HCl and vitamin A for brittleness, splitting and white spots. ♂

◗ Raw thyroid extract for spots or chipping.

BODYWORK

Note: nail enamels and supplies are among the most toxic environmental polluters. Fake nails or tips add weight to the nails annd prevent them from thickening naturally. Nail color dyes penetrate the nail to the skin, often causing allergic reactions. A simple manicure without polish - with beeswax spread on the nails and buffed to a shine can leave your nails naturally beautiful.

▶ If you polish your nails, don't keep them constantly polished. Allow them to "breathe " at least 1 day a week. To tint nails naturally: make a thin paste of red henna powder and water. Paint on and let dry in the sun. Rinse off. Pretty pink nails with no chipping.

▶ Acupressure treatment: Press 3x for 10 seconds each, the moon of each nail, to stimulate circulation.

▶ Use a green clay poultice to draw out a nail infection; use wild alum (cranesbill) paste with water to relieve inflammation from ingrown or hangnails.

Common Nail Signs And Causes: *White spots* - zinc, thyroid or HCl deficiency; *White spots* - zinc, thyroid and protein deficiency; *white bands on the nails* - zinc and protein deficiency; *discolored nails* - Vit. B12 deficiency, kidney or liver problems; *yellow nails* - liver problems; *poor circulation, lymph congestion, too much polish; *green nails* - bacterial infection under the nail; *too white nails* - liver malfunction, poor circulation, anemia, general mineral deficiency; *blue nails* - lung and heart problems, drug reaction, blood toxicity from too much silver or copper; *black bands on the nails* - chemotherapy or radiation reaction; *no half moons or ridged nails* - Vit. A, kidney disorder, protein deficiency; *splitting, brittle or peeling nails* - Vit. A & D deficiency, poor circulation, thyroid problems, iron, calcium or HCl deficiency; *thick nails* - poor circulation; *dark, spoon-shaped nails* - anemia, B12 deficiency; *pitted, fraying, split nails* - vitamin C and protein deficiency, eczema/psoriasis problems; *"hammered metal" looking nails* - hair loss; *down-curving nails* - heart and liver disorders; *white nails with pink tips* - liver cirrhosis.

283

NARCOLEPSY

Narcolepsy is a chronic sleep disorder characterized by erratic, recurrent, overwhelming drowsiness or sleep attacks at any time of the day or night. Sufferers are unable to control these sleep spells, but are easily awakened. Research indicates that there are two types of this order - DDD (dopamine dependent depression), and a type involving a B_6 deficiency of the dopaminergic system.

FOOD THERAPY

🌿 The diet should be low in fats and clogging foods, such as dairy products and animal proteins; high in light cleansing foods, such as leafy greens and sea vegetables.

🌿 See HYPOGLYCEMIA and THYROID HEALTH pages in this book for more information.

🌿 Brewer's yeast and other foods high in B vitamins, such as brown rice, on a regular basis.

🌿 Eat tyrosine-rich foods, such as wheat germ, poultry, oats and eggs.

VITAMINS/MINERALS

Note: when treating for DDD with tyrosine, do not use B_6 therapy.

▶ Enzymatic Therapy THYROID/ TYROSINE caps. 4 daily, as an anti-depressant, with ADRENAL COMPLEX 2 daily. ♀

▶ B Complex 150mg. daily, with extra B_6 200mg. daily, and CoQ 10 30mg. 2x daily.

▶ Effective anti-oxidants:
✦ Country Life DMG B_{15} daily as needed.
✦ Unipro DMG extract, under the tongue as needed.
✦ Pycnogenol 50mg. 4, 4x daily.

▶ Effective neurotransmitters:
✦ Octacosanol 1000mg. ♂
✦ Choline 600mg.
✦ Choline/Inositol

▶ Chromium picolinate 200mcg. daily, and magnesium 400mg. 2x daily.

▶ Omega 3 fish or flax oils 3-4x daily for sugar regulation, and a pre-digested amino acid complex for additional protein.

HERBAL THERAPY

🌿 Ginkgo biloba and/or St. John's wort extract as needed.

🌿 Excel Energy or Vital Force formulas, 1 to 2 tablets as needed, daily. ♂

🌿 Evening primrose oil caps 4 daily for prostaglandin formation and body "electrical" alignment.

🌿 Crystal Star potassium capsules with ADR-ACTIVE™ caps for thyroid and adrenal energy, 2 each daily. ♀
and/or
🌿 RAINFOREST ENERGY™ tea and capsules.

🌿 Solaray ephedra caps 1 as needed daily. ♀

BODYWORK

▶ Take regular daily exercise for circulation and tissue oxygen.

▶ Biofeedback and chiropractic adjustment have both been effective in correcting the "electrical-shorts" involved in brain-to-motor transmission.

Common Symptoms: Uncontrolled, excessive drowsiness, inappropriate, erratic periods of sleep, from which the sleeper is easily awakened; loss of muscle control with sleep palsy; hallucinations; insomnia; depression accompanying poor brain and adrenaline function.

Common Causes: Hypoglycemia; Vit. B_6 *or* tyrosine deficiency; low thyroid function and metabolism; heredity; constant exposure to physical or mental stress; brain infection, a blow to the head or a brain tumor; poor assimilation and use of body oxygen.

NERVE HEALTH

Nervous Tension ✧ Anxiety

The nervous system is the first to be affected by by stress and tension. Poor nerve health can spawn a host of physical disorders and mental conditions from undesirable defense mechanisms to full-fledged neuroses; from a feeling of apprehension and dread about the future to unrestricted, excessive anxiety.

FOOD THERAPY

See High Blood Pressure Diet suggestions for additional information.

☙ Diet improvement is a key factor in controlling nerve health..
  ♠ Add to the diet regularly: high fiber foods, fresh greens, vegetable proteins, and natural sulfur foods, such as oat bran, lettuce, cucumbers, and celery.
  ♠ B vitamin foods are important; eat plenty of brown rice, whole grains and leafy greens.

☙ Effective special foods:
  ♠ Brewer's yeast for calming B vitamins.
  ♠ Sun seeds and molasses for thiamine and iron.
  ♠ Carrot/celery juice for nerve restoration.
  ♠ Green drinks (pg. 54) for chlorophyll.
  ♠ Wheat germ oil 1 teasp. daily.
  ♠ Garlic capsules 6 daily

☙ Keep the diet is low in salt and saturated fats.

☙ Avoid acid forming foods, such as red meats, caffeine, carbonated drinks - the phophorus binds up magnesium, making it unavailable. *Magnesium is a key mineral in nerve health.*

VITAMINS/MINERALS

▶ Country Life MAXI B complex w/ taurine daily, and extra B₁ 500mg. and B₆ 100mg. daily.

▶ Ascorbate or Ester C 3-5,000mg. daily with bioflavonoids and rutin 500mg. each.

▶ Alta Health CANGEST with meals, and MANGANESE with B₁₂ sublingually.

▶ Twin Lab TYROSINE 500mg. 2x daily as needed.

▶ Rainbow Light CALCIUM PLUS with high magnesium, 4 daily.

▶ Nature's Plus MAGNESIUM/ POTASS./BROMELAIN caps. ♂

▶ Mezotrace SEA MINERAL COMPLEX 2-3 daily.

▶ Vitamin E 400IU daily or Phos. choline 1 daily.

▶ High omega 3 flax oil 3x daily.

HERBAL THERAPY

❧ Crystal Star RELAX™ caps and tea as needed,
  with
SYSTEM STRENGTH™ broth and/or hawthorne extract as nerve tonics.

❧ Crystal Star HEARTSEASE-H.B.P.™ caps with MINERAL SPECTRUM™ caps 2-4 daily.

❧ Effective nervines:
  ◆ Chamomile
  ◆ Peppermint/hops
  ◆ Rosemary
  ◆ Scullcap
  ◆ Reishi mushroom
  ◆ Ginseng/gotu kola ♂
  ◆ Bee pollen ♂
  ◆ Siberian ginseng extract
  ◆ Gotu kola
  ◆ Lobelia
  • Catnip ☺

❧ Deva Flowers ANXIETY drops as needed.

BODYWORK

➤ Tobacco and obesity both aggravate nerve disorders and tension. Lose weight and stop smoking.

➤ Reflexology points:

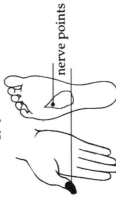

nerve points

➤ Wear acupressure sandals for a short period every day to clear reflexology meridians.

➤ Aromatherapy: Peppermint or cinnamon oil.

➤ Many relaxation techniques are effective:
  → A brisk walk with deep breathing every day for body oxygen.
  → Regular massage therapy treatments.
  → Crossword puzzles, video and computer games hobbies, artwork, etc. can all relieve tension and anxiety.
  → Laughter is the best relief of all.

Common Symptoms: Extreme nervousness and irritability, often with high blood pressure; inability to relax; lack of energy; chronic headaches and neck stiffness; dizziness, palpitations and heart disease proneness.
Common Causes: Too many refined foods, especially sugars; smoking; unrelieved mental or emotional stress; hyperthyroidism and metabolic imbalance; prostaglandin deficiency.

NEURITIS ▣ NEURALGIA

Neuritis is an inflammation of a nerve or nerves. It is usually a degenerating process, and often part of a degenerating illness, such as diabetes or leukemia. Neuralgia is sudden, sharp, severe pains shooting along the course of a nerve - often because of pressure on the nerve trunks, or poor nerve nutrition and an over-acid condition.

FOOD THERAPY

☙ Go on a short 24 hour liquid diet (pg. 44) to rebalance body acid/alkaline pH.
Then, for the rest of the week eat mostly fresh foods, with plenty of leafy greens, sprouts, celery, sea vegetables, and enzyme foods such as apples and pineapple. Take a glass of lemon juice and water every morning. Have a potassium broth or essence (pg. 53) every other day.
Drink 6 glasses of water with a slice of lemon, lime or cucumber daily.

☙ Make a mix and take 2 TBS. daily:
♣ Lecithin granules
♣ Sesame Seeds
♣ Brewer's yeast
♣ Wheat germ

☙ Avoid caffeine, hard liquor and soft drinks, that bind up magnesium.

☙ Keep salts, saturated fats, and sugars low.

☙ See "COOKING FOR HEALTHY HEALING" by Linda Rector-Page for a complete diet for nerve conditions.

VITAMINS/MINERALS

▶ Niacin therapy: 500-1500mg. daily to stimulate circulation, with
Bromelain 500mg. 2x daily
or
Quercetin Plus with bromelain 3-4 daily,
and
Ascorbate or Ester C with bioflavs. and rutin, 5000mg. daily, to rebuild connective tissue.

▶ Stress B Complex 100mg. with extra B6 250mg., pantothenic acid 500mg., and taurine 500mg.
and
Ener B12 internasal gel every other day.

▶ Effective homeopathic remedies:
✦ Hylands Nerve Tonic
✦ Calms or Calms Forte tabs
✦ Aranea Diadema - radiating pain
✦ Mag. Phos. - spasmodic pain.
✦ Hypericum if nerve injury.

▶ Country Life LIGATEND caps as needed, with Future Biotics VITAL K 3 teasp. daily.

▶ Chromium picolinate 200mcg. 2-3 daily.

▶ DLPA 750mg. as needed for pain.

HERBAL THERAPY

❧ Crystal Star RELAX CAPS™ as needed for rebuilding the nerve sheath, 2-4 daily.

❧ Evening primrose oil caps 4 daily, with the following tea daily to rebuild nerves.
Equal parts: St. John's wort, peppermint, lavender, valerian, lemon balm, blessed thistle.

❧ Effective nervine extracts:
◆ Lobelia
◆ Valerian/wild lettuce
◆ Passion flower
◆ Scullcap
◆ Ginkgo biloba, esp. for facial tics.

❧ Crystal Star ANTI-FLAM™ caps to relieve inflammation, 4 daily, BACK TO RELIEF™ or ANTI-SPZ™ caps as needed for pain.

❧ Crystal Star POTASSIUM-SOURCE™ capsules 4 daily as an effective source of sea vegetables.

BODYWORK

▶ Get some regular mild exercise every day for body oxygen and circulation.

▶ Use hot and cold hydrotherapy to stimulate circulation (pg. 49).

▶ Do 10 neck rolls as needed at a time to relieve nerve trauma.

▶ Chiropractic adjustment, shiatsu, and massage therapy are all effective in controlling nerve disorders.

▶ Reflexology points:

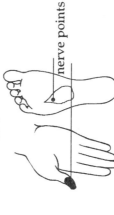
nerve points

▶ Apply B&T TRI-FLORA analgesic gel.

Common Symptoms: Muscle weakness and degeneration; burning, tingling, numbness in the muscles or nerve area; motor and reflex weakness; facial tics; nerve inflammation.
Common Causes: Spinal pinch or lesions; excess alcohol or prescription drugs; prostaglandin and/or B vitamin deficiency; diabetic reaction; herpes; poor circulation; multiple sclerosis-type weakness and numbness; kidney and gallbladder malfunction; arthritis; lupus; migraines; heavy metal poisoning.

NUMBNESS ■ NERVE PARALYSIS

Temporary suspension or permanent loss of function and sensation of the motor neurons.

FOOD THERAPY

➢ Go on a short 24 hour liquid diet (pg. 44) to lighten the circulatory load and clean out waste.

➢ Then, eat only fresh foods for 3-4 days to alkalize and clean the bloodstream. Follow with a modified macrobiotic diet (pg. 52) for 3-4 weeks, emphasizing whole grains and vegetable proteins, until condition clears.

➢ Make a mix and take 2 TBS. daily;
   ♦ Brewer's yeast or BioStrath liquid
   ♦ Unsulphured molasses

VITAMINS/MINERALS

➤ Rainbow Light CALCIUM PLUS caps with high magnesium, 4 daily.

➤ Ctry. Life RELAXER w. taurine.

➤ Green Foods GREEN MAGMA, 2 packets daily with 1 teasp. kelp granules added to each drink for nerve restoration.
   or
   Sun chlorella tabs, 15 daily. with 2 tabs kelp.

➤ Twin Lab CSA caps. as directed.

➤ Niacin therapy: 500mg. or more daily.
   with
   Vitamin C up to 5000mg. daily with bioflavonoids and rutin for nerve connective tissue.

➤ B Complex 100mg. daily with extra B6 500mg. if the extremities are periodically numb.
   or
   B6 250mg. 6-8x daily, if numbness is from nerve interference or a stroke.

➤ Enzymatic Therapy THYROID/TYROSINE caps, 4 daily, with HERBAL K KIQUID.

HERBAL THERAPY

❦ Crystal Star RELAX CAPS™ to rebuild nerve sheathing. with HEARTSEASE/CIRCU-CLIENSE™ tea daily.
   or
   HAWTHORNE™ extract as needed to strengthen circulation.

❦ Kukicha twig tea, 2 cups daily with cayenne/ginger caps 3 daily for 1-2 months,
   or
   Crystal Star GREEN TEA CLEANSER™ every morning and evening.

❦ Ginkgo biloba extract as needed 2 to 4 daily.

❦ Butcher's broom capsules, 2 to 4 daily.

❦ Crystal Star RECOVERY TONIC™ extract drops in water daily for severe cases.

❦ Effective teas: best taken at night.
   ◆ Ginger/oatstraw
   ◆ Gotu kola
   ◆ Scullcap

BODYWORK

➤ Apply cayenne/ginger compresses to the area.

➤ Apply B&T TRIFLORA analgesic gel.

➤ Use alternating hot and cold hydrotherapy (pg. 49).

➤ Acupuncture, massage therapy, shiatsu, and chiropractic adjustment have all shown excellent results with these conditions.

➤ Reflexology point:

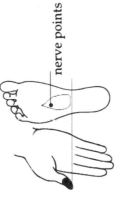

nerve points

Common Symptoms: Lack of feeling in various parts of the body; hands, legs, fingers and toes "going to sleep".
Common Causes: Poor circulation; thyroid deficiency; pinched nerve or spinal lesions; psychic inhibition, such as from hysteria; multiple sclerosis type nerve damage; poor diet with too many mucous-forming foods.

OSTEOPOROSIS ▧ OSTEOMALACIA

Osteoporosis means a decrease in bone mass and density. There is a lack of both calcium and other minerals, as well as a reduction of the non-mineral framework. Osteoporosis also involves hormonal, lifestyle, nutrition and environmental factors. Osteomalacia involves only a decrease in calcium in the bone. Both are preventable conditions. Nutritional therapy is a good choice for both treatment and prevention because it can offer the broadest base of protection against a wide array of factors.

FOOD THERAPY

Vegetarians have a lower risk of osteoporosis; they have denser, stronger bones - particularly after menopause, and in later life.

🍃 Avoid red meats, and reduce animal protein. These are high in phosphates that leach calcium. (*Contrary to popular belief, pasteurized milk is not a very good source of absorbable calcium, and can actually interfere with mineral assimilation.*)
♣ Have a fresh green salad daily. Take a high protein drink from vegetable sources 3 times a week.

🍃 Body Essentials SILICA GEL, 1 TB. in water daily for 6 mos.

🍃 Eat plenty of calcium, magnesium and potassium-rich foods; broccoli, sea vegetables, fish and seafood, eggs, yogurt, kefir, carrots, dried fruits, sprouts, miso, beans, leafy greens, tofu, bananas, apricots, molasses, etc.

🍃 Avoid sugar, caffeine and caffeine-containing foods, hard liquor, tobacco, and nightshade plants that interfere with calcium absorption.

🍃 See "COOKING FOR HEALTHY HEALING" by Linda Rector-Page for a complete bone-building diet.

VITAMINS/MINERALS

Calcium absorption is a key, and can be greatly improved with supplementation.

▶ Apply PSI PROGEST CREAM as directed. Helpful in both preventing and reversing bone loss, *with Germanium 100mg. daily.*

▶ NutriPathic CALC./COLLAGEN.

▶ Enzymatic Therapy OSTEOPRIME.

▶ Vitamin C or Ester C with bioflavs. up to 5000mg. daily for connective tissue, with Vit. D 1000IU, marine carotene 50,000IU, and zinc 30mg. daily.

▶ Alta Health SIL-X silica, 10 daily for 15 days, then 5 daily for 15 days, then 2 daily for 3-4 months, with MANGANESE with B12.

▶ Calcium citrate 1500mg, magnesium 1000mg. *and boron for absorption. Note: taking too much boron alone can actually cause bone loss.*

▶ Body Essentials SILICA gel internally as directed, *with Twin Lab CSA or DLPA 750mg. for pain, and Ener B internasal gel B12 every other day.*

▶ Mezotrace sea mineral complex, with Betaine HCl for absorption and vitamin K 100mg.

HERBAL THERAPY

🌿 Phyto-estrogens are a key for marrow development:
◆ Crystal Star BONZ™ formulas
◆ Licorice rt.
◆ Dong quai/damiana extract
◆ Crystal Star EST-AID™
◆ Black cohosh caps
◆ Vitex extract

🌿 Herbal mineral formulas are a key for bone health:
◆ Crystal Star MINERAL SPECTRUM™ caps, CALCIUM SOURCE™ caps and extract, SILICA SOURCE™ extract (dietary silica biologically engenders calcium production in the body).
◆ Horsetail/comfrey rt.
◆ Dandelion/nettles
◆ Sarsaparilla bk.

🌿 Herbal flavonoids are a key:
◆ Hawthorne berry extract
◆ Bilberry extract
◆ Crystal Star BIOFLAV., FIBER & C SUPPORT™ drink.

🌿 Solaray ALFAJUICE caps, with bee pollen caps 1000mg. 2x daily.

🌿 Evening primrose oil caps 6 daily, with Crystal Star SYSTEM STRENGTH™ drink.

BODYWORK

Note: Cotico-steroid drugs over a long period of time leach potassium from the system and weaken the bones. It is now also becoming known that calcium-containing antacids, such as TUMS are linked to severe bone pain and fracture and are sometimes considered a cause of bone disease through the reduction of stomach acids.

▶ New tests show smoking cigarettes causes damaging bone loss to women. Smoking a pack a day during adulthood results in bones up to 10% less dense and more subject to fracture than than those of non-smokers.

▶ Exercise is a nutrient in itself. Weight-bearing exercise is one of the best ways to build bone and prevent bone loss. Duration of exercise is more important than intensity.

▶ Get early morning sunlight on the body every day possible for vit. D.

▶ Avoid fluorescent lighting, electric blankets, aluminum cookware, non-filtered computer screens, etc. All tend to leach calcium from the body.

▶ Reflexology point:

spine

Commom Symptoms: Decrease in bone mass and density, usually without symptoms until a severe backache develops; porous and open spaces in the bones where supporting structure is lost; weight and height loss; easy bone breaks - spontaneous fracture of the hip or vertebrae; thin, brittle bones.
Common Causes: Menopause and a drop in estrogen levels; poor use of synthetic estrogen; mineral, (calcium and magnesium) protein and collagen deficiency; thyroid and parathyroid malfunction; poor Vitamin C use and assimilation; prostaglandin deficiency; too much cortisone and antibiotics; smoking; excess sugar and hard liquor consumption (especially for men); heavy metal and environmental pollutants, (especially cadmium); anxiety and emotional stress.

Important Facts To Help You Arrest & Avoid Osteoporosis & Post-menopausal Bone Loss

Bone and cartilage are an ever-changing infrastructure of the body. We know now that many factors, including excessive meat and caffeine consumption, preservatives and refined foods, lack of vitamin D from sunlight, and too little exercise, all contribute to bone porosity and lack of mineral absorption. Steroid and antibiotic abuse, tobacco, and too much alcohol all contribute to mineral depletion, and a weakening of body structure. Osteoporosis is a far more complex problem than was originally thought, involving not only calcium deficiency, but a drop in estrogen levels, thyroid and parathyroid malfunction, and poor collagen protein development among several other factors. High stress life styles and habits also inhibit mineral absorption.

But the fact remains that minerals are of prime importance to bone health. Organically grown foods and herbs are becoming the best way to get them. Over a third of our population, and more than 50% of the women, suffer from calcium deficiency alone. Mineral needs increase as the body ages and requires more digestive, HCl and enzyme help. Minerals and trace minerals cannot be made by the body, and must be taken in regularly through food and drink. Mineral rich nutrition provides the body's building blocks, the most basic elements needed for growth. Healthy bones act as reservoirs for the body's mineral needs. Minerals are also the bonding agents between you and your food. Without them the body is not able to absorb nutrients or utilize food. Dietary calcium from food, herbs and food source supplements is far superior in absorption and benefits, because it occurs naturally with estrogen forming, and other natural precursors to insure assimilation. Dietary silica for instance, biologically engenders calcium production in the body, and vitamin D deficiency, not older age, is a more usual cause of poor calcium absorption. The body uses dietary minerals through its own enzyme action, as a whole, not as a single partitioned element or an extracted substance, and this is a key to their effectiveness. Vegetarians traditionally have denser, better-formed bone structure, because the most usable minerals come from green leafy vegetables, sprouts, whole grains, soy foods, and vegetable complex carbohydrates. The two most concentrated sources of absorbable plant minerals - dried sea vegetables and herbs - are ideally suited to today's concerns for better, less processed foods and responsible environmental harvesting.

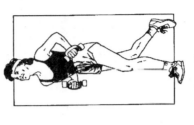

Osteoporosis can be treated and prevented nutritionally. It can be arrested and current bone mass maintained. But the program must be continued, or bone loss will continue. Life style, heredity, and body type all play significant parts in an osteoporosis risk profile.

Here are the higher risk factors:

◆ Female, small-boned, white or Asian, with a family history of osteoporosis.
◆ Post-menopausal white women.
◆ Lifelong low calcium and vitamin D intake.
◆ Removal of ovaries before menopause, or early menopause, before 45 years old.
◆ No child-bearing.
◆ Have reached an advanced age.
◆ Irregular or no menstrual periods.
◆ Consistently high consumption of hard alcohol, cigarettes, caffeine and animal proteins.
◆ Regular and consistent use of certain medications, such as corticosteroids.
◆ Long use of synthetic thyroid can result in osteoporosis. It can also aggravate breast and weight problems, result in cholesterol rise, and engender fatigue.

✳ Poor hormone production greatly increases the risk of osteoporosis regardless of age. Hormone and calcium deficiencies appear regularly in women with irregular menstrual cycles because of excessive running or exercise, or who are bulemic or anorexic. Over 50% of American women suffer from calcium deficiency alone. (Taking a calcium citrate supplement before a period can let you know if this is your problem. Calcium deficiencies show up premenstrually as back pain, tooth pain, and cramping. Calcium supplementation should help these symptoms disappear). See About Estrogen Replacement on page 272.

✳ You can test yourself for probable osteoporosis. Use pH paper (sold in most health food stores), and test your urine. A habitual reading below pH 7 (acid) usually leads to calcium and bone loss. Above pH 7 (alkaline) indicates a low risk system.

✳ Note: Few men suffer osteoporosis because of their increased testosterone supply. New research is centering on natural testosterone sources such as Smilax for arresting bone loss. Herbal extracts of sarsaparilla root are being used experimentally with hope of success.

♀ OVARIAN CYSTS ♀

Ovarian cysts are becoming common today, especially in women with menstrual difficulties (either not having periods, or bleeding excessively). These cysts are small tumors stimulated by too much estrogen, but they are not cancerous, (nor are they cancer precursors). They usually cease to grow after menopause, but may be painful, especially during intercourse, and can cause excessive menstrual bleeding. Natural therapy focuses on normalizing hormone levels and correcting a system environment that promotes cyst development. It has been quite successful, and allows you a choice before jumping into surgery. See Endometriosis, and Ovarian, Uterine and Cervical Cancer, page 167 for further information.

FOOD THERAPY

🍂 Follow a low fat, fresh foods vegetarian diet. High fats mean high estrogen production. Too much estrogen is the most common cause of cysts and their complications.

◆ Get adequate high quality protein daily for healing, from largely vegetable sources to avoid saturated fats: whole grains, sprouts, tofu, sea foods, sea veggies, low fat dairy, etc.

◆ Increase intake of B vitamin foods, such as brown rice, wheat germ and brewer's yeast.

◆ Add miso, sea vegetables, and leafy greens to alkalize the system.

◆ Avoid fried and salty foods, especially during menses.

◆ Avoid red meat, caffeine and refined sugars that can cause iodine deficiency.

◆ Avoid concentrated starches, full fat dairy products, and hard liquor on a continuing basis.

🍂 Keep the continuing diet high in fresh foods - about 50-60%). Drink only bottled water.

🍂 Take 4 teasp. wheat germ oil daily for tissue oxygen.

🍂 Have some fresh apple or carrot juice every day.

VITAMINS/MINERALS

▶ Nature's Plus Vitamin E 800IU or Am Biologics EMULSIFIED A & E.
with
Twin Lab marine carotene 100,000IU daily.
and
Ascorbate Vitamin C, Ester C with bioflavonoids, or QUERCETIN PLUS, 5000mg. daily.
and
Alta Health SIL-X silica for collagen regrowth.

▶ Cartilade SHARK CARTILAGE as an antiinfective.

▶ PSI PROGEST CREAM rubbed on the abdomen. Reduction in approx. 3 months.
with
Pancreatin 1300mg. for fat/protein metabolism

▶ Anti-oxidants are important:
✚ Sun CHLORELLA 20 daily
✚ Pycnogenol 50mg. 3x daily
✚ Germanium 100mg. daily

▶ Enzymatic Therapy RAW MAMMARY or RAW OVARY caps, or NU-CLEOPRO F caps.

HERBAL THERAPY

🌿 Crystal Star WOMAN'S BEST FRIEND™ caps, 4 daily for 3 months, with ANTI-FLAM caps as needed.
with
Evening primrose oil caps 4-6 daily for 3 months.
then
Crystal Star FEMALE HARMONY™ capsules 2 daily as a hormone balancer to prevent return.

🌿 Iodine therapy is part of the key - *often effective in 3-4 months*.
◆ ATOMODINE drops 2-3x daily.
◆ Crystal Star IODINE SOURCE™ caps/extract. (Take with vit. E for best results)

🌿 Effective hormone-balancing herbs:
◆ Vitex extract
◆ Sarsaparilla extract
◆ Dong quai/damiana extract
◆ Saw palmetto extract 2x daily

🌿 For a Type 2 PAP smear, begin the following program immediately:
◆ Green drinks/Sun CHLORELLA.
◆ Crystal Star WOMAN'S BEST FRIEND™ capsules 6 daily.
◆ Goldenseal/echinacea, or goldenseal/chaparral caps 1 wk. a month.
◆ Cartilade SHARK CARTILAGE.
◆ Evening primrose oil caps.

BODYWORK

▶ Avoid IUDs and X-rays as a partial cause of cysts.

▶ Reflexology point:

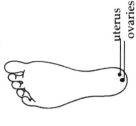

uterus
ovaries

▶ Pain in the heels, and swollen breasts at times other than menses, indicate ovarian cysts.

▶ Ovarian area:

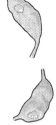

Common Symptoms: Acute or chronic pain in the fallopian tubes or ovaries; disturbance in the normal menstrual cycle, with unfamiliar pain and discomfort in the lower abdomen; painful intercourse; infertility; unusual abdominal swelling, gas and pain; fever and coated tongue.
Common Causes: IUDs and/or radiation and X-rays that change cell function and structure; prostaglandin and EFA deficiency; too much caffeine and saturated fat; high dose birth control pills or synthetic hormones causing too much estrogen; obesity; alcohol-induced diabetes; high stress lifestyle and over-acid diet producing poorly eliminated wastes.

Menstrual Cramps ◇ Swollen Breasts ◇ Lower Back Pain ◇ Pre-period Edema

FOOD THERAPY

Diet can be a key factor in preventing PMS. A vegetarian diet offers the most advantages.

❧ Follow a mild Liver Cleansing Diet, or a modified Hypoglycemia Diet for two months. (See those pages in this book).

❧ Get plenty of low fat protein from vegetable sources, such as whole grains, legumes, soy foods, sprouts, or sea foods. Or take a protein drink such as Nature's Plus SPIRUTEIN each morning.

❧ **Keep the diet low in fats, salt and sugar - high in greens and whole grains. Eat plenty of cultured foods, such as yogurt and kefir for friendly flora.**

❧ Avoid caffeine, caffeine-containing foods, red meat, sugars and saturated fat animal products. **Eliminate dairy products during PMS days.**

❧ Make a mix and take 2 TBS. daily:
♦ Brewer's yeast
♦ Toasted wheat germ
♦ Unsulphured molasses

❧ Drink only bottled water. Drink green tea, or Crystal Star GREEN TEA CLEANSER every morning to cleanse the body, and provide a mini detox.

VITAMINS/MINERALS

▶ **Prof. Ser. PROGEST CREAM - rub on abdomen, or homeopathic** *Mag. Phos.* **to relieve cramping.**

▶ Enzymatic Therapy RAW OVARY and RAW MAMMARY caps daily, or NUCLEOPRO F caps. (May also be chewed for almost immediate results.)

▶ Nature's Plus vitamin E 800IU 1 daily, with

Alta Health magnesium w. SL B12 2500mcg. and vit. B6 200mg. daily, or *Mag Phos. tabs* to relieve congestion.

▶ Effective brand products:
✦ Schiff PMS formula 1 & 2.
✦ Natrol SAF capsules.
✦ Country Life RELAXER and MAXINE caps.
✦ Rainbow Light FEM-GEN caps and WOMEN'S NUT. SYST. w. vitex.
✦ Zand PMS formula.
✦ Woman's Health RELEAF formula.

▶ ATOMODINE drops, or Source Naturals FRAC w. vitamin E 400IU to relieve breast swelling and soreness.

▶ For daily prevention:
B Complex 100mg., with extra B6, vitamin C with bioflavonoids and rutin, and bromelain 500mg. 2x daily.

▶ DLPA to alleviate mood swings.

HERBAL THERAPY

❧ **Evening primrose oil 4-6 daily, 1st month, then 4 daily the 2nd month.**
with
Crystal Star FEMALE HARMONY™ capsules 2 daily each month. Add 2 FIRST AID CAPS™, or 2 baberry capsules daily if flow is excessively heavy.

❧ Use Crystal Star RELAX CAPS™ for stress and tension. WOMAN'S BEST FRIEND™ caps to prevent cramping and pain. During the period use as needed, ANTI-SPZ™ caps 4 at a time, FLOW EASE™ tea, or CRAMP BARK COMBO™ extract.

❧ Effective extracts:
◆ Dong quai/damiana
◆ Chaste tree berries (vitex)
◆ Bilberry for flavonoids
◆ Cramp bark
◆ Echinacea

❧ Effective teas:
◆ Sliced fresh ginger for cramping
◆ Burdock rt. for hormone balance
◆ Licorice/Dong quai
◆ Cranesbill/red raspberry
◆ Chamomile tea for cramping.
◆ Dandelion to help liver function.

❧ Effective progesterone sources:
◆ Sarsaparilla
◆ Wild Yam
◆ Saw palmetto

BODYWORK

▶ Treat yourself to a good massage, sauna or shiatsu session before your period to loosen and release clogging mucous and fatty formations and to cleanse the system and improve circulation.

▶ Stop smoking and avoid secondary smoke. Nicotine inhibits good hormone function.

▶ Get plenty of fresh air and sunshine during your period. Take a brisk walk every day.

▶ Effective applications:
→ Ice packs to the pelvic area.
→ Fresh ginger rt. compresses over pelvic area, covered with a hot water bottle.

▶ For facial blemishes at period time, apply liquid chlorophyll as needed.

▶ Reflexology point:

uterus
ovaries

Common Symptoms: Mood swings, tension, irritability, and depression; argumentative, aggressive behavior; water retention, bloating, and constipation; headaches and lower back pain; sore, swollen breasts; nausea; heavy cramping and excessive menstrual flow; low biorhythm and low energy; food cravings for salt and sweets with extreme thirst; alcohol craving; nerve pain; acne and skin eruptions; light-headedness. If there are moth sores and bleeding gums with mood swings, there is probably a low progesterone or thyroid level.
Common Causes: Prostaglandin imbalance; estrogen excess or imbalance because of liver malfunction; glandular insufficiency (especially the thyroid); lack of regular exercise; poor diet with lack of B vitamins, and magnesium, calcium and protein deficiencies; endometriosis; poor circulation; too much salt, red meat, sugar and caffeine; stress and emotional tension

More Information About P.M.S.

The intricacies of a woman's body are very delicately tuned, and can become unbalanced or obstructed easily, causing pain, poor function, and lack of "oneness" that often results in physiological and emotional problems, especially during the menstrual cycle. Drugs, chemicals and synthetic medicines, standing as they do outside this natural cycle, often do not bring positive results for women. These substances usually try to add something to the woman's body, or act directly on a specific problem area. A highly nutritious diet, herbs as concentrated foods, and naturally-derived vitamin compounds, are identified and used by the woman's own individual enzyme action. These nutrients encourage the body to do its own work, providing balance and relief that is much more gratifying.

Premenstrual syndrome covers such a wide variety of symptoms (over 150 have been documented) that it is now estimated that up to 70% of all women between the ages of 20 and 50 experience varying degrees of PMS. Symptoms tend to get worse for women in their thirties and older, and are often magnified after taking birth control pills and after pregnancy because of hormone imbalances. With such a broad spectrum of symptoms, affecting every system of the body, there is clearly no one cause and no one cure. Indeed the medical establishment, with its highly focused treatment emphasis has not been successful in addressing PMS. Natural therapies and a holistic approach have proven more successful. Self care can tailor treatment to individual needs - and include diet changes, exercise, stress management and emotional support, as well as supplementation.

The suggestions outlined on the previous page usually take at least two months to effect complete relief, as the body works through both ovary cycles. The first month, there is noticeable decrease in P.M.S. symptoms; the second month finds them virtually gone. However, the problem is complex. So many body functions are tied into hormone secretions and glandular cycles. PMS can mean too much estrogen *or* progesterone. Don't be discouraged if you need 6 months or more to gently coax your system into balance. Continuing with the diet recommendations, and lower doses of the herb and/or vitamin choices even after most of the symptoms are gone makes sense toward preventing P.M.S. return.

There are several keys to controlling PMS:

☙ **Prostaglandin formation.** Prostaglandins are vital hormone-type compounds that act as transient hormones, regulating all body functions electrically. Supplementing the body's essential fatty acid supply through dietary means, with foods such as ocean fish, sea foods, olive, safflower or sunflower oils, or herbs such as evening primrose and flax oils, helps to balance prostaglandins. Conversely, excess saturated fats in the body, especially from fatty animal foods, inhibit both prostaglandin production and proper hormone flow.

☙ **Iodine therapy.** Iodine is essential to the health of the thyroid gland, and estrogen levels are controlled by thyroid hormones. If the thyroid does not receive enough iodine, insufficient thyroxine is produced and too much estrogen builds up. Take your choice of iodine therapy with vitamin E for best results.

☙ **Regular exercise** is a must. Aerobic, outdoor exercise is the best. We know it's hard to find the time to add one more thing to an already crowded day, but the benefits for controlling PMS are worth it. Exercise improves the way your body assimilates and metbolizes nutrients. It changes your food habits, and decreases craving for alcohol or tobacco. It makes you feel better by increasing the level of beta endorphins in the brain. It improves circulation to relieve congestion. It encourages regularity for more rapid elimination of toxins. Stretching and relaxation exercises such as yoga also help, as do switching from tampons to pads for many women.

☙ **Stress reduction techniques and relaxation time** are important. Daily self-massage of breasts and ovary areas helps relieve tension and relax reproductive organs. End your morning shower with a cool rinse to stimulate circulation and the lymphatic system to relieve congestion. Be gentle with your schedule during your premenstrual time. Give yourself a little slack, and take some time out to read, listen to music and relax. Acupuncture and massage therapy are both effective for PMS symptoms.

Menstruation is a natural part of our lives. PMS is not. The good news is that women can take control of PMS naturally and effectively.

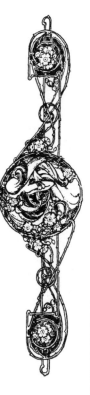

PAIN CONTROL

Pain is a mechanism to draw attention to a problem that the autonomic system cannot handle by itself. Pain signals us to consciously address the underlying cause. Pain is almost completely individual. It can stem from large pain centers that control certain areas of the body, and also from specific local areas that demand exact pinpointed action. There are different kinds of pain; physical, emotional, chronic, local, intermittent, throbbing, dull, spasmodic, sharp, shooting, etc. Every person feels and reacts differently to pain, so that you can treat the right area. **Pain can be your body's best friend.** It alerts you when something is wrong and needs your attention. It identifies the location, severity, and type of problem. **Pain can be your body's worst enemy.** Continuous, constant body trauma saps strength and spirit, causes irrational acts and decisions, and alters personality. Pain killers are obviously useful for these as well as other reasons. They allow you to think clearly, work and live, while addressing the cause of the problem. Chemical pain killing drugs, while strong, afford relief by masking pain, or deadening certain body mechanisms so that they cannot function. Herbal pain relievers are more subtle and work at a deeper level, to relax, soothe, ease and calm the distressed area. You can use the pain for information about your body, yet not be overwhelmed by the trauma to body and spirit that unrelieved suffering can bring. There are four basic pain centers in the body: 1) the cerebro-spinal area, controlling neural affliction, lower back pain and cramping; 2) the frontal lobe area, involved in earaches, toothaches, and headaches over the eyes; 3) the base of the brain, involved in migraines and tension headaches; 4) the abdominal area, affecting menstrual cramping, digestive and elimination pain. This page addresses chronic, lower back, joint and nerve pain. For many people natural therapies and herbs are superior to pharmaceutical drugs and their side effects.

FOOD THERAPY

🥕 Make sure the diet is rich in complex carbohydrates and vegetable proteins for strength: whole grains, broccoli, peas, brown rice, legumes, sea foods, etc.
Add high mineral foods to the diet for solid body blocks. Emphasize magnesium and calcium foods for bone and muscle strength. (See "COOKING FOR HEALTHY HEALING" by Linda Rector-Page for an effective high mineral diet.)

🥕 Have a green drink (pg. 54ff), and/or a green leafy salad every day.

🥕 Make a mix and take 2 TBS. daily:
♣ Brewer's yeast
♣ Cider vinegar and honey in water.

🥕 Include bioflavonoid-rich foods, and/or take Crystal Star BIOFLAV., FIBER & C SUPPORT™ drink for tissue integrity.

🥕 Avoid caffeine, salty foods and refined sugars that engender an over-acid condition.

VITAMINS/MINERALS

▷ DLPA 500-750mg. as needed daily, ♀ or

▷ Twin Lab CoQ 10 30mg. 2x daily or CSA for lower back pain as needed.
with
Quercetin with bromelain 500mg.

▷ Solaray CALCIUM CITRATE 1000mg.
with
Ascorbate vitamin C with bioflavonoids and rutin 5000mg. daily for connective tissue formation.

▷ Country Life LIGATEND capsules as needed daily, and/or RELAXER caps as needed .

▷ Enzymatic Therapy MYOTONE capsules for muscle pain and weakness.

▷ Twin Lab GABA PLUS caps daily.

▷ B Complex 100mg. with ENER B internasal B12.

▷ Mezotrace SEA MINERAL CMPLX., or Prof. Nutr. Dr. SUPER MINERALS.

HERBAL THERAPY

☙ Effective analgesic herbs:
◆ Valerian/wild lettuce - sedative and anti-spasmodic.
◆ White willow bk. - anti-inflammatory and analgesic.
◆ Cramp bark - cramping.
◆ Passion flower - gentle sedative.
◆ St. John's wort - nerve damage.
◆ Wild yam - anti-inflammatory.
◆ Yucca -anti-inflammatory.

☙ Crystal Star formulas for pain:
◆ ANTI-FLAM™ caps to relieve inflammation.
◆ BACK TO RELIEF™ caps for lower back, general and cerebro-spinal pain.
◆ ANTI-SPZ™ caps 4 at a time, or CRAMP BARK COMBO™ extract for spasmodic and muscle pain.
◆ STRESSED-OUT™ tea, STRESSED OUT™ and DEPRESS-EX™ extracts, and RELAX™ caps 2 at a time, as needed for nerve pain and tension.
◆ AR EASE™ caps and tea, and Rth TONE™ extract for joint pain.
◆ VALERIAN/WILD LETTUCE extract as a sedative for pain.
◆ ULCR™ caps and extract for stomach pain.

BODYWORK

➤ Chiropractic adjustment, shiatsu massage, biofeedback, acupuncture, and massage therapy are all effective in controlling pain.

➤ Effective compresses:
→ Plantain/marshmallow
→ Comfrey
→ Lobelia

➤ Effective oil rubs:
→ Mullein
→ Tea tree
→ TIGER BALM
→ Wintergreen/cajeput
→ B&T ARNI-FLORA gel.

➤ Acupressure: pinch and massage webs between the thumb and index finger to reduce pain.

➤ Reflexology point:

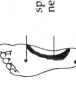

spine
nerves

Common Symptoms: Sharp shooting twinges or a dull ache; muscle wasting; poor reflexes; numbness; soreness in the sensory nerves.
Common Causes: Poor posture; poor nutrition with lack of green vegetables and calcium-rich foods; an over-acid diet that eats away protective mucous membrane and nerve sheathing; poor muscle development; adrenal and pituitary gland exhaustion; flat feet; obesity; internal or external tumors or growths.

PARASITES ◼ INTESTINAL WORMS
Giardia ✧ Amoebic Dysentery ✧ Stomach Bacterial Infection

Worm and parasite infestations can range from mild and hardly noticeable to serious and even life-threatening in a child. Worms are parasites that live and feed in the intestinal tract. Other parasites seem to be able to move all over the body, including the brain, weakening the entire system. Nutritional therapy is a good choice for thread and pin worms, but is very slow in cases of heavy infestation. Short term allopathic treatment is often more beneficial for masses of hook and tape worms and blood flukes.

FOOD THERAPY

☙ Go on an apple juice fast and mono diet for 4 days. (One day for a child) ☺
 ◆ Take 8 garlic caps daily during and chew fresh papaya seeds mixed with honey frequently.
 ◆ On the 3rd day, add papaya juice with 1 TB. wormwood tea, and 1 TB. molasses.
 ◆ On the 4th day, add 2 cups senna/peppermint tea with 1 TB. castor oil, and eat a handful of raw pumpkin seeds every 4 hours.
 ◆ After worms are gone, eat a high vegetable protein diet and lots of cultured foods, such as yogurt.

☙ A high resistance diet must be followed to prevent recurrence. Eat lots of onions and garlic. Avoid sweets, pasteurized milk and refined foods. Eat a green salad every day. No junk foods!

☙ Herbal fast to expel tapeworms: ☺
 Mix 4 oz. cucumber juice with honey and water. Take only this mixture for 24 hours. Follow with 3 cups senna/ pumpkin seed tea. Drink down all at once to use as a cathartic.

VITAMINS/MINERALS

▶ Take garlic oil capsules in the morning. Refrain from eating or drinking until bowels have moved. Repeat for 3 days.

▶ Am. Biologics DIOXYCHLOR as directed for giardia infestation.

▶ Nutri-biotic GRAPEFRUIT SEED extract internally as directed.

▶ Nature's Way HERBAL PUMPKIN formula. ♂

▶ Floradix HERBAL IRON liquid for strength during healing.
 with

▶ B Complex 50mg. daily. ♀ ☺

▶ Beta carotene 50,000IU daily as an anti-infective.

▶ Aloe vera juice 2-3 glasses daily.

▶ Dr. DOPHILUS or other multi-culture powder, 1/2 teasp. 3x daily before meals to rebuilding intestinal flora.

HERBAL THERAPY

☙ Take psyllium husk and/or Sonné bentonite in water 3x daily, and 2 cups daily senna tea to purge.

☙ Black walnut extract 4-6x daily.
 with
 Barberry tea as an anti-infective.

☙ Solaray GARLIC/BLACK WALNUT capsules. ♀

☙ Crystal Star VERMEX™ capsules, 4 daily with 2 garlic capsules, after every meal for 2 weeks, and 4 cups fennel tea daily.
 and/or
 Crystal Star ANTI-BIO™ caps 4 daily as an anti-infective and lymph flush.

☙ Effective vermifuge herbs:
 ◆ Black walnut
 ◆ Valerian
 ◆ Chaparral
 ◆ Wormwood/tansy
 ◆ Chamomile
 ◆ Pau de arco
 ◆ Echinacea rt.
 ◆ Mullein oil
 ◆ Myrrh extract

BODYWORK

▶ Garlic enemas daily as needed during healing.

▶ Apply zinc oxide to opening of anus. Then take a warm sitz bath using 1 1/2 cups epsom salts per gallon of water. Repeat for 3 days. Worms will often expel into the sitz bath.

▶ For crabs and lice; apply
 ↠ Thyme oil
 ↠ Sassafras oil
 ↠ Tea tree oil
 ↠ Myrrh extract and tea tree oil mixed.

Common Symptoms: Round worms: fever, cough and intestinal cramping. **Hookworms:** anemia, abdominal pain, diarrhea, lethargy, malnutrition and even under development in children. **Whipworms:** abdominal pain, diarrhea; **blood flukes:** cause lesions on the lungs and hemorrhages under the skin - typical in AIDS cases. **Protozoa,** such as amoebae cause arthritis-like pain, leukemia-like symptoms, and weaken the whole system. They can also coat the inside lining of the small intestine and prevent absorption of nutrients from food, causing life-threatening malnutrition. **Tapeworms:** intestinal obstruction, gas and distress (even from a single worm). Tapeworm eggs in the liver cause such illness that they have been mistaken for and treated with chemotherapy as if they were cancer. Giardia is the most prevalent parasite in the U.S. - the number one cause of water-borne disease. It causes diarrhea, weakness, weight loss, abdominal cramping, bloating and fever.
Common Causes: Lowered immune defenses allowing infestation; poor diet with too much sugar and refined carbohydrates (junk foods); too much red meat; poor hygiene; fungal and yeast overgrowth conditions; infested, uncooked, poorly cooked, or spoiled meat.

PARKINSON'S DISEASE

Parkinson's disease is a degenerative central nervous system dysfunction characterized by a fine, slowly spreading tremor, muscular weakness and body rigidity. Normal posture, walking gait and movement are affected. L-dopa, the drug of choice for Parkinson's has serious hallucinatory side effects.

FOOD THERAPY

🥄 Go on a completely fresh foods diet for 3 days to cleanse and alkalize the body. Use organically grown foods wherever possible.

♠ Then, follow a modified macrobiotic diet (pg. 52) for 3-6 months until condition improves.

♠ Use short 24 hr. juice fasts (pg. 44) with aloe vera juice each morning once every two weeks during healing to accelerate toxin release.

🥄 Live cell therapy from green drinks and chlorella has been notably successful in reducing symptoms. Take green drinks (pg. 55ff) frequently, at least twice a week, and/or Sun CHLORELLA once a day.

🥄 Drink only bottled water.

🥄 Make a mix and take 2 TBS. daily:
  ♣ Lecithin granules
  ♣ Brewer's yeast

🥄 Eat smaller meals more frequently. No large heavy meals.

🥄 See ANEMIA and M.S. DIET suggestions in this book for more information.

VITAMINS/MINERALS

If taking L-Dopa, do not take vitamin B6.

▶ Twin Lab GABA plus, or Co. Life RELAXER caps as needed.
  or
DLPA 500-750mg. as needed for depression.

▶ Pycnogenol 50mg. 3x daily, and Lysine 500mg. daily. (Parkinson's victims are historically low.)

▶ Tyrosine 500mg. 2x daily for L-Dopa production.
  with
Solaray EUROCALM to aid in serotonin formation.

▶ High Omega 3 flax or fish oils 3x daily, and/or phosphatidyl choline (PC 55) 2 daily.

▶ Vital Health FORMULA 1 advanced chelation w/ EDTA 2 packs daily.

▶ Niacin therapy: 500mg. 2x daily, with B Complex 100mg., extra B6 500mg. daily if not taking L-dopa, and Ener B internasal gel every other day.

▶ Nature's Plus Vitamin E 800IU with magnesium 500mg. ♀

▶ Enzymatic Therapy RAW BRAIN and ADRENAL COMPLEX.

HERBAL THERAPY

🌿 Evening primrose oil caps 4-6 daily, or Source Naturals MEGA GLA, with
Crystal Star RELAX CAPS™ to rebuild nerve sheath, and STRESSED OUT™ extract or WITHDRAWAL SUPPORT™ caps to ease shakiness.
  and
MENTAL CLARITY™ caps or ginkgo biloba extract for brain and tremor
  or
Then ADR-ACTIVE™ caps with SYSTEM STRENGTH™ drink to restore strength.

🌿 Ginseng/royal jelly vials daily. ♂
  or
Unsprayed bee pollen 2 teasp. daily. ♂

🌿 Solaray GINSENG/DAMIANA and CAYENNE/GINSENG formulas.

🌿 Hawthorne extract for increased circulation, and a feeling of well-being.

🌿 Effective teas:
  ◆ Pau de arco
  ◆ Crystal Star FEEL GREAT™
  ◆ Sun SIBERIAN GINSENG
  ◆ Sage

BODYWORK

▶ Chiropractic treatment, shiatsu, acupuncture and acupressure have had some success in reversing early Parkinson's.

▶ Take long warm baths. Crystal Star LOVE BATH FOR MEN has had some success.

▶ Use catnip enemas once a week to encourage liver/kidney function.

▶ Avoid aluminum (cookware, deodorants with aluminum chloride, condiments with alum, etc.) and heavy metals that lodge in the brain and nerve centers.

▶ Reflexology point:

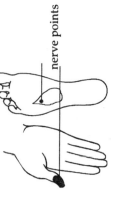

nerve points

Common Symptoms: Central nervous system dysfunction affecting normal posture and movement; brain abnormality; muscle rigidity and lethargic movement; speech difficulty; vision problems; expressionless face; numbness and tingling in the hands and feet; depression (which can show dramatic improvement with supplementation); continuous tremor.
Common Causes: Poor diet causing malnutrition; aluminum or heavy metal toxicity; over-use of some drugs; allergy reaction; nerve malfunction; poor diet allowing degeneration

PHLEBITIS

Blood Clots ✦ Embolism ✦ Thrombosis

Phlebitis is vein inflammation, usually in the legs. An embolism is the obstruction of a blood vessel by a foreign substance or blood clot. Thrombosis is the existence of a blood clot within the vascular system. Deep vein thrombosis is life-threatening because the clot can occlude a vessel and prevent blood supply to an organ or part. Get medical help immediately!

FOOD THERAPY

ò Have one glass of each every other day:
♦ Black cherry juice
♦ Fresh carrot juice
♦ Crystal Star ENERGY GREEN™ drink or other green drink (pg. 54ff).

ò Drink 6-8 glasses of bottled water daily.

ò Make a mix and take 2 TBS. daily:
♣ Lecithin granules
♣ Brewer's yeast

ò Avoid all starchy, fried and fatty foods. Avoid refined sugars, caffeine and hard liquor.

ò Eat plenty of onions, garlic and other high sulphur foods. Have an onion/garlic broth at least 2-3x week (pg. 58). Have a leafy green salad every ay.

ò See HEALTHY HEART DIET in this book for more information.

ò Crystal Star BIOFLAV., FIBER & C SUPPORT™ drink for venous integrity.

VITAMINS/MINERALS

▶ Nature's Plus vitamin E 800IU to keep body oxygen in good compound form.

▶ Bromelain 500mg. 2 daily, and/or Quercetin Plus as an anti-inflammatory for fragile veins.

▶ Twin Lab CSA capsules as directed for anti-thrombogenic and anti-coagulant activity.

▶ Free radical scavenging antioxidants:
♣ Biogenetics BIOGUARD PLUS 6 daily.
♦ Pycnogenol 50mg. 3x daily.
♦ Ascorbate vitamin C crystals with bioflavs and rutin, ¼ teasp. daily to bowel tolerance.
♣ Germanium 100mg. daily, or 150mg. SL.

▶ High omega 3 flax oils 3 daily. ♂

▶ Niacin therapy: 500mg. 3x daily, with
Chromium picolinate 200mcg. ♀ or Solaray CHROMIACIN daily.

▶ Enzymatic Therapy SPLEEN & LYMPH COMPLEX.

HERBAL THERAPY

ò Butcher's broom capsules or tea or Crystal Star HEARTSEASE/CIRCU-CLENZ™ tea with butcher's broom,
and
HEARTSEASE/HAWTHORNE caps or hawthorne extract 2-4x daily.

ò Crystal Star GREEN TEA CLEANSER™ or kukicha tea w. ANTI-FLAM™ as needed. ♀
and
Health Concerns POWER MUSHROOMS, or reishi mushroom capsules.

ò Evening primrose oil 4-6 daily, with
Crystal Star HEARTSEASE/ANEMIGIZE™ caps

ò Solaray CENTELLA VEIN, with hawthorne extract 3x daily.

ò Effective herbal bioflavonoids:
♦ Bilberry extract
♦ Echinacea extract
♦ Enzymatic Therapy HERBAL FLAVONOIDS caps. ♀

ò Take tienchi ginseng tea, and apply Crystal Star GINSENG SKIN REPAIR GEL W. C™.

BODYWORK

▶ Elevate legs whenever possible. Consciously stretch and walk frequently during the day. Keep weight down to relieve pressure on circulatory system.

▶ Tale a brisk half hour walk daily.

▶ Avoid smoking and secondary smoke. It constricts blood vessels and restricts oxygen use.

▶ Avoid chemical anti-coagulants and oral contraceptives unless absolutely necessary.

▶ Take alternating hot and cold sitz baths, and/or apply alternating hot and cold ginger/cayenne compresses to stimulate leg blood circulation.

▶ Effective applications:
→ B&T ARNICA GEL.
→ B&T CALIFLORA gel
→ Care Plus OXYGEL.

▶ Effective compresses:
→ Plantain
→ Witch hazel
→ Fresh comfrey leaf

Common Symptoms: Swelling, inflammation; redness and aching in the legs; pain and tenderness along course of a vein; swelling below obstruction.
Common Causes: Clogged and toxic bloodstream from excess saturated fats, especially from too much red meat and fried food; inactivity, lack of daily exercise, and sedentary life style; poor circulation from constipation, obesity or weak heart; oral contraceptive side effect; prolonged emotional stress.

PITUITARY, PINEAL & HYPOTHALAMUS GLANDS

The pituitary is called the "master gland" because it controls all gland secretions. It is a miraculous, pea-sized "micro-chip" that retards aging, releases energy, controls reproduction governs kidney function, blood sugar metabolism and water retention. Pituitary secretions affect all physical body growth and weight distribution functions. **The hypothalamus** has a unique rapport with the pituitary in dictating all gland functions, acting as a kind of relay station for the entire body. **Pineal gland** is the third eye of the body, a means of looking inward - and its development affects metaphysical understanding, and higher consciousness thinking. It is also of primary importance to the endocrine, skin pigmentation and lymphatic systems. Together they are the age barometer of the body. Sunlight is key to the health and activity of these glands, particularly as they use it to increase longevity.

FOOD THERAPY

🥬 Eat plenty of green leafy vegetables every day. Have a green drink (pg. 54ff) or Sun CHLORELLA drink, or Crystal Star ENERGY GREEN™ drink for blood & oxygen building, once a week.

🥬 Eat plenty of complex carbohydrates; broccoli, potatoes, sprouts, peas, dried fruits, whole grains and brown rice, etc.

🥬 Have plenty of fresh fruit juices.

🥬 Drink only bottled water.

🥬 Avoid beer, sweet wines, refined flour, sugar, heavy pastries, and canned foods. Avoid all MSG-containing foods and preserved foods.

VITAMINS/MINERALS

▶ Mezotrace sea mineral complex, 1 daily working up to 3-4 daily.

▶ Vitamin C or Ester C with bioflavonoids and rutin, 550mg. 4x daily. with Choline or phosphatidyl choline.

▶ Alta Health SIL-X silica capsules 2 daily, and MANGANESE w/ B₁₂.

▶ B Complex 100mg. daily, with extra B6 250mg. and PABA 1000mg. daily. and Argenine/ornithine caps 500/500mg. daily for growth hormone release and anti-aging. ♂

▶ Enzymatic Therapy RAW PITUITARY caps 4 daily. ♀

🐝 Ener B12 internasal gel every other day.

▶ Future Biotics VITAL K 3x daily.

HERBAL THERAPY

🌿 Crystal Star GINSENG 6 DEFENSE RESTORATIVE™ super tea or capsules 2x daily, with IODINE SOURCE™ caps or extract for brain potassium and iodine.

🌿 YS royal jelly and honey drink mix daily with Crystal Star SILICA SOURCE™ extract.

🌿 Effective teas:
- ◆ Alfalfa
- ◆ Burdock
- ◆ Horsetail/oatstraw
- ◆ Crystal Star MEDITATION™ tea
- ◆ Licorice rt.
- ◆ Saw palmetto ♂

🌿 Crystal Star ENDO-BAL™ for overall gland activity.

🌿 Solaray ALFAJUICE caps.

🌿 Solaray gotu kola / damiana caps 4 daily. ♂

BODYWORK

▶ Acupressure points: Press for 10 seconds, 3x each over the left eyebrow for pituitary stimulation; on the forehead where the eyebrows meet for pineal stimulation.

▶ Reflexology points:

pituitary
pineal

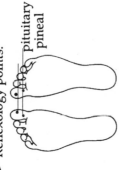

▶ Aromatherapy:
→ Bergamot oil

▶ Pituitary, pineal, hypothalamus area:

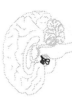

Common Symptoms: Fatigue; mental stress; lack of growth and/or poor growth; inability to understand metaphysical or higher consciousness concepts; gastritis and ulcers; obesity and water retention; recurrent diarrhea; poor enzyme and digestive action.
Common Causes: Excessive stress, emotional pressure and adrenal exhaustion; heavy metal toxicity (the pituitary is particularly vulnerable, and is affected first of all the glands); hypoglycemia; diabetic, pancreatic, and sugar regulation abnormalities; poor nutrition, especially protein deficiency.

BACTERIAL PNEUMONIA ▨ VIRAL PNEUMONIA ▨ PLEURISY

Pneumonias and pleurisy are inflammatory lung diseases caused by a wide spectrum of mico-organisms or chemical irritants. Bacterial pneumonia, usually caused by staph, strep or pneumo-bacilli responds to antibiotics, both medical and herbal. Viral pneumonia is an acute systemic disease, caused by a variety of virulent viruses, and does not respond to antibiotics. Herbal antivirals have shown some success. Pleurisy is an inflammation of the pleura membrane surrounding the lungs, and often accompanies pneumonia.

FOOD THERAPY

See Lung Disease page in this book for more suggestions.

🍃 Go on a mucous-cleansing liquid diet for 1-3 days during the first and acute stages. (pg. 42).

✿ Take a hot lemon and honey drink with water each morning.

✿ Have a fresh carrot juice a potassium broth (pg. 53) or Crystal Star SYSTEM STRENGTH™ broth daily.

✿ Drink plenty of fruit juices, herb teas and bottled water to thin mucous. Avoid alcohol.

✿ Then follow a largely fresh foods, cleansing diet for 1-2 weeks.

✿ Then eat a diet high in vegetable proteins, low in meat, dairy and animal fats, to allow lungs to heal easily. Add cultured foods, such as yogurt and kefir.

🍃 Take fresh grated horseradish root in a spoon with lemon juice. Hang over a sink immediately to expel large quantities of mucous.

🍃 Include Crystal Star BIOFLAV., FIBER & C SUPPORT™ daily for a month to 6 weeks of healing.

🍃 Apply a mustard plaster to chest to stimulate lungs and draw out poisons: Mix 1 TB. mustard pdwr., 1 egg, 3 TBS. flour and water to make a paste. Leave on until skin turns pink.

VITAMINS/MINERALS

▶ Ascorbate vitamin C crystals with bioflavanoids and rutin, $1/4$ teasp. every half hour to bowel tolerance, daily for 2 weeks; then every 2 hours for 2 weeks; then 3000mg. daily for another month.
with
Beta carotene 150,000IU or vit. A 75,000IU ☺ daily and vitamin E 400IU 2x daily, for the first 2 weeks.

▶ Effective anti-oxidants:
❋ Care Plus H2O2 OXYGEL rubbed on the chest daily, and/or taken internally, $1/2$ teasp. in a glass of water 2x daily for a week.
❋ CoQ 10 30mg. 3x daily.
❋ Pycnogenol 50mg. 6 daily.
❋ Germanium 150SL 2 daily.
❋ Vitamin E 1000IU daily.
❋ Unipro liquid DMG 2x daily. ♂

▶ Effective extracts:
❋ Rainbow Light blue/green algae
❋ Sun Chlorella WAKASA extract
❋ Raw lung and raw thymus
❋ Garlic 4-6x daily.

▶ Am. Biologics INFLAZYME FORTE as an anti-infective with a full spectrum pre-digested amino acid complex daily for extra protein, *and* a strong enzyme formula, such as Rainbow Light DETOX-ZYME.

HERBAL THERAPY

🌿 Crystal Star ANTI-BIO™ caps or extract (or ANTI-VI™ extract or tea for viral pneumonia) 6x daily to flush toxins, with FIRST AID CAPS™ to sweat out mucous.

🌿 Crystal Star RSPR™ caps and tea w. ANTI-HST™ extract after crisis has passed to heal lungs and encourage oxygen uptake.

🌿 Cayenne/ginger/goldenseal caps 6 daily. ♀
or
Excel Ephedra extract formulas for bronchial dilation. ♂

🌿 Effective extracts:
◆ Echinacea/goldenseal.
◆ Hawthorne as needed daily.
◆ St. John's wort extract caps. ♀
◆ Lomatium/hypericum. ♂
◆ Mullein/Lobelia. ☺

🌿 Effective bacterial pneumonia teas:
◆ Ephedra
◆ Comfrey/fenugreek
◆ Slippery elm
◆ Pleurisy root

🌿 Effective herbal diuretics:
◆ Uva Ursi/cornsilk combination
◆ Senna/dandelion combination

BODYWORK

Do not risk your health if you experience major difficulty in breathing. Short term heroic medicine may be necessary. We have found CIPRO to be broad spectrum, effective and less harmful to normal body functions than most primary medical drugs. Ask your physician.

▶ Get plenty of rest. Do conscious diaphragmatic breathing - esp. when recovering. Breathe in, pushing abdomen out, then from chest to completely fill upper and lower lungs.

▶ Apply a cayenne poultice: Mix $1/2$ teasp. cayenne, 1 TB. lobelia, 3 TBS. slippery elm and enough water to make a paste. Leave on 1 hour.

▶ Take an oxygen bath. Use 1-2 cups food grade H2O2 to a tub of water. Soak 20 minutes.

▶ Take hot and cold showers to stimulate lung circulation (pg. 49). Then use chest percussion with a cupped hand front and back to loosen matter.

▶ Reflexology points:

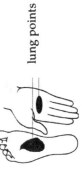

lung points

Common Symptoms: Inflamed lungs and chest pain; aggravated flu and cold symptoms; swollen lymph glands; difficult breathing; heavy coughing and expectoration; back, muscle and body aches; chills and high fever; sore throat; inability to "get over it"; fluid and lymph in lungs; great fatigue which remains for six to eight weeks even after recovery.
Common Causes: Low immunity from poor nutrition; a preceding respiratory infection from a virus or bacteria; clogged lymph nodes; chemical sensitivity or allergy, especially to pesticides and herbicides; body stress and fatigue, especially from a long day outdoors in winter.

POISONING, FOOD

Arsenic ◇ Salmonella ◇ Botulism

Even with all our government inspections, advanced packaging, refrigeration and chemical food preservers, poisoning from food still affects millions of people every year, and often leads to serious or chronic diseases. Natural protective food supplements can help you avoid many pathogenic organisms.

FOOD THERAPY

🌿 Take 1/2 cup olive oil very slowly through a straw to remove poison from the stomach area *or* take a glass of warm water with 1 teasp. baking soda.

♦ Take no milk, fruit juice, alcohol or vinegar until poison has moved out of the stomach.

♦ Eat largely fresh foods for a week after poisoning to rebalance the system.

🌿 Effective neutralizers:
♦ 1-2 heads of iceberg lettuce
♦ Bamboo shoots
♦ Strong black tea
♦ Burnt toast
♦ Lemon water
♦ 2 raw eggs
♦ Milk of magnesia
♦ Onions and garlic

🌿 Effective protectors against pesticides and poisons in food:
♦ high fiber foods, citrus fruits, wheat germ, whole grains, dark green and yellow vegetables.

🌿 Use Am. Biologics DIOXYCHLOR or NutriBiotic GRAPEFRUIT SEED extract in water as directed to decontaminate foods.

VITAMINS/MINERALS

▶ **Activated charcoal tabs to absorb poison; 3 to 5 every 15 minutes.**
and/or
Ascorbate vitamin C powder, 1/2 teasp. every 1/2 hour to bowel tolerance to flush and alkalize the tissues.

▶ Niacin therapy to sweat out poisons; 250-500mg. every hour until improvement is felt (about 3-4 capsules). ♂

▶ Protector supplements against food poisons:
✦ Acidophilus caps or powder before meals.
✦ Vit. E with selenium 400IU
✦ Vit. C with bioflavs and rutin
✦ Beta carotene 25-50,000IU
✦ Biogenetics BIOGUARD enzymes-SOD w/ catalase
✦ Glutathione 50mg.

▶ Natures Life CAL-MAG LIQUID, phos. free.

▶ Rainbow Light food sensitivity system if there are allergies.

🌿 Enzymatic Therapy LIVA-TOX capsules 3 daily.

HERBAL THERAPY

🌿 Crystal Star CLEANSING & PURIFYING™ tea as needed, several times daily.
and/or
ENERGY GREEN™ drink or Sun CHLORELLA drink or tabs, 5 to 10 every 4 hours to neutralize, with Bach Flower RESCUE REMEDY to rebalance the system.

🌿 Effective teas:
♦ Plantain
♦ Scullcap
♦ Elecampane
♦ Wormwood
♦ Yellow dock/nettles for arsenic poisoning.

🌿 Solaray MONTMORILLITE CLAY caps or bentonite clay powder as directed.

🌿 Herbal protectors:
♦ Garlic caps 2 with each meal.
♦ Kelp tabs 8-12 daily. ♀

🌿 Take a glass of aloe vera juice morning and evening for a week after poisoning to cleanse the digestive tract.
and use
Apple pectin caps. ♂

BODYWORK

➤ Use an emetic of *Ipecac*, or strong lobelia tea with 1/4 - 1/2 teasp. cayenne, to throw up poisons and empty the stomach.
→ Follow with white oak tincture to neutralize and normalize the stomach.

➤ Use a coffee or catnip enema to flush the bowel and stimulate liver detox function.

➤ Sweat out pesticides and poisons in a long, low heat sauna.

➤ Overheating therapy is effective. See P. Airola "How To Get Well" or page 49 in this book for correct technique.

Common Symptoms: Nausea and vomiting; cold sweats after eating; severe indigestion, abdominal pain and flatulence; severe headache; hot flushes followed by chills; diarrhea; red, rashed skin.
Common Causes: Harmful bacteria in food; pesticides and fungicides; food additives and preservatives; sulfites; food allergy reaction; MSG; breathing noxious fumes; lack of proper cleaning of cutting boards and food preparation areas in both restaurants and homes.

POISONING, HEAVY METALS

Lead ◇ Cadmium ◇ Mercury ◇ Radiation

Heavy metal poisoning is becoming a major problem of modern society. There seems to be no way to get away from toxic exposure. Periodic system detoxification needs to be a part of life so that the body can use its own cleansing mechanisms to maintain healthy immune response.

FOOD THERAPY

Note: Do not go on an all-liquid diet when trying to release heavy metals or chemicals from the body. They enter the bloodstream too fast and too heavily for the body to handle, and can poison you even more.

🍃 Go on a seven day brown rice and vegetable juice diet (pg. 44) to start releasing poisons from the body. Have one each of the following daily:
  ♦ a glass of fresh carrot juice
  ♦ a potassium broth (pg. 54)
  ♦ miso soup
  ♦ George's ALOE VERA JUICE.

🍃 Take a green drink (pg. 55ff) or Crystal Star ENERGY GREEN™ or SYSTEM STRENGTH™ drinks as detoxifiers and blood builders.

🍃 Eat organically grown fresh foods as much as possible. Avoid canned foods.

🍃 Make a mix and take 2 TBS. daily:
  ♦ Brewer's yeast
  ♦ Wheat germ
  ♦ Lecithin granules

🍃 Drink only bottled water. Avoid caffeine - it inhibits liver filtering function.

VITAMINS/MINERALS

▶ Glutathione 500mg. 2 daily
    with
Enzymatic Therapy LIVA-TOX caps.

▶ Protective antioxidants:
  ✿ Pycnogenol 50mg. 3x daily.
  ✿ CoQ10 10mg. 3x daily.
  ✿ Vit. E 400Iu w/ selenium

▶ Protective nutrients:
  ✿ Beta carotene 150,000IU
  ✿ Future Biotics VITAL K.
  ✿ Solaray SELENOMETHIONINE
  ✿ Alta Health SELENIUM PLUS
  ✿ Zinc 50-100mg. daily.
  ✿ Liquid chlorophyll 1 teasp. every 4 hours.

▶ Ascorbate vitamin C powder, 1/2 teasp. every hour to bowel tolerance daily as a tissue flush.
    with
Solaray CALCIUM CITRATE 6 daily, or Nature's Life CAL-MAG PHOS. FREE liquid.

▶ Biogenetics BIOGUARD PLUS S.O.D. w/catalase, 6 daily.

▶ Vital Health FORMULA 1 oral chelation/EDTA 2 pkts. daily. ♂

HERBAL THERAPY

See pages 40 on neutralizing the effects of chemotherapy and radiation.

🍃 Evening primrose oil caps 4 daily with 2 cysteine caps each time.

🍃 Yerba Prima aloe vera juice with herbs, 1 glass every 4 hours.

🍃 Pau de arco tea or milk thistle extract every 4 hours, or Crystal Star LIV-ALIVE™ tea.

🍃 Crystal Star HEAVY METAL™ or DETOX™ caps for 2-3 months, with CLEANSING & PURIFYING™ tea.

LIV-ALIVE™ and IODINE THERAPY™ caps 2-6 daily. ♀

🍃 Effective herbal protection:
  ◆ Astragalus extract ♂
  ◆ Kelp 8-10
  ◆ Garlic 6-8
  ◆ Siberian ginseng extract caps

🍃 Sun CHLORELLA or Green Foods GREEN MAGMA 10-20 daily, (especially to overcome radiation/chemotherapy toxins); spirulina, 8 daily for chemical toxins. Start at a low dose, and work up.

BODYWORK

▶ For chemical burns; apply a green clay poultice.

▶ Avoid antacids - they interfere with enzyme production, and the ability of the body to carry off heavy metals.

▶ Avoid smoking and secondary smoke, pesticides and fungicides, phosphorus fertilizers, fluorescent lights, aluminum cookware and deodorants, electric blankets; microwave ovens, and non-filtered computer screens whenever possible.

▶ Signs and signals that you may be chemically toxic:
  → You can smell things better than most people.
  → You can't tolerate alcohol well.
  → Perfumes and strong cleansers bother you.
  → There are many medications you can't take, and even some vitamins make you feel worse.
  → You feel worse in certain stores.
  → Your reaction time when driving is noticeably poorer in city traffic.

Common Symptoms: Seizures; schizophrenic-like, uncontrolled psychotic behavior as poisons react in the system; memory loss and senility; infertility and impotency; insomnia; small black spots along gum line; bad breath and body odor as the body tries to throw off the alien substances.
Common Causes: Improperly metabolized build up of industrial pollutants and other toxic chemicals in the body; nicotine; insecticides; dental fillings; over-treated water; copper paints and pipes; hair dyes; aluminum cookware and deodorants; smoke and smog; zinc depletion.

POISON OAK

Individual allergic reaction to this systemic poison can range from a mild, annoying itch to a life-threatening condition.

FOOD THERAPY

⚘ Apply cider vinegar, denatured alcohol, or a cornstarch paste to blisters to control itching and neutralize acid poisons.

⚘ Follow a fresh foods diet during acute blistering to cleanse systemic poisons out of the bloodstream.

⚘ Take several green drinks during acute phase (pg. 54ff).

⚘ Apply oatmeal to rash areas to neutralize toxins.

VITAMINS/MINERALS

▶ Ascorbate vitamin C crystals, ¼ teasp. every hour to bowel tolerance, til itching lessens, then reduce to ¼ teasp. 4x daily until clear.

▶ Wright Pathways NO SCRATCHUM.

▶ Nutribiotic GRAPEFRUIT SEED extract. Take internally. Apply locally.

▶ Effective topicals:
   ♣ Liquid chlorophyll
   ♣ Care Plus OXY GEL
   ♣ Vitamin E oil
   ♣ Nature's Life CAL-MAG liquid.

▶ Enzymatic Therapy CORTO-TONE caps, with DERMAZYME ointment.

▶ Homeopathic *Rhus Tox.*

▶ Hylands homeopathic poison oak tabs to build immunity against poison oak.

HERBAL THERAPY

❧ Effective topicals:
   ◆ Comfrey/aloe salve
   ◆ Tea tree oil ☺
   ◆ B & T CALIFLORA gel
   ◆ Calendula ointment
   ◆ Witch hazel
   ◆ Echinacea cream
   ◆ Plantain

❧ Crystal Star P.O. #1 and P.O. # 2 capsules alternately as directed. ☺

❧ Crystal Star ANTI-HST™ capsules 4-6 daily until clear, to help the liver produce natural antihistamines.

❧ Crystal Star ADRN™ extract or ADR-ACTIVE™ caps 2x daily, to strengthen the adrenal glands as a protection factor.

❧ Black walnut tincture. Apply locally. Take internally.

❧ Jewelweed tea. Apply locally. Take internally.

BODYWORK

➤ Take epsom salts baths.

➤ Swim in the ocean if possible, as effective neutralizing therapy.

➤ Effective applications: wash off in cold water first.
   ↠ Aloe vera gel or aloe ice gel. ♂
   ↠ Chinese WHITE FLOWER OIL.
   ↠ Pau de arco gel.
   ↠ Rubbing alcohol.

Common Symptoms: Itching, burning blisters on the skin that ooze, erupt and spread the systemic plant poisons.

♂ PROSTATE ENLARGEMENT & INFLAMMATION ■ BENIGN PROSTATIC HYPERTROPHY (BPH) ♂

With BPH, the disease is basically the symptoms - see below.
Note: Some studies are showing that a man should think twice before having a vasectomy, because of the increased risk of prostate cancer among vasectomized men. As sperm builds up in the sealed-off vas deferens, the body reabsorbs it and sometimes tries to mount an autoimmune response to its own tissue. In addition, the testes are a powerful focal point of the life force of a man. When something interferes with the movement of sperm, energy flow is blocked, eventually resulting in stagnation and degeneration. A vasectomy can also result in a liver blockage that leads to prostate inflammation, leg cramps, lower abdomen pain and irritability.

FOOD THERAPY

☙ Take lemon juice and water every morning to cleanse sediment; then cider vinegar and honey in water daily to prevent recurrence.

☙ Follow a fresh foods diet the first week of healing with lots of leafy green salads, sea vegetables, fresh fruits, juices and steamed vegetables.
♣ Then, add simply cooked whole grains, and sea foods for 3 weeks. Keep the diet very low in fats.
♣ Drink 6 to 8 glasses of water or cleansing fluids every day to keep the system free and flowing.

☙ Make a mix and take 4 tbs. daily:
♣ Lecithin granules
♣ Wheat germ
♣ Pumpkin seeds
♣ Oat bran
♣ Brewer's yeast flakes
♣ Sesame seeds
♣ Crumbled dry sea vegetables

☙ Avoid red meats, caffeine, hard liquor, carbonated drinks, and tomato juice during healing.
Avoid tobacco, and all fried, fatty and refined foods forever.

VITAMINS/MINERALS

▶ Zinc 100mg. daily for 1 month, then 50mg. daily for 1 month with B6 200mg.
with
Marine carotene 100,000IU to control infection; Nature's Plus vitamin E 800IU daily.

▶ Ascorbate vitamin C crystals, 1/2 teasp. every hour to bowel tolerance daily for 2 weeks, then 1/2 teasp. 4x daily for 2 weeks, then 3000mg. daily for 1 month.

▶ High omega 3 fish or flax oils 3x daily to lower cholesterol levels.
and
Bromelain 500mg. 2x daily for faster healing and enzyme therapy.

▶ Effective brand products:
✦ Enzymatic Therapy NUCLEO-PRO M caps for prevention.
✦ Nature's Life ZINC/COPPER caps
✦ Solaray PYGEUM or PROSTA-GEUM capsules.
✦ Co. Life PROSTA-MAX caps.

▶ Amino acid therapy:
✣ GABA for night time urination
✣ Glycine for sediment control
✣ Glutamine 500mg. daily.

HERBAL THERAPY

❧ Crystal Star PROX CAPS™ or PROX™ extract 4-6 daily as needed for 1 month, then 2-4 daily for 1 month, and RELAX™ caps to relax nerves and facilitate urination; take with
Evening primrose oil caps 4-6 daily for 1 month, then 2-4 daily for 1 month with bee pollen 2 daily.
and
ANTI-BIO™ or ANTI-FLAM™ as needed to reduce inflammation and infection;
then
MALE PERFORMANCE™ caps for area regeneration; IODINE SOURCE™ caps or extract for prevention, with vitamin E 400IU.

❧ Effective prevention herbs:
◆ Echinacea/goldenseal extract
◆ White oak bk.
◆ Kelp 6-8 daily
◆ Bee pollen 2-4 daily
◆ Pau de arco
◆ Saw palmetto berries
◆ Damiana
◆ Parsley rt.

❧ Sun CHLORELLA 20 tabs daily for prevention.

❧ Biotec CELL GUARD 6 daily for prevention.

BODYWORK

Sexual intercourse during prostatitis will irritate the prostate and delay recovery. After recovery sex life should be normal in frequency and in desire with a natural climax. Avoid prolonged sex or interrupted climax.

▶ Use chamomile tea enemas (pg. 49) once a week during healing to cleanse the body of harmful acids.
Or take warm chamomile sitz baths for 20 minutes at a time morning and evening.

▶ Apply ice packs to reduce pain.

▶ A brisk daily walk is important.

▶ Avoid chemical antihistamines. Overuse impairs liver function, that then results in prostate trouble.
Also note: the new Merck PROS-GUARD drug that shrinks the swelling of the prostate gland also decreases potency and libido, and in some cases stifles it entirely.

▶ Reflexology point:

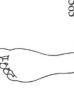

coccyx & prostate

Common Symptoms: Inflamed, swollen, infected prostate gland, under the scrotum and testes; frequent, painful desire to urinate with reduced flow of urine; incontinence in severe cases; fever; lower back and leg pains; impotence, and/or painful ejaculation; loss of libido; unusual sleepiness and/or fatigue.
Common Causes: Poor diet with too little fiber, and too many over-acid, or spicy foods; too much alcohol and caffeine; EFA and prostaglandin depletion; exhausted lymph system from too many over-the-counter antihistamines; internal congestion and poor circulation; lack of exercise; zinc deficiency; venereal disease.

RHEUMATIC FEVER

Rheumatic fever is a serious strep infection that affects small children. The severe inflammation can affect the heart or brain; pain and stiffness often settle in the joints. Rheumatic fever can be prevented if the strep virus is killed within ten to twelve days of infection, because it will not have become virulent enough in that time to overwhelm the body's own immune defenses. Homeopathic treatment is very effective in this initial phase, (see a homeopathic physician) and may be taken even if chemical antibiotics are already being used.

FOOD THERAPY

 Adhere to a fresh juice and liquid diet for the first bedridden stages of healing to reduce body work and strain.
 ♣ Take potassium broth or essence, and apple/alfalfa sprout juice daily during acute period.
 ♣ Take Vegex yeast broth and miso soup daily for B vitamins and strength.

 Then eat fresh and mildly cooked foods, including plenty of sea foods and vegetable protein from whole grains, tofu, sprouts, etc.

 Take only small meals.

 Drink only bottled water.

 Avoid all sugars, salty and refined foods during healing. Keep fats low. No fried foods. No caffeine or carbonated drinks during healing.

VITAMINS/MINERALS

Remember to reduce doses for children. ☺

 Ascorbate vitamin C crystals with bioflavonoids, 1/4 teasp. every hour in juice, to bowel tolerance during acute periods, then reduce dosage to 3-5000mg. daily. ☺
  with
 Beta carotene 50-100,000IU daily as an anti-infective, and

 Raw thymus extract. ☺

 Cartilade SHARK CARTILAGE caps 2 daily to as an antiviral.

 Effective anti-oxidants:
 ♣ Vitamin E 4-800IU daily. ♀
 ♣ Co. Life B₁₅ DMG SL
 ♣ Germanium 30mg. 3x daily.
 ♣ CoQ 10 30mg. daily

 Solaray SELENOMETHIONINE for liver health, and Dr. DOPHILUS powder 1/4 teasp. in water 3x daily.

 Ener B12 internasal gel every other day.

 High potency royal jelly 2 teasp. daily. ♂

HERBAL THERAPY

❦ Evening primrose oil caps 4 daily, with Crystal Star ANTI-BIO™ caps 4 daily for at least a month. Then HEARTSEASE HAWTHORN™ caps, *or* BODY REBUILDER™ and ADR-ACTIVE™ caps, with GINSENG 6 DEFENSE RESTORATIVE™ SUPER TEA to strengthen the system against recurrence.

❦ Garlic tabs 6 daily.

❦ Sun chlorella or Green Foods GREEN MAGMA granules, one packet daily.

❦ Lobelia or dandelion extracts. ☺

❦ Apply wintergreen oil compresses to chest. Take wintergreen/ white willow tea internally.

BODYWORK

➤ Plenty of bed rest is a key. Yoga and mild muscle-toning exercises, and/or massage therapy during confinement (which can last for several weeks) will prevent loss and atrophy of body strength.

➤ Take a catnip enema once a week to reduce fever.

➤ Do not use aspirin as an antiinflammatory. Notify dentist of rheumatic heart disorder if having an extraction or anesthesia for any reason.

Common Symptoms: Extreme weakness; heart weakness affecting joints and skin; shortness of breath; poor circulation and lack of blood flow.
Common Causes: Holes in the heart ventricles; inflammation of the main circulatory system; allergic reaction; low immunity, especially in children; often accompanied by acute viral disease; toxic exposure to harmful chemicals, environmental pollutants, or radiation.

SCHIZOPHRENIA ▓ PSYCHOSIS ▓ MENTAL ILLNESS

Tardive Dyskinisia

Schizophrenia is a form of psychosis that exhibits severe perception disorder, characterized by hallucinations, delusions, extreme paranoia, and disturbed thought content. Personal relationships are abnormal, work is almost impossible, and the schizophrenic often withdraws emotionally and socially. Anti-psychotic drugs can do more harm than good. **Tardive dyskinisia** is a side effect disorder, with slow, rhythmical, involuntary movements, caused exclusively by neuroleptic drugs used to treat schizophrenia and psychosis. It is bizarre in that the symptoms themselves are similar to a psychosis. Over 70% of the patients taking antipsychotic drugs develop this grim disorder. Natural therapies are very successful in reversing TD.

FOOD THERAPY

🍃 Start with a short liquid, juice and cleansing diet to normalize blood levels (pg. 42). Minimize fruit juices if hypoglycemia is involved.
♣ Then, eat largely fresh foods for the remainder of the week.
♣ Then, gradually add vegetable proteins, gluten-free grains (especially brown rice, millet and amaranth), sea foods, fish, nuts and seeds.
♣ Eliminate all refined sugars, red meats and preserved foods.

🍃 Make a mix and take 2 TBS. daily:
♣ Brewer's yeast
♣ Lecithin granules

🍃 Take Crystal Star BIOFLAV., FIBER & C SUPPORT ™ drink daily.

🍃 A diet for hypoglycemia has been very successful in controlling schizophrenia. See the Hypoglycemia Diet suggestions in this book for more information.

VITAMINS/MINERALS

◗ Ascorbate vitamin C powder with bioflavonoids and rutin, 1/2 teasp. every hour to bowel tolerance daily for the first month of healing. (Vitamin C is a natural tranquilizer. It will help in withdrawal from chemical tranquilizers and drugs.)

◗ Logic LITHIUM as directed.

◗ Niacin therapy: 1-3000mg. or Solaray CHROMIACIN daily. (A baby aspirin before taking will remove niacin flush). ♂

◗ Glutamine 1000mg. and tyrosine 1000mg. 2x daily.

◗ B Complex 150mg. with extra B6 500mg., B1 250mg. 3x daily, and B12 2500mcg SL daily. ♀

◗ Phosphatidyl Choline (PC55) 3x daily for anxiety and depression, with zinc 50mg. 2x daily, and Twin Lab GABA 500mg 2x daily. ♂

◗ Effective for tardive dyskinesia:
✦ Alta Health MANGANESE w. B12
✦ Niacin 500mg. 3x daily.
✦ B6 200mg. 2x daily.

HERBAL THERAPY

🍃 Evening primrose oil caps 4-6 daily for prostaglandin balance.

🍃 Crystal Star RELAX CAPS™ as needed for nerve rehabilitation; WITHDRAWAL SUPPORT™ caps for tardive dyskinesia.
with
IODINE SOURCE™ caps or extract, and/or DEPRESS-EX™ extract caps 6-8 daily.
and
ADR-ACTIVE™ caps or FEEL GREAT™ caps or tea for balance. ♀

🍃 ATOMODINE drops 2-3x daily, or kelp tabs 6-8 daily.

🍃 Effective teas:
♦ Sage ♂
♦ Gotu kola
♦ Prickly ash

🍃 Body balancing and calming herb:
♦ Sun CHLORELLA 20 tabs daily.
♦ Country Life MOOD FACTORS as needed. ♂

BODYWORK

➤ Get some exercise every day, especially running, walking or jogging. The oxygen will do wonders for your head.

➤ Regular massage therapy and spinal adjustment have had some success.

➤ Take ocean walks for sea minerals, or a visit to a mineral-rich spring and spa are effective.

➤ Avoid all pleasure drugs, and as many prescription drugs as possible. For many people, permanent brain change and psychosis can result.

Common Symptoms: Severe mental depression; lethargy; emotional swings, often to violent actions; delusions and hallucinations; detachment from reality.
Common Causes: Hypoglycemia; diabetes; severe gluten and/or dairy allergies; heavy metal toxicity, particularly too high copper levels; general poor nutrition with too many junk foods, and refined sugars causing constipation and autotoxemia; prescription and/or pleasure drug abuse; vitamin B12 deficiency; iodine deficiency; elevated histamine levels; hypothyroidism; glandular imbalance; when occurring in young children, schizophrenia is sometimes caused by a virus or other trauma experienced during the 2nd trimester of pregnancy.

SCIATICA

Neuritis of the sciatic nerve, characterized by sharp, shooting pain running down the back of the thigh. The inflammation is arthritic in nature - extremely sensitive to weather change and to the touch. See NEURITIS/NEURALGIA page for more information.

FOOD THERAPY

🍃 Take a potassium broth or essence (pg. 53) every other day for a month to rebuild nerve health.

🍃 Have a leafy green salad every day. Take a little white wine with dinner to relieve tension and nerve trauma.

🍃 Eat calcium and magnesium rich foods, such as green vegetables, sea vegetables, shellfish, tofu, whole grains, molasses, nuts and seeds.

🍃 Take a good natural protein drink, such as one from page 63, or Nature's Plus SPIRUTEIN daily.

🍃 Drink bottled mineral water, 6-8 glasses daily.

VITAMINS/MINERALS

▶ Country Life LIGATEND capsules as needed.
with
Vitamin E 400IU daily.

▶ Quercetin Plus 3-4 daily with bromelain 500mg. as an anti-inflammatory.

▶ Cal/mag/zinc 4 daily, with vitamin D 400IU.

▶ Homeopathic *Mag. Phos.* tabs.

▶ Ascorbate vitamin C or Ester C with bioflavonoids and rutin, 3-5000mg. daily for connective tissue development.

▶ DLPA 500-750mg. 2x daily as needed for pain.

▶ B Complex 100mg. with extra B1 100mg., B6 250mg., niacin 250mg., and Future Biotics VITAL K liquid 3 teasp. daily. ♀

HERBAL THERAPY

❦ Crystal Star RELAX CAPS™ as needed for rebuilding the nerve sheath, with ANTI-FLAM™ as needed for inflammation.
and
CALCIUM SOURCE™ caps or extract on a regular basis. ♀

❦ Mix wintergreen, cajeput, rosemary oils. Massage into area.

❦ Liquid chlorophyll 3 teasp. daily with meals.
or
Wakunaga KYO-GREEN one packet daily, for nerve rebuilding.

❦ Mezotrace sea mineral complex 4 daily.

❦ Garlic/parsley caps 4-6 daily.

BODYWORK

▶ Apply alternating hot and cold, or hops/lobelia compresses to stimulate circulation.

▶ Reflexology point:

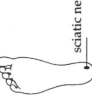

sciatic nerve

▶ Massage therapy and chiropractic adjustment are both effective.

▶ Apply ice packs or *wet* heat to relieve pain.

▶ Gentle morning and evening stretches, and daily yoga exercises are effective.

▶ Take hot epsom salts baths.

▶ Effective topical applications:
➤ Aloe MINERAL ICE gel, or ALOE ICE gel.
➤ Olive oil
➤ TIGER BALM
➤ Chinese WHITE FLOWER oil
➤ B & T TRIFLORA gel.

Common Symptoms: Severe pain in the leg along the course of the sciatic nerve - felt at the back of the thigh, running down the inside of the leg; lower back pain; muscle weakness and wasting; reduced reflex activity.
Common Causes: Compression of the sciatic nerve resulting from a ruptured disc or arthritis, an improper buttock injection; poor posture and muscle tone; poor bone and cartilage development; exhausted pituitary and adrenal glands; menopause symptoms; obesity; lack of exercise; high heels; protein and calcium depletion; not enough green vegetables; flat feet.

SEASONAL AFFECTIVE DISORDER

S.A.D. makes people sad. Work effectiveness is noticeably reduced, and relationships suffer. New studies are showing that it affects a large group of people, usually manifesting itself in the winter when sunlight is low. It is a result of the pineal gland not receiving enough light stimulation to stop secreting melatonin. The eating and energy loss aspects of this disorder also show a tie between psychological well-being and nutritional factors as they affect our nervous system and behavior. The natural healing community is just beginning to address SAD - the suggestions below have shown effectiveness.

FOOD THERAPY

Conscious diet improvement is the main key to reducing SAD symptoms.

❧ Make sure you are following a balanced diet with natural foods, rich in complex carbohydrates, and low in fats and sugars. Include B-vitamin and mineral-rich foods, such as brown rice and fresh vegetables. Whole grains, legumes and soy products will help control cravings.
♣ Take a brewer's yeast supplement daily, such as Lewis Labs, or BioStrath as a source of B vitamins and chromium.
♣ Add seafoods and especially sea vegetables to the diet for absorbable vitamin D and beta carotene.

❧ A diet for hypoglycemia has been effective. See the HYPO-GLYCEMIA DIET in this book for more information.

VITAMINS/MINERALS

▶ Take natural A & D supplements all during the winter.
♣ Am. Biologics EMULSIFIED A & D 2x daily.
♣ Twin Lab ALLERGY D, or A & D.
♣ Solaray A & D 25,000/1,000.

▶ B Complex 100mg. daily with extra B₁ 100mg. and B₆ 200mg. daily.
with
Chromium picolinate 200mcg. daily to control blood sugar levels and normalize brain chemistry.

▶ A well-balanced multi-vitamin/mineral such as Rainbow Light COMPLETE NUTRITONAL SYSTEM, Living Source MASTER NUTRIENT SYSTEM, or Country Life MAXINE and MAX for men and women.

▶ Rainbow Light CALCIUM PLUS w. high magnesium 2x daily. ♀

▶ Glutamine 500mg. 2x daily.

▶ Effective Homeopathic remedies: ☺
♣ *Sepia 30x*
♣ *Sulfur 30x*

HERBAL THERAPY

❧ Pineal/pituitary gland stimulation is a key factor:
◆ Rosemary ♀
◆ Crystal Star MEDITATION™ tea.
◆ Parsley/sage tea ♂
◆ Ginkgo biloba extract 3 x daily.

❧ Evening primrose oil 4 daily for brain electrical connections. ♀

❧ Effective herbal neurotrasmitter stimulants:
◆ Alfalfa
◆ Cayenne
◆ Dandelion

❧ Ginsengs are key whole body nutrients:
◆ Crystal Star SUPER GINSENG 6™ tea and capsules.
◆ Crystal Star ROYAL MU™ tea ♂
◆ Ginseng/gotu kola capsules.

❧ Effective herbal brain foods:
◆ Royal jelly 2 teasp. daily
◆ Kelp tabs 6 daily
◆ Gotu kola

BODYWORK

Shutting off melatonin secretion through exposure to light can prevent or reduce SAD symptoms. Indoor and fluorescent light is not effective. Full-spectrum light is necessary.

▶ Get some *outdoor* exercise every day, especially running, walking or jogging. Light is a nutrient that will do wonders for your pineal gland. The oxygen will do wonders for your head.

Common Symptoms: Unexplained depression and mood swings; unusual sleepiness, poor sleep and/or fatigue; increased appetite, carbohydrate craving and weight gain;
Common Causes: Not enough full spectrum light, especially during winter months; hormone imbalance that results in unusual diet cravings (especially sweets) and weight gain.

Reduced or inhibited sexual desire can stem from many reasons, both psychological and physical. For many of us these days, lack of time to turn our attention to our partners and body love seems to be the biggest problem. Both women and men today are beleaguered with family and home care, career responsibilities, sports and activities that require all our energy, and leave us only able to collapse at the end of every day. This page offers some natural sexual energy tonics to turn your thoughts and mood to love.

FOOD THERAPY

☙ Lack of normal libido can often be overcome simply by improving a poor diet. Junk foods, chemical and processed foods are a key factor in the body's not feeling "up to it". A whole and fresh foods diet definitely encourages more zest for life.

☙ Add mineral-rich foods to the diet: shellfish, leafy greens, sea vegetables, whole grains, nuts, legumes, and molasses.

☙ Avoid red meats; keep saturated fats, salt and sugar low. They all inhibit the free-flow of the system.

☙ While there are no real "aphrodisiac foods", there are some "vitality" foods that have the extra energy nutrients needed for healthy sex and desire: broccoli, whole grains, brewer's yeast, spinach, peas, oysters, salmon and other sea foods, eggs, cantaloupe, carrots, soy products and cinnamon.

VITAMINS/MINERALS

Male:

▶ Effective anti-oxidants:
 ♣ B15 DMG liquid or SL tablets.
 ♣ Germanium 150mg. SL daily.
 ♣ Zinc 50mg. 2x daily with lecithin caps for healthy seminal fluids.

▶ Liquid niacin before sexual intercourse seems to be effective for men.

▶ Carnitine 500mg. 2x daily, with Strength Systems ORCHIC TEST extract and SMILAX PLUS.

▶ Country Life MAX capsules daily.

Female:

▶ Vitamin E 800IU daily with lecithin caps, or Crystal Star WOMEN'S DRYNESS™ for vaginal fluids.

▶ PSI PROGEST cream.

▶ B15 DMG liquid or SL tablets.

▶ Tyrosine 500-1000mg., and/or phenylalanine 500mg, or Nature's Plus PIZZAZZ (liquid phenylalanine)

▶ Highest potency YS royal jelly 60,000-120,000mg. daily.

Both:

▶ Country Life ADRENAL w. TYROSINE tabs.

HERBAL THERAPY

Male:

❦ Yohimbe casules 750-1000mg. to stimulate testosterone (*Do not take yohimbe if you are taking diet products containing phenylpropanolamine, or have heart, kidney or liver disorders.*)

❦ Crystal Star LOVING MOOD EXTRACT FOR MEN, and/or LOVE CAPS MALE™ 2-4 daily as needed.

❦ Effective stimulants:
 ◆ BioForce ginsavena extract
 ◆ Highest potency YS royal jelly 60,000-120,000mg. daily.
 ◆ Scandinavia EXSATIVA
 ◆ PEP COBRA tabs
 ◆ Ginseng/Sarsaparilla caps

Female:

❦ Crystal Star LOVE CAPS FEMALE™ 2 daily, or dong quai/damiana extract for several days before a special weekend.

❦ Yohimbe 500mg. capsules. (See above for contra-indications.)

Both:

❦ Ginseng combinations:
 ◆ Jade Medicine SAGES GINSENG
 ◆ Ginseng/damiana, 4 as needed.
 ◆ Crystal Star CUPID'S FLAME™ or GINSENG 6 SUPER tea or caps.

BODYWORK

➤ Crystal Star LOVE BATHS FOR MEN & WOMEN.

➤ Exercise can increase sex drive, especially when you do it together. Regular exercise such as dancing, walking, and swimming stimulates circulation and increases body oxygen.

➤ Hypnotherapy has been effective when the problem is psychologically based.

➤ Many drugs, both pleasure and prescription, can have the side effect of impaired sex drive. Take a good look at any you may be using.

Common Symptoms: Impotence; frigidity; lack of normal sexual interest.
Common Causes: Dissatisfaction with one's life, age, looks, etc.; emotional stress and tension from job, relationship unhappiness, or life style; poor diet resulting in physical malfunction; lack of exercise; childhood abuse and trauma; prescription and/or pleasure drug reaction.

SEXUALLY TRANSMITTED DISEASES ■ VENEREAL DISEASE

Herpes Genitalis ✧ Syphilis ✧ Gonorrhea ✧ Chlamydia ✧ Venereal Warts - HPV (Human Papilloma Virus) ✧ PID (Pelvic Inflammatory Disease)

Diseases that are transmitted from an infected partner during intercourse or other contact with the sex organs. They are widespread and increasingly virulent in today's world, reaching epidemic proportions in some segments of society. Treatment must be swift and vigorous to avoid severe, degenerative, and sometimes life-threatening consequences. The following natural therapies have been effective as an alternative to massive doses of medical antibiotics which end up destroying much immune balance in the G.I. and genito-urinary tract. But, as with other modern opportunistic diseases, a strong immune system is the best treatment and the only defense. (See the following pages, page 208 and page 175 for more information.)

FOOD THERAPY

🍃 Follow a very cleansing liquid diet for 3-7 days (pg. 42) during acute stages. Take one each of the following juices daily:
   ✦ Potassium broth (pg. 53).
   ✦ Fresh carrot juice
   ✦ A green drink (pg. 54ff)
   ✦ Apple/parsley juice

🍃 Then continue with a cleansing fresh foods diet. Include several bunches of green grapes daily (an old remedy that still works).

🍃 Avoid refined, starchy, fried and saturated fat foods. Avoid red meats, pasteurized dairy products, and caffeine during healing.

🍃 For venereal warts:
   ✦ Apply aloe vera gel locally. Take George's ALOE VERA JUICE internally 2 glasses daily.

VITAMINS/MINERALS

▶ Beta carotene 150,000IU daily, with Vitamin C crystals $1/2$ teasp. every hour to bowel tolerance during acute phase, reduced to 5000mg. daily for a month.
   and
   Vitamin E 400IU 2x daily.

▶ Liquid Chlorophyll 3 t.easp. daily before meals, with echinacea extract.
   or
   Sun CHLORELLA 1 packet daily.

▶ Solaray MULTI-DOPHILUS powder, $1/2$ teasp. 6x daily.

▶ Raw thymus glandular daily.

▶ For venereal warts:
   ✦ Enzymatic Therapy ACID-A-CAL capsules.
   ✦ Raw thymus glandular daily.
   ✦ Germanium 100mg. as an effective wound-healing antioxidant.
   ✦ Lysine cream and lysine caps 1000mg. 3x daily.
   ✦ Cartilade SHARK CARTILAGE 2-4 daily as an anti-viral agent.
   ✦ Am. Biologics emulsified A & E.

HERBAL THERAPY

🌿 Crystal Star ANTI-BIO™ or ANTI-VI™ formulas 4-6 x daily, with Crystal Star WHITES OUT™ #1 & #2 capsules alternately as needed.

🌿 Effective extracts; may be applied locally and taken internally:
   ✦ White oak bark ♂
   ✦ Sarsaparilla ♂
   ✦ Black walnut
   ✦ Lomatium
   ✦ Gotu kola
   ✦ Mandrake - dilute tincture

🌿 Crystal Star DETOX™ capsules for 1 month, 2-4 daily. May also be opened and applied to sores.

🌿 Effective blood cleansing herbs:
   ✦ Pau de arco
   ✦ Red clover/burdock rt.
   ✦ Oregon grape/gentian/lobelia
   ✦ Calendula tea 3 cups daily

🌿 For venereal warts:
   ✦ Crystal Star ANTI-VI™ capsules 4 daily, with FIRST AID CAPS™ to raise body temperature during acute stages; one week off and one week on until improvement is felt.

BODYWORK

Strong doses of antibiotics are the usual medical treatment, but the most recent outbreaks (especially in teenagers) are showing resistance and non-response to these drugs.

▶ Overheating therapy is very effective in controlling virus replication. Even slight body temperature increases can lead to considerable reduction of infection. See Airola "How To Get Well" or page 49 in this book for effective technique.

▶ Bathe sores several times daily in a goldenseal/myrrh solution.

▶ For venereal warts:
   ↪ Care Plus H₂O₂ 3% dilute solution, (1 TB. in 8oz. of water) daily for a month; then rest for a month, and resume if necessary. If noticeable improvement has occurred in this first month, returning to this treatment may not be necessary. The body's defense forces will have taken over and can better continue on their own.

Note: If sores are also in the mouth, treat as for thrush. See Thrush Fungal Infection page in this book.

Common Symptoms: *Symptoms usually appear two to three weeks after sexual contact.* **Gonorrhea:** cloudy discharge for both sexes; frequent, painful urination, yeast infection symptoms; pelvic inflammation. **Syphilis:** *First contagious stage;* sores on the genitalia, rash and patchy, flaky tissue, fever, mouth sores and chronic sore throat. **Chlamydia:** thick, vaginal discharge in both men and women, urethritis; pelvic pain, sterility. Can cause birth defects if present during pregnancy. **PID:** microorganisms sexually transmitted, but infection can also enter during miscarriage treatment, childbirth, surgery, or endometrial biopsy. Symptoms extend from a discharge to a chronic dull ache and pain in lower abdomen. **Venereal Warts:** genital warts (HPV) - the most common STD; sexually transmitted, *extremely contagious.* Symptoms can be latent and unknown by infected party; can infect ovaries, fallopian tubes, cervix, and uterus. Chronic yeast infection with heavy, pus-filled discharge; pain during intercourse; painful, infected, and often bloody sores in the genital area; high fever when infected, often leading to brain damage. Linked to cervical cancer - triggered by co-factors of birth control pills, smoking, herpes and other STD's.

HERPES GENITALIS

Herpes is a highly infectious viral disease of the skin and mucous membranes around the genitals. Transmission is by direct contact with infected fluids from saliva, skin discharges, or sexual fluids. Incubation is two to ten days after exposure; a typical outbreak lasts from one to two weeks. After the initial infection, the virus never leaves, but becomes dormant in the nerve ganglia. Recurrent outbreaks may be triggered by emotional stress, poor diet, food allergies, menstruation, drugs and alcohol, sunburn, fever, or a minor infection. Men are more susceptible to recurrence than women. Outbreaks are opportunistic in that it takes over when immunity is low and stress is high. Optimizing immune function is of primary importance.

FOOD THERAPY

☙ Go on a short 3 day cleanse (pg. 42) to alkalize the body. Have plenty of fruit juices, and a carrot/beet/cucumber juice or potassium broth (pg. 53) each day. Take 2 teasp. sesame oil daily.

☙ Then keep the diet consciously alkaline with miso soup, brown rice and vegetables frequently. Add cultured vegetable protein foods such as tofu and tempeh for healing and friendly G.I. bacteria. Increase consumption of fresh fish (rich in lysine).

☙ **Avoid all sweets, alcohol, refined carbohydrates, and arginine-forming foods, such as nuts, corn, tomatoes, caffeine, cereals, gelatin desserts, and legumes. Reduce dairy intake, especially hard cheeses, and red meat.**

☙ Avoid citrus fruits during healing.

VITAMINS/MINERALS

▶ Apply lysine cream frequently. Take lysine 500mg. capsules 4-6 daily until clear.

▶ Dr. Diamond HERPANACINE capsules as directed, with raw thymus extract.

▶ Homeopathic *Cantharis* for symptom relief.

▶ DR. DOPHILUS 1 teasp. 6x daily.

▶ Quercetin Plus w. bromelain for instant inflammation relief.
   with
   B Complex 100mg. 2x daily, tyrosine 500mg., and extra pantothenic acid 500mg, and B12 2000mcg.

▶ Ascorbate vit. C or Ester C powder $1/4$ teasp. every hour in water up to 10,000mg. or to bowel tolerance daily during an attack.

▶ Beta carotene or emulsified Vitamin A 50,000IU daily, with Vit. E 400IU 3x daily. Also apply vitamin E oil directly. ♂

▶ Enzymatic Therapy ACID-A-CAL caps, with egg yolk lecithin capsules as directed.

HERBAL THERAPY

☙ Crystal Star HRPS™ capsules 4 daily, with ANTI-FLAM™ caps or extract, ♀ and/or ANTI-VI™ extract for 7 days to overcome virus.
   with
   LYSINE/LICORICE GEL™ applied topically as needed.

☙ Locally pat on sores Crystal Star THERADERM™ tea or CALENDULA GEL, ♀ or open a Crystal Star ANTI-BIO™ capsule and apply directly to sores. ♂

☙ Effective applications to lesions:
   ◆ Black walnut tincture
   ◆ Myrrh tincture
   ◆ Echinacea extract - also take 1 dropperful orally every 2 hrs.
   ◆ Aloe vera/goldenseal solution.

☙ Effective herbal neutralizers:
   ◆ Dandelion/sarsaparilla rt.
   ◆ Ligustrum
   ◆ Astragalus

☙ An effective herpes tea: dandelion rt, sarsaparilla rt, astragalus, ligustrum, echinacea rt.

☙ St. John's wort extract capsules as an antiviral.

BODYWORK

▶ Apply ice packs to lesions for pain and inflammation relief. Ice may also be applied as a *preventive measure* when the sufferer feels a flare-up coming on.

▶ Get some early morning sunlight on the sores every day for healing Vit. D.

▶ Take hot baths frequently for overheating therapy. (pg. 49)

▶ Wear cotton underwear.

▶ Practice stress reduction techniques to prevent outbreaks.

▶ Cortico-steroid drugs taken over a long period of time for herpes greatly weakens both the immune system and bone density.

▶ Effective applications:
   → Nutribiotic GRAPEFRUIT SEED EXTRACT spray.
   → Crystal Star LYSINE/LICORICE gel.
   → Lithium oitment or solution.
   → BioForce echinacea cream.
   → Body Essentials SILICA GEL.

▶ Acupuncture is effective for herpes.

Common Symptoms: Painful, fluid-filled rupturing blisters that leave red inflamed painful lesions on thighs, genitals, and face; discomfort urinating; vaginal or urethral discharge.
Common Causes: Transmitted from kissing, oral sex, intercourse; excess arginine in the body; too many drugs; an acid-forming diet; hormone imbalance related to the menstrual cycle.

STDs and Birth Control

Contraceptive methods and sexually transmitted diseases must be considered together. Unless you are in a long-term relationship, in which you are absolutely sure that your partner is faithful, you should take precautions against STDs. Even if you know your partner is monogamous you should be careful. Once a virus gets into your system, it never goes out. Sometimes people carry diseases from previous relationships and don't know it, or don't want to share the fact with a new partner. When considering your sexual lifestyle choices, remember that AIDS can kill you; herpes and HPV, (the virus that induces genital warts) are permanent. These STDs may become dormant, but they do not leave the body. Even others, that are not permanent, cause a great deal of pain and can leave you permanently infertile. There are risks and benefits to every method of contraception, but the risks of sexually transmitted disease, abortion or unwanted pregnancy are obviously greater. Both partners, but especially women, need to earnestly evaluate their life styles, sexual discipline and partner's attitudes to make a responsible health choice.

Barrier methods - condom, diaphragm, cervical cap and vaginal sponge - have become the most popular contraceptive devices since the advent of the AIDS epidemic. The latex (not lambskin) condom is the only method that offers almost complete protection from STDs. It encourages couples to share responsibility for birth and disease control. It should not, however, be used without a back-up , because the high failure rate from breakage, heat or wear is almost 15%. To guard against pregnancy, a spermicide should be used in conjunction with a condom.

Because the pill shifted the responsibility for contraception from men to women, condom use has, unfortunately, become less common - especially among teenagers, where the greatest STD infection is being experienced. Young, unsophisticated lovers tend to think of the condom as a barrier to sexual enjoyment rather than as a part of a mature, responsible relationship. The new female condoms, polyurethane ringed sheaths that fit over the cervix, have been conceived to address this problem. They are comfortable, the effectiveness rate is high, and they can be inserted ahead of time, but have the disadvantage of hanging slightly outside the vagina. However, they do give the woman the choice, if the man refuses to wear a condom - and they do protect against STDs.

The diaphragm, fitted correctly, used with spermicide, without any tiny holes or cracks is an effective, unobtrusive method of birth control, and does provide some protection against STDs. Unfortunately, many sensitive women get bladder infections from the rubbing of the diaphragm against the urethra, and yeast infections from the spermicide that must be used.

The cervical cap is used with spermicidal jelly to create a seal that prevents sperm penetration and inactivates sperm for contraception. It is effective for 48 hours at a time, and effective for birth control if inserted properly, but not effective against STDs.

The vaginal sponge is a simple device, impregnated with spermicide, that is inserted in the back of the vagina, and is effective for 24 hours. It is not a good choice for women who have had children, however, or for sensitive women who experience irritation from a large dose of spermicide. In addition, it has often become a cause of toxic shock syndrome when the women was unable to remove the sponge or when fragments remained.

Spermicides - creams, jellies, suppositories and foams put into the vagina to kill or immobilize sperm. They have some ability to kill sexually-transmitted viruses, but should always be used in conjunction with a barrier method of contraception.

Hormonal contraceptives - although today's pills have much lower doses of hormones, overcoming many of the life-threatening side-effects, increased risk of breast cancer is still a controversy, and many women are still sensitive to the synthetic estrogen impact. High blood pressure, migraine headaches, depression, water retention, thrush, gum inflammation and changes in skin pigmentation are still frequent short-term effects - and of course the pill does not protect against STDs. Hormone implants are surgically inserted into the skin of a woman's upper arm, and release very small doses of hormone into the bloodstream. Even in these substantially smaller amounts of synthetic hormone there are still some side effects of irregular menstruation, intra-period spotting, headaches, depression. They are effective birth control for five years, but do not protect against STDs.

Sterilization is the most common form of contraception in America, and also the most rapidly increasing, as the sexually active population ages past child-bearing years. A tubal ligation is a procedure where hormones, ovulation and menstruation continue as usual, but the egg disintegrates in the tubes and is absorbed by the bloodstream. Side effects are irregular bleeding, increased menstrual pain and excessively heavy periods, to the point in some cases that a hysterectomy becomes necessary to stop the bleeding. A vasectomy is a procedure where the tubes that carry the sperm to the penis are cut and tied. The man can continue to ejaculate semen without sperm, but many questions about side effects and long-term hormone imbalances are now being raised. (See page 302, Prostate Enlargement, for more information.) Neither sterilization form protects against STDs.

IUDs have fallen from favor because of their many complications, increased risk of infertility, and adverse health effects. The most recently discovered is that the string on an IUD acts as a wick for germs, thus spreading vaginal bacteria, including sexually transmitted diseases such as gonorrhea, into the uterus.

SHINGLES ▦ HIVES

Shingles are the eruption of acute, inflammatory, herpes-type blisters on the trunk of the body along a peripheral nerve. The condition is virally caused and the blisters are infectious. Since the virus is the same as that causing chicken pox, there is proneness to shingles if one had chicken pox as a child. Hives are the same type of itching blisters, but caused by an allergic reaction to a chemical or food. Both are very painful, inflammatory skin conditions. See Herpes, page 309 in this book for more information.

FOOD THERAPY

🍃 Go on a short 3 day cleansing diet to eliminate acid wastes and alkalize the blood (pg. 43).

♦ Take a carrot/beet/cucumber juice, and a natural cranberry juice each day. Take an apple juice or celery juice each night.

♦ Then, eat only fresh foods for 1-2 weeks, with lots of alkalizing salads and fruits.

🍃 Keep the diet consciously alkaline, with plenty of miso soup, brown rice, vegetables and leafy greens. Eat foods high in B vitamins, such as brown rice, green vegetables and brewer's yeast.

🍃 Include cultured foods, such as yogurt and kefir for friendly G.I. flora.

🍃 Avoid acid-forming foods, such as red meats, caffeine, fried foods, and carbonated drinks.

🍃 Eliminate food with preservatives, additives and colorings. Avoid refined foods, sugars, aspirin, tetracyclines, and meats that can contain nitrates and nitrites.

VITAMINS/MINERALS

▶ **Stress B complex 200mg. with extra B6 250mg. and B12 2500mcg.** with

Lysine 1000mg, and apply LYSINE PLUS cream to blisters.

▶ Quercetin with bromelain for instant action against inflammation. with

Phosphatidyl choline (PC 55)

▶ Propolis tincture or lozenges 2-3x daily.

▶ Ascorbate vitamin C or Ester C powder with bioflavs., 1/4 teasp. every hour in water up to 10,000mg. or bowel tolerance daily during an attack, then reduce to 5000mg. daily until blisters heal.

▶ **Emulsified A & D 50,000/1,000IU 2x daily,** with

Vit. E 400IU 3x daily. Apply E oil directly. ♂

▶ Enzymatic Therapy HERPILYN PLUS capsules. ♀

▶ DLPA 750mg. for pain.

HERBAL THERAPY

🌿 Crystal Star THERADERM™ or HRPS™ capsules. and

THERADERM™ tea, internally, and topically, patted on blisters to neutralize acids coming out through the skin. with

RELAX CAPS™ to rebuild strong nerve structure.

🌿 Crystal Star ANTI-VI™ tea 2-4 cups daily, with high omega 3 flax oil 3 teasp. daily.

🌿 Effective teas:
♦ Alfalfa
♦ **St. John's wort extract**
♦ Red clover/nettles
♦ Burdock rt.
♦ Reishi mushroom

🌿 Kelp tabs 6-8 daily with cayenne caps, 2 daily.

🌿 Effective topical applications:
♦ BioForce ECHINACEA cream
♦ **Aloe vera/golden seal solution or ointment.**
♦ **B & T CALIFLORA gel**
♦ Calendula gel
♦ Crystal Star LYSINE/LICO-RICE™ skin gel.

BODYWORK

▶ Effective topical applications to relieve pain:
→ Petroleum jelly.
→ Flax seed compresses.
→ B&T SSSTING STOP gel.
→ B & T TRIFLORA analgesic gel.

▶ Take epsom salt or oatmeal baths to neutralize acids.

▶ Get early morning sunlight on the body for healing vitamin D.

▶ Remember that cortico-steroid drugs taken over a long period of time for shingles, weaken the immune system, allowing future attacks.

▶ Relaxation and tension control techniques are effective. Stress creates an acid body condition, and erodes protective nerve sheathing.

▶ Avoid acetaminophen pain killers such as Tylenol, that can aggravate the blisters.

Common Symptos: Swollen red skin blisters, usually around the upper part of the body; pain radiating along one or several nerves preceding outbreaks; attacks last from 2 days to 2 weeks, leaving irritated nerves even after blisters are gone; accompanied by fever, weakness, chills and nausea.
Common Causes: Food allergies, esp. to milk , shellfish, wheat, MSG, food additives and preservatives; over-chlorined drinking water; stress; adrenal and/ or liver exhaustion; histimine reaction; acidosis and HCl depletion; poor circulation and constipation; too many prescription drugs; too much caffeine or hard liquor.

SHOCK ✳ TRAUMA

Shock is the condition that develops when blood flow is reduced below the levels needed to maintain vital body functions. Obviously, shock and trauma can happen during serious injuries or illnesses where a great deal of blood and other body fluids are lost. But it can also occur during severe infections, allergic reactions (such as anaphylactic shock), and malfunction of the nervous system (such as a severe reaction to a poisonous insect or snake bite).

Every significant injury is accompanied by some degree of shock, because the autonomic nervous system responds to the trauma of injury by altering blood flow. It is usually wise to treat any severely injured person for shock in addition to treating them specifically for the injury. If there is lots of bleeding, major burns, or a head wound, treatment for shock should be very high priority.

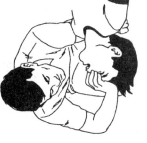

Have the person lie down with legs elevated slightly above the head. Don't bend the legs. Loosen clothing at neck, waist and chest. Protect the person from extremes of warmth and cold. If there is a chance of serious or life-threatening injury, do not move the person. Give small sips of fluids only if fully conscious - no solid food.

Get medical care immediately!

The following emergency measures are beneficial until medical help arrives:

✔ Deva Flowers FIRST AID remedy, homeopathic *Arnica Montana*, or Bach Flowers RESCUE REMEDY; 2-4 drops on the tongue every 5 minutes until breathing normalizes.
✔ Crystal Star RECOVERY TONIC™ drops on the back of the tongue every 10 minutes until breathing and heart rate normalize.
✔ Cayenne solution in water (1-3 teasp. or 2-4 capsules); give with an eyedropper on the back of the tongue if necessary every 10 minutes to restore normal heart rate.
✔ Consciousness-reviving herbs such as strong incense, camphor, bay oil or musk can be used under the victim's nose as aromatherapy for revival.
✔ Gingko biloba extract - a few drops in water, given on the tongue helps with stroke and allergic reactions such as dizziness, loss of balance, memory loss or ringing in the ears.
✔ Arnica drops are usually the first homeopathic remedy to give for injury; every half hour to 1 hour on the tongue.
✔ Bromelain 500mg, or Quercetin Plus with bromelain to control body trauma - open 1-2 capsules in water and give in small sips. Acts like aspirin, an anti-inflammatory without the stomach upset.
✔ Hops/valerian tincture, or valerian/wild lettuce; 5-6 drops in water. Give in small sips every 10-15 minutes for calmness.

Common Symptoms: General weakness; cold; pale skin; rapid weak heartbeat; heart attack or stroke; reduced alertness and consciousness; shallow, irregular breathing; confusion.
Common Causes: Major burns; heat prostration; major accident and injury; loss of blood; head injury; poisonous insect or snake bite; bone breaks, sprains, and falls.
✳ Thanks and credit to "Everybody's Guide to Homeopathic Medicines" for this section. It is needed for a family reference, and our experience has not included emergency shock trauma.

Cardiopulmonary resuscitation (CPR) is another important medical emergency procedure. If a person's heart or breathing has stopped, CPR is essential in order to avoid brain damage, which usually begins in 4 to 6 minutes after cardiopulmonary arrest.

1. Be sure the person is truly unconscious. If tapping, shouting or shaking does not wake him or her, call immediately for help, giving precise directions and telephone number.
2. Lay the victim flat on the back on a straight, firm surface. If you have to roll the person over, roll him or her toward you with one of your hands supporting the neck as you turn.
3. Open the airway so the tongue is not blocking it. If you feel the person may have a neck injury, use your fingers to move the tongue out of the airway. If not, use the following procedure. Place one of your palms across the forehead, and using your other hand, lift the chin up and forward. At the same time, gently push down the forehead. This head and chin-tilt movement lifts the chin but does not fully close the mouth. As the jaw is tilted, the tongue will move out of the mouth. Remove any dentures if present.
4. Check to see if the person is breathing. Opening the airway may be all that is needed. If no signs of breathing are detected, move the tongue out of the airway again.
5. Begin mouth-to-mouth resuscitation. Remove your hand from the forehead and pinch the person's nostrils together. Take a deep breath and place your open mouth over the victims mouth. Exhale completely into the person's mouth. Take your mouth away, inhale quickly, and repeat four times.
6. Check the pulse on the side of the neck. You should feel the pulse of the carotid artery here. Move your fingers around if you don't feel it at once, and keep trying for 10 to 15 seconds. If there is no pulse begin chest compression to maintain circulation until medical help arrives.

✔ Kneel next to the victim's chest, midway between the shoulder and waist.
✔ Find the tip of the breastbone, and place your hands one over the other, palms down on this point.

✔ Shift your weight forward, and with your elbows locked, bear down on the victim's chest, compressing it $1\frac{1}{2}$ to 2 inches.
✔ Compress the chest for about a half second, then relax for a half second. Compress again, and relax, etc.
Count "1 and 2 and 3 and 4 and 5". Each time you reach 5 you should have done 5 compressions.
✔ After you have done 15 compressions, take you hands off the chest and place them on the neck and forehead as before.
Pinch the nostrils and administer 2 strong breaths into the victim's mouth.
✔ Do 15 more chest compressions and administer 2 strong breaths again, check again for pulse and breathing.
✔ If neither pulse nor breathing have returned, resume until medical help arrives, the victim revives, or you can no longer continue.
Don't give up too soon!

SINUS PROBLEMS ■ SINUSITIS

The sinuses are thin, resonating air-filled chambers in the cartilage around the nose, on both sides of the forehead, between the nasal passages and the eye sockets and in the cheekbones. When sinus openings are obstructed, mucous and sometimes infected pus collect in the sinuses causing pain and swelling. Acute sinusitis is an inflammation of the mucous membranes lining the sinuses. Chronic sinusitis often causes nasal polyps and scar tissue. Natural healing methods revolve around relieving the cause of the clogging and inflammation. Suppressive over-the-counter sinus drugs can both trigger an infection by not allowing the draining of infective material, and aggravate it by driving the infection deeper into the sinuses.

FOOD THERAPY

☙ Go on a short 3 day mucous cleansing liquid diet. (pg. 42)
   ◆ Take a glass of lemon juice and water each morning to thin mucous secretions.
   ◆ Add an extra glass of fresh carrot juice the 1st day.
   ◆ Add a pineapple/papaya juice the 2nd day.
   ◆ Add a glass of apple juice the 3rd day.
Mix fresh grated horseradish root with lemon juice in a spoon. Take and hang over a sink to expel lots of mucous all at once.
Then, eat only fresh foods for the rest of the week to cleanse encrusted mucous deposits.

☙ Take an onion/garlic, or mucous cleansing broth (pg. 58) each day.

☙ Slowly add back whole grains, vegetable protein, and cultured foods to your own tolerance.

☙ Avoid heavy starches, red meats, pasteurized dairy products, caffeine and refined sugars.

☙ See "COOKING FOR HEALTHY HEALING" by Linda Rector-Page for a complete diet for respiratory health.

VITAMINS/MINERALS

▶ Vitamin C therapy: Use ascorbate or Ester C powder, 1/4 teasp. every hour to bowel tolerance daily during acute phase.
Also, dissolve crystals in water and drip into nose with an eye-dropper.

▶ Beta carotene 100,000IU, with Zinc picolinate 50mg.

▶ Enzymatic Therapy LIQUID LIVER caps, and RAW ADRENAL complex. ♂

▶ Nutrition Res. Nutribiotic GRAPEFRUIT SEED EXTRACT diluted as directed, as an anti-biotic nasal rinse.

▶ Boiron *Sinusitis* tabs.

▶ Propolis tincture drops ♂
       and/or
High potency royal jelly 2 teasp. daily. ♀

▶ B complex 100mg. with extra B6 250mg., pantothenic acid 500mg., and B12 2500mcg. sublingually.

HERBAL THERAPY

❧ Crystal Star ANTI-BIO™ caps *and FIRST AID CAPS™* 2-3x daily each for a week, *with* ALRG™ caps, ALR-HST™ tea, or ALRG/HST™ extract.

❧ BioForce SINUSAN drops or tabs.

❧ Zand DECONGEST HERBAL.

❧ Apply Tiger Balm or Chinese WHITE FLOWER OIL to sinuses.

❧ Unsprayed bee pollen 2 teasp. daily, *and/or* propolis extract.

❧ Effective herbs to clear sinuses:
   ◆ Comfrey/fenugreek
   ◆ Fenugreek/thyme
   ◆ Ephedra as a bronchodilator
   ◆ Echinacea extract drops
   ◆ Osha root as an anti-viral
   ◆ Crystal Star ANTI-VI™ extract.
   ◆ Lobelia
   ◆ Bayberry

BODYWORK

▶ Take a hot sauna for 20 minutes daily during acute phases.

▶ Steam face and head with eucalyptus/mullein steam.

▶ Apply a hot ginger compress.

▶ Acupressure points:
Massage under the big toes for 1 minute every day.
Squeeze ends of each finger and thumb hard for 20 seconds daily.

▶ Reflexology points:

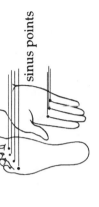

sinus points

▶ Mix 1 teasp. 3% H_2O_2 or several drops of tea tree oil in a vaporizer. Use at night for clear morning sinuses.

▶ When clearing the sinuses, blow one nostril to avoid spreading infection to the ears.

Common Symptoms: Difficult breathing; pressure headaches and a mucous-clogged head; runny nose and inflamed nasal passages; post-nasal drip with yellowish discharge coughed up; sore throat; indigestion because of mucous overload; facial pain and pain behind the eyes; loss of smell and taste; bad breath from low grade infection.
Common Causes: A viral or bacterial infection, often triggered by an allergy condition; too many mucous-forming foods, such as pasteurized dairy products and refined carbohydrates; too many salty, fatty foods; poor food combining; lack of green vegetables; constipation and poor circulation; lack of exercise and deep breathing.

SKIN BEAUTY & HEALTH

Beautiful skin is more than skin deep. The skin is the largest organ of nourishment and elimination. The acid mantle, or covering of the skin, inhibits the growth of disease-causing bacteria. Skin problems are one of the surest signs of poor nutrition. Improved nutrition is quickly mirrored by skin health.

FOOD THERAPY

🥬 Great skin starts with a good diet:

🥬 Eat plenty of mineral-rich foods, such as leafy greens, bell peppers, broccoli sesame and sunflower seeds, fish and sea vegetables.

🥬 Eat plenty of cultured foods, such as yogurt, tofu and kefir.

🥬 Eat plenty of cleansing foods, such as fresh fruit and cucumbers.

🥬 Eat vitamin C, E and beta carotene-rich foods such as sea foods, and fresh vegetables.

🥬 Drink 6 glasses of bottled water every day. Take a glass of George's ALOE VERA JUICE each morning.

🥬 Drink watermelon juice whenever it is available. It is rich in skin nourishing natural silica, and keeps the system flushed and alkaline.

🥬 Eliminate red meats, fried, fatty and fast foods. Reduce salt, caffeine, dairy foods and heavy starches.

🥬 Make a mix and take 2 TBS. daily:
- ◆ Sesame seeds
- ◆ Wheat germ
- ◆ Molasses
- ◆ Brewer's yeast

🥬 Kitchen cosmetic face lifts: Apply, leave on 30 minutes and rinse off.
- ◆ Yogurt to balance Ph
- ◆ Oatmeal to exfoliate
- ◆ Honey for external enzyme therapy
- ◆ Eggs for wrinkles.

VITAMINS/MINERALS

Vitamins feed the skin, and supplement nutrition deficiencies that show up in the skin.

▶ Effective collagen support:
- ✦ Alta Health SIL-X silica 4 daily.
- ✦ Pycnogenol 50mg. daily.
- ✦ Ascorbate vitamin C or Ester C with bioflavonoids, 3000mg. daily.
- ✦ Collagen tabs or powder.
- ✦ Nutrapathic CALCIUM/COLLA-GEN tabs.

▶ Essential fatty acid liposomes:
- ✦ **Body Essentials SILICA GEL. Use internally and externally.**
- ✦ Vitamin E 800IU daily.
- ✦ Vitamin A & D 25,000/1,000
- ✦ Jason ESTER C lotion.
- ✦ M.I.S.T. collagen moisture spray.
- ✦ Am. Biol. emulsified A & E oil.
- ✦ Am. Health PEARL CREME.

▶ Dr. DOPHILUS caps at meals, with B6 250mg. and Mezotrace SEA MINERAL COMPLEX tabs 1 daily.

🍀 High potency YS or Premier 1 royal jelly, and/or Superior GINSENG/BEE SECRETION.

▶ Natural, quick vitamin facial - once a week: Prick open and squeeze out 1 vitamin A&D 25,000IU, and 1 vitamin E 400IU capsule. Grind up 1 zinc 30mg. tablet and 1 PABA 100mg. tab. Mix with 2 teasp. wheat germ oil and smear on face. Let dry and rinse off.

▶ High omega 3 flax oil caps 3 daily

HERBAL THERAPY

Herbs are wonderful for beautiful skin. They are packed with absorbable minerals, anti-oxidants, fatty acids and bioflavonoids to cleanse, hydrate, heal, alkalize, and balance glands and hormones.

🍀 Essential fatty acid sources:
- ◆ Evening primrose oil caps 4 daily.
- ◆ Borage seed oil 4 daily.
- ◆ Black currant oil 4 daily

🍀 **Crystal Star BEAUTIFUL SKIN™ tea. Use internally and externally - pat on problem spots.**

🍀 Effective blood cleansing herbs:
- ◆ Crystal Star SKIN THERAPY # 1
- ◆ Sage
- ◆ Burdock rt.
- ◆ Crystal Star PAU DE ARCO/ECHINACEA extract.

🍀 Effective anti-oxidant herbs:
- ◆ Rosemary
- ◆ Chaparral
- ◆ Dandelion rt.

🍀 Effective bioflavonoid sources:
- ◆ Bilberry extract
- ◆ Rosehips
- ◆ Crystal Star BIOFLAV., FIBER & C SUPPORT.

🍀 Effective healing/hydrating herbs:
- ◆ Calendula
- ◆ Rosehips/lemon juice
- ◆ Chamomile
- ◆ Witch Hazel
- ◆ SKIN THERAPY #2

BODYWORK

▶ Use a gentle, balancing mask once a week, such as Crystal Star NATURAL CLAY TONING™ mask, Reviva LIGHT SKIN PEEL, or Zia SUPER HYDRATING mask, or PAPAYA PEEL.
→ Follow with a blend of aloe vera gel and vitamin E oil.

▶ Get 20 minutes of early morning sunlight on the skin every day possible for Vitamin D.

▶ **Cosmetic acupuncture and acupressure treatments are effective.**

▶ Get regular aerobic exercise to increase circulation and tone.

▶ Effective exfoliant/cleansers for glowing skin:
→ Loofa sponge, ayate cloth, dry skin brush.
- → Cucumber/papaya skins
- → Oatmeal and seaweed baths
- → Crystal Star LEMON SALT GLOW
- → Honey/almond/oatmeal scrub

▶ Effective cleansers/balancers:
- → Zia SEA TONIC with aloe
- → Crystal Star HOT SEAWEED bath.
- → Aubrey JOJOBA CLEANSER
- → Olive oil soap
- → Tea tree oil soap

▶ Good softening agents:
- → Jojoba oil
- → Sesame oil

Common Symptoms: Unbalanced skin and acid mantle, with sores, spots, cracks, oiliness or dryness, scaling, itching, chapping, redness and rashes.
Common Causes: Emotional stress; poor diet of excess refined foods and sugars; too many saturated fats; caffeine overload; food allergies; too high copper levels causing blotching; poor digestion and assimilation; PMS; irritating cosmetics; essential fatty acid and bioflavonoid depletion; liver malfunction.

More Natural Therapy For Skin Problems

❦ **For white hard bumps on the upper arms and chest:** Emulsified vitamin A 25,000IU 2 daily, zinc picolinate 50mg. daily, and Ester C 550mg. with bioflavoncids and rutin 2-3 daily. High omega 3 flax oil 3x daily. Use a dry skin brush or an ayate cloth, and brush the areas morning and night until the skin is pink from increased circulation. This gives your skin oxygen, sloughs off dead cells and speeds up cell renewal. Apply a non-greasy lotion to the areas.

❦ **For vitiligo (a genetic immune system disorder causing depigmentation of the skin):** Some effectiveness has been shown when treated as for radiation poisoning (see that page in this book). The newest treatment is phenylalanine 1000mg. one hour before exposure to UV light. Also, Solaray TURMERIC capsules 4 daily; vitamin C 3-5000mg. daily w. bioflavonoids; Alta Health SIL-X silica tabs; PABA 1000mg. with 2 TBS. molasses daily as an iron source, pantothenic acid 1000mg.; vitamin E 400IU with selenium; Biotec AGELESS BEAUTY capsules 6 daily; Crystal Star IODINE SOURCE™ and ADR-ACTIVE extracts to address glandular deficiencies. Smart, Inc COLLAGEN tabs; Sun CHLORELLA 1 packet daily, with egg yolk lecithin and ginkgo biloba extract. Calendula gel is an effective topical. Beware of long use of cortico-steroids given for vitiligo. There is some repigmentation, but higher risk of skin cancer.

❦ **For scleroderma (a runaway healing process where the body inexplicably begins and continues to produce too much collagen and connective tissue, replacing normal cell structure, and causing scar tissue to build up on skin, lungs and circulatory organs. It begins with discolored skin, followed by lesions and swelling):** Take regular baths with aloe vera gel added to the water. Apply calendula gel to lesions. Get regular aerobic exercise to increase perspiration, stimulate metabolism, and rid the body of carbon dioxide build-up. Stop smoking and avoid secondary smoke. Add vitamins A 25,000IU 4x daily, C with bioflavonoids, 5000mg. daily, B6 250mg. daily, and zinc 30mg. daily. Keep nutrition at the highest possible level with concentrated nutrient supplements, such as NutriTech ALL 1 and a protein drink every day. Add green drinks and fresh carrot juice at least twice a week.

❦ **For liver spots/age spots:** High potency Premier one or YS royal jelly 2 teasp. daily, Biotec AGELESS BEAUTY to release rancid fats, Reviva BROWN SPOT REMOVER, PABA 100mg. with pantothenic acid 1000mg, high omega 3 flax oil 3 teasp. daily. Alpha Hydroxy-acids; chamomile tea applications or CamoCare CHAMOMILECONCENTRATE; lemon juice several times daily. Crystal Star ADR-ACTIVE™ caps for spots and freckling. Always use SPF 15 or greater sun screen . Even minimal sun exposure is enough to sustain spots.

❦ **For dry and damaged skin:** Apply aloe vera gel mixed with vitamin E oil, or aloe ice gel; rub face with the inside of papaya skins; high omega 3 flax oil 3 teasp. daily, evening primrose oil capsules 4 daily, Camocare Concentrate. Phyto-estrogen plants, such as dong quai, vitex, black cohosh can help stimulate better estrogen supply for the skin. Zia ESSENTIAL extract.

❦ **For oily, shiny skin:** Make an oatmeal/almond meal mask with water. Rub on and rinse. Mix 1 egg white, beaten until foamy with 1 squeezed lemon. Apply for 5 minutes and rinse. Use astringent herbs such as, yarrow, sage, rosemary and lavender to dry excess surface oil, decrease perspiration, and slow down oil production. Zia OIL CONTROL extract.

❦ **For strawberries /excess pigmentation:** Reduce too high copper levels by adding more zinc and iron-rich foods. Reduce clogging waste with an herbal laxative. Apply B&T CALIFLO-RA ointment, take pantothenic acid 1000mg. and B6 500mg.

❦ **For poor skin tone and color:** Crystal Star LEMON SALT GLOW™, ALOE ICE gel, jojoba oil, Crystal Star SYSTEM STRENGTH™ drink mix.

❦ **For free radical scavenging and protection from environmental pollutants:** Twin Lab SUPER GERMANIUM WITH SUMA capsules 3-4 daily, Biotec AGELESS BEAUTY capsules 6 daily, Vitamin E with selenium 400IU, egg yolk lecithin capsules, ginkgo biloba extract, cosmetics and skin care products with azuline.

❦ **To balance skin ph:** Twin Lab GERMANIUM w. SUMA caps, Jason SUMA moisturizer, Crystal Star BEAUTIFUL SKIN™ tea, cider vinegar baths, lemon juice to restore acid mantle.

❦ **For skin eruptions and blemishes:** Apply a drop of lavender, lemon grass or tea tree oil to the spot several times daily. Apply Crystal Star BEAUTIFUL SKIN™ tea or gel.

❦ **For rosacea (severe chronic skin eruptions):** Apply calendula gel to spots. Apply Crystal Star BEAUTIFUL SKIN™ tea or gel. Apply GRAPEFRUIT SEED extract as recommended above; also take GRAPEFRUIT SEED extract capsules internally daily as an effective anti-biotic treatment for the skin. Add a strong GLA source, such as borage oil, or Source Naturals MEGA-GLA 240, B complex 100mg. daily, beta carotene 100,000IU daily, and high omega 3 flax oil 3x daily. Add an herb combination such as Crystal Star THERADERM™ caps or BEAUTIFUL SKIN™ tea, containing burdock rt., sarsaparilla rt., echinacea rt., and Oregon grape rt. Drink pau de arco tea 3 to 4 cups daily as an anti-infective. Dr. Diamond HERPANACINE capsules as directed.

❦ **For little red dots on the skin:** Generally a liver malfunction, or a mineral deficiency. Reduce fats and concentrated protein in the diet. Add B complex vitamins 100mg. daily. Take Crystal Star MINERAL SPECTRUM™ caps 2 daily, IODINE SOURCE™ caps for thyroid stimulation and minerals, or Mezotrace SEA MINERAL complex tabs.

❦ **For wrinkling and dry cracks:** Zia PAPAYA PEEL, Revivia LIGHT SKIN PEEL, 1 teasp. aloe gel mixed with 1 pricked vitamin E 400IU capsule. Rub face with papaya skins, and add apples, papaya and citrus fruits to the diet.

❦ **Natural make-up removers:** Make a mix of apricot, avocado, almond and sesame oils; good for all skin types - makes your skin feel wonderful.

AGING & DRY SKIN ■ WRINKLES

The relative health of your collagen determines the contour of your skin, that is, how wrinkled and lined it is. Dermal collagen decreases by 1% per year after age 20. Aging of the skin occurs when collagen becomes hard and crosslinked with neighboring collagen fibers. This prevents it from holding water and plumping up. Instead, it collapses on itself; binds with other collagen fibers, and forms a kind of fish net below the surface of the skin. You perceive it as wrinkles. The cause of the crosslinking is oxidation, or free radical formation. Free radicals attack cell membranes, collagen proteins and elastin proteins and genetic cell material, allowing wrinkles, sagging contours, sallow complexion due to waste retention and skin cancer.

FOOD THERAPY

☙ The diet should consciously include plenty of vegetable protein, such as whole grains, seafoods, sprouts and soy foods; mineral-rich foods, such as leafy greens, onions, root and cruciferous vegetables and molasses; and foods rich in beta carotene, vitamin E and C, such as carrots, greens, sea vegetables and broccoli.

☙ **Take 8 glasses of water daily. Take 2 glasses of George's ALOE VERA JUICE w. herbs. Have a glass of Crystal Star BIOFLAV. FIBER drink.**

☙ Avoid refined sugars, red meats, and caffeine containing foods. All are very drying to the skin.

☙ Make a mix and take 2 TBS. daily:
  ✦ Lecithin granules
  ✦ Wheat germ
  ✦ Brewer's yeast
  ✦ Molasses

☙ Natural anti-wrinkle facials:
  ✦ Rub the insides of fresh papaya skins on the face.
  ✦ Mix 1 whipped egg white and 2 TBS. cream. Pat on face; let dry 20 minutes. Rinse off.
  ✦ Apply a mix of tincture of benzoin, vegetable glycerine, honey and cologne drops. Leave on 15 min. Rinse off.
  ✦ Lemon juice.

VITAMINS/MINERALS

▶ Natural products with anti-wrinkle effects:
  ✦ North Pacific ALPHA HYDROXY LOTION and LIQUID.
  ✦ Zia PAPAYA PEEL and ESSENTIAL HYDRATING extract.
  ✦ **Urist RETINOL EXTRA.**
  ✦ 1 teasp. aloe vera gel mixed with 1 pricked vitamin E 400IU capsule.
  ✦ Reviva collagen ampules.
  ✦ **Nayad (hyaluronic acid)**
  ✦ Nature's Life RNA/DNA.
  ✦ RevivaBody Essentials SILICA gel.
  ✦ Reviva LIGHT SKIN PEEL and NIGHT CREAM & DAY CREAM.
  ✦ High potency royal jelly ampules.
  ✦ Biotec AGELESS BEAUTY capsules
  ✦ MIST collagen moisturizer spray.

▶ Effective anti-oxidants/free radical scavengers:
  ✦ Twin Lab SUPER GERMANIUM with suma.
  ✦ Biotec AGELESS BEAUTY
  ✦ Vitamin E 800IU w/ selenium
  ✦ Vitamin C 3-5000mg. daily.
  ✦ Ginkgo biloba extract

▶ Essential fatty acids for liposomes:
  ✦ Pycnogenol 50mg. 3x daily.
  ✦ Alta Health SIL-X silicatabs.
  ✦ Jason AGE DEFENSE moisturizer.

▶ B Complex 100mg. with extra PABA 1000mg. and bromelain 500mg. daily.

HERBAL THERAPY

Estrogen is a tissue builder, laying down collagen that shores up skin and renews skin elasticity.

❧ Effective phyto-estrogen herbs:
  ◆ Crystal Star EST-AID™ caps.
  ◆ Dong quai/damiana.
  ◆ Vitex extract.

❧ Iodine therapy: Atomodine drops in water daily with vitamin E 400IU, or Crystal Star IODINE SOURCE™ caps or extract, or SYSTEM STRENGTH™ drink.

❧ CamoCare FACIAL THERAPY.

❧ **Evening primrose or borage oil caps 4 daily with vitamin E 400IU daily esp. for eye skin wrinkling.**

❧ Steam face with hydrating/ aromatherapy herbs:
  ◆ Chamomile flowers
  ◆ Eucalyptus leaves
  ◆ Rosemary leaves

❧ Pat on topical toners:
  ◆ Nettles
  ◆ Nature's Life GINSENG cream
  ◆ Witch hazel.

❧ Apply a facial mix: 1 teasp. vegetable glycerine, 1 teasp. rosewater, 1 teasp. witch hazel, 3 TBS. honey. Leave on 15-20 minutes.

BODYWORK

▶ **Regular daily use of sunscreens greatly reduces aging skin signs.**

▶ Avoid smoking and all forms of tobacco. Tar and nicotine deprive of oxygen, causing shriveling/wrinkles.

▶ Apply Care Plus H2O2 OXYGEL to wrinkles before bed as a source of absorbable oxygen.

▶ **Cosmetic acupuncture and acupressure treatments for facial rejuvenation are effective.**

▶ Effective softening massages:
  ➜ Jojoba oil
  ➜ Sesame oil
  ➜ Wheat germ oil
  ➜ Vitamin E oil
  ➜ Aloe vera gel

▶ Use a gentle balancing mask once a week, such as Crystal Star CLAY TONING MASK.
  ➜ Follow with a blend of aloe vera gel and vitamin E oil.

▶ For elasticity and tone:
  ➜ Facial exercises
  ➜ Massage therapy to release toxins from the lymph system and tone facialmuscles.
  ➜ Crystal Star SYSTEM STRENGTH™ DRINK.

Common Causes: Free radical damage caused by smog and environmental pollutants, too much sunlight, stress, poor diet, liver exhaustion, etc.; skin dehydration often caused by hormone (estrogen depletion); poor diet with too much tobacco, fried foods, caffeine, and alcohol; broken capillaries; weak vein walls.

SKIN SCARS ▧ STRETCH MARKS

FOOD THERAPY

☙ Wheat germ oil. Apply locally. Take 2 teasp. daily internally.

☙ Have a green drink at least three times a week during first healing stages. (pg. 54ff).
♠ Take a Crystal Star BIOFLAV., FIBER & C SUPPORT™ drink for the first month of healing.

☙ Apply sesame oil.

☙ Apply avocado oil. Eat avocados for skin elasticity.

☙ Eat a high vegetable protein diet for faster healing. Include plenty of whole grains, sprouts, tofu, and a protein drink every morning, such as Nature's Plus SPIRU-TEIN.

VITAMINS/MINERALS

▶ Alta Health SIL-X silica caps, 4 daily, Crystal Star SILICA SOURCE™ capsules or Body Essentials SILICA GEL. Silicon skin healing treatments usually take from 3 to 4 months, depending on severity of the scar.

▶ Apply vitamin E oil. Take E 400IU internally daily.

▶ Vitamin C therapy, for collagen production and connective tissue growth:
Ascorbate C powder with bioflavonoids and rutin - take up to 5000mg. daily; also mix with water into a solution and apply directly.

▶ Enzymatic Therapy DERMA-ZYME ointment and HERBAL FLAVONOIDS caps.

▶ Germanium 25-30mg. for wound healing, for at least a month.

▶ A & D oil capsules. Take 25-50,000IU internally daily. Puncture a capsule and apply directly 2-3x daily.

▶ Unipro BCAAs as a protein source to accelerate healing tissue.

HERBAL THERAPY

❦ Crystal Star GINSENG SKIN REPAIR GEL with vitamin C™ for 2 to 3 months.

❦ Crystal Star ENERGY GREEN™ drink for blood and tissue building.

❦ Sun CHLORELLA or Green Foods GREEN MAGMA granules, 1 packet daily.

❦ Effective applications:
♦ Aloe vera gel
♦ Calendula gel
♦ Tea tree oil
♦ B&T CALIFLORA gel
♦ Comfrey/aloe salve
♦ Golden seal salve
♦ BioForce ECHINACEA cream

❦ Highest potency YS or Premier 1 royal jelly 2 teasp. daily, and apply locally.

❦ Superior GINSENG/BEE SE-CRETION. ♀

BODYWORK

▶ Get regular exercise daily for muscle and skin tone, and body oxygen.

▶ Massage the scar thoroughly when rubbing your choice of topical application, to bring up healthy circulation and skin tone.

▶ Effective applications:
→ Heritage SCAR MASSAGE.
→ Mountain Ocean MOTHER'S BLEND cream.
→ Aubrey SCARS/EVENING PRIMROSE OIL.
→ Reviva Collagen and Elastin ampule concentrates.

Common Symptoms: Non-healing or slow healing skin wounds, often with continuing redness, roughness, and irregular weals.
Common Causes: Protein deficiency; vitamin A & D deficiency; zinc and other mineral deficiency; poor overall nutrition.

SKIN CANCERS ▨ ULCERATIONS

Skin cancer is an undeclared epidemic of our time. It is the most common of all cancers (one in every three cancers is skin cancer). Over *500,000 new cases* are diagnosed each year in the U.S. alone, affecting one in every seven Americans, and affecting more men than women. Over 90% of all skin cancers are caused by UV radiation from the sun - radiation that is increasing in toxicity as the earth's protective ozone layer is steadily depleted. Unfortunately, overexposure to the sun as a cause of melanoma (the most dangerous form of skin cancer), is far more harmful to a child's skin than to an adults. Fortunately, almost all skin cancer is preventable, and it is curable when treated in its earliest stages.

FOOD THERAPY

ə. Keep the diet simple and alkaline during healing. Add more fresh fruits and vegetables. Consciously add vegetable protein sources for faster healing: whole grains, soy foods, sea foods and cultured foods.

❧ Include beta carotene-rich foods for both healing and prevention: carrots, sweet potatoes, other yellow-orange vegetables and sea vegetables.
❧ Include vitamin C-rich foods for collagen and interstitial tissue health.
❧ Include silicon-rich foods to build health connective skin tissue: vegetables, whole grains and seafoods.

ə. Take 1 teasp. *each* in a glass of aloe vera juice 2x daily:
♦ Wheat germ oil
♦ Brewer's yeast

ə. Drink 6-8 glasses of bottled water daily to keep acid wastes flushed.

ə. Avoid saturated fats, sugars, caffeine and caffeine-containing foods.

VITAMINS/MINERALS

▶ Basal cell carcinomas: *Open, ulcerous sores, forming slowly spreading chronic reddish patches; small mole or shiny lump growths, usually in areas exposed regularly to the sun. Do not metastasize.*
✦ Care Plus H2O2 OXY GEL, or Am. Biologics DIOXYCHLOR.
✦ PSI Progest cream - also for open ulcerations.
✦ Calendula gel
✦ PABA 500-1000mg.
✦ Enzymatic Therapy DERMA-ZYME ointment. ♀

▶ Squamous cell carcinomas: *Pink, opaque nodules or wart-like growth, under the skin on the face or head. Fast growing. Can metastasize.*
♣ Beta carotene 100,000IU
♣ Vit. E 400IU w/ selenium
♣ Tea tree oil
♣ Germanium solution in water.

▶ Malignant melanomas: *Small or large brown-black or multi-colored patches or irregular nodules that grow rapidly, metastasize and can be lethal.*
♣ Calendula gel
♣ Vitamin C solution
♣ Care Plus H2O2 OXY GEL or Am. Biologics DIOXYCHLOR.

▶ Ascorbate or Ester C powder, 1/2 teasp. hourly to bowel tolerance during healing, for collagen production and connective tissue growth.

HERBAL THERAPY

❧ Highest potency YS or Premier 1 royal jelly 2 teasp. daily.

❧ Solaray turmeric capsules 4 daily with burdock tea 2 cups daily.

❧ Apply Crystal Star GINSENG, GERMANIUM SKIN REPAIR GEL with vitamin C™, and GREEN TEA CLEANSER™ each morning.

❧ Evening primrose oil caps or Source Naturals MEGA GLA caps 4-6 daily,

❧ Effective internal herbs:
♦ Pau de arco 4 cups daily
♦ Burdock tea 2 cups daily
♦ Propolis tablets
♦ Ginkgo biloba extract
♦ Aloe vera juice
♦ Gotu kola extract for skin ulcers
♦ Crystal Star GINSENG 6 SUPER TEA™.

▶ Bromelain 500mg. with omega 3 flax oil 3x daily. ♀

❧ Effective applications:
♦ BioForce ECHINACEA cream
♦ Goldenseal/myrrh solution
♦ Calendula gel
♦ Aloe vera gel, or ALOE ICE 24 HOUR RENEWAL GEL.

BODYWORK

▶ Prevention watchwords:
→ Use an SPF sun screen of 15 or higher regularly and liberally. Always apply after going in the water. Apply extra if you are going to be around snow, concrete, sand and water.
→ Avoid all pleasure drugs, especially cocaine. Drugs constrict the blood vessels and leave the skin to shrivel and die without nutrients .
→ Cortico-steroid drugs over a long period of time for skin problems, can greatly weaken the immune defenses and allow cancers to take hold.

▶ Get early morning sunlight on the skin every day for 15 minutes. Early sun can help heal ulcerations. Midday sun aggravates them.

▶ Effective applications:
→ Hot comfrey compresses
→ Dry mustard plaster
→ Tea tree oil
→ Propolis tincture ♂
→ Green clay poultice
→ B & T CALIFLORA gel

▶ Apply Care Plus OXY GEL to affected area, and on to soles of feet. Usually a noticeable change in 3 weeks.

Common Symptoms: A skin growth that appears or increases suddenly in size, and appears partly translucent, tan, brown, black or multi-colored; A mole that changes in size, shape, color or texture and becomes irregularly shaped; a lesion or growth that continues to itch, hurt, scab, ulcerate, erode or bleed; an open sore that does not heal, or heals and then re-opens. **Common Causes:** Too much UV radiation from the sun because of ozone depletion; too many antibiotics, especially in children; malfunctioning sebaceous glands; allergies to sugars, wheat or pasteurized dairy; too much saturated fat and red meat, causing over-acid system; B vitamin depletion; fungus infection; Candida albicans; inherited thin sensitive skin.

SKIN DAMAGE FROM SUNBURN ▧ HEATSTROKE

For every sunburn you get that blisters, you double your risk of skin cancer. Even on a cloudy day, 80% of the sun's harmful UV rays come through. Sun damage is cumulative over a lifetime. Practice good sun sense so that you don't fry now and pay later. See preceding page for more information.

FOOD THERAPY

ఞ Effective natural electrolyte replacements:
♦ Celery juice
♦ Lemonade
♦ Mineral water
♦ Suck on limes
♦ Potassium broth (pg. 53)
♦ Effervescent C 2 packets daily
♦ Drink 6-8 glasses of water daily to rehydrate from within.

ఞ Add plenty of complex carbohydrates and vegetable proteins to the diet for skin renewal.

ఞ **Add 1 TB. chia seed to your protein drink.**

ఞ Apply yogurt, honey, black tea, or vinegar to relieve burn areas.

ఞ Apply grated apple to burned eyelids for immediate relief.

ఞ Make a mix and take 2 TBS. daily:
♦ Brewer's yeast
♦ Wheat germ
♦ Lecithin

ఞ Mix 1 teasp. vinegar and 1/2 cup sunflower oil and pat on burns.

VITAMINS/MINERALS

Prevention is the key. If your tissues are loaded with carotene A, vitamin C, E w/ selenium and B complex, whether from food or a good food source supplement, your skin will stand much less chance of being damaged from the sun.

◗ Effective anti-oxidants help protect skin from free radical attacks:
♣ Ascorbate vitamin C with bioflavonoids 1/4 teasp. in water every hour during acute stage; pat a C solution on burned areas frequently.
♣ Vitamin E 400IU daily internally. Prick a capsule and apply externally with an A & D capsule.
♣ Beta carotene for both anti-oxidant and anti-cancer activity.
♣ Pycnogenol 50mg. 3x daily.

◗ **Tyrosine 500mg. 2x daily as a tan activator and to improve the skin's resistance.**

◗ Homeopathic *Nat. Mur.* tabs. ♀

◗ B Complex 100mg. daily with extra PABA caps 1000mg. and PABA cream with zinc oxide. ♂
and
Raw adrenal extract. ♀

HERBAL THERAPY

ఞ **Drink aloe vera juice regularly. Apply aloe vera gel as needed.**

ఞ Crystal Star GINSENG SKIN REPAIR GEL™ with vitamin C™.

ఞ High potency royal jelly 2 teasp. daily for healthy skin regrowth. ♀

ఞ Effective applications:
♦ Comfrey/aloe salve
♦ Jojoba oil ♀
♦ Tea tree oil
♦ Green clay poultice
♦ B&T CALIFLORA gel ☉
♦ Calendula gel

ఞ Effective anti-oxidant herbs:
♦ Rosemary
♦ Chaparral
♦ Ginkgo biloba

ఞ Crystal Star SYSTEM STRENGTH™ drink for electrolyte minerals, or Mezotrace SEA MINERAL COMPLEX 2-3 daily.

ఞ Apply a wheat germ oil, vitamin E oil, comfrey leaf, and honey poultice.

BODYWORK

▶ **Regularly use a broad-spectrum, SPF 15 or more sunburn prevention cream or oil.** Wear a lip balm with sunscreen.

▶ Sun sense burn prevention:
→ Minimize exposure to mid-day sun, between 10a.m. and 3p.m.
→ Wear sunglasses with 100% UV filters to protect your eyes.
→ Drink plenty of water before, after and during exposure to replenish and moisturize your skin from within.
→ Avoid antibiotics, diuretics, hypoglycemia medicine, retinoic acid cosmetics, soaps w. hexachlorophene, Phenergan in creams. All increase sun sensitivity.

▶ For heat stroke: apply ice packs and wrap in a cold wet sheet. Get medical help immediately. Treat for shock (pg. 312).

▶ If burns are severe, see Burns page in this book. Apply cold compresses, or take a cool bath immediately (do not use soap or hot water).
→ Take an electrolyte drink, or a little salty water. No alcoholic beverages - they dehydrate.

Common Symptoms: Sunburn and dehydration; over-reaction to heat and sun exposure; headache; numbness; high blood pressure; often confusion and delirium; rapid pulse and shock condition, which, if serious, can lead to brain damage.
Common high risk factors: Having had frequent sunburns as a child; living at high altitude; being a man; being on immuno-suppressive therapy; using sun lamps or a tanning bed; having light-colored eyes and hair; having fair or freckled skin; moving from a northern climate to the south; working all day outdoors.

SMOKING, SECONDARY SMOKE, CHEWING TOBACCO
How To Stop

Each cigarette takes 8 minutes off your life; a pack a day takes 1 month off your life each year; 2 packs a day, takes 12-15 years off your life. Cigarettes have over 4000 known poisons, any of which can kill in high enough doses. One drop of pure nicotinic acid can kill a man. Depending on the age that you quit, your life expectancy can increase from 2-5 years. Secondary or passive smoke, and chewing tobacco are just as dangerous, especially for women. Passive smoke reduces fertility, successful pregnancies, and normal birth weight babies. It has been shown to increase the instance of cervical, uterine and lung cancer. Don't be discouraged. Quitting is hard work, but it gets easier every day, as the body loses dependence on nicotine.

FOOD THERAPY

There must be a lifestyle and diet change for there to be permanent success.

☙ Start with a 3 day liquid cleansing diet (pg. 42), with fresh fruit and vegetable juices and miso soup to neutralize and clear the blood of nicotinic acid and to fortify blood sugar. Then, follow with a fresh foods only diet for the rest of the week, with carrot juices, plenty of carrots and celery, leafy green salads, and lots of citrus fruits to promote body alkalinity. (pH 7 and above readings definitely show decreased desire for tobacco.) Include lots of vegetable proteins.

☙ Take a cup of green tea or Crystal Star **GREEN TEA CLEANSER™** daily to reduce body carcinogens.

☙ Eat smaller meals more frequently.

☙ Avoid junk foods and sugar that aggravate cravings.

☙ See Hypoglycemia Diet suggestions in this book for more information.

VITAMINS/MINERALS

◗ Enzymatic Therapy NICOTABS for at least 2 months.

◗ Anti-oxidants are a key:
  ❖ Vitamin E w/ selenium
  ❖ Ascorbate vitamin C powder, 1/2 teasp. in water every hour to bowel tolerance during acute stages of withdrawal, then reduce to 5000mg. daily.
  ❖ Glutathione 50mg. for secondary smoke.
  ❖ Solaray Germanium 150SL daily.
  ❖ CoQ 10 30mg. 2x daily.

◗ For nico-toxicity, take each 2x daily:
  ❖ 1 Cysteine capsule
  ❖ 1 Glutamine capsule
  ❖ 2 Vitamin C 1000mg. tablets
  ❖ 2 Evening primrose capsules
  ❖ 10 Sun CHLORELLA tabs

◗ Niacin therapy: 500-1000mg. daily. ♂

◗ Brain stimulants to replace nicotine stimulation:
  ❖ Phosphatidyl choline
  ❖ Choline/inositol ♂

◗ Folic acid 800mcg. with B12 2000mcg. to prevent cell/lung tissue damage.

HERBAL THERAPY

❧ Solaray **TURMERIC** caps to neutralize cancer-causing compounds.

❧ Crystal Star NICOSTOP™ tea, 2 cups taken over the day in sips to keep tissues flooded with elements that discourage the taste for nicotine.
  and
  RELAX CAPS™ or GINSENG 6 caps to rebuild nervous system, calm withdrawal tension. DEEP BREATHING™ tea to keep lungs clear.

❧ Make a tobacco addiction fighting tea to lessen desire, support nervous system, strengthen adrenals, and cleanse lungs and bronchi:
  One part each:
  Oatstraw and seed, lobelia seed and tops, licorice, calamus rt, sassafras.

❧ Effective extracts:
  ◆ **Crystal Star SUPER LICORICE™**
  ◆ **Echinacea**
  ◆ Valerian/wild lettuce
  ◆ Lobelia

❧ Effective teas:
  ◆ Sassafras Bark ♂
  ◆ Crystal Star SUPER GINSENG 6 DEFENSE RESTORATIVE™
  ◆ Oats/Scullcap ♀

BODYWORK

▶ Do deep breathing exercises for more body oxygen whenever you feel the urge for tobacco until the desire decreases - about 4 minutes.

▶ To help curb craving for chewing tobacco, chew licorice root sticks, calamus root or cloves for oral gratification.

Common Symptoms: Chronic bronchitis; constant hacking cough; difficult and shortness of breath; lung and respiratory depletion and infection; emphysema and dry lungs; often eventual lung cancer and other degenerative diseases; adrenal exhaustion and fatigue; poor circulation affecting vision; high blood pressure; premature aging and wrinkled, dehydrated skin with no color or elasticity; stomach ulcers; osteoporosis; low immunity; etc., etc., etc.
Common Causes: System stress and disease from nicotine poisoning; emotional insecurity; hypoglycemia; dietary deficiencies; nicotine addiction.

SNAKE BITE ■ POISONOUS SPIDER BITE

Get emergency medical help immediately! The methods below are to be used only until this help arrives. Shock and convulsions may occur. See Shock & Trauma page in this book for more emergency information. (pg. 312)

FOOD THERAPY

🍂 Wash bite with soap and water. No ice compresses.

🍂 Give the victim only small sips of water. No alcoholic drinks. The poison will spread faster.

🍂 Plant onions and garlic around the house to keep snakes away.

🍂 Make a tobacco and saliva poultice and apply to bite.

VITAMINS/MINERALS

In a life-threatening situation, where the victim may go into shock or convulsions, massive doses of vitamin C may save the person's life.

▶ Calcium ascorbate vitamin C powder, 1/4 teasp. in water every 15 minutes as a detoxifier during acute reaction phase.

▶ Niacin therapy: up to 500mg. daily *after poison is out of the body,* to dilate and tone blood vessels.

▶ Vitamin E 400IU. Take internally; prick capsule and apply locally.

▶ Vitamin A & D 25,000IU - take internally; prick capsule and apply locally.

HERBAL THERAPY

In a life-threatening situation, where the victim may go into cardiac arrest, cayenne may save the person's life.

🌿 Cayenne, 2 capsules or 8-10 drops of cayenne extract in warm water, or Crystal Star RECOVERY TONIC™ extract as a shock preventive to strengthen the heart.

            then

    Take ANTI-HST™ caps to help prevent a histamine reaction.

🌿 Take yellow dock tea with echinacea extract every hour until swelling goes down.

🌿 Effective applications:
- ◆ Aloe / comfrey salve
- ◆ Aloe vera gel
- ◆ Comfrey extract
- ◆ Calendula gel or lotion

🌿 Effective compresses:
- ◆ Plantain
- ◆ Rue
- ◆ Fresh comfrey leaf
- ◆ Slippery elm
- ◆ **Apply black cohosh solution as an antidote to venom.**

🌿 Apply Chinese WHITE FLOWER OIL.

BODYWORK

▶ Keep victim still and calm. Immobilize the bite area and keep it lower than the heart.

▶ Until medical help arrives, put a constricting band 2-4" above the bite. Do not cut off circulation. Move band up if swelling reaches it.

▶ If swelling is rapid and pain severe, make a small cut with a sharp knife up and down, not across, through each fang mark. Use suction by mouth or a suction cup for at least 30 minutes, repeatedly. Spit out blood. Rinse mouth immediately.

Common Symptoms: Slow upward spreading red lines as poison moves toward the heart; swelling, sometimes severe pain and nausea; sweating, increased heartbeat; dizziness, weakness and fainting; breathing difficulty.

321

SORE THROAT ▦ STREP THROAT
Swollen Glands ✧ Laryngitis ✧ Hoarseness

This is basically a symptomology suggestion page. See Colds & Flu, and Viral, Staph and Bacterial Infection pages for more information on addressing the cause.

FOOD THERAPY

☙ Go on a short 24 hr. liquid cleansing diet (pg. 44), or a 3 day mucous cleansing diet (pg. 42).
♣ Take lemon juice and honey in water, and a potassium broth (pg. 53) each morning. Take citrus juices throughout the day.
♣ Then eat mainly fresh foods during healing. Have plenty of leafy greens.
♣ Follow a cleansing diet for at least another week to overcome low grade infection; eat some steamed vegetables, tofu, fresh fruits, and brown rice every day.

☙ Avoid all dairy foods, sugars and fried fatty foods during healing.

☙ Effective gargles:
♣ **Lemon juice and brandy**
♣ **Black tea**
♣ Sea salt water
♣ Cider vinegar and water

☙ Hot parsley compresses on throat.

☙ For laryngitis and hoarseness:
♣ Take 1 teasp. cider vinegar and 1 teasp. honey in a small glass of water every hour until relief.
♣ Effective juices: Papaya, apple, carrot, aloe vera.
♣ Effective gargles: Lemon juice and water, liquid chlorophyll in water, a green drink, pg. 54.
♣ Take garlic syrup. Soak a chopped garlic bulb in 1 pt. honey and water overnight; take a teasp. every hour.

VITAMINS/MINERALS

▶ Zinc gluconate or propolis lozenges every few hours as needed. ☺

▶ Alacer EMERGEN-C every few hours. Hold in the mouth as long as possible for best absorption, and/or Vitamin C chewable 500mg. every hour during acute stages.

▶ Nutribiotic GRAPEFRUIT SEED extract throat spray and/or capsules.

▶ For chronic low-grade strep infection: take Enzymatic Therapy IMMUNO-PLEX caps w. vitamin C 5000mg. daily, raw thymus SL, Lysine 500mg. and zinc lozenges as needed daily.

▶ Solaray MULTIDOPHILUS or Nature's Plus JUNIOR DOPHILUS chewables for strep infection.☺

▶ Hylands *Hylavir* and C *Pkus* tabs. ☺

▶ Enzymatic Therapy VIRAPLEX caps and/or ORAL-ZYME lozenges. ♀

▶ For laryngitis and hoarseness:
✚ Alacer EMERGEN-C. ♂
✚ Zinc gluconate lozenges.
✚ Propolis lozenges. ♂
✚ Enz. Ther. ORAL-ZYME lozenges
✚ Vit. E 400IU daily as a preventive.

▶ Nutribiotic GRAPEFRUIT SEED ex-

HERBAL THERAPY

☙ Crystal Star ANTI-BIO™, ANTI-VI™ or FIRST AID CAPS™ formulas as depending on cause, 6 daily, with COFEX™ tea as needed.

☙ Cartilade SHARK CARTILAGE caps as an anti-strep factor, with garlic capsules 6 daily.

☙ BioForce SANTASAPINA throat drops, or SANTASAPINA or DROSINULA syrup. ☺

☙ Effective tinctures:
◆ Zand HERBAL INSURE
◆ Crystal Star SUPER LICORICE™
◆ Licorice root ♂
◆ Wild cherry
◆ Myrrh gum

☙ Effective teas:
◆ Horehound
◆ Slippery elm
◆ Crystal Star COFEX™ tea

☙ Effective herbal lozenges:
◆ Zand HERBAL INSURE
◆ Olbas

☙ For laryngitis and hoarseness:
◆ Satori VOCAL RESCUE spray
◆ Crystal Star SUPER LICORICE™
◆ Tea tree oil, 3 drops in water as a gargle.
◆ CamoCare CHAMOMILE throat spray and gargle. ♀

BODYWORK

▶ Effective applications:
↝ Hot ginger compresses.
↝ Massage w. Care Plus OXYGEL.
↝ Eucalyptus steams.
↝ Color therapy glasses: wear blue.

▶ Effective gargles:
↝ Goldenseal/myrrh solution
↝ Fenugreek/honey
↝ Liquid chlorophyll in water

▶ Take hot 20 minute saunas daily.

▶ Stick tongue out as far as it will go. Hold for 30 seconds. Release and relax. Repeat 3 times to increase blood supply to the area.

▶ Drip black walnut extract in throat.

▶ Take a catnip enema to cleanse infection from a strep throat. ☺

▶ For laryngitis and hoarseness:
↝ Apply ginger/cayenne compresses to the throat.
↝ Soak in a hot mineral or epsom salts bath.
↝ Stop smoking and avoid secondary smoke.
↝ Reflexology point:

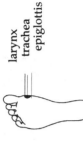

larynx
trachea
epiglottis

Common Symptoms: Sore, aching, inflamed, throat and tonsils; swollen throat tissues; difficult talking; laryngitis (inability to speak above a whisper because of swollen throat tissues).
Common Causes: Viral or strep infection; tonsilitis; beginnings of a cold or flu; consequence of smoking; lack of sleep; too many mucous-forming foods; adrenal exhaustion; stress.

SPORTS INJURIES

Torn Ligaments ✧ Sprains ✧ Muscle Pulls

A **strain** or pulled muscle is any damage to the tendon that anchors the muscle. A **sprain** is caused by a twisting motion that rips or tears ligaments that bind up the joints. It takes much longer to heal than a strain. **See sports Nutrition section on page 96 for more information.**

FOOD THERAPY

Athletes nutritional needs are considerably greater than those of the average person, (about 2000-6000 calories and 4-6 meals a day.) They need to have enough nutritional fuel to reach peak performance and avoid easily occurring injuries. Remember that protein is the least efficient energy source. If glycogen stores are too low, the body will use too much protein for energy and not for growth and repair.

• A basic diet should consist of about 65-70% complex carbohydrates - from vegetables, fruits, whole grains and legumes; 20-25% protein - from nuts, seeds, soy foods, poultry, seafood, and low fat dairy products; and 10-15% fats from quality sources - unsaturated vegetable oils, nuts, seeds, low fat dairy, butter, and fish.

• Eat chromium-rich foods such as lobster, low fat cheeses, brewer's yeast, and organ meats. Eat silicon-rich foods such as rice, oats, green grasses and leafy greens.

• Drink mineral water every day. Take an electrolyte replacement - Knudsens RECHARGE, or Twin Labs CARBO FUEL powder after exercise.

• Effective foods for massaging into injury:
♦ Cider vinegar/sea salt paste
♦ Hot linseed or flax oil
♦ Cayenne/vinegar solution
♦ Wheat germ oil

VITAMINS/MINERALS

▶ **Effective anti-inflammatories:**
♣ Quercetin Plus with bromelain 500-750mg. 2-4 caps daily.
♣ Pycnogenol 50mg. 2x daily
♣ Ctry. Life LIGATEND 4 daily. ♀
♣ Enzymatic Therapy ACID-A-CAL
♣ Strength Systems FIRST AID. ♂

▶ Vitamin C crystals, 1/2 teasp. in water, or Alacer Emergen-C every hour during acute stress for collagen and connective tissue healing.

▶ Effective homeopathic remedies:
♣ *Arnica Montana* for disclocations, sprains, bruises
♣ *Ruta Graveolens* for pulled tendons
♣ *Rhus Tox.* for swelling
♣ Boiron *Sporteniene*

▶ Twin Lab CSA caps with zinc 75mg. daily for healing and pain relief. ♂

▶ Vitamin E 800IU daily with methionine 500mg. for torn cartilege.

▶ Biogenetics BIOGUARD PLUS 6 daily for arthritis-like symptoms.

▶ Chromium picolinate 200mcg, Nutrition 21 CHROMAX 2, or Solaray CHROMIACIN caps.

▶ DLPA 500-750mg. as needed with CoQ 10 60mg. for pain relief.

HERBAL THERAPY

☙ Alta Health SIL-X silica tabs 4-6 daily, or Body Essentials SILICA GEL for new collagen and interstitial tissue regrowth. ♀

☙ Crystal Star HIGH PERFORMANCE™ caps 2-4 daily to provide long range energy and pre-vent lactic acid buildup. ANTI-FLAM™ caps to take down inflammation, and ADR-ACTIVE™ with BODY REBUILDER™ caps ♀.

☙ Ginseng and sports medicine: ♂
✦ Siberian ginseng extract for lactic acid build-up, increased oxygen use and glycogen storage.
✦ Panax extract vials - use one week on and one week off for best results.
✦ Crystal Star GINSENG 6 SUPER ENERGY™ tea and/or capsules - a non-overheating Am. ginseng source
✦ Ho-Shou-Wu for muscle, ligament, nerve healing
✦ Crystal Star GINSENG SKIN REPAIR w. C™ for abrasions, cuts, wounds and blisters.
✦ RAINFOREST ENERGY tea and capsules for long range performance.
✦ Ctry. Life ENERGIX vials. ♂
✦ Zand ACTIVE HERBAL ext. ♀

☙ Performance-enhancing herbs: ginkgo, cayenne, guarana, yohimbe.

BODY WORK

▶ Elevate the injured area:
→ Apply ice packs immediately. Leave on for 30 minutes. Remove for 15 minutes. Repeat process for 3 hrs. This procedure decreases bleeding from injured vessels by causing them to constrict.
→ Wrap the sprain or strain with an elastic bandage (over the ice if necessary) to limit swelling.
→ Apply alternating hot and cold packs the next day to stimulate circulation and relax cramps.
→ Consciously rest the injured area so that the injury is not extended, and healing is faster.

▶ Take a lavender or rosemary foot bath for sore feet.

▶ Make a healing topical paste, and apply. Mix one part each goldenseal, comfrey root and slippery elm powders in 2 parts aloe vera gel.

▶ Effective applications:
→ Calendula gel for blisters
→ St. John's wort salve - muscle pain
→ MINERAL ICE or ALOE ICE
→ Hylands *Arnicaid*
→ Tiger balm
→ B&T ANALGESIC rub
→ Tea tree oil
→ DMSO w. aloe vera
→ Chinese WHITE FLOWER oil
→ CamoCare PAIN RELIEF cream
→ Care Plus OXYGEL
→ Homeopathic *Arnica* gel

Common Symptoms: Wrenched knees; twisted ankles; sprained wrists; shin splints; tennis elbows; torn ligaments; muscle pulls; arthritis-like symptoms; bruises; tendon inflammation; Achilles heel; shooting pains in the ankles, feet and knees.

323

STOMACH UPSET

😊 Colic ◇ Hiccups 😊

This page and information is dedicated to all the long-suffering parents who have spent many sleepless nights with colicky, hurting babies - natural relief at last.

FOOD THERAPY

🍃 If you are nursing, watch your diet very carefully. The baby's digestion is still dependent on yours. Avoid cabbage, brussels sprouts, onions, garlic, yeast breads, fried foods and fast foods. Refrain from red meat, alcohol, refined sugar and caffeine until the child's digestion improves.

🍃 Avoid giving cow's milk to a colicky baby. Chronic upset stomach in an infant indicates an allergy to dairy products. Goat's milk or soy milk are both better alternatives.

🍃 Give papaya juice or apple juice.

🍃 Give lemon and *processed* honey in water.

VITAMINS/MINERALS

▶ Natren LIFE START $1/4$ teasp. in water or juice 2-3x daily.

▶ Solaray BABY LIFE for mineral and B Complex deficiency.

▶ Solaray BIFIDO-BACTERIA POWDER for infants.

▶ Hyland's Homeopathic *Colic* tabs or *Biliousness* tabs.

▶ Homeopathic *Mag. Phos.* tabs.

▶ Small doses of papaya enzymes.

▶ B Complex liquid dilute doses in water about once a week.

HERBAL THERAPY

🍃 Apply warm ginger compresses to the stomach and abdomen.

🍃 Turmeric powder $1/4$ teasp. in juice or water.

🍃 Fennel tea or catnip tea, 1t. in water with a little honey.

🍃 Peppermint or spearmint tea with a pinch of ginger.

🍃 Catnip/peppermint tea.

🍃 Dill seed tea.

BODYWORK

▶ Give a catnip enema once a week, or as needed for instant gas release.

▶ Reflexology point:

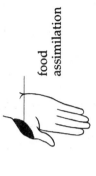

food assimilation

Common Symptoms: Excess gas and abdominal discomfort; incessant crying; burping hiccups.

Common Causes: Poor diet with too many acid-forming foods, or poor food combination; introduction of protein foods too soon (this will often form lifelong allergies and colic); mother's tension and acidity during breast feeding; mineral deficiency in the milk formula; enzyme deficiency; Candida albicans yeast overgrowth; poor food absorption; chronic constipation.

STRESS

Everyone is affected by varying degrees of stress. It is experienced by those who work in polluted atmospheres, by those who are immobilized at control desks with machines or instruments demanding continual attention, by those who travel coast to coast constantly, by those with mundane, boring jobs, etc. At best, stress causes useless fatigue; at worst it is dangerous to health. Profound stress, such as that caused by job loss or the loss of a loved one can take a serious physical toll. But the human body is designed to handle stressful situations, if not indeed to thrive and be challenged by some of them. The goal should not be to avoid all stress, but to maintain a high degree of health so that one handles and survives stress well. Poor health cannot be blamed on stress. We fall prey to stress *because of poor health*.

FOOD THERAPY

🍃 Good nutrition is a good answer to stress and tension. As stress increases, protein needs go up. Under extreme stress the amount of protein used up in one day is that supplied by a gallon of milk. Protein and mineral-rich foods are the best choice, such as vegetable proteins from whole grains, sea vegetables, seafoods, soy foods eggs and sprouts. Have fresh carrot juice and fresh fish or seafood at least once a week.

🍃 Add magnesium-rich foods from green vegetables and whole grains.

🍃 Make a mix and take 2 TBS. daily:
   ✦ Brewer's yeast
   ✦ Wheat germ
   ✦ Sunflower seeds
   ✦ Molasses
   ✦ High Omega 3 flax oil

🍃 Observe good food combining to relieve indigestion caused by stress. Take a glass of wine before dinner. No liquids with meals.

🍃 Don't eat on the run, while working between meals, or while watching TV

🍃 Drink only bottled water.

VITAMINS/MINERALS

▶ Fight stress with anti-oxidants:
   ✦ Ascorbate vitamin C with bioflavonoids, 500mg. every 4 hours during acute periods.
   ✦ Natures Plus germanium w. suma
   ✦ CoQ 10 15-30mg. daily.
   ✦ Beta-carotene 25,000, 3x daily
   ✦ Zinc 30mg. ♂

▶ Stress B Complex 100mg. 2-3x daily, with extra B6 250mg. and pantothenic acid 1500mg.
   with
YS royal jelly, ginseng and honey tea, or royal jelly ½ teasp. daily. ♀
   or
Ctry. Life RELAXER tabs under the tongue for fast reief. ♂

▶ Effective mineral supplements:
   ✦ Magnesium/potassium/bromelain caps ♂, or homeopathic *Mag. Phos.* ♀
   ✦ Mezotrace SEA MINERAL CPLX.
   ✦ Rainbow Light EVERYDAY CALCIUM. ♀

▶ Effective supplements for nerves
   ✦ DLPA 500-750mg. as needed daily
   ✦ Evening primrose oil 2-4 daily
   ✦ Source Naturals MEGA GLA caps
   ✦ Hylands *Calms and Calms Forte*
   ✦ Twin Labs GABA PLUS w. taurine

HERBAL THERAPY

🌿 Feed your nerves:
   ◆ Crystal Star RELAX CAPS™ 2-4 daily, or STRESSED OUT™ extract.
   ◆ Wisdom of the Ancients YERBA MATÉ tea.
   ◆ Gotu kola
   ◆ Scullcap
   ◆ Chamomile

🌿 Feed your adrenals;
   ◆ Crystal Star ADR-ACTIVE™ caps or ADRN™ extract.
   ◆ Licorice extract

🌿 Add herbal minerals for stability:
   ◆ Crystal Star CALCIUM SOURCE™caps or extract, or MINERAL SPECTRUM™ caps
   ◆ Kelp tabs 8 daily

🌿 Body balancers against stress:
   ◆ Siberian ginseng
   ◆ Astragalus
   ◆ Suma
   ◆ Ho-Shou-Wu
   ◆ Reishi mushroom tea

🌿 Effective calmatives:
   ◆ Valerian/wild lettuce
   ◆ Hops/valerian
   ◆ Bach Flower RESCUE REMEDY
   ◆ Medicine Wheel SERENE extract
   ◆ Passion flower ♀
   ◆ Crystal Star RELAX™ tea
   ◆ Zand VALERIAN HERBAL

BODYWORK

You have to unwind before you can unleash.

▲ Go on a short vacation. Take a long weekend. It will do wonders for your head.
Work addiction is the health hazard of our time. Build adequate rest and exercise into your life.

▲ Do deep breathing exercises every day and get regular aerobic exercise for tissue oxygen.

▲ Consciously take a rest and relaxation period every day. Listen to soft music. Meditate.Do 3 minutes of neck rolls when you are stressed out.

▲ Hypnotherapy, aromatherapy with chamomile oil, massage therapy and shiatsu have all shown effective results against stress.

▲ Have a good laugh every day.

▲ Don't smoke. Nicotine constricts the blood vessels, causing increased body stress.

Common Symptoms: Four levels of stress symptoms: 1) losing interest in enjoyable activities, sagging of the corners of the eyes, creasing of the forehead, becoming short-tempered, bored, nervous; 2) tiredness, anger, insomnia, paranoia, sadness; 3) chronic head and neck aches, high blood pressure, upset stomach, looking older; 4) skin disorders, kidney malfunction, susceptibility to frequent infections, asthma, heart disease, mental breakdown.
Common Causes: Emotional and/or psycholgical problems; overuse of drugs or prescription medicines; work addiction; fatigue, lack of rest; too much tobacco, caffeine or alcohol; allergies; hypoglycemia; mineral depletion; noise, air, environmental pollutants; overcrowding; unemployment or job pressure; poverty; marital, social problems.

TASTE & SMELL LOSS

While there is a broad variety of reasons for this dysfunction, the natural healing focus on overcoming nutritional deficiencies has been able to successfully address many of the root causes. In most cases, if total atrophy has not developed, at least partial taste and smell can be restored.

FOOD THERAPY

A mineral-rich, low fat, low salt diet is a key factor.

- Make sure the diet is low in salt and refined sugars.

- Use herbal salt-free seasonings.

- Keep the diet free of mucous-clogging foods, such as heavy starches, red meats and pasteurized dairy foods.

- Have some brown rice, miso soup, and sea vegetables every day for 3 months to boost minerals and B vitamins.

- See the Low Salt Diet (pg. 74) for more information.

VITAMINS/MINERALS

- Zinc, up to 100mg. daily. Most people with sensory loss have a zinc deficiency.

- ENER B₁₂ internasal gel every other day. ♀

- B complex 100mg. daily, with extra B6 100mg.
  with
  Ester C 550mg. with bioflavonoids 4-6 daily. ♀

- Marine carotene up to 100,000IU daily,
  with
  Solaray CAL/MAG CITRATE capsules 4-6 daily. ♀

- Glutamine 500mg. 2 daily,
  with
  Mezotrace SEA MINERAL complex tabs 3 daily. ♂

- Enzymatic Therapy LIQUID LIVER with Siberian ginseng capsules 3-4 daily. ♂

HERBAL THERAPY

- Crystal Star MINERAL SPECTRUM™ capsules 4 daily, or SYSTEM STRENGTH™ drink daily, for at least 3 months to increase natural foundation minerals in the body.

- Kelp tabs 6 daily.

- Ginkgo biloba extract 3-4x daily. ♂

- Twin Lab propolis extract 3-4x daily. ♂

- Siberian ginseng extract capsules 2 daily,
  or
  Superior ginseng/royal jelly vials 1 daily. ♂

BODYWORK

- Use a catnip or chlorophyll enema to cleanse clogging mucous.

- Regular exercise with deep breathing to keep passages clear.

- Reflexology point:

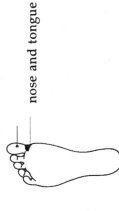

nose and tongue

Common Causes: Zinc and other mineral deficiency; too many antibiotics, causing zinc excretion; side effect of chemotherapy; deviated septum; chronic low grade throat and sinus infection; poor circulation and mucous clogged system; atrophied nerve endings; over-the-counter cold medicines; chemical diuretics; high blood pressure medicine; gland imbalance and poor hormone secretions; hereditary proneness.

See Children's Remedies in this book for more information, page 112.

FOOD THERAPY

🍃 Effective food applications on gums:
  ♠ Garlic oil if there is infection.
  ♠ Sea salt and honey mix.
  ♠ Wine or brandy if there is swelling.
  ♠ Clove oil if there is redness and swelling.

🍃 Include vitamin A-rich vegetables, vitamin D-rich eggs, fish and sea vegetables and high bioflavonoid foods in the child's diet.

🍃 Give a dilute solution of Crystal Star BIOFLAV., FIBER & C SUPPORT™ drink several times a week.

🍃 Feed plenty of chilled foods; fresh fruits, yogurt, etc. to relieve discomfort.

🍃 Give lots of cool water daily.

VITAMINS/MINERALS

▶ Natra-Bio *Teething* drops.

▶ Hylands *Teething* tablets.

▶ Homeopathic *Chamomilla*. Rub *Plantago Majus tincture* directly on tender gums.

▶ Ascorbate vitamin C powder with bioflavonoids - make a weak solution in water. Give internally and apply to gums every few hours.

▶ Chewable Mezotrace CHILDREN'S SEA MINERAL complex. (Break in half or dissolve in juice.)

▶ Hyland's *Calc.-Phos.* tabs (break in half, or dissolve in juice)

▶ Apply aloe vera gel to gums as needed.

HERBAL THERAPY

🌿 Rub on lobelia extract.

🌿 Rub on peppermint oil.

🌿 Rub on myrrh extract.

🌿 Rub on bilberry extract drops as an anti-inflammatory.

🌿 Make a weak goldenseal solution in water. Give internally with an eye dropper on the back of the tongue. Rub on gums as an anti-infective.

🌿 Effective weak teas:
  ◆ Slippery elm
  ◆ Chamomile
  ◆ Raspberry
  ◆ Catnip
  ◆ Peppermint
  ◆ Fennel

🌿 Soak yarrow flowers in bran and water for 3 days. Strain and rub on gums as needed.

🌿 Let the child chew on natural licorice or cold raw carrot sticks.

BODYWORK

▶ Make a weak tea tree oil solution with water, and rub on gums if there is swelling and infection.

▶ Let the child play in the sun for 15 to 20 minutes every morning for full-spectrum vitamins - especially sunlight vitamin D.

▶ Reflexology points:

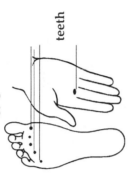

teeth

Common Symptoms: Sore, inflamed gums where teeth are pushing through the skin; often slight fever and infection; crying and discomfort.

TENDONITIS ▦ FIBROMYALGIA

Muscle Cramps ◇ Leg Cramps ◇ Joint Inflammation

Tendonitis is the painful inflammation of a tendon, usually resulting from a strain, and developing as a dull or dragging sensation after exercise. Fibromyalgia indicates pain in the fibrous connective tissue components of the muscles, tendons and ligaments. See Sports Injuries and Bursitis pages in this book for more information.

FOOD THERAPY

🥬 Concentrate on fresh foods (at least 50% of the diet) during healing. Include plenty of vegetable proteins for faster healing, and magnesium-rich foods for muscle tension. Add a weekly potassium broth (pg. 53) for electrolyte replacement.

🥬 Eat high vitamin C foods, particularly a drink of lemon juice, honey and water at night, and grapefruit or pineapple juice in the morning.

🥬 Make a mix and take 2 TBS. daily:
♦ Brewer's yeast
♦ Wheat germ
♦ Lecithin

🥬 Avoid acid-forming foods, such as red meats, caffeine and carbonated drinks. Restrict intake of fats and sugars.

For fibromyalgia:
♦ Eliminate common food allergens such as milk, corn, wheat, eggs and nightshade vegetables such as tomatoes, potatoes, peppers and eggplant.

🥬 See the Arthritis Diet in this book for more suggestions.

VITAMINS/MINERALS

▶ DLPA 500-750mg. for pain relief.

▶ Quercetin Plus with bromelain 500mg. 2-4x daily as an effective anti-inflammatory.
with
Ctry. Life Magnesium/potassium/bromelain caps 2 daily.

▶ Effective anti-inflammatories:
♣ Country Life LIGATEND tabs.
♣ Am. Biologics INFLAZYME FORTE.
♣ Enzymatic Therapy ACID-A-CAL, with MYOTONE or COR-TOTONE.

▶ Homeopathic *Arnica Montana* with a salve of *Ruta Graveolens*.

▶ Mezotrace SEA MINERAL COMPLEX 4 daily, *with* vitamin E 400IU.

▶ Alta Health SIL-X silica caps 4 daily, with MANGANESE & B12 lozenges 2 daily.

▶ Future Biotics VITAL K, *with* high omega 3 flax oil 3x daily. ♀

▶ For fibromyalgia:
♣ Bromelain 500mg. 2x daily.
♣ Pancreatin 1300mg. before meals.

HERBAL THERAPY

🌿 Crystal Star RELAX CAPS™ to rebuild nerve sheath,
with
ANTI-FLAM™ caps or extract for inflammation, ANTI-SPZ™ or CRAMP BARK COMBO™ extract as needed for pain. ♂

🌿 Crystal Star BONZ™ and/or ADR-ACTIVE™ caps to rebuild adrenal cortex.

🌿 Liquid chlorophyll 3 teasp. daily with meals, or Crystal Star energy green drink, or Sun CHLORELLA 15 tabs daily.

🌿 Lobelia extract drops. ☺

🌿 Rub on Care Plus OXYGEL or aloe vera gel.

🌿 Crystal Star HIGH PERFORMANCE™ capsules 2-4 *before* stressing the muscles to prevent lactic and uric acid buildup. SILICA SOURCE™ extract for collagen formation.

🌿 For fibromyalgia:
♦ Solaray TURMERIC compound.
♦ Butcher's broom tea or caps.
♦ Milk thistle seed extract for liver sensitivity to solvents.
♦ St. John's wort extract for sleep.

BODYWORK

▶ Apply ice packs immediately. Elevate legs and slap them hard with open palms to stimulate circulation.

▶ Effective applications:
→ DMSO liquid w. aloe vera
→ B&T TRIFLORA ANALGESIC
→ TIGER BALM
→ Chinese WHITE FLOWER oil

▶ Effective compresses:
→ B&T ARNIFLORA GEL
→ Calendula gel
→ Comfrey
→ Hot burdock tea

▶ Massage affected areas well and frequently. Massage therapy and shiatsu are both effective treatments.

▶ Use alternating hot and cold compresses on affected areas to increase circulation, and take down swelling.

▶ For fibromyalgia:
→ Exercise with walking, low-impact aerobics and swimming.
→ Regular massage therapy treatments.

Common Symptoms: Cramping and soreness during and after muscle exertion; painful joints and nerve endings; limited range of motion; leg cramps at night.
Common Causes: Calcium, magnesium, and general mineral deficiency; poor diet, high in acid-forming foods, low in green vegetables and whole grains; too much saturated fat and sugar; HCl depletion; poor circulation. Stress, insomnia, cleaning solvent compounds and cold, damp weather aggravate fibromyalgia.

THYROID HEALTH

See hyperthyroid and hypothyroid pages in this book for additional information.

The thyroid is the thermostat of the body. It produces hormones which work to keep the metabolic rate stable, and keep energy-producing and energy-using processes in balance. Thyroid hormone is the body's carburetor. If it is depleted or deficient, the rest of the body functions poorly. To determine your thyroid condition, take your basal temperature for 10 minutes on rising in the morning. It should be between 97.8 and 98.2 for health. Below this, and a sluggish thyroid still exists. Temperature will return to normal as nutritional therapies become effective. (See basal thyroid test in the Appendix for more detailed information.)

FOOD THERAPY

� Follow a diet with at least 50% fresh foods for a month to rebalance the system for better metabolism.

🌞 Eat iodine-rich foods:
 ♣ Sea vegetables, sea foods and leafy greens.

🌞 Eat vitamin A-rich foods: yellow vegetables, eggs, carrots, dark green vegetables, raw dairy.

🌞 Make an equal mix and take 2 TBS. daily:
 ♣ brewer's yeast
 ♣ wheat germ

🌞 Avoid refined foods, saturated fats, sugars, white flour products and red meats.

🌞 Avoid brussels sprouts, cabbages, etc. They have anti-thyroid substances.

🌞 Cancer of the thyroid has been linked to highly fluoridated water.

VITAMINS/MINERALS

▶ **Nutri-Pak thyroxin-free double strength thyroid.**

▶ Emulsified A 25,000IU 3x daily, or beta carotene 100,000IU daily, with Vitamin E 400IU daily.
 and
 Ester C with bioflavonoids 3000mg. daily.

▶ CoQ 10 30mg. daily.

▶ Magnesium/potassium/bromelain caps 2 daily, and zinc 75mg. daily. ♂

▶ Taurine 500mg. with lysine 500mg. 2x daily.

▶ Enzymatic Therapy THYROID/TYROSINE caps. ♀

▶ B Complex 100mg. with extra B2 100mg., B1 500mg., and B6 250mg.

▶ Raw glandulars for thyroid health:
 ♣ Raw thyroid
 ♣ Raw pituitary
 ♣ Raw adrenal substance

HERBAL THERAPY

The thyroid needs body iodine to produce its hormones. An imbalanced thyroid invariably causes over-production of estrogen and all of its attendant problems for women. Herbal iodine sources are effective without side effects or imbalances.

🌿 Crystal Star IODINE SOURCE™ caps or extract 3x daily.
 or
 META-TABS™ 2x daily, with ADRN™ extract 2x daily.

🌿 Sun CHLORELLA, or Wakasa GOLD DRINK or Crystal Star SYSTEM STRENGTH™ daily.

🌿 Heritage atomodine. ♀
 with
 Nature's Plus Vit. E 800IU.

🌿 Evening primrose oil caps 4 daily.

🌿 **Kelp tabs 6-8 daily, with c-ayenne caps 3 daily.**

🌿 Siberian ginseng extract under the tongue 2x daily. ♂

BODYWORK

▶ Take a half hour brisk walk daily to oxygenate and stimulate circulation.

▶ Sunbathe in the morning. Sea swim/wade whenever possible.

▶ Acupressure point: Press hollow at the base of the throat to stimulate thyroid, 3x for 10 seconds each time.

▶ Reflexology point:

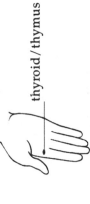

thyroid/thymus

▶ Avoid fluorescent lights when possible. They deplete calcium and vitamin A in the body.

▶ Color therapy: for hypothyroid- wear orange glasses 20-30 min; switch to blue for 5 minutes. Reverse for hyperthyroid.

Common Symptoms: Weak, sluggish system; dry, cold skin; slow thinking; chronic fatigue; weight gain because of poor metabolism.
Common Causes: Iodine depletion, often from X-rays or low dose radiation tests, such as mammograms; pituitary and thyroid malfunction; air and environmental pollutants that deplete vitamin A in the body; overuse of diet pills and other drugs; vitamin A, E and zinc deficiency.

TONSILLITIS

The tonsils are part of the lymphatic tissue of the pharynx, acting to strain out and process poisons from the body. Tonsillitis is the inflammation of a tonsil and may be caused by a variety of streptococcal organisms. While the infection itself may not be serious, it always indicates a deeper immune response attack, and can lead to very serious problems, such as rheumatic fever and nephritis.

FOOD THERAPY

🍃 Go on a 24 hr. (pg. 44) or 3 day liquid cleansing diet (pg. 43) to clear out body toxins.

◆ Then eat only fresh foods for the rest of the week during an attack.

◆ Have lemon juice and water each morning with plenty of other high vitamin C juices throughout the day, such as orange, pineapple, and grapefruit juice.

◆ Have a fresh carrot juice, and a potassium broth or essence (pg. 53) once a day.

◆ Get plenty of vegetable protein for healing.

🍃 Have an onion/garlic broth each day. (pg. 57).

🍃 Avoid sugars, pasteurized dairy products, and all junk foods until condition clears.

🍃 **Drink 6-8 glasses of bottled water daily to keep the body flushed.**
Sip aloe vera juice as needed for soothing.

VITAMINS/MINERALS

▷ Zinc gluconate throat lozenges as needed. ☺

▷ Spray throat with Nutribiotic GRAPEFRUIT SEED extract spray as needed.

▷ Nature's Plus CHEWABLE ACEROLA C 500mg. with bioflavonoids, 1-2 every hour during acute stages.
   and
Beta carotene 100,000IU daily as an anti-infective.

▷ Enzymatic Therapy VIRAPLEX caps 4 daily, with ORAL-ZYME lozenges as needed.

▷ Raw thymus extract for increased immune strength.

▷ Solaray pantothenic acid 1500mg. with B6 250mg. to take down swelling. ♀

▷ Propolis lozenges or tincture as needed. ♂

HERBAL THERAPY

❦ Anti-inflammatories are a key to relief:
   ◆ Crystal Star ANTI-FLAM™ caps or extract as needed.
   ◆ Crystal Star ASPIR-SOURCE™ caps to relieve head and throat pain. ☺
   ◆ Licorice root or Crystal Star SUPER LICORICE extract.
   ◆ Solaray TURMERIC caps.

❦ Crystal Star ANTI-BIO™ caps 4-6 daily to flush lymph glands and clear infection.
   with
FIRST AID CAPS™, 4-6 daily during the acute phase.

❦ Crystal Star COFEX™ TEA as a soothing throat coat.

❦ Effective extracts and drops:
   ◆ Echinacea to clear lymph
   ◆ Garlic oil
   ◆ Gotu kola
   ◆ Black walnut
   ◆ Lobelia if there is fever ☺
   ◆ Mullein ⊛

❦ Use mullein or lobelia tea as a throat compress.

BODYWORK

➤ Take a garlic or catnip enema during an attack to clear body poisons. ☺

➤ Ice the throat with a towel wrapped over crushed ice.

➤ Wear blue color therapy glasses 20-30 minutes at a time.

➤ Effective gargles:
   → Weak tea tree oil solution in water every 2-3 hours.
   → Slippery elm tea.
   → Liquid chlorophyll 1 teasp. in water.
   → Goldenseal/myrrh solution.

➤ Take hot mineral salts baths frequently.

➤ Reflexology point:

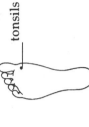
tonsils

➤ Get plenty of bed rest during acute stage.

Common Symptoms: Swollen tonsils and lymph glands; difficulty swallowing; fever, chills, and tender sore throat; aches and pains in the back and extremities; bad breath because of the infection; ear infection and hearing difficulty because of the swollen glands.
Common Causes: A strep infection; poor diet that aggravates a sporadic infection, with too many starches, sugars, and pasteurized dairy foods; not enough green vegetables and soluble fiber foods; constipation causing toxic build-up; food allergies, particularly to wheat and dairy; poor digestion, and non-assimilation of nutrients.

Plaque-causing bacteria can be formed and begin damaging teeth and gums within 12 hours if the teeth have not been properly cleaned. It is important to brush at least twice a day and to floss or water pick just before going to bed. Various kinds of sweeteners, especially sucrose, and refined carbohydrates are known to significantly increase plaque accumulation.

FOOD THERAPY

❧ Eat crunchy teeth-cleaning fresh vegetables; celery, carrots, broccoli, cauliflower, apples, etc.

❧ Eat lots of green leafy vegetables and high fiber foods. Have a large fresh salad every day.

❧ Eat cashews or chew cardamom seeds. The oil in either fights decay by interfering with production of plaque acid, and by washing away cavity-causing bacteria.

❧ Avoid soft, gooey foods, and dairy products such as ice cream or soft cheeses that leave a film on the teeth.

❧ **Reduce dietary fats. A high fat diet results in high lipid levels in the saliva and a higher risk of tooth decay.**

❧ **Rub strawberry halves on the teeth. Leave on 1/2 hour. Rinse and brush.**

❧ Wash and rinse the mouth often with cider vinegar or lemon juice. Scrub teeth with lemon

VITAMINS/MINERALS

▶ Enzymatic Therapy ACID-A-CAL caps 4 daily.

▶ Twin Lab PROPOLIS TINCTURE. Take under the tongue and hold as long as possible.

▶ Alta Health SIL-X silica daily.

▶ Cal/mag/zinc 4 daily, with beta carotene 25,000IU 4 daily.

▶ Ascorbate vitamin C crystals with bioflavs. and rutin 1/4 teasp. 4x daily in water. Swish and hold in mouth before swallowing for best results.

▶ CoQ 10, 10mg. 3x daily.

▶ Solaray CAL/MAG 500/500mg. with vitamin D 1000IU for tooth strength.

▶ Massage gums with vitamin E oil; take internally 400IU daily.

▶ For salivary duct stones:
♣ Potassium iodide drops for 1-3 months.
♣ Ascorbate vitamin C or Ester C, 3000mg. daily.

HERBAL THERAPY

❦ Add 3 drops tea tree oil to water and use as a mouthwash.

❦ Solaray ALFAJUICE capsules 4 daily,

or

Sun CHLORELLA 1 packet daily, for concentrated green food.

❦ Crystal Star MINERAL SPECTRUM caps 4 daily for a month to build tooth enamel. ♀

❦ Effective teas:
◆ Dandelion root
◆ White sage
◆ Parsley

❦ For salivary duct stones:
◆ Rinse mouth with a solution of equal parts goldenseal root tea and white oak bark tea to reduce pain, swelling and bleeding.
◆ Rinse mouth with ginger root solution, and apply ginger root compresses to affected area.
◆ Rinse mouth with Atomodine solution in water for natural potassium and iodine.

BODYWORK

▶ Floss daily, and brush well *after every meal* if you have a tendency to tartar build-up.

▶ Mix equal parts of cream of tartar and sea salt, or baking soda and sea salt. Brush teeth to remove tartar.

▶ Use papain powder or baking soda as a tooth powder. Both actually help to kill harmful bacteria, and are less abrasive than commercial toothpastes.

▶ Dissolve 1 TBS. of food grade 3% H$_2$O$_2$ in an 8oz. glass of water, and use as a mouthwash daily for a month.

▶ Use Nutribiotic GRAPEFRUIT SEED EXTRACT in water as a mouthwash.

▶ Chew all food well for jaw growth and to prevent corrosion.

▶ Use toothpaste and chew gum that has Xylitol as a sweetener. It has been shown not to cause plaque formation.

Common Symptoms: Bad breath; noticeable sticky film on the teeth; bad mouth taste. Salivary stones cause swelling and pain in the jaw just in front of the ear, and a stone-like growth that blocks saliva.
Common Causes: Too many refined carbohydrates and sugars; excess red meat, caffeine and soft drinks that cause constipation and acid in the system; vitamin and fresh food deficiency.

TOOTHACHE ▨ WISDOM TOOTH INFECTION ▨ TMJ

Many dentists now realize that you need to see a nutritionist along with a dentist if you have chronic toothaches and infection. Diet, nutrition and lifestyle changes are indicated - not just more brushing and flossing. Current natural healing wisdom about wisdom teeth - grow them in straight; eat right so they don't decay; clean them well and keep them. They help the immune system of the mouth to work. TMJ is a chronic syndrome that links various dental and other health problems to poor jaw alignment.

FOOD THERAPY

🍂 Eat primarily fresh foods during acute stages to speed healing, with plenty of leafy greens and green drinks (pg. 54ff).
  🍂 Then, to prevent recurring tooth problems, eat lots of crunchy, crisp foods, such as celery, and other raw vegetables, nuts and seeds, and whole grain crackers.

🍂 Eat calcium-rich foods: greens and shellfish.

🍂 Ice the jaw for pain. Take a little wine or brandy and hold on the aching area as long as possible.
  or
🍂 Mix 20 drops of clove oil with 1 oz. brandy. Apply with a cotton swab to toothache area.

🍂 Avoid soft, gooey foods. No sweets, soft drinks or sodas, if your teeth are not strong.
  🍂 Go light on acid citrus juices. They are great for your insides, but not for your teeth.

VITAMINS/MINERALS

▶ Take liquid chlorophyll in a small amount of water. Swish and hold in mouth as long as possible. ♂

▶ Nature's Plus CAL/MAG 500mg. each, 4 daily, with boron 3mg. daily for better tooth growth.
  or
Nature's Life LIQUID CALCIUM PHOS. FREE with vitamin D.

▶ Take CoQ 10, 30mg. daily on a regular basis as a preventive.

▶ B Complex 100mg. with extra B6 100mg., niacin 100mg., and vitamin A 10,000IU 2x daily.

▶ Enzymatic Therapy ORAL-ZYME lozenges as needed.

▶ DLPA 500mg. as needed for pain. ♀

▶ Effective homeopathic remedies:
  ✤ NatraBio *Teeth & Gums* tincture.
  ✤ *Chamomilla* - neuralgic aches.
  ✤ *Belladonna* - wisdom tooth pain.
  ✤ For TMJ - *Cal. Phos., Mag. Phos.,* and *Rhus Tox.*
  ✤ *Belladonna* - ache with pressure
  ✤ *Hypericum* - pain after extraction.

▶ Alta Health SIL-X silica caps 4 daily.

HERBAL THERAPY

🌿 Apply clove oil directly to painful tooth as needed.

🌿 Take and apply directly:
  ◆ Valerian/wild lettuce extract.
  ◆ Black walnut extract
  ◆ Twin Lab PROPOLIS extract
  ◆ Lobelia tincture ☺

🌿 Crystal Star ANTI-BIO™ caps or extract during infection period,
  and
Solaray TURMERIC caps, or Crystal Star ANTI-FLAM™ CAPS, 4 as needed for inflammation pain.

🌿 Crystal Star ASPIRSOURCE™ capsules for nerve pain.
  and
CALCIUM SOURCE™ and SILICA SOURCE™ caps for building strong teeth.

🌿 Other effective capsules:
  ◆ Kava Kava
  ◆ Cayenne/ginger
  ◆ Echinacea/myrrh

🌿 Effective mouth rinses:
  ◆ Sassafras
  ◆ Hops/chamomile
  ◆ Slippery elm

BODYWORK

▶ Acupressure: Squeeze the sides of each index finger at the end. Hold hard for 30 seconds.

▶ Effective compresses:
  ↠ Hot comfrey
  ↠ Ginger root

▶ Effective applications:
  ↠ Chinese WHITE FLOWER oil
  ↠ Propolis tincture
  ↠ Eucalyptus oil

▶ Rinse the mouth with a solution of equal parts goldenseal and white oak bark tea to take down pain and swelling.

▶ Reflexology point:

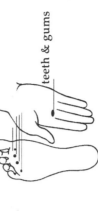
teeth & gums

▶ Chew food very well. Brush and floss well at night. These activities are exercise for the teeth and gums.

Common Symptoms: Sore jaw and/or gums; dull or shooting pains; tooth or root nerve pain from a cavity; tooth and jaw crowding from wisdom teeth coming in too big, misaligned, etc.; pain from bruxism (tooth grinding at night); periodontal disease, and/or bleeding gums. TMJ symptoms include headaches, ringing in the ears, sinus pain, hearing loss, depression, and facial neuralgia.

Toxic shock is a virulent, often fatal staphylococcal infection that takes over the body incredibly quickly when immunity is depressed. A victim can be deathly ill in a matter of hours. Despite what many women think, toxic shock syndrome has not disappeared, still victimizing one in 100,000 menstruating women every year. While absorbency ratings and safety procedures for dyes and fibers have improved, tampon absorbency is still the most important factor associated with toxic shock. Research has shown that continuous high absorbency tampon use significantly alters vaginal flora, rendering a woman more vulnerable to vaginal infections and ulcerations where the toxic virus can take over. A strong immune system is the best and only defense. See Shock & Trauma procedures, page 312, and Building & Strengthening Immunity on page 249 for more information.

FOOD THERAPY

The following diet recommendations are to prevent recurrence, and to strengthen the immune system after emergency treatment and the hospital stay.

❧ The body will have suffered major deterioration. Optimum, concentrated nutrition must be followed for recovery. Make sure you are including several fresh vegetable juices and green drinks every day (pg. 53ff), or one such as Crystal Star ENERGY GREEN™ drink.

❧ Include plenty of high vegetable **protein sources for faster recovery; plenty of whole grains, soy foods, sprouts and sea foods; complex carbohydrates for strength, and cultured foods for G.I. flora.**

❧ Make a mix and take 2 TBS. daily:
♦ Wheat germ
♦ Brewer's yeast flakes
♦ Unsulphured molasses

VITAMINS/MINERALS

▶ **Anti-oxidants are a key:**
♦ Germanium 100-150mg. SL daily, or dissolve 1 gm. in 1 qt. water, and take ¼ cup daily.
♣ CoQ 10 30mg. 3x daily, with bromelain 1000mg. daily.
♦ Vitamin C or Ester C powder with bioflavonoids and rutin, ½ teasp. every 2 hours to bowel tolerance all during the healing period for collagen and interstitial tissue regrowth.
♦ Biotec CELL GUARD enzymes 6 daily.

▶ Highest potency YS or Premier 1 royal jelly 3 teasp. daily.

▶ Alta Health SIL-X silica tabs for collagen and tissue formation, with Future Biotics VITAL K liquid, and Floradix HERBAL IRON liquid 3x daily.

▶ Mezotrace SEA MINERAL complex 4 daily.

▶ Molasses 2 TBS. with PABA 1000mg. and pantothenic acid 1000mg. for hair regrowth.

HERBAL THERAPY

❧ Crystal Star rebuilding formulas - 2 of each daily:
♦ ADR-ACTIVE™ with BODY REBUILDER™ caps
♦ GINSENG 6 SUPER ENERGY caps and DEFENSE RESTORATIVE™ super tea
♦ POTASSIUM SOURCE™ caps
♦ SILICA SOURCE™ extract
♦ HEARTSEASE/HAWTHORNE caps with vitamin E
♦ HEARTSEASE/ANEMI-GIZE™ caps
♦ Hawthorne extract
♦ SYSTEM STRENGTH™ drink

❧ Sun CHLORELLA or Green Foods GREEN MAGMA 2 packets daily, Solaray ALFAJUICE caps, 6 daily.

❧ Crystal Star GREEN TEA CLEANSER™, or bancha leaf or kukicha twig tea for cleansed blood and balanced body pH.

❧ Apply alternating hot and cold compresses to collapsed veins or numb extremities:
♦ Cayenne/ginger compresses for the hot application; plain ice water

BODYWORK

Get emergency medical help immediately if you suspect toxic shock. It it can rapidly become life-threatening. Emergency help can keep the victim alive if received in time. Natural therapies can help bring them back to health.

▶ Take precautions:
→ Use lower absorbency tampons.
→ Alternate their use with pads.
→ Don't leave tampons in over night.

▶ Avoid all pleasure drugs as a preventive measure. The immune system is affected first.

▶ Change tampons frequently, or avoid them altogether.
→ No super absorbent tampons at all.

▶ Natural alternatives to tampons:
→ Sea sponges - may be trimmed to fit, can be washed and re-used, and are inexpensive.
→ The Keeper - a menstrual cup.
→ Non-chlorine-bleached pads with no dioxins.
→ Re-usable, washable cotton pads.
After tampon use, douche with a solution of GRAPEFRUIT SEED extract - 10 drops in 1 qt. water as a precautionary measure.

Common Symptoms: High fever, nausea, vomiting, diarrhea, dizziness, a painless sunburn-like rash; drifting in and out of consciousness. The symptoms happen so fast and are so extreme, the victim has almost no time to examine or judge them. Only someone close to the victim can see the virulence and react.
Common Causes: Use of pleasure drugs, debilitating in their own right, with the chance of harmful poisons in the processing techniques; "New Age" eating on a long-term basis (low protein, primarily fruits and cleansing foods), with no substance to grow or live on; vitamin B depletion and deficiency; malnutrition, leaving the body with lowered immunity, wide open for a virulent virus to take over.

TUMORS

Malignant

Malignant tumors should be addressed as soon as possible to control spreading to other tissues. Immune enhancement is the key in natural treatment. A whole foods diet and natural supplementation program has been successful in both reducing and in some cases, completely eliminating tumors.

FOOD THERAPY

🍃 Begin with a short liquid cleansing diet (pg. 43). During the first month of healing have at least one each of the following juices daily:
  ♣ Potassium broth (pg. 53)
  ♣ A green drink (pg. 54)
  ♣ Cranberry juice
  ♣ Pineapple juice

🍃 Then, eat primarily fresh foods for a month.
  ♣ Add whole grains, high fiber foods and steamed vegetables during the 4th week.

🍃 Keep the system clean and clear and the liver functioning well with a diet high in greens, and low in dairy products and saturated fats.
  ♣ Avoid heavy starches, refined sugars, and all fried foods.
  ♣ Drink only distilled bottled water - 6-8 glasses daily to keep toxic wastes quickly clear of the body.

🍃 Take George's ALOE VERA JUICE with herbs *and* apply aloe vera gel twice daily.

VITAMINS/MINERALS

▶ Quercetin Plus with bromelain 2 daily, and vitamin K 100mg. 2 daily to inhibit growth.

▶ Ascorbate vitamin C with bioflavonoids, $\frac{1}{2}$ teasp. every 2-3 hours to bowel tolerance during healing.
  with
  Marine carotene 100,000IU

▶ Germanium with suma 50mg. daily. ♀ or Solaray TRI-O₂ 2 daily. ♂

▶ Sun CHLORELLA or Green Foods GREEN MAGMA, 2 packets in water daily.

▶ Cartilade or Ecomer SHARK CARTILAGE capsules.

▶ Natren LIFE START II, $\frac{1}{2}$ teasp. with meals, and Enzymatic Therapy IMMUNOPLEX caps as directed. ♀

▶ Phosphatidyl choline (PC 55) 4 daily and carnitine 500mg. 2 daily to help liver process toxic wastes better.

▶ B Complex 150mg. daily, with extra B6 250mg., pantothenic acid 500mg. and folic acid 400mcg. to help deter spread of cancerous cells.

HERBAL THERAPY

🌿 Iodine therapy: Crystal Star IODINE SOURCE™ caps or extract, or Heritage ATOMODINE drops 3-4x daily, or kelp tabs 8-10 daily, with Nature's Plus vitamin E 800IU.

🌿 Crystal Star ANTI-BIO™ caps or extract if there is infection,
  with
  Evening primrose oil caps 6 daily or Source Naturals MEGA GLA 240mg. especially for tumors caused by radiation/chemical carcinogens.

🌿 Effective tumor-reducing herbs:
  ♦ Comfrey tea 4-5 cups daily. ♂
  ♦ Pau de arco/butternut for natural quercetin. ♀
  ♦ Reishi mushroom capsules ♂
  ♦ Chamomile
  ♦ Suma extract
  ♦ Red clover ☺

🌿 Siberian ginseng extract 3-4x daily to retard growth.
  with

🌿 Effective herbal applications:
  ♦ Crystal Star GINSENG SKIN REPAIR GEL™ with germanium and vitamin C for several months.
  ♦ Pau de arco gel.
  ♦ Calendula gel, esp. when it is too late for an operation.
  ♦ Care Plus H₂O₂ OXYGEL for 2 months twice daily.

BODYWORK

▶ See Skin Cancer page in this book for more information.

▶ Effective packs:
  → Blue violet
  → Mullein/lobelia
  → Fresh comfrey leaf
  → Green clay poultices
  → Chaparral; also take 4 capsules daily.

Common Symptoms: Growing and mutating lumps and nodule - internally or externally - often inflamed, weeping, and painful; many times with adhesions to other tissue.
Common Causes: Poor diet with years of excess acid and mucous-forming foods; environmental, heavy metal, or radiation poisoning; X-rays and low grade radiation tests, such as mammograms, causing iodine deficiency and thyroid malfunction; viral infection such as Epstein-Barr, herpes simplex and Kaposi's sarcoma.

ULCERS - STOMACH, PEPTIC & DUODENAL

A peptic ulcer is an open sore, an erosion of the lining in either the stomach (a gastric ulcer), or the duodenum (the first part of the small intestine). When too much acid is secreted by the body (typical of duodenal ulcers) or the body's protective devices fail (typical of gastric ulcers), peptic ulcers result. Current estimates show that approximately 14 million Americans now have or have recently had, an ulcer. Ten thousand people die of peptic ulcer complications every year. Herbal remedies and vegetable juices are both gentle and succesful for ulcerated tissue.

FOOD THERAPY

🍃 Go on a short 3 day liquid diet to cleanse and alkalize the G.I. tract. Take 2-3 glasses of your choice of juices daily:
♣ Potassium broth (pg. 53)
♣ Green drinks (pg. 54)
♣ Cabbage/celery/parsley juice
♣ Apple/alfalfa sprout juice with 1 teasp. spirulina powder added.

🍃 Then, add easily digestible, fresh alkaline foods, such as leafy greens, steamed vegetables, whole grains and non-acidic fruits.
Include cultured foods, such as yogurt, kefir and buttermilk for friendly G.I. flora.

🍃 Avoid sugars, pasteurized dairy products, red meat, heavy spices, and refined foods. Reduce alcohol (a little white wine is ok). Eliminate fatty foods. They interfere with buffering activity of protein and calcium.

🍃 Drink 2-3 glasses mineral water daily. Avoid cola drinks - they provoke acid production.

🍃 Diet watchwords:
♣ Chew all food slowly and well.
♣ Eat small meals throughout the day. No large, heavy meals.
♣ Avoid late night snacks.

VITAMINS/MINERALS

▶ Enzymatic Therapy DGL chewable tabs with Sun CHLORELLA tabs 15 daily, or liquid chlorophyll 3 teasp. daily with meals.
and/or
IBS capsules as directed.

▶ High potency YS or Premier One royal jelly 2 teasp. daily. ♀

▶ Ascorbate vitamin C or Ester C, 3000mg. daily, for 3 months, with
♣ Vitamin E 400IU 2x daily
♣ Emulsified A 100,000IU daily
♣ Zinc 30mg. daily.

▶ Stress B Complex 100mg. with extra pantothenic acid 500mg. ♀

▶ Natren LIFE START #2, 1/2 teasp. before meals.

▶ Enzymatic Therapy RAW ADRENAL complex caps. ♀

▶ Propolis tincture as needed. ♂

▶ Omega 3 flax oil 3 teasp. daily. ♀

▶ Glutamine 500mg. daily.

HERBAL THERAPY

🌿 Crystal Star ULCR™ capsules or extract, with meals as needed.
and
RELAX™ caps or ANTI-SPZ™ caps as needed to calm and rebuild nerve structure. Take ANTI-BIO™ caps 4-6 daily if there is infection.

🌿 Yerba Prima aloe vera juice with herbs daily.

🌿 Effective extracts:
◆ Nature's Way ANTSP ♂
◆ Golden seal/myrrh
◆ Ginkgo biloba
◆ Licorice, or Crystal Star SUPER LICORICE™ ♂

🌿 Effective soothing/healing teas:
◆ Comfrey/mint
◆ Slippery elm
◆ Comfrey/fenugreek
◆ Chamomile/red sage

🌿 Effective anti-infective, anti-inflammatory herbs:
◆ Solaray TURMERIC capsules
◆ Solaray COOL CAYENNE caps
◆ Goldenseal/cayenne
◆ Wakunaga KYO-GREEN
◆ Garlic/parsley

BODYWORK

Avoid hard liquor, smoking, caffeine, and aspirin - key culprits in aggravating ulcers.

▶ Calcium carbonate antacids, such as TUMS and ALKA-2 actually produce increased gastric acid secretions when medication is stopped, and may cause kidney stones. Sodium bicarbonate antacids, such as Alka-Seltzer and Rolaids elevate blood pH levels interfering with metabolism and they can increase blood pressure. Aluminum-magnesium antacids, such as Maalox and Mylanta can cause calcium depletion and contribute to aluminum toxicity.
Tagamet and Zantac drugs (1 billion dollars in sales yearly) suppress HCl formation in the stomach, inhibit bone formation, and cause eventual liver damage. Both drugs also interfere with the liver's ability to metabolize and excrete toxic chemicals, making a person vulnerable to poisons from pesticides, herbicides, etc. Take DGL (deglycyrrhizinated licorice) to normalize after these drugs.

▶ Take a catnip or garlic enema once a week during healing to detoxify the G.I. tract.

▶ For duodenal ulcers: a mild olive oil flush: 2 TBS. oil through a straw before going to bed for a week.

Common Symptoms: Open sores or lesions in the stomach/duodenum walls, causing burning, nausea and diarrhea; pain right after eating for a stomach ulcer - two or three hours later for a duodenal ulcer. If the vomit is bright red, and the feces are very dark, it is a duodenal ulcer.
Common Causes: Prolonged stress and nervous tension creating an acid system; poor food combination and too many acid-forming foods; eating too fast; commercial antacids; food allergies; too many sugary foods, caffeine, alcohol and tobacco; anemia; Candida albicans; hypoglycemia.

♀ UTERINE FIBROIDS ♀

Uterine fibroids are benign growths that appear on the uterine wall. They consist of twisted muscle tissue, and are stimulated by too much estrogen. Size ranges from tiny to the dimensions of a grapefruit. They usually cease to grow after menopause, but may be painful, can cause excessive menstrual bleeding and sometimes infertility or miscarriage. Natural therapy focuses on diet improvement to rebalance hormone levels and alleviate complications. See also Ovarian Cysts, page 290 and Endometriosis, page 208.

FOOD THERAPY

🍃 Follow a low fat, fresh foods vegetarian diet (about 50-60% fresh foods) to rebalance gland functions and relieve symptoms. High fats mean high estrogen levels. Too much estrogen is a common cause of cysts and fibroids. Pain and excessive bleeding have disappeared within a matter of weeks with the change to a low fat, vegetarian diet.

♣ Get adequate high quality protein daily (about 60-70 grams) from largely vegetable sources to avoid saturated fats: whole grains, sprouts, tofu, sea foods, low fat dairy, etc.

♣ Increase intake of B vitamin-rich foods, such as brown rice, wheat germ and brewer's yeast.

♣ Avoid red meat, caffeine and refined sugars that can cause iodine deficiency.

♣ Add miso, sea vegetables, and leafy greens to alkalize the system.

♣ Avoid fried and salty foods, especially during menses.

♣ Avoid concentrated starches, full fat dairy products, and hard liquor on a continuing basis.

🍃 Take 4 teasp. wheat germ oil daily for tissue oxygen.

🍃 Have some fresh apple or carrot juice every day during healing.

VITAMINS/MINERALS

▶ Nature's Plus Vitamin E 800IU during healing.
with
Twin Lab marine carotene 100,000IU daily.

▶ High Omega 3 fish oils or squalene, shark liver oil 3x daily.

▶ Ascorbate Vitamin C, or Ester C with bioflavonoids, 5000mg. or Quercetin Plus 2 daily.
with
NutraPathic CALCIUM/COLLAGEN for collagen regrowth.

▶ If you have a Type II PAP smear, follow these steps:
✤ Green drinks, 1 daily.
✤ Goldenseal/chaparral 4 daily.
✤ Cartilade SHARK CARTILAGE 3 daily.
✤ Crystal Star WOMAN'S BEST FRIEND™ 6 daily for 3 months.
✤ Folic acid 800mcg. 2 daily for 3 months.

▶ Sun CHLORELLA 20 and germanium 100mg. daily as antioxidants.

▶ Enzymatic Therapy
✤ RAW MAMMARY caps
✤ RAW OVARY caps
✤ NUCLEOPRO F caps

HERBAL THERAPY

🌿 Crystal Star WOMAN'S BEST FRIEND™ capsules, 4 daily for 3 months.
with
Evening primrose oil caps 4-6 daily for 3 months.
then
Crystal Star LIV-ALIVE™ capsules 2 daily as a mild liver cleanse.

🌿 Iodine therapy is effective in treating frequent accompanying thyroid disorders - often successful in 3-4 months. (Take with vit. E for best results.)
◆ Atomodine drops 2-3x daily.
◆ Crystal Star IODINE SOURCE™ caps or extract.

🌿 Effective extracts:
◆ Echinacea
◆ Sarsaparilla (as a source of progesterone)
◆ Dong quai/damiana
◆ Crystal Star SILICA SOURCE™.

🌿 Crystal Star ANTI-SPZ™ caps, 4 at a time, or CRAMP BARK COMBO™ extract for cramping.

BODYWORK

▶ Be careful of jumping into surgery. Many worrisome cysts/fibroids/tumors are not cancer, and will not become cancer.

▶ Avoid IUDs and X-rays as causes of fibroid tumors.
→ Remember that synthetic estrogen increases the risk of uterine cancer.

▶ Reflexology point:

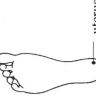 ← uterus and ovaries

Common Symptoms: Often symptomless; irregular bleeding or heavy menstrual flow, with unfamiliar back and abdominal pain; urinary problems, or pressure on the bladder, colon or abdominal veins; painful intercourse; infertility; inability to sustain pregnancy; fever and coated tongue.

Common Causes: IUDs and/or radiation and X-rays that change cell function and structure; underactive thyroid; prostaglandin and EFA deficiency; too much caffeine and saturated fat; high dose birth control pills and synthetic hormones that cause too much estrogen; obesity, because body fat converts a woman's male hormones into estrogen; hypertension; alcohol induced diabetes; high-stress lifestyle and over-acid diet producing acid wastes in the body that are poorly eliminated.

♀ VAGINAL YEAST INFECTION ■ VAGINITIS ♀

Leukorrhea ✧ Trichomonas ✧ Gardnerella ✧ Vulvitis

Trichomonas - caused by a parasite, found in both men and women, usually contracted through intercourse. **Leukorrhea** - a yeast type infection occurring during low resistance times and when normal vaginal acidity is disrupted. **Gardnerella** - a bacterial infection that thrives when vaginal pH is disturbed. **Vulvitis** - an inflammation of the vulva, caused by allergic reaction, irritation, bacterial or fungal infection. Natural therapies are very successful for most vaginal yeast infections, but a long-term cure is not likely unless dietary/lifestyle changes are made. See Candida albicans diet and healing suggestions in this book for more information.

FOOD THERAPY

🌿 The diet should be primarily fresh foods during healing. Have a large green salad with alfalfa sprouts every day. Keep meals very light, without heavy starches, fatty foods, sugars, or dairy products.

🌿 Eat plenty of fermented foods, such as yogurt and kefir, for friendly G.I. flora, especially if you have been taking antibiotics.

🌿 Acidify the system: drink 3-4 glasses of cranberry juice *from concentrate* daily.

🌿 Avoid red meats, hard liquor, sugar and caffeine while clearing.

🌿 Effective food douches:
  ◆ Cider vinegar - 2 TBS. to 1 qt. water. Add 1/4 teasp. cayenne if desired
  ◆ Diluted mineral water.
  ◆ Baking soda 2 teasp./honey 1 teasp. in 1 qt. water.
  ◆ Chlorophyll liquid 1 teasp. in 1 qt. water.

VITAMINS/MINERALS

▶ Beta carotene 100,000IU daily with Vit. E 400IU 2x daily for prevention.

▶ Vitamin C (ascorbic acid) crystals, 1/2 teasp. every 2 hours during healing, up to 5000mg. daily. A weak water solution may be used as a douche.

▶ B Complex 100mg. daily, with extra B6 100mg., and Vitamin K 100mg. 3x daily.

▶ Acidiphilus therapy: Dr. DOPHILUS 1/2 teasp. or contents of 5 capsules in 1 TB. yogurt. Smear on a tampon and insert upon retiring. Douche in the morning with 1/4 teasp. or contents of 3 caps in water.

▶ Effective brand products:
  ✿ Probiologics CERVAGYN.
  ✿ W.H.I. FEMICINE and YEAST GUARD.
  ✿ Providone IODINE DOUCHE.

▶ Nutrition Resource NUTRIBIOTIC GRAPEFRUIT SEED concentrate 20 drops in 1 gal. water as a douche.

HERBAL THERAPY

🌿 Effective extracts: both as douches in water, and under the tongue.
  ◆ Black walnut hulls
  ◆ Pau de Arco
  ◆ Garlic
  ◆ Ginkgo biloba

🌿 Crystal Star WHITES OUT™ # 1 and #2 capsules as directed, especially for more severe problems. with
Schiff GARLIC/ONION caps 6 daily and watermelon seed tea.

🌿 Crystal Star WOMAN'S BEST FRIEND™ caps 6 daily, with Crystal Star WHITES OUT DOUCHE™ for 3-6 days.

🌿 Sun CHLORELLA 1 packet daily. Also effective as a douche solution.

🌿 Effective vaginal herbal suppository: Mix powders of cranesbill, goldenseal, echinacea root, white oak bark, and raspberry with enough cocoa butter to bind. Insert at night. Seal with a napkin. Esp. for chronic vaginitis that is more than a yeast infection.

HERBAL THERAPY

▶ Effective douches: Add 1 oz. herbs to 1 qt. water. Steep 30 min., strain.
  → Calendula flowers
  → Pau de arco
  → Tea tree oil
  → White oak bark
  → Squaw vine
  → Mild white clay
  → Witch hazel bark and leaf
  → Sage/vinegar
  → 3% H₂O₂ 1 TB. in 1 qt. water.

▶ Insert tea tree oil suppositories.

▶ Apply cottage cheese or yogurt to a tampon, or acidophilus powder to a sanitary napkin and insert to rebalance vaginal pH.

▶ For vulvitis: Crystal Star FUN-GEX™ gel. Don't use fluorinated cortisone creams. They cause thinning and atrophy of the skin.

▶ For gardnerella and trich: Drink cranberry juice, insert tea tree oil suppositories for 14 days, alternate salt water and vinegar douches for a week, and take vitamins B complex and C daily.

Common Symptom: Leukorrhea: In general, there is itching, irritation, and inflammation of the vaginal tissues; foul discharge, itching and burning, chafing of the thighs, frequent urination. **Trichomonas:** severe itchiness and thin, foamy, yellowish discharge with a foul odor. **Gardnerella:** especially foul, fishy odor, creamy white discharge, moderate itchiness. **Vulvitis:** itching, redness and swelling, sometimes with fluid-filled blisters resembling genital herpes.
Common Causes: Often a condition, not a disease, in which vaginal pH is imbalanced. Causes range from long exposure to antibiotics, weakened immune system, and hormone imbalances. The active chemical in many spermicidal creams and foams, nonoxynol-9, increases recurrent cyctitis and Candida yeast infections. It also kills friendly lactobacilli that protect the vagina against disease causing micro-organisms.

337

VARICOSE VEINS ■ SPIDER VEINS

Varicose veins develop when a defect in the vein wall causes dilation in the vein and damage to the valves. When the valves are not functioning well, the increased pressure results in bulging. Women are affected four times as frequently as men. Vein fragility increases with age due to loss of tissue tone, muscle mass and weakening of vein walls.

FOOD THERAPY

❧ Go on a short 24 hour (pg. 44) liquid diet to clear circulation.
♠ Then, eat only fresh foods for the rest of the week, with plenty of green salads and juices. Add a glass of cider vinegar and honey each morning.
♠ Then follow a vegetarian, high fiber diet for the rest of the month. *Varicose veins are rarely seen in parts of the world where unrefined, high fiber diets are consumed.* Include sea foods, beans, whole grain cereals, brown rice, and steamed vegetables.

❧ Have one of the following juices every day:
♦ Pineapple
♦ Carrot
♦ Citrus
♦ Green drink (pg. 54ff)

❧ Make a mix and take 2 TBS. daily:
♦ Lecithin granules
♦ Brewer's yeast
♦ Wheat germ

❧ Reduce dairy products, fried foods, prepared meats, red meats, and saturated fats of all kinds.
Avoid salty, sugary and caffeine-containing foods.

❧ Crystal Star BIOFLAV., FIBER & C SUPPORT™t drink with acerola cherries for venous integrity.

VITAMINS/MINERALS

▷ Quercetin Plus with bromelain 500mg. 4 daily.
♣ Pycnogenol caps 50mg. 6 daily.
    and/or

▷ Vitamin C crystals with bioflavonoids and rutin, 1/2 teasp. every 2 hours to bowel tolerance daily for 1 month, for connective tissue and collagen formation.
    with
Vitamin E 400IU and zinc 30mg. daily.

▷ Nature's Plus vitamin E 800IU daily, and apply a mix of 1/4 teasp. vitamin E oil and 2 TBS. liquid lecithin. (The feet and legs will tingle and feel hot as if thawing out).

▷ Enzymatic Therapy HEMTONE caps 3 daily, and RAW ADRENAL complex capsules.

▷ B15 DMG sublingual daily. ♂

▷ Sun CHLORELLA 1 packet daily.

❧ BioForce *Varicose Veins* tincture.

HERBAL THERAPY

❧ Crystal Star VARI-TONE™ tea, 2-3 cups daily.

❧ Effective flavonoid-rich extracts:
♦ Ginkgo biloba
♦ Gotu kola
♦ Hawthorne
♦ Bilberry
♦ Enzymatic Therapy HERBAL FLAVONOIDS extr. caps 4 daily. ♀

❧ Butcher's broom tea and compresses for circulation increase. ♂

❧ Solaray CENTELLA VEIN capsules.

❧ Effective fibrinolytic spices:
♦ Capsicum 4 daily
♦ Ginger rt. 6 daily
♦ Schiff GARLIC/ONION capsules

❧ Crystal Star HEMR-EASE™ or HEARTSEASE/HAWTHORNE™ caps 3 daily, and/or CHO-LO FIBER TONE™ drink or capsules morning and evening.

❧ Effective compresses:
♦ White oak bark. (Also take 8 white oak capsules daily.)
♦ Witch hazel
♦ Plantain
♦ Bayberry bark
♦ Marshmallow root

BODYWORK

➤ Walk every day, and swim as much as possible, for the best leg exercises.
→ Elevate the legs when possible.
→ Massage feet and legs every morning and night with diluted myrrh oil.
→ Go barefoot, or wear flat sandals.
→ Walk in the ocean whenever possible for strengthening sea minerals.
→ Walk in the early morning dew-covered grass.

➤ Apply calendula lotion or gel, or Crystal Star CEL-LEAN™ gel. Elevate legs while application soaks in.

➤ Take mineral or epsom salts baths.

➤ Use alternating hot and cold hydrotherapy (pg. 49).

➤ Apply H2O2 3% OXYGEL to the legs and feet, 2x daily for 2 months.

➤ Effective compresses:
→ Cider vinegar
→ Fresh comfrey lf.
→ Calendula tea
→ B&T CALIFLORA gel

➤ Apply aloe vera gel 2x daily.

➤ Do not use knee high hosiery. The elastic band at the top impedes circulation.

Common Symptoms: Dilated, swollen, painful, bulging leg veins; legs feel heavy, tight and tired; thin red, unsightly spider veins; muscle cramps.
Common Causes: Low-fiber, meat and dairy based diet with too many refined foods; vitamin E, C, and A deficiency; EFA, essential fatty acid deficiency; constipation and straining at stool; pressure on the veins from excess weight or pregnancy; weakness of vascular tissue; poor posture and circulation; liver malfunction; long periods of standing or heavy lifting; damage to veins from inflammation and blood clots in the vein.

VERTIGO ▦ DIZZINESS ✧ Meniere's Syndrome

Inner Ear Malfunction ✧ Meniere's Syndrome

Vertigo is a result of equilibrium (inner ear) disturbance with the sensation of moving around in space, or of having objects move around you. Meniere's syndrome is a recurrent and usually progressive group of symptoms that include ringing and pressure in the ears, and dizziness. Rest, relaxation and proper nutrition are the key to preventing attacks.

FOOD THERAPY

🥄 The diet should be low in saturated fats and cholesterol, high in vegetable proteins and B vitamin foods, such as brown rice, broccoli, tofu, sea foods, and sprouts.

🥄 Make a mix and take 2 TBS. daily on a fresh salad:
  ◆ Brewer's yeast
  ◆ Wheat germ (or 2 teasp. wheat germ oil)

🥄 Avoid salty foods, chemical-containing foods and preserved foods.

🥄 Avoid caffeine, especially full-strength coffee.

🥄 Avoid all alcohol, marijuana, cocaine, hallucinogens, and balance-changing drugs.

🥄 Have a potassium broth or essence once a week (pg. 53).

VITAMINS/MINERALS

▶ B Complex 100mg. with extra B6 100mg, B12 2000mcg. SL and pantothenic acid 500mg.

▶ Rosehips vitamin C or Ester C with bioflavonoids and rutin, up to 5000mg. daily.

▶ Vitamin E 800IU daily.

▶ Glutamine 500mg. daily.

▶ DMG B15 sublingual daily.

▶ Niacin Therapy to clear circulation blocks, 250mg. 3x daily. ♂

▶ Rainbow Light FOOD SENSITIVITY SYSTEM capsules with meals, and CALCIUM PLUS capsules with high magnesium 4 daily.

▶ Twin Lab CHOLINE 600mg. 2-3x daily. ♂

▶ Enzymatic Therapy RAW ADRENAL complex caps.

HERBAL THERAPY

🌿 Ginkgo biloba extract drops as needed to promote circulation to the brain, for at least 1 mo.
  and
Crystal Star RELAX CAPS™ for nerve rebuilding, and MEDITATION TEA™ to restore mental stability.

🌿 Crystal Star ADRN-ALIVE™ 2 daily.

🌿 Make a tea for excess fluid elimination: 1 part each - uva ursi, parsley leaf, red clover, fennel seed, flax seed.

🌿 Effective circulation herbs:
  ◆ Butcher's broom capsules or tea, or Crystal Star HEARTSEASE/CIRCU-CLEANSE™ tea with butcher's broom.
  ◆ Catnip
  ◆ St. John's wort
  ◆ Cayenne/ginger capsules
  ◆ Peppermint if there is nausea

🌿 Bee products are a specific:
  ◆ Superior royal jelly/ginseng vials ♂
  ◆ High potency YS or Premier One royal jelly 2 t.easp. daily
  ◆ Ginseng/honey in water as a daily drink. ♀

BODYWORK

▶ Take preventive measures: Remove stress from your life as much as possible. Practice stress management techniques such as meditation, soft music and body stretches.
Get plenty of good quality sleep.

▶ Acupressure point: pinch between the eyebrows 3x for 10 seconds each time during an attack.
  or
Press top of the arm, just above the wrist line for 15 seconds at a time.

▶ Chiropractic adjustment and shiatsu massage have shown effective improvement.

▶ Attain ideal body weight for better body balance.

▶ Reflexology points:

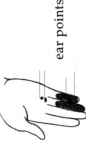

ear points

Common Symptoms: Starting with ear pain and pressure, and a feeling of lightheadedness, the victim has a feeling of falling and lack of steadiness; lightheadedness upon standing quickly; off-balance feeling.
Common Causes: Poor circulation; lack of tissue oxygen; chronic stress and anxiety; hypoglycemia; B vitamin deficiency.

WARTS ■ MOLES

Moles are congenital, discolored growths elevated above the surface of the skin. They are harmless unless continually irritated. Warts are single or clustered soft, irregular skin growths found on the hands, feet, arms and face, ranging in size from a pinhead to a small bean. Usually caused by a virus, they are contagious and will spread if picked, bitten, touched or nicked through shaving.

FOOD THERAPY

☙ Add **vitamin A rich foods to the diet**, such as yellow and green fruits and vegetables, eggs, and cold water fish.

☙ Add **sulphur-containing foods**, such as asparagus, garlic and onion family foods, fresh figs, citrus fruits and eggs.

☙ Include **high vitamin C foods** with bioflavonoids, and a concentrated source, such as Crystal Star BIO-FLAV., FIBER & C SUPPORT™ drink.

☙ Add yogurt and other cultured foods to the diet.

☙ Take a green drink (pg. 54ff) or Crystal Star ENERGY GREEN™ drink with sea vegetables, every day for a month.

☙ Effective applications:
  ♣ Mixture of lemon juice, sea salt, onion juice and vitamin E oil.
  ♣ Garlic oil 2x daily and apply a paste of garlic cloves directly.
  ♣ Papaya skins
  ♣ Wheat germ oil
  ♣ Raw potato
  ♣ Castor oil 2x daily.

VITAMINS/MINERALS

The high dosages recommended here should be used for no longer than 2-3 months at a time.

▶ **Beta carotene or emulsified A** 100,000-150,000IU as an anti-infective. (Nothing seems to happen for 1-2 months, then growths seem to disappear in a week or so, all at once).

▶ **Vitamin C crystals with bioflavonoid**; take internally, 1/2 teasp. in water every 4 hours daily. Apply locally to affected area. Also important for immunity against warts.

▶ Nature's Plus Vitamin E 800IU daily. (Also prick a capsule and apply.) with zinc 75IU daily.

▶ Cysteine 500mg. 2x daily.

▶ For wart and moles caused by a virus: (not HPV-caused warts)
  ♣ Enzymatic Therapy VIRAPLEX
  ♣ Rough up the wart with the smooth side of an emory board and apply a drop of 3% H_2O_2 to kill the virus.

▶ Alta Health SIL-X tabs 3-4 daily. ♀

▶ B Complex up to 200mg. daily, with extra B_6 250mg. daily.

HERBAL THERAPY

☙ Crystal Star ANTI-BIO™ caps or extract if there is inflammation or bacterial infection. Use ANTI-VI™ extract and *apply* ANTI-VI™ tea directly for warts.

☙ **Apply tea tree oil religiously for 1-2 months, 3-4 times daily. Wonderful results.** ☺

☙ Enzymatic Therapy LIQUID LIVER w. Siberian ginseng caps.
and
Apply Crystal Star GINSENG SKIN REPAIR™ GEL with germanium and vitamin C.

☙ Effective applications:
  ✦ B&T CALIFLORA ointment
  ✦ Aloe vera gel
  ✦ Jojoba oil
  ✦ Wintergreen oil
  ✦ NatureWorks Swedish Bitters
  ✦ Cinnamon oil drops
  ✦ Crystal Star CALENDULA GEL
  ✦ Nettles extract

☙ Garlic/parsley caps 6 daily.

BODYWORK

▶ For plantar warts: soak foot in the hottest water you can stand about 30 minutes daily for a month.
  → Then apply H2O2 OXYGEL or 3% solution. Rough up the wart with the smooth side of an emery board, and apply 1 drop 2-3x daily. Wart or mole will slowly shrink and slough off. Do not squeeze or pick.

▶ Hypnosis therapy has been successful in controlling warts and moles.

▶ **Apply Nutrition Resource Nutri-Biotic GRAPEFRUIT SEED extract full strength, or spray 2-3x daily.**

▶ Effective applications:
  → A paste of charcoal and water
  → Lysine cream applications, and take lysine capsules 500mg. 3-4x daily.

▶ Avoid smoking. It cuts off oxygen to the tissues.

Common Symptoms: Flat or raised nodules on the skin surface, with a rough, pitted discolored surface, sometimes causing pain and discomfort when rubbed or chafed; if virally caused, warts are often contagious.

Common Causes: Vitamin A and mineral deficiencies; viral infection; widespread use of anti-biotics and vaccinations that depress normal immunity.

WATER RETENTION ☒ BLOATING ☒ EDEMA

Water retention is often a problem of *not enough* water. Dieting can take away foods that previously provided water. Medical diuretics and other drugs can dehydrate. You may just not be drinking enough. If the body does not have sufficient water, fluid levels go out of balance, and it begins to retain more water in an effort to compensate. Note: Be careful of overusing chemical/medical diuretics. They can cause potassium and mineral loss, and eventually muscle weakness and fatigue. See PMS pages for more information about pre-period edema.

FOOD THERAPY

☙ **Reduce salt intake.**
Avoid starchy, sugary, foods. Reduce meats and dairy foods that demand more water to dissolve.

☙ Drink at least 6-8 glasses of bottled water daily for free flowing functions, waste removal, and appetite suppression.

☙ Eat largely fresh foods for 3 days to increase the body's food water content without density. Have a leafy green salad every day with plenty of cucumbers, parsley, and celery.

VITAMINS/MINERALS

If taking prescription diuretics, be sure to include a potassium supplement in your daily diet.

◗ Vitamin C crystals with bioflavs. and rutin, $1/2$ teasp. in water or juice every 2-3 hours until relief. Then 3-5000mg. daily for prevention.
with
B Complex 100mg. daily with extra B6 250mg. 2x daily.
and
Future Biotics VITAL K 2-4 teasp. daily.

◗ Bromelain 500mg. daily.

◗ Enzymatic Therapy ACID-A-CAL caps 3 daily.
with
Betaine HCl 3x daily.

◗ Lecithin 1900gr. 4 daily.

◗ Enzymatic Therapy LYMPH/SPLEEN tabs. ♀

HERBAL THERAPY

❧ Crystal Star BLDR-K™ caps or TINKLE CAPS™, 4-6 daily, and/or BLDR-K™ flushing tea.
and

❧ CEL-LEAN™ caps 3-4 daily for 1-3 months for enhanced liver function.

❧ Effective extracts:
◆ Hawthorne extract as needed to increase circulation. ♀
◆ Echinacea extract with burdock tea to flush lymph glands and balance hormones.
◆ Bilberry

❧ Effective diuretic teas:
◆ Cornsilk/dandelion ♀
◆ Juniper/uva ursi ♂
◆ Parsley
◆ Cleavers
◆ Fenugreek
◆ Wisdom of the Ancients YERBA MATÉ tea
◆ Stone root

❧ Crystal Star TINKLE TEA™ 2x daily as needed.

BODYWORK

➤ Take hot 20 minutes saunas, often.

➤ Crystal Star POUNDS OFF™ bath as a strong diaphoretic.

➤ Exercise every day to keep circulation and body metabolism free-flowing.

➤ Elevate head and shoulders for sleeping.

Common Symptoms: Swelling of hands, feet, ankles and stomach; PMS symptoms; headache and bloating.
Common Causes: Too much salt, red meat or MSG; kidney or bladder infection; oral contraceptives reaction; hypothyroidism; PMS symptoms; adrenal exhaustion; protein and B Complex deficiency; hormonal changes, especially estrogen output; climate changes; allergies; poor circulation; potassium depletion; corticosteroid drug reaction; obesity; constipation; lack of exercise.

WEIGHT LOSS ▨ EXCESS FAT RETENTION

Weight control today is often a strategy of prevention lifestyle - an attitude of keeping weight down. As fried and fatty foods have increased in our civilized diets, and the demand for physical labor has decreased, there has been a 500-800% increase in obesity in the 20th century. Most people today are appearance motivated to lose weight, looking for the "miracle magic bullet" to slimness and body tone, but everyone is slowly realizing that a good nutritional diet has to be front and center for permanent results. All signs indicate that the 90's will be a decade where weight loss is a component of a sound nutritious eating plan, rather than a try at the latest fad. People are becoming more motivated for health reasons to lose weight and want to change their way of eating to insure both looks and health.
Weight loss is not easy in today's life style. Reaching your ideal weight is a victory. Keeping it requires vigilance, especially in light of today's processed food offerings and fast life-style. But it can be successful on a long-term basis, and without side effects. It is a real achievement! Don't Weight!

FOOD THERAPY

The four keys to an effective weight control diet: low fat, high fiber from complex carbohydrates, regular exercise, plenty of water.

🍃 **Changing diet composition is the importance of cutting back on fat cannot be overstated.** You can eat two to three times more volume of low fat foods than high fat foods, and still lose weight. Fat is not all bad. It is the chief source of energy for the body, and essential for good body function in small amounts. The average overweight person often has **too high blood sugar and too low fat levels.** This causes constant hunger - the delicate balance between fat storage and fat utilization is upset, and the body's ability to use fat for energy decreases. Eating fast, fatty, fried, or junk foods particularly aggravates this imbalance. The person winds up with "empty calories" and more cravings. Fat becomes non-moving energy, and fat cells become fat storage depots. **Saturated fats are the hardest for the liver to metabolize. Stay away from them to control fat storage.**

🍃 Water can get you over weight loss plateaus. Drink it, and all liquids before eating to suppress appetite.

🍃 Small amounts of caffeine after a meal can raise thermogenesis (calorie burning) increasing metabolic rate.

🍃 See "COOKING FOR HEALTHY HEALING" by Linda Rector-Page for complete weight loss diets for both kids and adults.

VITAMINS/MINERALS

Take all regular supplements after meals to avoid appetite stimulation.

▶ For carbohydrate metabolism, take B Complex vitamins while dieting.

▶ For compulsive eating, take tyrosine 500mg. 2-3x, w/ zinc 30mg. 1 daily.

▶ For better thermogenesis of fat calories - carnitine 500mg. 2x daily; arginine/ornithine 1000mg. at bedtime.

▶ For effective appetite suppression - phenylalanine 500mg. before meals. *Do not take if sensitive to phenylalanine.*

▶ For metabolic and circulation sluggishness, take CoQ 10 30mg. daily.

▶ Effective weight loss supplements:
✦ Enzymatic Therapy thyroid/tyrosine caps with carnitine 500mg. for metabolic increase.
✦ Enzymatic Therapy RAW PITUITARY, MAMMARY, THYROID/TYROSINE for sluggish gland and pear-shaped problems.
✦ Source Naturals SUPER AMINO NIGHT caps ♂ at night and carnitine 500mg. and methionine 500mg. in the morning; or Quantum NIGHT TRIM and DAY TRIM.♀
✦ Lewis Labs WEIGH DOWN with chromium for appetite control and retaining muscle while losing fat.
✦ Strength Systems LIQUID FAT BURNERS - a lipotropic/carnitine formula.
✦ Kal DIET MAX plan.
✦ Nature's Plus FRUITEIN, SPIRU-TEIN, ENER-G drinks.

HERBAL THERAPY

See next page for effective Crystal Star weight loss formulas for specific problems.

🌱 Effective herbal supplements for weight loss:
◆ Bromelain 500mg. 3x daily for maximum metabolism
◆ Congleton DIET PEP, SUPER PEP and LADY PEP capsules.
◆ Rainbow Light SPIRULINA HERBAL DIET COMPLEX caps for appetite control.
◆ Wisdom of the Ancients YERBA MATÉ tea to control appetite.
◆ Esteem Plus DAYTIME, and TRIM & FIRM NIGHTIME caps for metabolic increase.
◆ Energy Balance LEMON FAST for body cleansing.
◆ Gymnema sylvestre caps to reduce sugar cravings.
◆ Laci LeBeau SUPER DIETERS TEA, or DIETER'S TREASURE tea for effective flushing.
◆ Spirulina, chlorella, and bee pollen for high proteins, energy and balance.
◆ High Omerga 3 flax oil to overcome binging and an addictive need for food.
◆ Wild yam caps for highest natural DHEA - appetite suppression.
◆ Crystal Star TIGHTENING & TONING HERBAL WRAP™ program for cellulite loss.
◆ Nutrapathic FAT METABOLIZER caps as directed with CALCIUM/COLLAGEN caps to help keep flesh firm and unwrinkled.

BODYWORK

No diet will work without exercise; with it, almost every diet will.

▶ Daily exercise is the key to permanent, painless weight control. Even if eating habits are changed very little, you can still lose weight by expending more energy with a brisk hour's walk, or 15 minutes of aerobic exercise. One pound of fat has 3500 calories. A 3 mile walk burns up 250 calories. In about 2 weeks you will have lost a pound of real fat, not water weight. That amounts to 3 pounds a month and 30 pounds a year without changing your diet. It's easy to see how cutting down even moderately on fatty, sugary foods in **combination with exercise can quickly provide the look and body tone desired.**
Exercise promotes an "afterburn" effect, raising the metabolic rate from 1.00 to 1.05-1.15 per minute for up to 24 hours afterwards. So calories are used up at an even faster rate *after* exercise.
Weight training exercise increases lean muscle mass, replacing fat-marbled muscle tissue with lean muscle. Muscle tissue uses up calories for energy. The greater the amount of muscle tissue you have, the more calories you can burn. This is particularly important as aging decreases muscle mass.
Exercise *before* a meal raises blood sugar levels and thus decreases appetite, often for several hours afterward. Exercise *after* eating raises heart and metabolism rates so that food is used by the system instead of just "sitting there".

Six Specific Programs for Common Weight Loss Problems

Crystal Star conducts a continuing review of diet and weight loss products, at both a manufacturing and a consumer level. The following products have proven their worth as viable aids to the weight loss process.

✓Try to lose 1% of your body weight per week. More than that and the body does not adjust properly. You will probably end up regaining the weight.

✓Don't worry about the pounds and the calories. Worry about the inches and the fat. Muscle is heavy. Adding exercise to your life and correcting your diet composition will take inches off a lot faster than pounds. Forget pounds and calories. Look at yourself in the mirror. Watch your clothing size go down!

The best way to use the recommendations below is first to identify the most prominant or chronic weight control problem, especially if there seems to be more than one. Best results will be achieved by working on the worst problem first. As success and improvement are realized in this primary area, secondary problems are often overcome in the process. If lingering problems still exist, they may be addressed in additional supplementation after the first program is well underway and producing noticeable results. The following categories represent the most common weight loss obstacles. After identifying your personal difficulty, choose the products within the problem area that most appeal to you. Since natural products are often working with the body to rebalance gland and hormone functions, product activity may be subtle and long-range for more permanent results. Overdosing is often not productive, nor will it increase activity.

Lazy Metabolism & Gland/Thyroid Imbalance
◆Crystal Star META-TABS™ CAPS - 2 daily.
◆Crystal Star RAINFOREST ENERGY™ tea and capsules.
◆Crystal Star ZING™ capsules with natural caffeine - 1 to 2 daily.
◆Enzymatic Therapy PEAR-SHAPED program - raw pituitary, raw mammary, thyroid/tyrosine.
◆MCT's medium chain triglycerides.
◆Sassafras and burdock tea; bee pollen capsules or granules 2x daily.
◆Carnitine, 250mg. with CoQ 10, 30mg. - 2x daily each.
◆Evening primrose oil, borage oil, or Source Naturals MEGA GLA 240.
◆Esteem Plus DAYTIME & NIGHTIME capsules.
◆Enzymatic Therapy THYROID/TYROSINE caps with carnitine capsules 500mg. - 2 caps 2x daily.

Cellulite Deposits & Liver Malfunction
◆Crystal Star CEL-LEAN™ diet support caps, CEL-LEAN™ release tea, CEL-LEAN™ gel/wafers.
◆Crystal Star CEL-LEAN™ HERBAL BODY WRAP PROGRAM - as needed.
◆Crystal Star BIOFLAVONOID, FIBER & C SUPPORT™ drink.
◆Crystal Star BITTERS & LEMON CLEANSE' extract - morning and before bed.
◆Enzymatic Therapy CELLU-VAR cream and caps as directed.
◆Source Naturals SUPER AMINO NIGHT caps - 2 to 4 at night before bed.

Overeating & Eating Too Much Fat
◆Crystal Star APPE-TIGHT™ caps, and/or SCALE DOWN DIET™ extract.
◆Crystal Star RAINFOREST ENERGY TEA™.
◆Crystal Star LIGHT WEIGHT™ MEAL REPLACEMENT PROGRAM.
◆Crystal Star ZING™ capsuleS with natural caffeine - 1 to 2 daily.
◆Bromelain 500mg. 2 to 3x daily.
◆Lewis Labs WEIGH DOWN DRINK, w. extra chromium picolinate capsules.
◆Wakunaga PERFECT SHAPE meal replacement drink.
◆Carnitine capsules, 500mg. with Rainbow Light TRIM-ZYME capsules.
◆Quantum NIGHT TRIM caps with high ornithine - before bed.
◆Crystal Star SCALE DOWN™ diet extract several times daily.
◆Strength Systems FAT BURNERS capsules - as directed.
◆Phenylalanine capsules, 500mg., with tyrosine capsules, 500mg. - 2 daily.
◆Rainbow Light SPIRULINA HERBAL DIET COMPLEX.
◆Enzymatic Therapy WILD YAM EXTRACT capsules with high DHEA.

Poor Circulation & Lack of Energy
◆Crystal Star RAINFOREST ENERGY™ tea and capsules.
◆Crystal Star ZING™ capsules, with unprocessed caffeine.
◆Crystal Star BIOFLAV., FIBER & C SUPPORT™ drink and capsules.
◆Crystal Star GREEN TEA CLEANSER™.
◆Crystal Star GINSENG 6 SUPER ENERGY™ capsules and/or ADRN™ extract.
◆Full-spectrum amino acid complex to stimulate HGH.
◆Enzymatic Therapy LIQUID LIVER with siberian ginseng.
◆Twin Lab DIET FUEL.
◆Congleton DIET PEP and SUPER PEP capsules.
◆Excel SLOW RELEASE ANTI-FATIGUE capsules.
◆Source Naturals GUARAÑA capsules - 1 to 2 daily.

Poor Elimination - Detoxification of the Colon, Bowel, Kidney & Bladder
◆Crystal Star LEAN & CLEAN DIET™ capsules and tea.
◆Crystal Star SUPER LEAN & CLEAN DIET™ capsules and tea.
◆Crystal Star HOT SEAWEED BATH™.
◆Crystal Star CHO-LO FIBER TONE™ capsules or drink morning and evening for one month to six weeks.
◆Crystal Star BITTERS & LEMON CLEANSE™ EXTRACT - morning and before bed.
◆Energy Balance LEMON FAST concentrate.
◆Crystal Star GREEN TEA CLEANSER™ every morning.
◆Crystal Star TINKLE CAPS™ and POUNDS OFF™ bath.
◆Crystal Star ALKALIZING ENZYME HERBAL BODY WRAP™
◆Crystal Star FIBER & HERBS COLON CLEANSE™ caps and LAXA-TEA™.
◆Laci LeBeau SUPER DIET TEAS.

Sugar Craving & Body Sugar Imbalance
◆Crystal Star SUPER LEAN™ diet capules and tea.
◆Chromium picolinate to control cravings and balance blood sugar levels.
◆Crystal Star LIGHT WEIGHT™ MEAL REPLACEMENT program.
◆Lewis Labs WEIGH DOWN DRINK, w. extra chromium picolinate capsules.
◆Crystal Star CHO-LO FIBER TONE™ capsules or drink morning and evening.
◆Gymnema sylvestre caps before meals.
◆Bee pollen capsules with royal jelly and ginseng.

There are often many reasons you may not be losing the weight you want. All of the following conditions hamper the body's ability to use food for fuel and energy, encouraging it instead to store it as fat: sluggish thyroid; lazy metabolism; glandular malfunction causing a pear-shaped figure; overeating; brown fat; cellulite; habit hunger; stress eating; bloating and puffiness from excess fluid retention; constipation; poor liver function and circulation; hyperinsulinism; poor assimilation of foods, such as dairy or wheat products; food sensitivities and intolerances. **Eating too much food, lack of exercise, diet composition and lifestyle are the major weight control factors.**

For weight loss to be real and permanent four essential things must happen:

❶ **The body must be detoxified. Toxins are stored in the fat cells.**
Success in permanent weight loss depends on body cleansing and detoxification. During the first liquid diet stage in this program, the body begins heavy elimination and the breaking down of fat cells so it can remove toxic wastes and fat deposits. Wastes are discarded faster than new tissue is made. Unneeded tissue (weight) is lost.

❷ **The craving for excess sweets and salts must be overcome.**
A chromium deficiency can greatly affect the body's perceived needs for sugary, salty foods. Stress, aging and chromium-depleted soils caused by chemically-dependent agricultural practices, strip body chromium. A diet rich in high chromium foods, such as brewer's yeast, whole wheat, cornmeal, mushrooms, apples, prunes, melons and seafoods can help overcome cravings for foods that put on weight.

❸ **Continual hunger and appetite must be curbed by better use of nutrients and body balance.**
Low fat, mineral-rich, complex carbohydrates are the key. You can eat two to three times more volume of these foods and still lose weight. They signal the insulin/serotonin synthesis reaction in the *appestat* center of the brain to communicate a feeling of fullness, even in the presence of less food intake.

❹ **Metabolism must be increased, so that the calories taken in are burned and used efficiently.**
Metabolic processes often cause weight gain. And all metabolisms are different. Men lose weight easier on a diet of fresh and cooked vegetables.

❋ *Living the thin life is not a lifelong deprivation sentence. Once basic metabolic processes have re-aligned and stabilized, and desired weight has been maintained for several months, you can have overeating days without losing weight control. Just balance them with undereating days, such as when you will be eating out, or with company, so that ideal weight can be sustained. Living thin just means knowing what it takes from you personally to maintain your weight, so that it becomes automatic and intuitive.*

A Successful Two Stage Weight Loss Diet

Stage One: The Modified Liquid Diet for Intense Weight Loss - with all fresh foods and juices. Liquid fasting sounds like a "fast" way to lose weight, and sometimes it is, if you get enough nutrients from fresh fruit and vegetable juices. Unfortunately, there are three inherent problems with a liquid fast for weight loss. 1)The body tends to form **more fat** at first when it receives no solid food at all. It feels threatened by the drastic decrease in its usual nutrients and tries to protect itself by forming fat for survival. 2) Fasting can be dangerous unless you are using organically grown foods. The pesticides and sprays on much of the commercial produce that we eat are very quickly absorbed into the blood stream when there is no food to slow them down. They can lodge in the bones and cause toxic reactions. 3) A fast means that the body is cleansing and discarding wastes more rapidly than new tissue is being formed, i.e. weight loss. A temporary degree of discomfort may be felt in terms of headache, bowel looseness or loss of energy. These symptoms are usually just initial detoxification sign, and a small price to pay for getting rid of long accumulated fat cells. **Weight loss cannot occur until these cells are gone.** Drinking six to eight glasses of pure water a day speeds along the initial flushing and release process. After a few days, as toxic waste is eliminated, the symptoms will be also cease.

Stage Two: Eating Right & Light Diet - *with regular exercise.* For permanent weight control, a biochemical change is necessary. This diet emphasizes four keys for lasting weight loss: 1) low fats 2) soluble dietary fiber from complex carbohydrates 3) regular exercise 4) plenty of water. (Thirst is often mistaken for hunger. Drinking water will save many calories throughout the day.) All red meats and full-fat dairy foods are omitted. All junk and processed foods are avoided. These can destroy the fat-metabolizing body system you have encouraged, causing poor nutrition, which in turn causes constant hunger, and the desire to eat "empty calorie" foods.

❋ *Stage One: The Modified Liquid Diet for Intense Weight Loss; 7 to 10 Days*
The following liquid diet is for intense weight loss periods. It is moderate, with plenty of nutrition, and is most effective when used for one to three weeks at a time, with light eating in between.

Note: Take only fruits and fruit juices until noon, to use up the body's own glycogen reserves and stimulate optimal metabolic action. Eat small, frequent, *grazing* meals. Exercise for 5 minutes before eating to raise blood sugar levels and decrease appetite.

On rising: take a glass of lemon juice and water with 1 tsp. honey, or Crystal Star GREEN TEA CLEANSER™ to flush fats and clean the kidneys.
Breakfast: have some fresh fruit, and a glass of apple or pineapple/papaya juice with 1 TB. psyllium husks, Crystal Star CHO-LO FIBER TONE™ or Sonné liquid bentonite for natural fiber and continued flushing of the bowel;
or a glass of aloe vera juice with herbs.

Mid-morning: have a glass of carrot/beet/cucumber juice to cleanse and scour the kidneys;
or a fresh carrot juice;
or a green drink such as Sun CHLORELLA or Green Foods GREEN ESSENCE in water.
Lunch: have a meal replacement drink, such as Nature's Plus SPIRUTEIN, Crystal Star LIGHT WEIGHT™, or Lewis Labs Biochrome WEIGH DOWN;
or a meal replacement supplement, such as Rainbow Light SPIRULINA HERBAL DIET COMPLEX or ESTEEM PLUS capsules.
Mid-afternoon: have some crunchy raw vegies with kefir cheese, or an all vegetable puree;
and a bottle of mineral water or herb tea, such as peppermint or licorice root tea, or Crystal Star CLEANSING & PURIFYING™ tea or LEAN 'N' CLEAN DIET™ tea.
Dinner: have a green leafy salad with sprouts, cucumbers, celery, carrots and a lemon/oil dressing;
and a cup of miso soup with sea vegetables snipped on top; or a cup of VEGEX yeast broth.
Before bed: have a glass of cranberry or apple juice with 1TB. liquid bentonite or psyllium:
or another glass of aloe vera juice with herbs for the night's cleanse.

Note: Take a short walk before retiring, to stimulate metabolic activity during the night. Stay cool. Cold temperature stimulates higher metabolism rates.

✤

Stage Two: Eating Right, Light, & Low Fat for Weight Control

This diet should be used for at least three months to assure that your system is realigned and stabilized in your new way of eating. It gives you the skills to develop long-term weight management - so you won't gain it back. Keep eating plenty of raw, fresh foods. They take more time to eat so that you eat less. They don't need fattening sauces to taste good. They add more high fiber bulk than cooked foods. Their high vitamin/mineral content satifies your body's needs with less food. The following weight control diet is high in vegetable and whole grain fiber, with complex carbohydrates to improve metabolism, and gland-enhancing foods to increase the amount of excreted calories by the body, and signal a feeling of fullness to allay hunger.

Note: Eat small meals more frequently instead of big sit-down meals. Eat only one main meal a day.

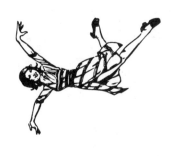

On rising: take 2 lemons squeezed in a glass of water, or Crystal Star GREEN TEA CLEANSER™.
Breakfast: take a cleansing/building protein drink such as Nature's Plus SPIRUTEIN, NutriTech ALL 1, or Crystal Star BIOFLAV., FIBER & C SUPPORT™ drink for vitamins and brain food without muscle wasting;
and some fresh fruits.
Mid-morning: have some yogurt with fresh fruit;
or a small bottle of mineral water;
or an herb tea, such as Crystal Star HIGH ENERGY™ or LEAN & CLEAN DIET™ tea, or a mint tea.
Lunch: have a fresh leafy green salad with lemon/oil or yogurt dressing;
with baked tofu, a baked potato or brown rice, and a low fat sauce or dressing; or use high omega 3 flax oil in place of butter.
or a light vegetable, black bean, lentil or miso soup, with steamed vegies and a soy/ginger sauce;
or whole grain or vegetable pasta salad, with seafood or salad vegies and a light sauce.
Mid-afternoon: have crunchy raw vegies or whole grain crackers with kefir cheese or a yogurt dip;
and a green drink such as Sun CHLORELLA or a refreshing herb tea or bottled mineral water;
and/or a hard boiled egg with a little sesame salt, and rice cakes with kefir cheese.
Dinner: have a large dinner salad with seafood and vegies, nuts and seeds, and a cup of light soup;
or a Chinese stir fry with lots of greens, onions, mushrooms, clear soup and brown rice;
or baked or broiled fish or seafood with some steamed vegies and brown rice or millet.
or some roast turkey with light cornbread, and a salad with poppyseed dressing;
or a whole grain or vegie pasta dish with vegetables and a light sauce; and a cup of soup.
❧ A little white wine with your main meal will improve digestion and circulation, and make dieting more pleasant.
T.V/Evening snack: have some unbuttered spicy popcorn. It's good for you and its airiness will fill you up and keep you from wanting heavier or 'habit' foods.

Before bed: a cup of VEGEX yeast broth; **or** a glass of apple or papaya juice, or a cup of mint tea.

Water & Weight Loss: Water is a prime factor for success.
Every effective weight loss plan should include six to eight glasses of bottled water throughout the day. No-calorie seltzers and mineral waters can also help fill this quota. When the body gets enough water, it works at its peak, fluid and salt retention decrease, glandular activity improves, the liver metabolizes more fats, and hunger is curtailed. All of this leads to greater weight loss. Enough water can also carry you through the plateau experience during a weight loss program. Since dieting takes away foods that were providing

tissue hydration; if you don't drink enough water, fluid levels go out of balance, and the body retains too much fluid in an effort to compensate. Besides fluid retention, lack of water leads to poor muscle tone, sagging skin, constipation and even weight gain. When calories are severely limited, water is pulled out of the tissues to metabolize stored sugars for fuel. Three to four pounds of water are lost for every pound of fuel burned. You become lighter, but you aren't losing fat. You are losing water and muscle tissue, the very things that can give you the look and health you are dieting for.

Weight Control for Kids ☺

Until the 1960's weight gain and weight control weren't much of a problem for kids. But ever since the fifties, over-refined and junk foods have changed parents' metabolism and cell structure. Hereditary factors from these parents of the fifties and sixties have passed immune defense depletion, and food assimilation problems to the kids of today. And that's in addition to the wide variety of junk and non-food foods, peer pressure, lack of exercise, and T.V. advertising that the kids themselves are constantly exposed to. Weight problems are mushrooming with American children. For all the current adult consciousness and attention to diet, recent statistics show that our children and teenagers are the fattest they have ever been! Obesity rates for young children jumped 54% between 1960 and 1981, and 30% for teenagers. They jumped another 50% between 1981 and 1988.

The 1985 study by the President's Council on Physical Fitness showed two very discerning facts: that 85% of the children and teenagers tested failed basic fitness tests, and that as many as 90 percent of American children already have at least one risk factor for a degenerating disease. Poor lifestyle eating habits, with too much fat, salt, sugar and calories, and lack of exercise are at the base of this poor performance. Snacks, lunch foods and meals can be satisfying and delicious without adding significant amounts of sugar, fat or salt. In fact, young children need two or three snacks daily to have a nutritious diet, because their stomachs don't hold all they need in just three meals. Kids need mineral-rich building foods, fiber-rich energy foods, protein-rich growth foods. Changing the type of food eaten without restricting the amount, can result in easy and spontaneous weight loss. Plenty of fresh fruit, unbuttered, spicy popcorn, and sandwich fixings are good defense against junk foods.

Breakfast can be a key. Both kids and adults who eat a high fiber breakfast don't feel as hungry at lunchtime, and eat an average of 200 fewer calories during the day. Your kids need you for good information, and as good diet role models to help them establish positive healthy eating habits. The following diet can serve as an easy weight control guideline for kids. It has passed many tests on both over-weight and "couch potato" kids with foods that they like and will eat.

On rising: give a vitamin/mineral drink such as NutriTech EARTHSHAKE or Nature's Plus SPIRUTEIN or FRUITEIN (lots of flavors), or 1 teaspoon liquid multi-vitamin in juice (such as Floradix CHILDREN'S MULTI-VITAMIN/MINERAL).
Breakfast: have a whole grain cereal with apple juice or a little yogurt and fresh fruit;
and if more is desired, whole grain toast or muffins, with a little butter, kefir cheese or nut butter;
add eggs, scrambled or baked or soft boiled (no fried eggs);
or have some hot oatmeal or kashi with a little maple syrup, and yogurt if desired.
Mid-morning: snacks can be whole grain crackers with kefir cheese or low fat cheese or dip, and a sugarless juice or sparkling mineral water;
and/or some fresh fruit, such as apples with yogurt or kefir cheese,
or dried fruit, or fruit leather;
or fresh crunchy vegies, like celery, with peanut butter or a nut spread;
or a no-sugar dried fruit, nut and seed candy bar (you can easily make your own) or a dried fruit and nut trail mix, stirred into yogurt.
Lunch: have a fresh vegie, turkey, chicken or shrimp salad sandwich on whole grain bread, with low fat or soy cheese and mayonnaise.
Add whole grain or corn chips with a low fat vegie or cheese dip;
or a hearty bean soup with whole grain toast or crackers, and a small salad or crunchy vegies with garbanzo spread;
or a baked potato with a butter, kefir cheese, or soy cheese, and a green salad with Italian dressing;
or a vegetarian pizza on a chapati or whole grain crust;
or whole grain spaghetti or pasta with a light sauce and parmesan cheese;
or a Mexican bean and vegie, or rice or whole wheat burrito with a light natural no-sugar salsa.
Mid-afternoon: have a sparkling juice and a dried fruit candy bar, or fruit juice-sweetened cookies;
or some fresh fruit or fruit juice, or a kefir drink with whole grain muffins and kefir cheese;
or a hard boiled egg, and some whole grain chips with a vegie or low fat cheese dip;
or some whole grain toast and peanut butter or other nut butter.
Dinner: a light pizza on a whole grain, chapati or egg crust, with vegies, shrimp, and soy or low fat mozzarella cheese topping;
or whole grain or egg pasta with vegetables and a light tomato and cheese sauce;
or a baked Mexican quesadilla with soy or low fat cheese and some steamed vegetables or a salad;
or a stir fry with crunchy noodles, brown rice, baked egg rolls and a light soup;
or some roast turkey with cornbread dressing and a salad;
or a tuna casserole with rice, peas and water chestnuts and toasted chapatis with a little butter.
Before bed: a glass of apple juice or vanilla soy milk or flavored kefir.
✓ A snack of unbuttered, spicy, savory popcorn is good and nutritious anytime. See the index for several delicious suggestions.

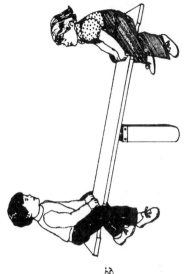

APPENDIX
A short, hands-on reference for healing techniques and self tests

❖ **Taking Your Basal Body Temperature:**
Body temperature reflects metabolic rate - largely determined by hormones secreted by the thyroid gland. Functionality of the thyroid can be measured by basal body temperature. You will need a thermometer.
1. Shake down thermometer to below 95ºF and place it by your bed before going to sleep at night.
2. On waking, place the thermometer in your armpit for a full 10 minutes. Make as little movement as possible. Lie and rest with your eyes closed for the best results.
3. After 10 minutes, read and record the temperature and date.
4. Record temperature for at least 3 mornings. Menstruating women must perform the test on the 2nd, 3rd, and 4th days of menstruation. Men and post-menopausal women can perform the test ant time. Normal basal body temperature is between 97.6º and 98.2º.

❖ **Ascorbic Acid Flush:**
This procedure is useful for accelerating detoxification programs, changing body chemistry to neutralize allergens and fight infections, promoting more rapid healing, and as a protective and preventive measure against illness.
1. Use ascorbate vitamin C or Ester C powder with bioflavonoids for best results.
2. Take $1/2$ teasp. every 20 minutes to bowel tolerance (diarrhea results).

  Note: Use $1/4$ teasp. every hour for a very young child; $1/2$ teasp. every hour for a child six to ten years old.
3. Then reduce amount taken slightly to just below bowel tolerance, so that the bowel produces a mealy, loose stool, but not diarrhea. The body will continue to cleanse at this point. You will be taking approximately 8-10,000mg. daily depending on body weight and make-up. Continue for one to two days for a thorough flush.

❖ **Bentonite Clay Colonic Cleanse:**
Bentonite clay is a mineral complex substance that has powerful absorption qualities to pull out impurities that are in suspension in the body. It helps to prevent proliferation of pathogenic organisms and parasites and sets up an environment for rebuilding healthy tissue. It is effective for lymph congestion, cellulite in the fatty tissues, blood cleansing and reducing toxicity from environmental pollutants. It may be used orally, anally, or vaginally. It works by going to the place where the problem lies, lodging there, sometimes for several days, while it darws out the toxic materials, and then drains and eliminates them through evacuation. For best results, avoid refined foods, especially sugars and flour, and pasteurized dairy products during this cleanse.
1. To take as an enema, mix $1/2$ cup clay to each enema bag of water.Use 5 to 6 bags *for each enema set* to replace a colonic. Follow the normal enema procedure as on page 49, or the directions with your enema apparatus.
2. Massage across the abdomen while expelling toxic waste into the toilet.
Note: Bentonite clay packs are also effective applied to varicose veins and arthritic areas.

❖ **Coca's Pulse Test:**
Dr. Arthur Coca, an immunologist, discovered that foods to which people are allergic produce a dramatic increase in the heartbeat - 20 or more beats a minute above normal. The pulse rate in a normal person is remarkably stable. It is not affected by digestion, ordinary physical activity, or normal emotional influences. Unless one is suffering from a cold, respiratory infection or a sunburn, deviation in normal pulse rate is probably due to an allergy. By performing Coca's "Pulse Test", one can find and eliminate foods that harm.
1. Take your pulse when you wake in the morning. Using a watch with a second hand, count the number of beats in a sixty-second period. A normal pulse readingis 50-70 beats per minute.
2. Take your pulse again after eating a suspected allergy food. Wait 15-20 minutes and take your pulse again. If the pulse rate has increased more than 10 beats per minute, omit the food from your diet

❖ **Muscle Testing:**

Simple muscle kinesiology attributes may often be able to determine an individual's response to a food or substance. Muscle testing is now being used by many people before buying a healing product to estimate the product's effectiveness for their particular body needs and make-up. You will need a partner for this procedure.

1. Hold your arm out straight from your side, parallel to the ground. Have a partner take hold of the arm with one hand just below the shoulder, and one hand on the forearm. Your partner should then try to force your arm down towards your side, while you exert all your strength to hold it level. Unless in ill health, or a greatly weakened condition, you will be able to withstand this pressure and keep your arm level.

2. Then, simply hold the item that you desire to test against your diaphragm (under the breastbone) or thyroid (the point where the collarbone comes together below the neck). The item may be in or out of normal packaging, or in its raw state, as with an individual food.

3. While holding the item as above, put your arm out straight from your side as before and have your partner try to press it down again. If the substance or product is beneficial for you, your arm will retain its strength, and your partner will be unable to force it down. If the substance or product is not beneficial, or would worsen your condition, your arm can be easily pushed down by your partner.

❖ **Herbal Vaginal Packs:**

A female vaginal cleansing herbal combination may be used as a vaginal pack placed against the cervix, or as a bolus inserted in the vagina. These substances are essentially internal poultices to draw out toxic wastes from the vagina, rectum or urethral areas. They are effective for cysts, benign tumors, polyps and against cerival dysplasia and uterine tumors. It takes 6 weeks to 6 months for complete healing, depending on the problem and severity. Two formula combinations are given.

1. Mix either combination with warmed cocoa butter to form finger-sized suppositories. Place in waxed paper in the refrigerator to chill and harden slightly.

2. A suppository may then be smeared on the end of a cotton tampon and inserted; or inserted as is, along with the use of a sanitary napkin to catch drainage.
Either method should be used at night and rinsed out in the morning with white oak bark or yellow dock root tea to rebalance vaginal pH.

3. Repeat for 6 days. Rest for one week. Resume and repeat.

Formula #1: Mix 1 part *each* with cocoa butter to form a suppository.
Squaw vine, Marshmallow root, Slippery elm, Goldenseal root, Pau de arco bark, Comfrey root, Mullein, Yellow dock root, Chickweed, Acidophilus powder.

Formula #2: Mix 1 part *each* with cocoa butter to form a suppository.
Cranesbill powder, Goldenseal root, Red raspberry leaf, White oak bark, Echinacea root, Myrrh gum powder

❖ **Therapeutic Sitz Bath:**

The sitz bath is a mild form of the alternating hot and cold hydrotherapy described on page 49. It may be used as a healing technique for a patient who cannot take a full shower. It is especially beneficial for increasing circulation in the pelvic and urethral area.

1. Fill a bathtub with water to cover the hips when seated. Start with water about 100º and increase the temperature by letting hot water run slowly and continuously into the tub, until the temperature reaches approximately 112º. Place your feet at the faucet end of the tub so that they are soaking in slightly hotter water as the water drips in.

2. Soak in the bath for 20-30 minutes. Cover the upper body with a towel, and place a cool, wet washcloth on the forehead if desired.

3. Take a quick cool water rinse in the shower, or splash the body with cool water before drying off to further stimulate circulation.

4. Epsom salts, Crystal Star HOT SEAWEED BATH, Breh or Batherapy bath salts, ginger powder, comfrey or chamomile may be added to the bath water for therapeutic results.

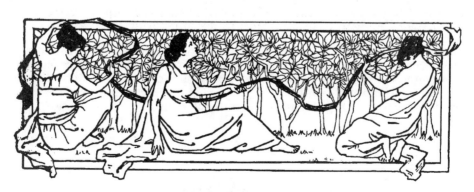

About Crystal Star Herbal Nutrition

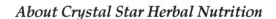

Crystal Star Herbal Nutrition is an exceptional herbal supplier that you can be proud and confident to offer and to use for therapeutic strength medicinals. Clearly, more and more people are increasing their use of herbs as natural alternatives to drugs.

Our company is a complete, high quality resource for herbal medicines that promote optimum health. Many herbal preparation methods are represented, including extracts, capsules, teas, baths, gels, Eurospa products, potpourris and aromatherapy salts.

Crystal Star has a firm commitment to excellence. Quality is never an accident. It is always the result of high intention, sincere effort, intelligent direction, skillful ability, and a willingness to pay for the difference. There is a world of disparity between fairly good and the best, between mediocrity and superiority.

For therapeutic success herbs must be BIO-ACTIVE and BIO-AVAILABLE. Crystal Star uses the finest quality herbs that we can find because we work with the these naturally-occurring, biochemical properties. High quality is not only a desired attribute, it is a mandatory element. Our superior plants usually cost far more than standard stock, but sell for proportionately far less - a true value for the alternative health consumer.

Most of our herbs are organically grown or wildcrafted in the fresh air of the California and Oregon foothills, and on coastal botanical farms. All of our wild-harvested plants are gathered ecologically in compliance with strict land-stewardship ethics. Our oriental herbs are of the highest quality. All of our combinations are formulated and filled in small batches. Our teas are blended on a weekly basis to assure you of freshness and the most potent product you can buy.

❧ Here are some of the checkpoints we use at Crystal Star Herbal Nutrition to insure top quality and potency:
1) **We buy organically grown or wildcrafted herbs whenever available.**
2) We buy fresh-dried locally grown herbs immediately upon harvest whenever possible. This assures the shortest transportation time and freshest quality for our stock.
3) **We buy small amounts of herbs more often, rather than large amounts that may lose potency before they are used.**
4) We choose our herbs for aromatic strength, lively color and good texture. If the leaves and flowers crumble, are brown, or lack "life" in the dried state, we do not buy them.
5) **We know and trust our herb suppliers and consistent quality sources. The herb world is small. Botanical importers and distributors are few. Integrity, or lack of it, becomes quickly known.**
6) We buy the best. In the medicinal herb world, price is generally a fair measure of quality. Even herbs that seem outrageously priced are usually worth it in terms of healing value, and a little goes a long way.
7) **We store our herbs in dark-colored sealed containers, away from light and heat. For the short time the herbs are in our warehouse they are kept cool and closed.**

Crystal Star is a small personal company without a large staff, marketing division or advertising program. The extra money we spend goes toward herbal education and research, and into the quality of our ingredients. We feel that our product results speak for themselves better than any advertising campaign we might devise.

SUPER TEAS

Super teas are a new concept in holistic and alternative healing. They are made from premium wildcrafted herbs and represent the highest in therapeutic activity and energy. The combinations are intricately balanced and advanced in formulation, to address today's more complex problems and needs.

GINSENG 6 DEFENSE RESTORATIVE™ TEA
Ingredients: Chinese White Ginseng, American Ginseng (Aralia),Tienchi (Japanese Ginseng), Suma (Brazilian Ginseng), Korean Ginseng, (opt.) Echinacea Angustifolia, Echinacea Purpurea, Pau de Arco Bark, Siberian Ginseng, Prince Ginseng, Astragalus Rt., St. John's Wort, Reishi Mushrooms, Ma Huang, Fennel Seed.
Directions: Two to three cups daily for one to two months after major illness or surgery.

ANTI-VI™ SUPER TEA
Ingredients: Osha Root, St. John's Wort, Echinacea Purpurea, Prince Ginseng, Astragalus Bk., Peppermint, Pau De Arco.
Directions: Take two to three cups daily as needed during high risk seasons. For best results, take alternately for one week on and one week off.

RAINFOREST ENERGY TEA™
Ingredients: Guarana Seed, Kola Nut, Suma, Yerba Maté, Cinnamon.

LEAN & CLEAN SUPER DIET™ TEA w. SUGAR BLOCK
Ingredients: Flax Seed, Centella, Fennel Seed, Uva Ursi, Senna Lf. & Pod, Lemon Peel, Gymnema Sylvestre, Burdock Rt., Fenugreek Sd., Parsley Lf., Bladderwrack, Bancha Leaf, Hibiscus, Red Clover.
Directions: Take two to three cups daily as needed for one month during a weight loss dieting program.

GREEN TEA CLEANSER™
Ingredients: Bancha Lf., Gotu Kola, Burdock Rt., Fo-Ti, Kukicha Twig, Hawthorne Berry, Orange Peel, Cinnamon.
Directions: Two cups may be taken in the morning or evening as a daily cleanser, or after meals as a digestive stimulant.

MEDICINAL TEAS

ALR-HST TEA™
Ingredients: Rosehips, Unsprayed Bee Pollen, Horehound, Peppermint, Roses & Rosebuds, Anise Seed, Ginger Rt., Orange Peel, Cloves, Burdock Rt., Ephedra, Honey Crystals.

AR-EASE TEA™
Ingredients: Devil's Claw, Oregon Grape Rt., Red Clover, Ginkgo Biloba, Prickly Ash, Ginger Rt., Gravel Rt., Shavegrass, Licorice Rt., Slippery Elm, Flax Seed.

ASTH-AID™ TEA
Ingredients: Marshmallow Rt., Mullein, Fenugreek Sd., Wild Cherry Bark, Rosemary, Ginkgo Biloba, Angelica Rt., Lobelia, Cinnamon, Passion Flower.

BEAUTIFUL SKIN TEA™
Ingredients: Licorice Rt., Burdock Rt., Rosemary, Dandelion Lf., Rosehips, Sarsaparilla Rt., Chamomile, Parsley Lf., Fennel Seed, Thyme.

BLDR-K FLUSH™
Ingredients: Juniper Berry, Cornsilk, Uva Ursi, Plantain, Parsley Lf., Cleavers, Dandelion Lf., Ginger Rt., Marshmallow Rt.

BONZ TEA™
Ingredients: Horsetail, Alfalfa, Dandelion Lf. & Rt., Oatstraw, Licorice Rt., Burdock, Marshmallow, Dulse, Nettles.

CEL-LEAN RELEASE™ TEA
Ingredients: Lemon Powder & Peel, Rosehips, Hawthorne Berries, Bilberry, Hibiscus.

CHILL CARE™ TEA
Ingredients: Peppermint, Elder Flwrs. & Brys., Coltsfoot, Hyssop, Licorice Rt., Yarrow, Boneset, Safflowers, Cloves, Rosehips, Ginger Rt., Cinnamon, Honey Crystals.

CHINESE ROYAL MU
Ingredients: Prince Ginseng Rts, Licorice Rt., Marshmallow Rt., Dandelion Rt., Sarsaparilla Rt., Burdock Rt., Cardamom Pods, Star Anise, Ginger Rt., Orange Peel, Cloves, Cinnamon.

❦ CLEANSING & PURIFYING TEA™
Ingredients: Red Clover, Hawthorne Lf. & Flwr., Pau de Arco Bk, Alfalfa Lf., Nettles, Sage, Horsetail Herb, Yerba Santa, Gotu Kola, Milk Thistle Seed, Echinacea Purpurea, Blue Malva, Lemon Grass.

❦ COFEX™
Ingredients: Wild Cherry Bk., Licorice Rt., Slippery Elm, Cinnamon Bk., Ginger Rt., Fennel Seed, Orange Peel, Cardamom.

❦ CONCEPTIONS™ TEA (formerly FRTL-TEA™)
Ingredients: Wild Yam, Damiana, Dong Quai, Sarsaparilla Rt., Yellow Dock Rt., Burdock Rt., Bladderwrack, Royal Jelly, Black Cohosh, Fo-Ti, Licorice Rt., Ginger Rt., Scullcap.

❦ CRAN-PLUS TEA™
Ingredients: Pau de Arco Bk., Cranberry Pwd., Rosehips, Damiana Lf., Echinacea Purpurea, Burdock Rt., Myrrh Gum, Lemon Balm, Cinnamon Chips, Hibiscus Flwrs.

❦ CREATIVI-TEA™
Ingredients: Prince Ginseng Rootlets, Damiana, Gotu Kola, Kava Kava, Muira Puama, Licorice Rt, Cloves, Juniper Berry, Spearmint.

❦ CUPID'S FLAME™
Ingredients: Damiana, Prince Ginseng Rt., Sarsaparilla, Licorice Rt., Fo-Ti, Gotu Kola, Saw Palmetto Berry, Kava Kava, Angelica Rt., Ginger Rt., Muira Puama, Allspice.

❦ DEEP BREATHING™ TEA
Ingredients: Wild Cherry Bk, Sage, Mullein, Parsley Lf., Safflowers, Thyme, Blackberry Lf., Ginger Rt., Pleurisy Rt., Ephedra Extract.

❦ EYE BRIGHT HERBAL™ TEA
Ingredients: Eyebright, Bilberry Lf., Passion Flwr., Plantain, Elder Flwr., Rosemary, Goldenseal Leaf, Red Raspberry.

❦ FEEL GREAT TEA™
Ingredients: Red Clover, Alfalfa, Hawthorne Lf. & Flwr., Spearmint, Dandelion Rt., Dulse, Sage, Licorice Rt., Lemon Grass.

❦ FEMALE HARMONY™
Ingredients: Red Raspberry Lf., Licorice Rt., Burdock Rt., Nettles, Rosebuds, Spearmint, Rosehips, Lemon Grass, Strawberry Lf., Sarsaparilla Rt.

❦ FIRST AID TEA FOR KIDS™
Ingredients: Chamomile, Lemon Balm, Catnip, Fennel Sd., Cinnamon, Acerola Cherry.
Directions: For infants - one quarter to one half cup 2 to 6 times daily; for 1 to 6 years - 1 cup, 2 to 6 times daily.

❦ FLOW EASE™
Ingredients: Cramp Bark, Spearmint, Sarsaparilla Rt., Ginger Rt., Angelica Rt., Chamomile, Squaw Vine.

❦ FLOW ON TEA™
Ingredients: Pennyroyal, Motherwort, Juniper, Angelica Rt., Blue Cohosh, Lovage, Canada Snakeroot, Tansy.

❦ FLOW- XS TEA™
Ingredients: White Oak Bark, Shepherd's Purse, Borage Seed, Oatstraw, Burdock Rt., Bayberry Bark, Lemon Peel, Milk Thistle Seed, Nettles, Dulse.

❦ GOOD NIGHT TEA™
Ingredients: Chamomile, Spearmint, Scullcap, Passion Flwr., Hops, Orange Blossoms, Rosehips & Rosebuds, Lemon Grass, Blackberry Lf., Catnip.

❦ HEALTHY HAIR & NAILS™
Ingredients: Horsetail Herb, Fenugreek Seed, Rosemary, Alfalfa Lf., Lemon Grass, Nettles, Dandelion Rt., Parsley Lf., Peppermint, Coltsfoot, Sage Lf.

❦ HEARTSEASE/CIRCU-CLEANSE™
Ingredients: Hawthorne Lf. & Flwr., Pau de Arco, Bilberries, Kukicha Twig, Ginger Rt., Heartsease, Ginkgo Biloba Lf., White Sage, Red Sage, Calendula Flwr., Yellow Dock Rt., Peppermint, Licorice Rt., Astragalus.

❦ HEARTSEASE/H.B.P.
Ingredients, Hawthorne Lf., Bry. & Flr., Scullcap, Dandelion Rt., Prince Ginseng Rt., Ginger Rt., Hibiscus, Rosehips, Valerian.

❧ HERBAL DEFENSE TEA™
Ingredients: Red Clover, Burdock Rt., Hawthorne Lf. & Flwr., Licorice Rt., Prince Ginseng Rt., Astragalus, Suma, Sage, Schizandra Bry., Boneset, Lemon Grass, Marshmallow Rt.

❧ HI ENERGY TEA™
Ingredients: Gotu Kola, Prince Ginseng, Damiana, Kava Kava, Red Clover, Raspberry, Peppermint, Cloves.

❧ INCREDIBLE DREAMS™
Ingredients: Fresh-dried Mugwort, Kava Kava, Rosemary, Lemon Grass, Raspberry Lf., Alfalfa, Spearmint.

❧ LAXA-TEA™
Ingredients: Papaya Lf., Fennel Sd., Ginger Rt., Hibiscus, Lemon Balm, Peppermint, Parsley, Calendula, Senna Ext..

❧ LEAN & CLEAN DIET™ TEA
Ingredients: Flax Seed, Fennel Seed, Uva Ursi, Parsley Lf., Senna Lf. and Pod, Lemon Peel, Cleavers, Chickweed, Hibiscus, Burdock Rt., Red Clover.

❧ LIV-ALIVE™
Ingredients: Dandelion Rt., Watercress, Yellow Dock Rt., Pau de Arco, Hyssop, Parsley Lf., Oregon Grape Rt., Red Sage, Licorice Rt., Milk Thistle Seed, Hibiscus.

❧ MEDITATION™ TEA
Ingredients: Cardamom Seed, Cinnamon, Fennel Seed, Cloves, Ginger Rt., Peppercorns.

❧ MIGR-TEA™
Ingredients: Feverfew, Valerian, Wild Lettuce, Cultiv. Lady Slipper, Ginkgo Biloba, Niacinamide-30mg.

❧ MOTHERING TEA™
Ingredients: Red Raspberry, Nettles, Horsetail, Spearmint, Ginger Rt., Alfalfa, Lemon Grass, Shavegrass, Strawberry Lf., Fennel Seed.

❧ NICO-STOP™
Ingredients: Lobelia, Licorice Rt., Chamomile, Peppermint, Sarsaparilla Rt., Oats.

❧ X-PECT-T™
Ingredients: Licorice Rt., Mullein, Pleurisy Rt., Marshmallow Rt., Rosehips, Ephedra, Calendula, Bonsest, Ginger Rt., Peppermint, Fennel Seed.

❧ RELAX TEA
Ingredients: Lemon Balm, Lemon Grass, Spearmint, Licorice Rt., Rosemary, Passion Flower, Yerba Santa, Orange Peel, Cinnamon, Rosebuds.

❧ RESPR TEA™
Ingredients: Fenugreek Sd., Hyssop, Horehound, Ginkgo Biloba, Rosehips, Boneset, Marshmallow Rt., Lobelia, Peppermint, Ephedra, Anise Seed, Honey Crystals.

❧ STRESSED-OUT TEA™
Ingredients: Catnip, Rosemary, Chamomile, Peppermint, White Willow, Gotu Kola, Feverfew, Blue Violet, Blessed Thistle, Wood Betony.

❧ SUGAR STRATEGY LO™
Ingredients: Prince Ginseng Rt., Licorice Rt., Unsprayed Bee Pollen, Dandelion Rt., Gotu Kola, Alfalfa Lf., Peppermint, Nettles.

❧ THERADERM™ TEA
Ingredients: Burdock, St. John's Wort, Dandelion Rt., Borage Seed, Calendula, Licorice Rt., Chamomile, Yellow Dock Rt., White Sage, Red Clover Blossoms.

❧ TINKLE™ TEA
Ingredients: Uva Ursi, Senna Lf., Parsley Lf., Fennel Seed, Dandelion Lf., Lemon Peel, Dulse, Ginger Rt.

❧ VARI-TONE™
Ingredients: Hawthorne Lf., Berry and Flower, Bilberry Lf., Ginkgo Biloba Lf., Gotu Kola, Myrrh, White Oak Bark, Lemon Peel, Butcher's Broom, Rosehips, Calendula, Eucalyptus Lf., Senna.

❧ WOMENS STRENGTH ENDO™ TEA
Ingredients: Sage, Motherwort, Blessed Thistle, Blue Vervain, Rosemary, Dong Quai, Damiana.

THERAPEUTIC BATHS & DOUCHES
All baths and douches include a re-usable muslin bath bag.

❦ **HOT SEA WEED BATH™**
Ingredients: Kelp, Dulse, Bladderwrack, Kombu, Watercress, Sea Palm
Note: Overheating therapy and iodine therapy are two of the most effective treatments in natural healing. They are powerful and should be used with care. If you are under medical supervision for heart disease or high blood pressure, check with your physician to determine if a seaweed bath is all right for you.

❦ **POUNDS OFF™ BATH**
Ingredients: Jaborandi, Pennyroyal, Orange Blossoms, Thyme, Angelica Rt., Elder Flowers, Kesu Flower.
FOR EXTERNAL USE ONLY. Stay in the bath for thirty to forty minutes for best results.

❦ **WHITES OUT DOUCHE™**
Note: For vaginal use only. Use on a temporary basis only, so that the vagina can rebuild its own balance and pH.
Ingredients: Comfrey Lf. & Rt., Juniper Bry., Myrrh Gum, Goldenseal Lf., Pau de Arco, Witch Hazel Lf. & Bk., Buchu Lf., Oat-straw, Squaw Vine, White Oak Bk.

❦ **MOTH FREE™ HERBAL SACHET**
A potent blend to save natural fiber clothes. Repels moths and harmful insects in closets and drawers. Three sachets to a box.
Ingredients: Cedarwood, Rosemary, Lemon Grass, Lavender, Basil, Bay, Natural Fiber Cellulose.

CAPSULE COMBINATIONS

❧ **ADR-ACTIVE™**
Ingredients: Licorice Rt., Sarsaparilla, Bladderwrack, Irish Moss, Uva Ursi, Rosehips Vitamin C, Ginger Rt., Capsicum, Astragalus, Pantothenic Acid-25mg. Vitamin B6 -20mg., Betaine HCl.

❧ **ALRG™ CAPS**
Ingredients: Marshmallow Rt., Burdock Rt., Mullein, Chaparral, Ephedra Extract, Parsley Rt., Goldenseal Rt., Capsicum, Acerola Cherry Fiber, Pantothenic Acid-30mg.

❧ **ANTI-BIO™**
Ingredients: Echinacea Angustifolia Root & Leaf, Echinacea Purpurea Root & Leaf, Golden Seal Root, Myrrh, Capsicum, Marshmallow, Chapparal, Yarrow, Elecampane, Turmeric.

❧ **ANTI-FLAM™**
Ingredients: White Willow, Echinacea Ang. & Purp., St. John's Wort, White Pine, Gotu Kola, Red Clover, Devil's Claw, Alfalfa Ext., Burdock, Dandelion, Chamomile, Uva Ursi, Ginger.

❧ **ANTI-HST™**
Ingredients: Unsprayed Bee Pollen, Marshmallow Rt., White Pine Bark, Ephedra Extract, Goldenseal, Burdock Rt., Juniper Berry, Parsley Rt., Acerola Cherry, Rosemary, Mullein, Capsicum, Lobelia, Pantothenic Acid 20mg, Vit. B6 20mg.

❧ **ANTI-SPZ™**
Ingredients: Cramp Bark, Black Haw, Rosemary, Kava Kava, St, John's Wort, Chaste Tree Berries, Valerian, Passion Flower, Red Raspberry, Kelp, Lobelia, Wild Yam.

❧ **APPE-TIGHT™ DIET CAPS**
Ingredients: Chickweed, Gotu Kola, Kelp, Fennel Seed, Guar Gum, Licorice Rt., Black Walnut, Ephedra, Lecithin, Hawthorne Berry, Safflowers, Echinacea Rt., Papain, L-Ornithine-25mg., Vit. B6-20mg.,Kola Nut, Niacin-10mg.

❧ **AR EASE™**
Ingredients: Yucca, Guggul, Chaparral, Devil's Claw Rt., Alfalfa, Buckthorn Bk., Black Cohosh, Burdock Rt., Bilberry, St. John's Wort, Rose Hips Ext., Dandelion Rt. & Lf., Slippery Elm Bk., Licorice Rt., Yarrow, Parsley Rt. & Lf., Hydrangea, Hawthorne Leaf & Flwr., Turmeric, Pantothenic Acid-15mg., DLPA -10mg., Vit. B6-10mg.

ASPIR-SOURCE™
Ingredients: White Willow, Wood Betony, Rosemary, Violet, Scullcap, Raspberry, Valerian, Eur. Mistletoe, Ginger Rt., Vervain.

ASTH-AID™ CAPS
Ingredients: Bupleurum, Elecampane, Bee Pollen, White Pine Bk., Royal Jelly, Scullcap, Chaparral, Ginger, Ephedra Ext., Acerola Cherry Fiber.

BACK TO RELIEF™
Ingredients: Wild Lettuce, Valerian, White Willow, St. John's Wort, Mag.-40mg., Capsicum, DLPA 20mg.

BLDR-K™ COMFORT
Ingredients: Juniper Berry, Parsley Rt., Goldenseal Rt., Uva Ursi, Marshmallow Rt., Dandelion Lf., Stone Rt., Mullein Lf., Ginger Rt., Hydrangea, Vit. B_6 - 25mg., Lobelia.

BODY REBUILDER
Ingredients: Unsprayed Bee Pollen, Rosehips/ascorbate vitamin C, Barley Grass, Hawthorne Berry, Flower & Lf., Siberian Ginseng, Alfalfa, Amino Acid compound, Spirulina, Sarsaparilla Rt., Red Raspberry Lf., Desiccated Liver, Kelp, Parsley Rt., Carrot Calcium Crystals, Goldenseal, Mullein Lf., Wild Cherry Bk., Zinc Gluconate-20mg.

BONZ™
Ingredients: Carrot Calcium, Barley Grass, Black Cohosh Rt., St. John's Wort, Parsley Lf. & Rt., Rosehips Vitamin C, Alfalfa, Sarsaparilla, White Oak Bk., Plantain Lf., Oatstraw, Borage Seed, Dandelion Lf. & Rt., Chapparal, Dulse, Licorice Rt., Burdock Rt., Marshmallow Rt., Nettles, Slippery Elm, Zinc-10mg, Yellow Dock.

BWL-TONE-IBS CAPS™
Ingredients: Peppermint, Aloe Vera Powder, Marshmallow Rt., Slippery Elm, Pau de Arco, Ginger Rt., Wild Yam, Lobelia.

CALCIUM SOURCE CAPS
Ingredients: Watercress, Oatstraw, Dandelion Leaf, Alfalfa, Rosemary, Borage Seed, Pau de Arco, Carrot Extract.

CAND-EX™
Ingredients: Pau de Arco, Veg. Acidophilus, Black Walnut Hulls, Garlic, Barberry, Rosehips Vitamin C, Sodium Caprylate, Spirulina, Cranberry, Burdock Rt., Licorice Rt., Echinacea Purp., Echinacea Ang., Rosemary, Peppermint, Dong Quai, Damiana, Thyme, Calcium Citrate-30mg., DLPA-10mg., Zinc-10mg.

CEL-LEAN CAPS™
Ingredients: Fenugreek Sd., Gotu Kola, Garlic, Quassia Chips, Black Cohosh, Red Sage, Golden Seal Rt., Lecithin, Bilberry, Milk Thistle Seed, Fennel Seed, Turmeric, Kola Nut, Kelp, Choline-25mg., Vitamin B6-15mg.

CHOL-EX™
Ingredients: Lecithin, Hawthorne Berry, Rosehips Extract, Guar Gum, Apple Pectin, Siberian Ginseng, Plantain, Fenugreek Seed, Vegetable Acidophilus, Barley Grass, Capsicum, Psyllium Husk Powder, Vitamin B6-10mg., Niacin-10mg.

CHOL-LO FIBER TONE™ CAPSULES
Ingredients: Organic Oat Bran, Organic Flax Seed (high in Omega 3 and 6 oils), Psyllium Husk, Guar Gum, Apple Pectin, Veg. Acidophilus, Organic Fennel Seed, Acerola Cherry Fiber, Grapefruit Seed Ext. (as a preservative).

CLUSTER CAPS™
Ingredients: Feverfew flowers leaf and herb, Valerian, Niacin-50mg. Wild Lettuce, Cult. Lady Slipper Rt., Ginkgo Biloba Lf,Capsicum, Goldenseal.

COLD SEASON DEFENSE™
Ingredients: Garlic, Rosehips Extract, Ascerola Cherry Fiber, Ascorbate Vit. C, Bayberry Bk., Unsprayed Bee Pollen, Veg. Acidolphilus, St. John's Wort, Parsley Rt., Ginger, Rosemary, Boneset, Capsicum, Potass.Chl.-10mg., Zinc-10mg.

DETOX!™
Ingredients: Red Clover, Licorice Rt., Burdock Rt., Pau de Arco, Echinacea Rt., Ascorbate Vit. C, Garlic, Kelp, Alfalfa, Milk Thistle Seed, Sarsaparilla, Astragalus, Yellow Dock Rt., Butternut Bark, Goldenseal Rt., Prickly Ash, Buckthorn Bk.

EASY CHANGE™
Ingredients: Black Cohosh, Cultiv. Lady Slipper, Cramp Bark, False Unicorn, Sarsaparilla Rt, Dong Quai, Damiana Lf., Squaw Vine, Uva Ursi, Red Raspberry Lf., Blessed Thistle, Bayberry Bk., Carrot Extract, Pennyroyal, Ginger Rt.

Ingredients: Sarsaparilla Rt., Siberian Ginseng, Fo-Ti, Licorice Rt., Irish Moss, Barley Grass Powder, Black Cohosh, Saw Palmetto, Dong Quai, Gotu Kola, Kelp, Alfalfa, Ginger Rt., Spirulina, Glutamine-10mg.

❧ EST-AID™
Ingredients: Bk. Cohosh, Sarsaparilla, Licorice, False Unicorn, Dong Quai, Wild Yam, Squaw Vine, Damiana, Blessed Thistle.

❧ EYEBRIGHT HERBAL™
Ingredients: Eyebright, Bilberry, Ginkgo Biloba, Parsley Rt., Goldenseal Rt., Passion Flower, Bayberry Bk., Hawthorne Lf. & Flwr., Red Raspberry, Capsicum, Angelica Rt.

❧ FEEL GREAT™
Ingredients: Siberian Ginseng, Unsprayed Bee Pollen, Gotu Kola, Sarsaparilla Rt., Licorice Rt., Suma, Golden Seal Rt., Barley Grass, Spirulina, Schizandra Berries, Black Cohosh, Ginkgo Biloba Lf., Hawthorne Berry, Lf., & Flwr., Am. Ginseng, Alfalfa, Kelp, Wild Cherry Bk., Nutritional Yeast, Rice Protein Powder, Capsicum, Choline-10mg., Zinc-10mg.

❧ FEMALE HARMONY™
Ingredients: Dong Quai, Damiana, Burdock Rt., Sarsaparilla Rt., Licorice Rt, Red Raspberry Lf., Oatstraw, Nettles, Dandelion Rt., Yellow Dock Rt., Rosemary, Hawthorne Lf. & Flwr., Peony Rt., Ma Huang, Ephedra, Angelica Rt., Fennel Seed, Ginger Rt., Roships, Chaste Tree Berries, Rehmannia, Chamomile, Cinnamon.

❧ FIBER & HERBS COLON CLEANSE™
Ingredients: Butternut Bark, Cascara Sagrada, Rhubarb Rt., Barberry Bk., Psyllium Husk, Organic Fennel Seed, Licorice Rt., Ginger Rt., Irish Moss, Capsicum.

❧ FIRST AID CAPS™
Ingredients: Bayberry, Rosehips, Vitamin C, White Pine Bk., White Willow, Ginger Rt., Cloves, Capsicum.

❧ FIVE WEEK FORMULA™ (special order only)
Ingredients: Red Raspberry Lf., Squaw Vine, Pennyroyal, Bilberry, Black Cohosh Rt., Blessed Thistle, False Unicorn, Lobelia.

❧ GINSENG 6 SUPER ENERGY CAPS™
Ingredients: American Ginseng, Unsprayed Bee Pollen, Siberian Ginseng, Gotu Kola, Fo-Ti, Prince Ginseng, Suma Rt., Kirin Ginseng, Dong Quai, L-Glutamine-10mg., Alfalfa Extract.

❧ HEARTSEASE/ANEMI-GIZE™
Ingredients: Beet Rt., Alfalfa, Dandelion Lf. & Rt., Yellow Dock, Bilberry, Parsley Rt., Nettles, Burdock Rt., Dulse, Siberian Ginseng, Capsicum.

❧ HEARTSEASE/HAWTHORNE™
Ingredients: Hawthorne Leaf, Berry & Flower, Siberian Ginseng, Motherwort, Bilberry, Capsicum, Ginkgo Biloba, Lecithin, D-Alpha Vit. E-25IU, Butcher's Broom, Niacin-15mg., Choline-15mg.

❧ HEARTSEASE/H.B.P™
Ingredients: Garlic, Hawthorne Rt., Bry, & Flr., Siberian Ginseng, Bilberry, Capsicum, Ginger Rt., Parsley Rt., Dandelion Rt. & Lf., Goldenseal Rt., Vit. B6-15mg.

❧ HEAVY METAL CAPS™ (special order only)
Ingredients: Ascorbate Vitamin C, Kelp, Bladderwrack, Bugleweed, Astragalus, Irish Moss, Licorice Rt., Parsley Rt., Prickly Ash, Potassium Chl.- 25mg.

❧ HEMR-EASE™
Ingredients: Stone Rt., Slippery Elm, Rose Hips, Ascorbate Vitamin C, Butcher's Broom, Goldenseal Rt., Bilberry Lf., Mullein, Cranesbill, Witch Hazel Lf.

❧ HERBAL DEFENSE TEAM™ CAPS
Ingredients: Echinacea Rt., Pau de Arco, Garlic, Ascorbate Vitamin C-50mg., Astragalus, Unsprayed Bee Pollen, Hawthorne Lf. & Flwr., Suma, Bayberry Bk., Acerola Cherry Fiber, Barley Grass, Goldenseal Rt., Schizandra Bry., Yarrow, Burdock Rt., Elecampane, Red Sage, Kelp, Capsicum, Potassium Chl.-10mg., Zinc-10mg.

❧ HERBAL ENZ™
Ingredients: Ginger Root, Fennel, Vegetable Acidophilus, Cramp Bark, Peppermint, Spearmint, Catnip, Papaya, Turmeric.

❧ HRPS™
Ingredients: Astragalus, L-Lysine, Yellow Dock Rt., Echinacea Rt., Red Sage, Myrrh Gum, Wild Yam, Sarsaparilla Rt., Oregon Grape Rt., Marshmallow Rt., Vit. E-15IU, Poria Mushroom.

❧ HI PERFORMANCE™
Ingredients: Siberian Ginseng, Unsprayed Bee Pollen, Sarsaparilla Rt., Gotu Kola, Licorice Rt., Spirulina, Barley Grass, Dandelion Rt., Wild Yam, Alfalfa, Yarrow, Ginger Rt., Capsicum, Arginine-15mg., Ornithine-15mg., Zinc-15mg.

❧ IODINE SOURCE™ CAPS
Ingredients: Kelp, Kombu, Dulse, Organic Alfalfa, Watercress, Borage Seed, Irish Moss, Spirulina, Nettles.

❧ IRON SOURCE™ CAPS
Ingredients: Beet Rt., Yellow Dock Rt., Dulse, Borage Seed, Parsley Lf., Rosemary Lf., Dandelion Lf., Alfalfa.

❧ LEAN & CLEAN DIET CAPS™
Ingredients: Spirulina, Senna Lf. & Pod, Kelp, Unsprayed Bee Pollen, Bancha Green Tea, Cascara Sagrada, Alfalfa Seed, Fennel Seed, Ginger Rt., Guar Gum, Uva Ursi, Vit. B_6-20mg., L-Phenalalanine-10mg.

❧ LIV-ALIVE™
Ingredients: Beet Rt., Milk Thistle Sd.,Oregon Grape Rt., Dandelion Rt., Wild Yam, Yellow Dock Rt., Licorice Rt., Ginkgo Biloba, Barberry Bk., Gotu Kola, Ginger Rt., Wild Cherry Bk., Choline-10mg., Inositol-10mg.

❧ LOVE CAPS™ FEMALE
Ingredients: Dong Quai Rt., Damiana, Sarsaparilla Rt., Licorice Rt., Gotu Kola, Burdock Rt., Parsley Lf., Ginger Rt., Ma Huang, Guarana, Yohimbe Bk.
Note: Contains small amounts of yohimbe bk. Do not use if taking high blood pressure medicine or if there is heart arrhytmia.

❧ LOVE CAPS™ MALE
Ingredients: Sarsaparilla Rt., Damiana, Siberian Ginseng, Saw Palmetto, Kava Kava, Guaraña, Wild Yam, Ma Huang, Muira Puama, Gotu Kola, Ginger Rt., Yohimbe Bk., Zinc-10mg., Niacin-18mg.
Note: Contains small amounts of yohimbe bk. Do not use if taking high blood pressure medicine or if there is heart arrythmia.

❧ MALE PERFORMANCE™
Ingredients: Unsprayed Royal Jelly, Siberian Ginseng, Sarsaparilla Rt., Saw Palmetto, Wild Yam, Dandelion Rt., Damiana, Muira Puama, Licorice, Yellow Dock, Gotu Kola, Am. Ginseng, Fo-Ti, Capsicum.

❧ MINERAL SPECTRUM™ CAPS
Ingredients: Watercress, Yellow Dock Rt., Nettles, Organic Alfalfa, Irish Moss, Kelp, Parsley Lf. & Rt., Borage Seed, Dulse, Dandelion Lf. & Rt., Barley Grass, L-Glutamine-10mg.

❧ MENTAL CLARITY™
Ingredients: Korean White Ginseng, Fo-Ti, Siberian Ginseng, Ginkgo Biloba, Kelp, Gotu Kola, Rosemary, Prickly Ash, Schizandra, Capsicum, L-Phenalalanine-40mg., Glutamine-25mg., Choline-15mg., Zinc-15mg.

❧ META-TABS™
Ingredients: Irish Moss, Kelp, Parsley Rt. & Lf., Watercress, Mullein, Sarsaparilla, Carrot Ext.-30mg, Glutamine-15mg., Lobelia.

❧ MIGR-EASE™
Ingredients: Valerian, Wild Lettuce, Feverfew, European Mistletoe, Gentian Rt., Licorice Rt., DLPA-15mg.

❧ NIGHT CAPS™
Ingredients: Valerian Rt., Scullcap, Passion Flower, Kava Kava, Hops, Carrot Crystals, GABA-20mg., Taurine -30mg., Vit. B_6 -20mg., Niacin -10mg.

❧ P.O. #1
Ingredients: Echinacea Ang., Echinacea Purp., Yellow Dock Rt., Chaparral, Capsicum, Black Walnut Hulls, Lysine - 40mg.

❧ P.O. #2
Ingredients: Jewel Weed, Mugwort, Grindelia, Red Raspberry Lf., Black Cohosh Rt.,Lobelia, Kava Kava.

❧ PROS-CAPS™
Ingredients: Licorice Rt., Goldenseal Rt., Saw Palmetto Berry, Parsley Rt., Juniper Berry, Gravel Rt., Carrot Crystals, Uva Ursi, Marshmallow Rt., Hydrangea Rt.,Ginger Rt., Capsicum, Zinc-25mg., Vitamin E-15IU.

❧ RAINFOREST ENERGY™ CAPS
Ingredients: Guarana, Kola Nut, Suma, Bee Pollen, Astragalus Bk., Capsicum, Ginger, L-Glutamine-30mg.

❧ RELAX CAPS™
Ingredients: Black Cohosh, Cultivated Lady Slipper, Scullcap, Kava Kava, Black Haw, Hops, Valerian Rt., European Mistletoe, Wood Betony, Oatstraw, Lobelia.

❧ RSPR CAPS™
Ingredients: Mullein, Wild Cherry Bk., Pleurisy Rt., Plantain, Ginkgo Biloba Lf., Horehound, Licorice Rt., Slippery Elm, Acerola Cherry, Marshmallow Rt., Chickweed, Kelp, Cinnamon, Capsicum, Ephedra Extract.

❧ SKIN THERAPY™ #1
Ingredients: Burdock, Red Clover, Dandelion Rt., Echinacea Rt., Chamomile, Licorice Rt., Yellow Dock Rt., L-Glutamine-20mg., Vit. B6-25mg.

❧ SKIN THERAPY™ #2
Ingredients: Burdock Rt., Yellow Dock Rt., Chaparral, Dandelion Rt., Chickweed, Alfalfa, Sarsaparilla, Rosemary, Licorice Rt., Wild Yam, Ginger, Bilberry, L-Glutamine-10mg., Zinc Gluconate-10mg.

❧ STN-EX™
Ingredients: Dandelion Rt., Parsley Rt., Milk Thistle Seed, Marshmallow Rt., Hydrangea Rt., Gravel Rt., Wild Yam, Licorice Rt., Lemon Balm, Lecithin, Ginger Rt.

❧ SUGAR STRATEGY HIGH™
Ingredients: Cedar Berries, Dandelion Rt., Licorice Rt., Guar Gum, Elecampane, Mullein, Kelp, Wild Yam, Uva Ursi, Horseradish, Bilberry, Capsicum, Glutamine-25mg., Panto. Acid-25mg., Zinc-10mg., Mang.-5mg.

❧ SUGAR STRATEGY LOW™
Ingredients: Licorice Rt., Spirulina, Dandelion Rt., Cedar Berry, Alfalfa, Barley Grass, Gotu Kola, Wild Yam, Horseradish, Suma, Guar Gum, Amino Acid Compound-25mg.

❧ SUPER LEAN DIET™ CAPS
Ingredients: Gotu Kola, Gymnema Sylvestre, Chickweed, Guarana, L-Lysine-25mg., Ornithine-50mg., DL-Phenylalanine-10mg. Carnitine-50mg., Bromelain-40mg., Glycine-25mg., Chromium-200mcg., B6-10mg. Rosehips/Ascorbate vit. C w. bioflavs, GTF Chromium 10mg.

❧ SUPERMAX™
Ingredients: Unsprayed Bee Pollen, Spirulina, Siberian Ginseng, Suma, Gotu Kola, Barley Grass, Alfalfa, Desiccated Liver, Full Spectrum Amino Acid Compound-20mg., Kelp, Pantothenic Acid-25mg.

❧ THERADERM CAPS™
Ingredients: Burdock, Dandelion, Clevers, Turmeric, Echinacea Rt., Yellow Dock Rt., St. John's Wort, Kelp, Nettles, Lysine-30mg.

❧ TINKLE CAPS™
Ingredients: Uva Ursi, Cornsilk, Dandelion Rt. & Lf., Parsley, Juniper, Cleavors, Ginger Rt., Marshmallow, Vit. B6-40mg., Kelp.

❧ U.L.C.R. COMPLEX™
Ingredients: Goldenseal Rt., Slippery Elm, Licorice Rt., Myrrh Gum, Bilberry, Calendula Flr., Capsicum.

❧ VERMEX™
Ingredients: Black Walnut Hulls, Garlic, Pumpkin Seed, Butternut Bark, Cascara Sagrada, Mugwort, False Unicorn, Gentian Rt., Slippery Elm, Wormwood, Fennel Seed.

❧ WHITES OUT #1
Ingredients: Goldenseal Rt., Myrrh Gum, Pau de Arco, Echinacea Rt., Vegetable Acidophilus, Ginkgo Biloba.

❧ WHITES OUT # 2
Ingredients: Burdock Rt., Bayberry, Dandelion Rt., Black Walnut Hulls, Gentian, Uva Ursi, Parsley, Juniper Bry., Squaw Vine.

❧ WITHDRAWAL SUPPORT™
Ingredients: Scullcap, Siberian Ginseng, Valerian Rt., Ascorbate Vit, C-50mg., Chaparral, Kava Kava, Rt., Wood Betony, Licorice Rt., DLPA-25mg., Capsicum, Niacin-20mg.

❧ WOMAN'S BEST FRIEND™
Ingredients: Goldenseal Rt., Cramp Bark, Squaw Vine, Red Raspberry Lf., Rosehips, False Unicorn, Sarsaparilla Rt., Uva Ursi, Dong Quai, Blessed Thistle, Ginger Rt., Peony Rt., Rehmannia, Lobelia.

SINGLE HERB EXTRACTS

- **BILBERRY -** *Vaccinium Myrtillus*

- **BIO-VI -** *Usnea Extract*

- **BLACK WALNUT HULLS** - *Juglans Nigra*

- **CHLORELLA/GINSENG**

- **DONG QUAI/DAMIANA -** *Angelica Sinensis 50%, Turnera Diffusa 50%*

- **ECHINACEA 100% Root, Leaf & Stem -** *Echinacea Angustifolia 50%, Echinacea Purpurea 50%*

- **GINKGO BILOBA LEAF**

- **HAWTHORNE 100% Leaf, Flwr. & Berry** - *Crataegus Oxyacanthus*

- **MILK THISTLE SEED -** *Silybum Marianum*

- **PAU DE ARCO/ECHINACEA 100% -** *Tabebuia Impetiginosa 70%, Echinacea Angustifolia 30%*

- **SIBERIAN GINSENG -** *Eleuterococcus Senticosus*

- **SUPER SARSAPARILLA**

- **SUPER LICORICE 100% -** *Glycyrrhiza Glabra*

- **VALERIAN/WILD LETTUCE 100% -** *Valeriana Officinalis 50%, Lactuca Elongata 50%*

- **VITEX, *CHASTE TREE BERRIES* -***Vitex Agnus-Castus*

CUSTOM EXTRACT COMBINATIONS

ADRN-ACTIVE™
Ingredients: Licorice Rt., Bladderwrack, Sarsaparilla Rt., Irish Moss.

ALRG-HST™
Ingredients: Ma Huang, Mullein, Marshmallow Rt., Goldenseal Rt., Burdock Rt., Wild Cherry Bk., Licorice, Cinnamon.

ANTI-BIO™
Ingredients: Echinacea Angust. root, leaf & herb, Echinacea Purp. root, leaf & herb, Goldenseal Rt., Myrrh Gum, Pau De Arco.

ANTI-FLAM
Ingredients: Curcumin Ext., St. John's Wort, Butcher's Broom, White Willow, Bromelian.

ANTI-VI™
Ingredients: Lomatium Dissectum, St. John's Wort.

Directions: Use this formula is at fairly high dosage for a short term. 10 to 30 drops in $1/2$ cup of water 1 to 3 times a day for 10 days or less, is sufficient. It is not for long-term use. Do not use in conjunction with acidophilus culture which works against the antiviral properties.

BITTERS & LEMON CLEANSE™
Ingredients: Oregon Grape Rt., Gentian, Cardamom Sd. Lemon Peel, Dandelion Rt., Senna Lf., Peppermint.

BLDR-K FLUSH™
Ingredients: Cornsilk, Juniper Bry., Dandelion Rt., Uva Ursi, Goldenseal Rt., Parsley Rt. & Lf., Marshmallow Rt., Ginger Rt.

BRNX™ EXTRACT
Ingredients: Mullein, Grindelia, Usnea Barbata, Osha Rt., Coltsfoot, Licorice Rt., Goldenseal, Lobelia.

CALCIUM SOURCE™ EXTRACT
Ingredients: Watercress, Horsetail Herb, Alfalfa, Oatstraw, Rosemary, Dandelion Lf., Borage Seed.

CRAMP BARK COMBINATION™
Ingredients: Black Haw, Kava Kava, Cramp Bark, Rosemary, Lobelia Herb & Seed.

DEPRS-EX™
Ingredients: Scullcap, Cult. Lady Slipper, Rosemary, Catnip, Valerian, Peppermint, Hops, Wood Betony, Celery, Cinnamon.

DIAR-EX™
Ingredients: Aloe Vera, Bayberry Bk., Myrrh, Ginger Rt., Slippery Elm, Catnip, Cardamom. DIARR-EX is gentle and effective for children taken in water.

EPILEX™ EXTRACT
Ingredients: Bupleurum, Cinnamon, Ginger Rt., Catnip, Scullcap, Ginkgo Biloba Lf.

EST-AID™
Ingredients: Black Cohosh, Peony Rt., Licorice Rt., Dong Quai., Sarsaparilla Rt., Oatstraw, Burdock Rt., Damiana, Red Raspberry, Rosemary.

HERBAL DEFENSE TEAM™
Ingredients: Echinacea Rt., Garlic, Hawthorne Lf., Berry & Flwr., Siberian Ginseng, Goldenseal Rt., Rosehips Vitamin C.

IODINE SOURCE™EXTRACT
Ingredients: Kelp, Kombu, Dulse, Wakame, Watercress, Irish Moss, Horsetail Herb, Alfalfa.

IRON SOURCE™ EXTRACT
Ingredients: Yellow Dock Rt., Nettles, Dulse, Borage Seed.

LIV ALIVE™ EXTRACT
Ingredients: Oregon Grape Rt., Milk Thistle Seed, Dandelion Rt., Yellow Dock Rt., Ginkgo Biloba Lf., Red Sage, Licorice Rt., Wild Yam, Fennel Seed, Cascara Sagrada.

LOVING MOOD EXTRACT FOR MEN™
Ingredients: Siberian Ginseng, Damiana, Wild Oats, Dandelion Rt., Capsicum, Licorice Rt., Yohimbe Bk.

MIGR EXTRACT™
Ingredients: Feverfew, Siberian Ginseng, Ginkgo Biloba, Echinacea, Capsicum.

MINERAL SOURCE™ COMPLEX
Ingredients: Horsetail Herb, Yellow Dock Rt., Nettles, Alfalfa, Watercress, Irish Moss, Parsley Rt. & Lf., Dandelion Lf. & Rt.

PRE-MEAL ENZ™ DROPS
Ingredients: Fennel, Ginger Rt., Papaya Seed, Turmeric, Peppermint, Spearmint, Cramp Bark, Catnip Lf.

PROX™ TONIC
Ingredients: Saw Palmetto Berry, White Oak Bark, Echinacea Angustifolia Root, Pau de Arco Bark, Goldenseal Rt., Marshmallow Root, Uva Ursi.

RECOVERY TONIC™
Ingredients: Capsicum, Siberian Ginseng, Hawthorne Berry, Honey.

RTH TONE™
Ingredients: Devil's Claw, Yucca, Siberian Ginseng, White Willow, Echinacea Rt., Capsicum.

SCALE DOWN DIET EXTRACT™
Ingredients: Chickweed, Gotu Kola, Licorice Rt., Dulse, Spirulina, Lemon Peel, Fennel, Ma Huang, Senna.

SILICA SOURCE™
Ingredients: Extracts of Organic Horsetail Herb, Organic Oatstraw, in a base of Organic Carrot.

NIGHT ZZZs™
Ingredients: Valerian Rt., Wild Lettuce, Scullcap, Passion Flower, Hops Flr.

STRESSED-OUT™ EXTRACT
Ingredients: Black Cohosh, Wood Betony, Black Haw, Kava Kava, Scullcap, Carrot Calcium.

● **SUPER MAN'S ENERGY TONIC™**
Ingredients: Sarsaparilla Rt., Saw Palmetto Berries, Suma Rt., Siberian Ginseng, Gotu Kola, Capsicum.

● **TRAVEL EASE™**
Ingredients: Ginger, Ginkgo Biloba, Passion Flower, Catnip, St. John's Wort, Lavender, Peppermint.

● **U.L.C.R. COMPLEX™**
Ingredients: Goldenseal Rt., Slippery Elm Bk., Organic Licorice, Myrrh Gum, Calendula Flr., Capsicum.

● **WOMEN"S DRYNESS™**
Ingredients: Dendrobium, Organic Licorice Rt.

● **ZINC SOURCE™**
Ingredients: Echinacea, Spirulina, Gotu Kola, Bilberry Lf. and Bry., Peppermint, Yellow Dock, Alfalfa, Barley.

THE HERBAL SPA PRODUCTS

Because these are all natural herbal treatments rather than cosmetics, they have the color and smell of fresh herbs. Some separation may occur. Stir before using.

❧ **TIGHTENING & TONING BODY WRAP™**
Ingredients: The Wrap Gel: Extracts of Cranesbill, Angelica and White Oak Bark as skin-tightening astringents; Hawthorne Leaf & Flower with high flavonoids to cleanse, tone and help form new tissue; Rosemary as an herbal oxygenator for the skin; Marshmallow Rt. as a soothing herbal calcium and silicon source for tissue formation; Lemon Balm as a systemic "spring cleaning" herb; - in a base of Olive, Rice Bran and Grapeseed Oils, with Lecithin; Aloe Vera Gel, Vegetable Glycerine and Beeswax, with Vitamin E powder, Spice Extracts and Ascorbate Vitamin C as life preservers.
Ingredients: The Bio-Drink:Lemon Peel, to cleanse and alkalize the system; Hawthorne Berries, to add stronger flavonoids and act as a circulatory toning agent; Rosehips, to provide bioflavonoids with Vitamin C; Hibiscus, for additional flavonoids and to enhance assimilation.
Ingredients: The Capsules: Ginger, to stimulate circulation to the extremities; Niacinamide, a non-flushing stimulant that dilates blood vessels and capillaries; Vegetable Acidolphilus, to alkalize the body and increase enzyme activity.

❧ **ALKALIZING ENZYME BODY WRAP™**
Ingredients: The Wrap Gel: Extracts of Bladderwrack, Alfalfa, Ginger Rt., Dandelion Root, Spearmint, Capsicum, Cinnamon; in a base of Aloe Vera Gel, Olive Oil, Rice Bran Oil, Grapeseed Oil, Lecithin, Cocoa Butter, Vegetable Glycerine, Vegetable Acidolphilus & Beeswax.
Ingredients: The Drink: Miso Granules, Dulse, Barley Green, Turmeric, Ginger.
Ingredients: The Capsules: Spirulina, Alfalfa, Vegetable Acidolphilus.

   ✧Both herbal wrap processes are relaxing, and perfectly safe. However, if you have any special individual health problems or questions, see your health care professional before beginning a wrap.

❧ **CEL-LEAN™ CONTOUR GEL & CLEANSING WAFER KIT**
Ingredients: Gel Lotion: Extracts of Bladderwrack, Gotu Kola, Rosemary, Uva Ursi, Lemon Peel, Butcher's Broom, Plantain, Eucalyptus, Cayenne and Vanilla, in a base of Aloe Vera Gel, vegetable cellulose, distilled water, vegetable glycerine, with grapefruit seed extract, ascorbate vitamin C and vitamin E as life preservers, and essential oils for fragrance.
Wafer Ingredients: Lemon juice powder, Lemon Peel, Hibiscus, Rosehips, Hawthorne Berry.

❧ **LEMON SALT GLOW™ -** *A Total Body Exfoliant For The Skin*
Ingredients: Sun -dried Sea Salt, Aloe Vera Gel, Lemon Peel Granules, Almond Oil, Lemon Oil.

❧ **WHITE CLAY & HERBS TONING MASQUE**
Ingredients: White French Clay, Organic Calendula Flowers, Golden Seal Rt., Lemon Peel, Chamomile Flowers, Fennel Seed, Eucalyptus, Rosemary, and Spearmint.

❧ **HOT SEAWEED BATH™**
Ingredients: Kelp, Bladderwrack, Kombu, Dulse, Watercress and Sea Grasses.

PHYTO-THERAPY GELS

Therapeutic topical gels represent a new category of Crystal Star products. These gels are made in our own FDA-approved clean room from fresh and fresh-dried ingredients. They exemplify the highest quality and active ingredient potency available. We use only natural transfer media to get the therapeutic benefits to the problem. The gels may be used on the skin as needed.

❧ **GINSENG SKIN REPAIR GEL™ with germanium and vitamin C**
Ingredients: Wild American Ginseng, Siberian Ginseng and Suma, White Pine Bark, Ascorbate Vit. C, Calendula, Germanium.

❧ **BEAUTIFUL SKIN™ GEL with royal jelly and propolis**
Ingredients: Licorice Rt., Burdock Rt., Rosemary, Rosehips, Sarsaparilla, Sage, Chamomile, Parsley, Fennel Seed, Thyme, Dandelion, Unsprayed Royal Jelly, Propolis and Ginseng Extracts.

❧ **HEMR-EASE™ GEL**
Ingredients: Stone Rt., Slippery Elm, Rosehips, Ascorbate Vit. C, Goldenseal, Bilberry, Mullein, Cranesbill, Butcher's Broom, Witch Hazel.

❧ **LYSINE/LICORICE ROOT HEALING GEL™ with myrrh**
Ingredients: Extracts of Licorice and Myrrh with 800 mg. Lysine.

❧ **FUNGEX GEL™ with una de gato and grapefruit seed extract**
Ingredients: Pau de Arco, Gentian Rt., Myrrh, Goldenseal Rt., Witch Hazel, Lomatuim, Grapefruit Seed, Vitamin D.

❧ **ORGANIC CALENDULA GEL**
Ingredients: Organic Calendula Flower Extract, Veg, Glycerine, Chamomile Extract, Aloe Vera Powder, Agar-Agar, Grapefruit Seed Extract, Ascorbate Vit. C with Bioflavonoids.

❧ **RAINFOREST RECOVERY™ GEL**
Ingredients: Una de Gato Bk., Pau De Arco Bk. and Calendula Flowers.

THE DRINK MIXES

✻ **ENERGY GREEN™**
Ingredients: Barley Grass, Unsprayed Bee Pollen, Siberian Ginseng, Alfalfa, Apple Pectin, Dulse, Oats, Acerola Cherry Fiber, Sarsaparilla, Licorice Rt., Dandelion Rt. & Lf., Gotu Kola, Lemon Juice powder; in a base of pure rice protein powder.
Special Note: While exact amounts of micro-nutrient such as an enzyme or trace mineral are difficult to obtain without single-batch assays, measureable elements that you may consistently expect in this drink are as follows: *Amino Acid Profile:* Isoleucine, Leucine, Lysine, Methionine, Threonine, Phenylalanine, Tryptophan, Alanine, Arginine, Aspartic Acid, Cysteine, Cystine, Glutamic Acid, Glycine, Histidine, Ornithine, Proline, Serine, Tyrosine, Valine. *Vitamin Profile:* Beta Carotene A, B Complex from Rice, C from Rosehips, Vit. D. *Mineral Profile:* Iodine, Calcium, Magnesium, Potassium, Iron, Chromium, Zinc. *Food Profile:* Whole Cell Proteins, Complex Carbohydrates, Soluble Fiber, Chlorophyll and Bioflavonoids.

✻ **SYSTEM STRENGTH™**
Ingredients: The Food Blend: Miso Broth Powder, Soy Protein Powder, Brewer's Yeast, Vegetable Acidophilus, Cranberries.
The Sea Vegetable Blend: Macrobiotic Quality Dulse, Wakame, Kombu, Sea Palm.
The Herbal Blend: Alfalfa, Barley Grass, Watercress, Oatstraw, Yellow Dock Rt., Dandelion Lf., Borage Seed, Licorice Rt., Fennel Seed, Pau de Arco, Nettles, Parsley Rt. & Lf., Red Raspberry Lf., Horsetail, Siberian Ginseng, Rosemary.
Special Note: As with Energy Green™ above, exact amounts of individual micro-nutrients such as enzymes and trace minerals are almost impossible to obtain, but measureable elements you may consistently expect from this drink are as follows: *Amino Acid Profile:* Isoleucine, Leucine, Lysine, Methionine, Threonine, Phenylalanine, Tryptophan, Alanine, Arginine, Aspartic Acid, Cysteine, Cystine, Glutamic Acid, Glycine, Histidine, Ornithine, Proline, Serine, Tyrosine, Valine. *Vitamin Profile:* Beta Carotene A, B Complex from Soy and Brewer's Yeast, C from Cranberries, D. *Mineral Profile:* Naturally occuring Iodine, Calcium, Magnesium, Potassium, Silica, Iron, Manganese, Chromium, Copper, Zinc. *Enzyme Profile:* Whole complex from Acidophilus and Miso. *Food Profile:* Whole Cell Proteins, Complex Carbohydrates, Soluble Fiber, Chlorophyll and Bioflavonoids.

✻ **CHOL-LO FIBER TONE™**
Ingredients for both capsules and drink blend: Organic Oat Bran, Organic Flax Seed, Psyllium Husk, Vegetable Acidolphilus, Guar Gum, Acerola Cherry, Organic Fennel Seed, Orange or Cherry Oil, Epimers of vitamin E, (a food anti-oxidant).

Crystal Star Formulas

❋ **BIOFLAVONOID, FIBER & C SUPPORT™ DRINK**
Ingredients for both drink and wafers: Whole Pear Fiber, Cranberries and Cranberry Extract, Acerola Cherry, Rose Hips, Bilberry, Apple Pectin, Lemon and Orange Peels, Ginkgo Biloba Lf., Hawthorne Berries, Buckwheat Fiber, Hibiscus Flowers.

❋ **LIGHT WEIGHT™ MEAL REPLACEMENT PROGRAM**
LIGHT WEIGHT™ Drink Ingredients: *The complex carbohydrate/protein/fiber blend;* Pure Rice Protein, Organic Oat Bran, Guar Gum, Bee Pollen, Apple Pectin. *The cleansing/pH balancing/mineral blend;* Spirulina, Sweet Barley Grass, Acerola Cherry, Citrus Bioflavonoids, Aloe Vera, Senna Lf. & Pod, Fennel Seed, Red Raspberry Lf., Buckwheat Powder, *The co-enzyme therapy blend;* Wild Yam, Pineapple, Papaya, Ginger Rt., Vegetable Acidophilus. *The sweetening blend;* Honey Crystals, Vanilla.
LIGHT WEIGHT™ Capsule Ingredients: Ornithine-100mg., DL-Phenylalanine-100mg., Glycine-10mg., Carnitine-100mg., Lysine-75mg., Tyrosine-50mg., Gymnema Sylv., Ginger, Gotu Kola, Lecithin, Chromium-100mcg. Chickweed, Bromelain.
LIGHT WEIGHT™ comes in all natural cherry vanilla, and pineapple orange flavors.

THE ANIMAL MIX
Ingredients: Brewer's Yeast, Alfalfa, Lecithin, Kelp, Wheat Bran & Germ, Comfrey Lf., Spirulina, Garlic, Soy Protein powder, Dandelion Rt., Sodium Ascorbate Vit.C, Whey Acidophilus, Psyllium Husk, Rosemary.

CRYSTAL STAR PRODUCTS FOR AREAS OF PARTICULAR INTEREST

Women's Products
Cran-Plus™ Tea
Female Harmony™ Capsules and Tea
Vitex Extract
Flow Ease™ Tea
Flow On™ Tea special order only
Easy Change™
Dong Quai/Damiana Extract
Est-Aid™ Capsules and Extract
Flow-XS Tea™
Love Caps™ Female
Whites Out Capsules and Douche
Woman's Best Friend™ Capsules
Women's Dryness™ Extract
Conceptions™ Tea
Mothering Tea™

Products for Weight Loss, Water Retention & Cellulite
Lean & Clean™ Super Diet Tea
Super Lean™ Diet Capsules
Light Weight™ Meal Replacement Program
Tightening & Toning™ Herbal Body Wrap
Cel-Lean™ Tea and Capsules
Cel-Lean™ Contour Gel & Wafer Kit
Lean & Clean Diet™ Tea & Capsules
Appe-Tight Diet™ Capsules
Meta-Tabs™ Capsules
Scale Down™ Diet Extract
Tinkle™ Tea and Capsules
Pounds Off™ Bath
Rainforest Energy Tea & Capsules™

Products for Detoxification & Cleansing
Cleansing & Fasting Tea™
Green Tea Cleanser™
Detox Capsules and the Body Detox Kit
Echinacea Extract
Pau de Arco/Echinacea Extract
System Strength™ Drink Mix
Heartsease/Circu-Cleanse™ Tea
Liv-Alive Flush™ Tea, Extract and Capsules
Milk Thistle Seed Extract
Laxa-Tea™
BWL-Tone™
Candid-Ex™ Capsules
Alkalizing Enzyme Herbal Body Wrap
Cho-Lo Fiber Tone™ Capsules & Drink Mix
Fiber & Herbs Colon Cleanse™
Chol Ex™ Capsules
Withdrawal Support™ Capsules
Stnx™ Caps
Vermex™ Capsules

Men's Products
Love Caps™ Male
Male Performance™
Loving Mood™ Extract for Men
Pros- Caps™ and Prox™ Extract
Super Man's Energy Tonic™

Products for Athletic Performance
High Performance™ Capsules
SuperMax™ Caps
Siberian Ginseng Extract
Super Man's Energy Tonic™
Ginseng Super 6 Energy Caps™ and Tea

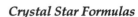

Immune Enhancers
Ginseng 6 Defense Restorative Super Tea™
Herbal Defense Team™ Capsules, Extract & Tea
Anti-Bio™ Caps and Extract
Bioflavonoid, Fiber & C Support™ Drink
Cold Season Defense Caps™
Resistance Support Caps™
Echinacea 100%™ Extract
Pau De Arco/Echinacia™ Extract

Products For Infection & Congestion
Anti-Bio'™Capsules & Extract
Anti-Flam™ Capsules
Asth-Aid™ Tea & Capsules
X-Pect T™
BLDR-K Flush™ Tea, Capsules and Extract
Deep Breathing™ Tea
Rspr™ Caps and Tea
Black Walnut Hulls Extract
Anti-Vi™ Extract & Super Tea

Products for Colds & Flu
Anti-Bio™ Capsules and Extract
Anti-Vi Super Tea™ & Extract
First Aid Caps™
Chill Care™ Tea
Cold Season Defense™
Cofex™ Tea
Anti-HS'T™ Capsules & Extract
Bioflavonoid, Fiber & C Support™ Drink

Pain Relievers
Migr™ Tea & Capsules
Anti-Flam™ Capsules
Headache Defense™ Extract
Back to Relief™ Capsules
Cramp Bark Combo™ Extract
AR Ease™ Caps & Tea
Cluster Caps™
Rth Tone™ Extract
Anti-Spz™ Capsules
AspirSource™ Capsules
Anti-Flam™ Capsules

Products for Stress & Tension
Stressed Out™ Tea & Extract
Heartsease H.B.P.™ Capsules
Relax™ Caps and Tea
Night ZZZs™ Extract
Withdrawal Support™ Caps
Night Caps™
ADR-Active™ Capsules & Extract
Valerian/Wild Lettuce Extract
Deprs-Ex™ Extract

Products for Digestion & Nutrient Assimilation
Sugar Strategy Low™ Tea & Capsules
Sugar Strategy High™ Capsules
Bitters & Lemon Cleanse™ Extract
Herbal Enz™
Diar-Ex™ Extract
Pre-Meal Enz™ Drops
U.L.C.R.™ Capsules & Extract

Energizers
Ginseng 6 Super Energy™ Caps and Tea
Creativi-Tea™
Cupid's Flame™
Feel Great™ Capsules and Tea
Rainforest Energy™ Tea
Rainforest Energy™ Capsules
High Energy Tea™
Mental Clarity™ Capsules
Energy Green™ Drink
ADRN™ Extract

Products for Allergy Control
ALRG™ Capsules
ALR-Hst Tea™
Anti-HST™ Capsules
X-Pect-T™
ALRG-HST™ Extract

Products for Beauty & Body Improvement
Beautiful Skin Tea™
Eyebright Herbal Tea
Licorice/Lysine Healing Gel™
Calendula Gel
Ginseng Skin Repair Gel w. C
Skin Therapy' # 1 & # 2 Capsules
Healthy Hair & Nails
Theraderm™ Caps & Tea
Vari-Tone™ Tea
Eyebright Herbal™ Capsules
Hot Seaweed Bath™
Lemon Salt Glow™
White Clay & Herbs Toning Mask

Effective Products for Children
Anti-Bio™ Capsules & Extract
Anti-Vi Super Tea™ & Extract
First Aid Caps™
Echinacea Extract
Epilex™ Extract
First Aid Tea for Kids™
Chill Care™ Tea
System Strength™ Drink Mix
Cold Season Defense™
Cofex™ Tea
Epilex™ Extract
Anti-HS'T™ Capsules & Extract
Bioflavonoid, Fiber & C Support™ Drink
Asth-Aid™ Tea & Capsules
Deep Breathing™ Tea
RSPR™ Caps & Tea
Vermex™ Capsules

RESOURCES & BIBLIOGRAPHY

❖The staff and clients of Country Store Natural Foods, whose self-healing efforts and accomplishments have contributed invaluable concrete information and evidence.

❖Aromatherapy Healing Wheel, Naturally Exotic Co., Weaverville, CA.

❖Best Ways Magazine

❖Better Health Through Natural Healing: Dr. Ross Trattler, D.C.

❖Better Nutrition for Today's Living Magazine

❖Cooking For Healthy Healing: Linda Rector-Page, N.D., Ph. D.

❖Country Life: Nutritional Literature, by Marcia Zimmerman

❖Dr. Pitcairn's Complete Guide To Natural Health For Dogs & Cats: Dr. R.H. Pitcairn, DVM

❖EastWest Natural Health Magazine

❖Encyclopedia of Natural Medicine: Michael Murray, N.D., & Joseph Pizzorno, N.D.

❖Enzymatic Therapy: Nutritional Formulas For The Right Body Chemistry, and Health Counselor

❖Everybody's Guide To Homeopathic Medicines: S. Cummings & Dana Ullman

❖Food & Healing: Anne-Marie Colbin

❖The Healing Nutrients Within: E.R. Braverman, M.D. & Carl C. Pfeiffer, M.D., Ph. D.

❖The Holistic Herbal: David Hoffman

❖How To Get Well: Paavo Airola

❖The How To Herb Book: V.J. Keith & Monteen Gordon

❖Let's Live Magazine

❖Nutrition Almanac: Lavon J. Dunne

❖Nutrition News: Riverside, Calif.

❖Nutritional Herbology: Mark Pedersen

❖Stories The Feet Have Told Through Reflexology: Eunice D. Ingham

❖Vegetarian Times Magazine

❖The Way Of Herbs: Michael Tierra

❖Whole Foods Magazine

Where we get what we recommend...

The following listing is included at the request of many readers of previous editions of "HEALTHY HEALING". It is for your convenience and assistance in obtaining further information about a product or its effectivness. The list is unsolicited by the companies named. We realize that there are many other fine companies and products that are not included here, but the ones mentioned have a solid, successful history of testing by us and the stores that have so generously shared their product experiences with us. We feel that you can count on these companies and products to perform with the highest quality and best results.

- All 1, Nutritech, Inc. SantaBarbara, CA., 93103.
- Alta Health Products, Pasadene, CA., 91107.
- Bio-Biotanica, Inc., Hauppauge, N.Y., 11788.
- BioForce of America, Ltd., Kinderhooh, N.Y., 12106.
- Biogenetics Food Corp., Naples, Fla., 33942.
- Boericke & Tafel, Inc., Santa Rosa, CA., 95407.
- Care Plus Products, Milwaukee, WI>, 53208.
- Cartilage Technologies, 2105 Luna Rd., Suite 320, Carrollton, TX., 75006.
- Country Life, Hauppauge, N.Y., 11788.
- De Souzas Food Corp., Banning, CA., 92220.
- Enzymatic Therapy, Inc., Green Bay, Wisconsin, 54305.
- Excel/Key Products Co., 3280 W. Hacienda, Suite 205, Las Vegas, N.Y., 89118.
- Floradix, imported by Miracle Exclusives, Inc., Locust Valley, N.Y., 11560.
- Food Science Labs, 20 New England Dr., Essex Junction, VT., 05453.
- George's Aloe Vera, Stafford, TX., 77477
- Golden Pride/Rawleigh, Inc., West Palm Beach, Fla., 33407.
- Green Foods Corp., Torrance, CA., 90503.
- Health Concerns, Alameda CA., 94501.
- Health Plus, Inc., Chino, CA., 91710.
- Heritage Products, Virginia Beach, VA., 23458
- Hyland's, Standard Homeopathic Co., Los Angeles, CA., 90061.
- Kyolic, Wakunaga of America, Mission Viejo, CA., 92691.
- Logic, International Mktng., Com., P.O. Box 4444, Pahrump, Nev., 89041.
- Madaus Murdock, Inc. - Nature's Way, P.O.Box 4000, Springville, UT., 84663.
- McZand Herbal, Inc., Santa Monica, CA., 90409.
- Natren, Inc., Westlake Village, CA., 91361.
- Natrol, Inc., Chatsworth, CA. 91311.
- Nature's Life, Cypress, CA., 90630.
- Nature's Plus, Farmingdale, N.Y., 11735.
- Nature Works, Inc., Agoura Hills, CA., 91301.
- New Chapter/New Moon, Brattleboro, Vt., 05301.
- NuAge Labs Ltd., 4200 Laciede Ave., St. Louis, Mo., 63108.
- NutriBiotic, Lakeport, CA., 95453.
- NutriCology, 400 Preda St., San Leandro, CA., 94577-0489.
- Nutritional Specialties, Inc., Pasadena, CA., 91106.
- Parametric Associates, Inc., St. Louis, Mo., 63126.
- Planetary Formulas, Soquel, CA., 94501.
- Professional Nutrition, Santa Barabara, CA., 93109.
- Quantum, Inc., Eugene, OR., 97402.
- Rainbow Light, 207 McPherson St., Santa Cruz, CA., 95060.
- Schiff Products, Inc., Moonachie, N.J., 07074.
- Solaray, Inc., 2815 Industrial Dr., Ogden, UT., 84401.
- Sonné Organic Foods, Inc., Natick, Mass., 01760.
- Source Naturals, Inc., Scotts Valley, CA., 91365.
- Strength Systems, Newington, CT., 06111.
- Sun Chlorella, Schamburg, Ill., 60193.
- Twin Labs, Ronkonkoma, N.Y., 11779.
- U.A.S. Labs, Minneapolis, Minn., 55431.
- Viobin Corp., Monticello, Ill., 61856.
- World Organics, Fountain Valley, CA., 92728.

INDEX

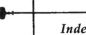

Index

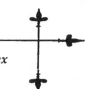

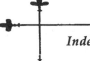

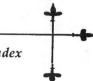